THE NETTER COLLECTION

OF MEDICAL ILLUSTRATIONS

Reproductive System

3rd Edition

VOLUME 1

A compilation of paintings prepared by **FRANK H. NETTER, MD**

Edited by

Roger P. Smith, MD
Adjunct Professor, Department of Obstetrics and Gynecology
Virginia Tech Carilion School of Medicine
Roanoke, Virginia

Paul J. Turek, MD
Director, The Turek Clinic
Former Professor and Endowed Chair
University of California, San Francisco
San Francisco, California

Additional Illustrations by

Carlos A.G. Machado, MD

CONTRIBUTING ILLUSTRATORS
John A. Craig, MD
Tiffany S. DaVanzo, MA, CMI
DragonFly Media
Paul Kim, MS
Kristen W. Marzejon, CMI
James A. Perkins, MS, MFA

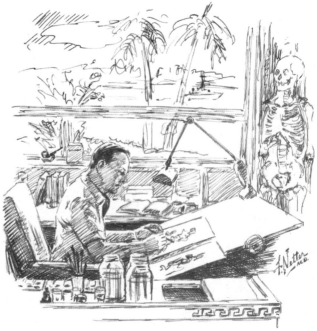

Self portrait by Dr. Netter

Elsevier
1600 John F. Kennedy Blvd.
Suite 1600
Philadelphia, Pennsylvania

THE NETTER COLLECTION OF MEDICAL ILLUSTRATIONS:
REPRODUCTIVE SYSTEM, VOLUME 1, THIRD EDITION   ISBN: 978-0-323-88083-1

Notices

Knowledge and best practice in this field are constantly changing. As new research and experience broaden our understanding, changes in research methods, professional practices, or medical treatment may become necessary.

Practitioners and researchers must always rely on their own experience and knowledge in evaluating and using any information, methods, compounds, or experiments described herein. In using such information or methods they should be mindful of their own safety and the safety of others, including parties for whom they have a professional responsibility.

With respect to any drug or pharmaceutical products identified, readers are advised to check the most current information provided (i) on procedures featured or (ii) by the manufacturer of each product to be administered, to verify the recommended dose or formula, the method and duration of administration, and contraindications. It is the responsibility of practitioners, relying on their own experience and knowledge of their patients, to make diagnoses, to determine dosages and the best treatment for each individual patient, and to take all appropriate safety precautions.

To the fullest extent of the law, neither the Publisher nor the authors, contributors, or editors, assume any liability for any injury and/or damage to persons or property as a matter of products liability, negligence or otherwise, or from any use or operation of any methods, products, instructions, or ideas contained in the material herein.

Publisher: Elyse O'Grady
Senior Content Strategist: Marybeth Thiel
Publishing Services Manager: Catherine Jackson
Project Manager: Rosanne Toroian
Book Design: Patrick Ferguson

Printed in India

Last digit is the print number: 9 8 7 6 5 4 3 2 1

Working together
to grow libraries in
developing countries

www.elsevier.com • www.bookaid.org

"Clarification is the goal. No matter how beautifully it is painted, a medical illustration has little value if it does not make clear a medical point."

Frank H. Netter, MD

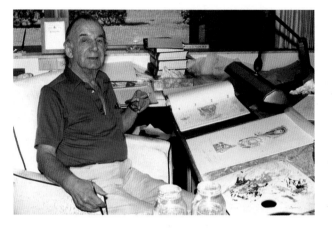

Dr. Frank Netter at work.

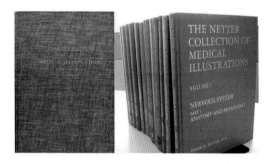

The single-volume "Blue Book" that preceded the multivolume *Netter Collection of Medical Illustrations* series, affectionately known as the "Green Books."

The Netter Collection
OF MEDICAL ILLUSTRATIONS
3rd Edition

Dr. Frank Netter created an illustrated legacy unifying his perspectives as physician, artist, and teacher. Both his greatest challenge and greatest success was charting a middle course between artistic clarity and instructional complexity. That success is captured in *The Netter Collection,* beginning in 1948 when the first comprehensive book of Netter's work was published by CIBA Pharmaceuticals. It met with such success that over the following 40 years the collection was expanded into an 8-volume series—with each title devoted to a single body system. Between 2011 and 2016, these books were updated and rereleased. Now, after another decade of innovation in medical imaging, renewed focus on patient-centered care, conscious efforts to improve inequities in healthcare and medical education, and a growing understanding of many clinical conditions, including multisystem effects of COVID-19, we are happy to make available a third edition of Netter's timeless work enhanced and informed by modern medical knowledge and context.

Inside the classic green covers, students and practitioners will find hundreds of original works of art. This is a collection of the human body in pictures—Dr. Netter called them *pictures,* never paintings. The latest expert medical knowledge is anchored by the sublime style of Frank Netter that has guided physicians' hands and nurtured their imaginations for more than half a century.

Noted artist-physician Carlos Machado, MD, the primary successor responsible for continuing the Netter tradition, has particular appreciation for the Green Book series. "*The Reproductive System* is of special significance for those who, like me, deeply admire Dr. Netter's work. In this volume, he masters the representation of textures of different surfaces, which I like to call 'the rhythm of the brush,' since it is the dimension, the direction of the strokes, and the interval separating them that create the illusion of given textures: organs have their external surfaces, the surfaces of their cavities, and texture of their parenchymas realistically represented. It set the style for the subsequent volumes of *The Netter Collection*—each an amazing combination of painting masterpieces and precise scientific information."

This third edition could not exist without the dedication of all those who edited, authored, or in other ways contributed to the second edition or the original books, nor, of course, without the excellence of Dr. Netter. For this third edition, we also owe our gratitude to the authors, editors, and artists whose relentless efforts were instrumental in adapting these classic works into reliable references for today's clinicians in training and in practice. From all of us with the Netter Publishing Team at Elsevier, thank you.

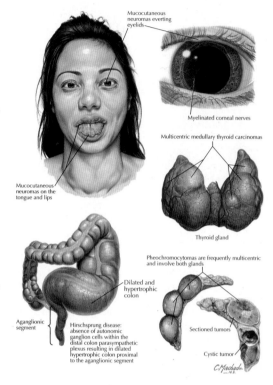

An illustrated plate painted by Carlos Machado, MD.

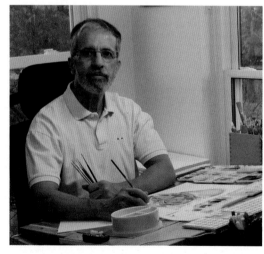

Dr. Carlos Machado at work.

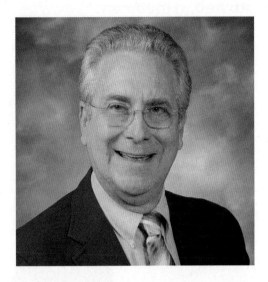

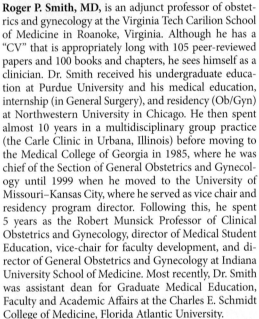

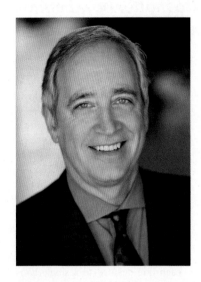

Roger P. Smith, MD, is an adjunct professor of obstetrics and gynecology at the Virginia Tech Carilion School of Medicine in Roanoke, Virginia. Although he has a "CV" that is appropriately long with 105 peer-reviewed papers and 100 books and chapters, he sees himself as a clinician. Dr. Smith received his undergraduate education at Purdue University and his medical education, internship (in General Surgery), and residency (Ob/Gyn) at Northwestern University in Chicago. He then spent almost 10 years in a multidisciplinary group practice (the Carle Clinic in Urbana, Illinois) before moving to the Medical College of Georgia in 1985, where he was chief of the Section of General Obstetrics and Gynecology until 1999 when he moved to the University of Missouri–Kansas City, where he served as vice chair and residency program director. Following this, he spent 5 years as the Robert Munsick Professor of Clinical Obstetrics and Gynecology, director of Medical Student Education, vice-chair for faculty development, and director of General Obstetrics and Gynecology at Indiana University School of Medicine. Most recently, Dr. Smith was assistant dean for Graduate Medical Education, Faculty and Academic Affairs at the Charles E. Schmidt College of Medicine, Florida Atlantic University.

He is married, with one son who is a graduate of the University of Southern California and is associate dean of Admission for Pomona College and a second son who is a graduate of Denison University in Granville, Ohio, who teaches history to high school students in Davidson, North Carolina. Dr. Smith is a collector of antique gumball machines, author of a collector's column on the history of vending machines, and a semiprofessional magician as well.

Paul J. Turek, MD, FACS, FRSM, is Director of The Turek Clinic, an innovative men's health practice in San Francisco and Los Angeles. Before retiring from the University of California San Francisco (UCSF), he held the Academy of Medical Educators Endowed Chair in Urology Education and was professor of urology, obstetrics, gynecology and reproductive sciences. While at UCSF, he directed the highly competitive Andrology Fellowship Program, directed the Medical Student Clerkship, authored the National Medical Student Curriculum in Urology and founded PROGENI, the Program in the Genetics of Infertility. Dr. Turek attended Yale College, followed by Stanford University Medical School. Following his urology residency at the University of Pennsylvania, Dr. Turek undertook fellowship training at Baylor College of Medicine in reproductive microsurgery. He has authored over 200 publications in genetic infertility, the stem cell basis for cancer and spermatogenesis, and men's health epidemiology. In addition, he has published on several innovative and now popular surgical techniques in male reproductive medicine and is a noted microsurgeon. He is an active member of the American Urological Association and the American Society of Andrology and is a Fellow of the American College of Surgeons, the Royal College of Physicians (UK), and the Société Internationale d'Urologie. He is past president of the American Society of Andrology and the Society of Male Reproduction and Urology. He has authored an award-winning blog on Men's Health (TurekonMensHealth.com) for over a decade and has also written for WebMD. His hobbies include longboard surfing and vintage cars.

"The challenge, therefore, was to absorb and assimilate the new learning and to exhibit it in a form easily understandable, attractive and so instructive that the essential points could be readily visualized and the more important details grasped without need for search in specific or original publications."

Frank H. Netter, MD
Introduction, *The Netter Collection of Illustrations, Reproductive System,* 1954

No student of medicine, past or present, is unaware of the extraordinary series of medical illustrations created by Dr. Frank Netter, the master artist-surgeon. This incredible body of work has since been carried forward after Dr. Netter's passing by the talented Carlos Machado, MD, and others, all remarkably gifted medical illustrators. Physicians old and young have looked at these images time and again for the last 5 decades, returning to them as comfortable sources of clear and clinically succinct information. For many of us, it was this volume that was bought for us by our parents as our first textbook in medical school and is still cherished to this day.

The Netter series of illustrations underwent 19 printings over 56 years but had never undergone a substantive revision until 2011. The privilege of editing this monumental tome has been both daunting and revealing. Dr. Netter's art is utterly timeless, highly exact, and informed to the point of being prescient. How do you improve on a masterpiece? On the other hand, medicine has been changing dramatically since this volume first appeared and since its last revision. This demands that entirely new and previously unimagined medical knowledge be brought to the readership. Similar to restoring a da Vinci painting or translating a Nabokov novel, editing this volume has highlighted for us both the magnitude of change in medicine and the timelessness of Dr. Netter's art. Consistent with Dr. Netter's philosophy, we have chosen to let the art do most of the speaking and have limited the text to providing context, clarification, and clinical application.

French writer Jean-Baptiste Alphonse Karr first wrote: "The more things change, the more they stay the same." We would also submit that the more things stay the same, the more they change. In producing this third edition, it has become clear to us that unchanging anatomic principles serve as a dependable springboard for medical innovation. This is no more aptly illustrated by reviewing the newly included gender reassignment surgery section in this edition. Well-founded anatomic principles have allowed the creatives among us to push tissue sculpting and neo-organ formation to almost metaphysical limits: witness the creation of a neophallus from a forearm skin graft or the use of microfluidic technology to help reintroduce the principle of natural selection into the arena of sperm selection for assisted reproduction. We are again honored to present to you, through the timeless artistic imagery that is the hallmark of the Netter's series, the well-known and the newly discovered anatomic and physiologic principles that continue to inspire us in reproductive medicine.

It is our hope that this work will be as treasured and as valued as the original, even if it remains clinically relevant for only a fraction of the time. Join us as we celebrate the beauty, logic, mystery, complexity, and artistic richness of clinical medicine illustrated in this third edition of the Netter Collection.

Roger P. Smith, MD
Paul J. Turek, MD, FACS, FRSM

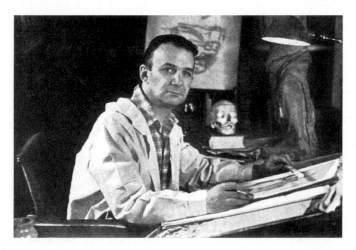

For over 12 years it has been my privilege to be what may be called a "regular" in the preparation of the nearly 660 pictures that, under CIBA's sponsorship, Dr. Netter has painted for the medical profession. As a member of a group proposing the program, as a bystander in the numerous conferences with our consultants, as a reviewer of the sketches and finished paintings, and, finally, as editor of this volume, my contacts with Frank Netter have been so frequent and so manifold that I feel qualified to say here a few words about the man and his methods.

Netter's expressional power with brush and color, his craftsmanship, needs no further comment. The pictures themselves are, in this respect, the most eloquent witnesses. What the pictures, however, do not reflect to the mere spectator is the amount of work and study expended before the artist starts the process of transmitting onto paper his ideas about an anatomic or pathologic problem or his concepts of the multitudinous facts and details. The simplicity and unsophisticated portrayal of the subject matter make it seem that these plates have come into existence with miraculous ease but, in reality, nothing but the artist's formative act of painting is spontaneous.

Never satisfied with the mere reporting of facts or with an unimaginative copying of nature, as can be done with pencil and camera alike, Netter's creative forces are generated only after a complete, intellectual assimilation of a subject, its scientific background and its theoretical, as well as practical, significance. Rarely does he permit himself a shortcut, because he incessantly questions the correctness of his own memory. He starts all over again. Whether essential or bordering on the trivial, all anatomic details are recapitulated. All available texts and other publications, particularly the pertinent literature of the past 25 years, are read, checked, rechecked, and compared. It is actually like classwork, with the main difference that our "student" performs his task with the support of an enormously widened horizon and boundless experience, especially with regard to the relationship of form and function.

Though, as disclosed in the sessions with the consultants, a certain degree of scientific curiosity guides this prying into the original sources, the mainspring is his irresistible compulsion to penetrate and to comprehend as a physician before liberating the creative forces of the artist. In this way Netter's final achievements cause the sensation of a well-rounded concept and a vivid reproduction in contrast to an inanimate representation of endless details. Some of the pictures, of course, demand less thought and absorption of knowledge than do others. This, however, is of minor influence on the total energy expended on the scholarly approach, because, at least in a collection of pictures such as those in this book, Netter endeavors to dramatize a complete narrative of an organ and its structural relationship to normal, as well as disturbed, function. The single entities, for example, of a specific disease, become a part of the whole story rather than a detached object.

Netter's concentration during such a "study period" is so intense that it works like a lock for other brain activities—a sometimes rather painful discovery for those surrounding him, as well as for an editor. It is rather difficult to approach him or to get action in any affair other than the one occupying his mind. But once Netter has mastered all the intricacies of the project-in-the-making, he is immediately available for the next one, into which he plunges, then, without pause. The "appropriation process" for a new topic starts, usually, in the first conference with the chosen consultant. There, the primary outline of a chapter is made, and the number and order of pictures are anticipated, though the ultimate number and order are never the same as originally conceived. Specimens and countless slides are examined. Netter, on these occasions, mostly looks on and listens. Rarely is he observed to make a written note during these consultations and, if he puts something on paper, it is usually a rough sketch. This technique is used also in his reading. Where others make excerpts and abstracts, Frank Netter uses the pencil to draw a few lines.

While the zealous submersion in books and articles goes on, subsequent meetings with the consultants follow at intervals of a month or two. But the character of these meetings changes markedly after the first conference. Usually during the second session, when Netter arrives with a pack of sketches, his acquired familiarity with the field of the expert asserts itself. Mutual trust and respect between the consultant and Netter develop with remarkable speed. The sincere and friendly relations, without which I do not think Frank Netter could work, are attributable, in part, to his professional knowledge and to the acuteness of his mind but, essentially, to his human personality, his amiability, and his sound sense of humor.

During the years of indecision—long past—when he did not know whether to turn to a medical career or follow his inborn talents as a painter, Netter succeeded in amalgamating physician and artist. With a genuine seriousness and readiness to accept the responsibility connotive of a physician and the impelling urge of an artist, he has now surrendered to his life's task—to depict the human body and the causes and processes of its ailments in a forcefully instructive, easily comprehensible, unconventional, and artistic form.

E. Oppenheimer, MD

An attempt to determine the natal hours of modern scientific anatomy is as unavailing as would be an effort to set an exact date for the beginning of the Renaissance era. The changes of mind, intellect, and interest, of conceptual thinking, which we in our time admire in retrospect, began slowly and developed only over a span of 2 centuries. One can, however, scarcely go wrong in stating that the momentum for scientific research was at no time (except perhaps our own) as poignant as in the 15th and 17th centuries. This was the period in which philosophers, scientists, physicians, and the great artists alike became not only interested in but devoted to the study of forms and structures inside the human body. The motives of an Andrea del Verrocchio (1435–1488), of a Donatello (1386–1466), of a Leonardo da Vinci (1452–1519), of a Michelangelo Buonarroti (1475–1564), of a Raffaello Santi (1483–1520)—just to name a few of the best-known Renaissance artists—for drawing anatomic subjects are difficult to explain. Whether it was sheer curiosity, a fashionable trend, scientific interest, or other reasons that prompted them to leave to posterity these magnificent works of art concerned with the muscles, bones, and internal parts of *Homo sapiens*, one can be sure that these drawings were not meant to accompany or to clarify the anatomist's dissections and descriptions. Nevertheless, the painters of that period can be designated as the creators of medical illustration, because it may safely be assumed that the first useful instrument that provided a general and more popular knowledge of the inner structures of the human body was not the knife of the dissecting anatomist or his description written in Latin but the pencil of the artist. Health, standing second only to nutrition in the minds of people of all times, must have been a "hot news" topic half a millennium ago as it is in our day, in which the so-called science writer has taken over the function of making accessible to contemporary intellectuals what the language or idiom of the scientist has left inaccessible.

With the exception of Leonardo, whose geniality and universal inquisitiveness in every field of science led him to be far ahead of his contemporaries, none of the many excellent artists who took a fancy to drawing or painting anatomic subject matter contributed to the factual knowledge of anatomy or medicine, but it became a landmark of extraordinary significance when Andreas Vesalius (1514–1564) wrote his *De Corporis Humani Fabrica* and found in John de Calcar (1499–1546), Flemish painter and pupil of Titian (1477–1576), the congenial artist who supplemented the great anatomist's revolutionizing work with his magnificent illustrations, the first true-to-life reproductions of the structures of the human organism. The "Magna Carta" of anatomy, as posterity has called Vesalius's opus, was engendered by an ideal union of scientist and artist as two equal partners, as far as creative power, each in his own field, goes.

The mystery of the propagation of life occupied the minds and emotions of mankind from the time the deities of fertility demanded devotion and sacrifice. One naturally is inclined, therefore, to expect that in ages progressive in science, such as the Renaissance, the knowledge of the generative tract, or, more generally, the search to elucidate procreative processes, would be exposed to special benefit and encouragement. This, however, seems not to be the case, perhaps because specialization was a thing of naught to Renaissance mentality. The advances in knowledge of the anatomy of the reproductive system during the time of Vesalius and the 300 years after him were as respectable as those in the lore of all other sciences, but not more so. Remarkable contributions and disclosures were reported, as witnessed by the many anatomic designations which still carry the names of their discoverers, such as Gabriello Fallopio (1523–1562), Thomas Wharton (1614–1673), Regnier de Graaf (1641–1673), Anton Nuck (1650–1692), Edward Tyson (1650–1708), Caspar Bartholin (1655–1738), Alexis Littré (1658–1726), William Cowper (1666–1709), James Douglas (1675–1742), Kaspar Friedrich Wolff (1733–1794), Johannes Müller (1801–1852), and others, names that will be encountered on many pages of this book. But anatomy of the genital organs and the physiology (or pathology) of reproduction were not favored by the appearance of a Harvey who revolutionized the physiology of circulation and, with it, of medicine in general.

It is from this historical aspect the more surprising to observe that under our own eyes, as a matter of fact within scarcely more than a single generation, so many new phenomena have come to light, and discoveries so revolutionizing have been made that our concepts and knowledge of the physiology and pathology of reproduction have undergone fundamental changes. Endocrinologic research has presented to us the story of the mutual relationship between the pituitary gland and the gonads and of the activities and functions of the secretion products of these organs on the genitals and other parts of the body. The impact of these scientific accomplishments on the practice of medicine, particularly for the interpretation of genito-urinary and gynecologic diseases, has been tremendous. In addition to the progress in endocrinology, we have lived to see simultaneously the rise of chemotherapy, which inaugurated a magic alteration in the character, management, and prognosis of the formerly most frequent diseases of the reproductive structures.

This progress is not, of course, as everybody knows, the result of the genius of one or of a few single individuals; it is the yield of the efforts of an endless number of scientists from all parts of the world and—in view of the foregoing paragraphs—it should also be remembered that the speed and the intensity with which this progress has been achieved have not been restricted solitarily to the science of reproductive physiology or pathology of the genital organs but belong to the scientific tide of our times, as can be noticed in all branches of science.

These chips of thoughts have been uttered here, because those about the early artist-illustrators occupied my mind in the few hours of leisure permitted me during the preparation of this book, and those about the recent changes in our specific topic suggested themselves continuously during the preparation of the new and the checking of the older plates. The situation the advancements in our knowledge have caused, as indicated sketchily in the foregoing, presented a specific task and, concurrently, a straightforward challenge. Despite my intentions and efforts, shared, I am sure, by all responsible practicing physicians, to "keep informed," many of the facts, facets, connections, concepts, etc., which experimental biology and medicine have brought to light were novelties to me, as they must have been or have been to a generation of still-active physicians—those who studied medicine during the time of my school days or even before. The challenge, therefore, was to absorb and assimilate the new learning and to exhibit it in a form easily understandable, attractive, and so instructive that the essential points could be readily visualized and the more important details grasped without need for search in specific or original publications.

The subjects of the pictures were selected on the basis of what seemed to be of the greatest clinical import and interest. Although we aimed to secure a reasonably complete coverage, it is obvious that not everything could be included. With the newer knowledge crowding in so rapidly upon the old and from so many sources—chemistry, biology, anatomy, physiology, pathology, etc.—with the accumulation of so many pertinent data, the book could have grown to twice its size. Would we, with greater completeness, have better served the student or busy practitioner with his difficulties in following and correlating? It was the opinion of all concerned that this would not have been the case and that the adopted restriction would prove more helpful. Actually, the book grew much larger than was originally anticipated, particularly because it was felt that certain "correlation" or "summation" plates—for example, pages 5, 105, 115, 120, 162, 175, 211, 213, 214, and 241—were necessary for the mission we flattered ourselves this book could fulfill.

In view of the steadily increasing number of plates, it was natural that at some time during the preparation of the book the question should be seriously discussed and considered whether the treatise on the male and female reproductive systems should appear as separately bound books or in one volume under the same cover. The decision fell in favor of a single volume containing the exhibit of both genital tracts, because separation into two volumes would have seriously counteracted my earnest striving for integration of the knowledge on the two tracts. It was also felt very strongly that the small monetary advantage that would have been gained by those distinctly interested in only one part of the book—in all probability a small minority—would be more than compensated by the educational benefit conferred by the contiguity of the topics and the amalgamation of the two parts.

Whereas in the series of illustrations published in earlier years, the gross anatomy of an organ was reviewed in direct association with the pictures on the pathology of that organ, it will be found that for the purpose of this book the anatomy of the organs follows the description of the anatomy of the whole system. In other words, Section II and Section VI contain, respectively, the accounts of the male and the female genital tracts in toto, succeeded by more detailed depictions of the parts. This arrangement was thought to be more expedient from the didactic and more logical from the organizational points of view. As a consequence of this method, it will be noted that Section VI, in contrast to the other sections, each of which was compiled and prepared with one consultant, lists numerous collaborators, each describing the anatomy of that part of the tract for which he was consultant in the sections on the diseases. The danger of inconsistencies or lack of uniformity in one section that might have been incidental to this concurrent effort of a plurality was happily circumvented by the splendid adaptability of each individual coauthor. Duplication of features within the paintings was avoided by appropriate planning. Repetitions, occurring when the essays were submitted, could be eliminated without any difficulty, although a few were allowed to remain intentionally, mostly because it seemed warranted to discuss certain points from different aspects.

In Section VI we have also inserted pictures not originally painted for the series collected in this book. Neuropathways of Parturition (page 105) seemed, however, to fit in with the illustrations of the innervation of the female genital tract and to make a desirable supplement. I am greatly obliged to Dr. Hingson for his approval of the use of this picture together with his rearranged explanatory text.

From Dr. Decker's article in CIBA CLINICAL SYMPOSIA (4:201, August–September 1952), we took one plate demonstrating the technique of Culdoscopy (page 123) and, in abbreviated form, his description. The culdoscopic views used in Sections X and XII are from the same source. I drew them from actual observations through the culdoscope in Dr. Decker's clinic. His cooperative courtesy and permission are gratefully acknowledged.

The plates on diagnostic topics, I would like to emphasize, are by no means intended as instructions for the execution of such procedures, nor are they or the concomitant texts proposed as precepts for the evaluation of the results. It would not have been difficult to add more diagnostic features and to describe with brush and pen a great many technical details and also a great many varieties of diagnostic results. This was considered definitely beyond the scope and purpose of this book. The same holds true for the illustrating of operative procedures. The four plates pictorializing the surgical approaches to the prostate (pages 58–61) were included because Dr. Vest and I were convinced they would satisfy a need of the non-urologists and would acquaint them with the urologic reasonings underlying the urologist's proposals for the management of the recommended patient. No such necessity seemed to exist for the great variety of surgical techniques in the field of gynecology. It is great fun for an artist to paint surgical procedures in their various phases, particularly when properly directed by an experienced surgeon. I did not surrender to such temptation, because it would have jeopardized the adopted principal purpose of the book, which, in short, is to promote the understanding of medical facts and problems but not to show how things are done. For the same reason we omitted from this volume topics concerned with obstetrics, despite the fact that pictures of this kind were available, as I had made some for CIBA in whose CLINICAL SYMPOSIA (4:215, October 1952) they appeared.

Several pictures dealing with the development of the reproductive systems or organs were added, because the interpretation and understanding of most congenital anomalies and also of some pathologic conditions are difficult, if at all possible, without at least a cursory idea of the embryology of the generative organs. A brief, admittedly oversimplified survey of the formation of the fetal internal and external genitalia, therefore, seemed in order (pages 2 and 3). With these plates, as with those demonstrating in rudimentary fashion the development and implantation of the ovum and fetal membranes (pages 217 and 218), nothing was further from my mind than to introduce the reader into the complex details that embryologic research has brought to light. The scientific importance of these details is beyond question, but they have—at least to my knowledge and at this moment—no direct bearing on the interest of the majority of those for whom this book has been prepared.

To mention all the deliberations and reflections that, in the course of several years, shaped this book is impossible, but I would like to say a few words more to express my appreciation to each of the consultants. I agree wholeheartedly with the editor's statement in the preface that this volume in its present form could not have been executed without their unerring and intense devotion. The support I received from their knowledge and experience and from the material they placed at my disposal was vitally essential for the entire project.

Dr. Vest, who patronized Sections I through V and Section XIV, is one of my steadfast, unwavering collaborators and has become a long-tried, but still critical, friend. For over a decade I have been fortunate enough to enjoy not only his giving freely of his expert information but also his remarkable comprehension of what is didactically important and unimportant. I deeply regret that with the completion of this series of illustrations I will have to forego his cooperation for the present, and I await anxiously that time that will enable me again to have him participate in my efforts, when we are ready for the illustrations of the urinary tract.

For the plates covering the complex topic, testicular failure (pages 73–79), in Dr. Vest's Section V, we received stimulus and help from Dr. Warren O. Nelson (University of Iowa), who not only offered his proficient advice derived from his long-time special study of the anatomy, physiology, and pathology of the human testis but provided us also with a great number of slides from his impressive collection. From this source stem also the microscopic views on pages 73 and 82.

The treatment of the subject matter on testicular failure presented a delicate problem, because no final concept of the various conditions has been agreed upon. The knowledge in this field is still in an evolutionary state, but by the importance these conditions assume nowadays in the practice of medicine, we were forced, so to say, to take a stand and to compromise with the general principle maintained in this book, namely, to avoid controversial matters. It is realized that the concept we submit in the presentation of testicular failure might not find approval with all investigators, and the reader should understand that in due course new findings may be recorded which may substantially change the information now available.

In connection with Dr. Vest's sections, I would like, furthermore, to thank Dr. J. E. Kindred (University of Virginia) for his generosity in permitting me to make free use of his own drawing of the phases of spermatogenesis, which I followed in great detail, in preparing the schematic picture on page 25.

A sizeable part of the book—altogether 44 plates—were under the consultative sponsorship of Dr. Gaines, whose active interest in my work also dates back over a decennium. His participation in this book began with his contribution to Section VI, continued with Section VII and ended with his collaborative effort and preparation of the learned text for Section XI. Diseases of the Ovary represents surely, with regard to organizational arrangement and factual information, one of the most complicated chapters of morbid anatomy and histopathology. Dr. Gaines' decisive counseling in the selection of the conditions to be portrayed and his support of my aim to demonstrate exemplary rather than specific entities were of indispensable help, which I would like to recognize with my profound thanks. A certain restraint was necessary, naturally, in all sections but in none more essential than in Section XI, where a limitless possibility to demonstrate more and more specimens of cysts or tumors can readily be envisaged.

The series on major anatomy and pathology of the breast, prepared and issued in 1946, has been in such demand since its appearance that it seemed advisable to insert Section XIII in this volume, dealing with the entire reproductive system. Dr. Geschickter, to whom I was indebted for his counsel when the pictures were made, gladly agreed to check the plates and to revise the texts. Except for the substitution of one microscopic view and omission of one plate, the series of paintings remained unchanged and was found to meet modern requirements. Dr. Geschickter's attending to overhauling the texts—a rather troublesome task—is deeply appreciated.

For the composition of the chapter on diseases of the uterus (Section IX) and the cyclic function of this organ (part of Section VI), it was my great fortune to have the collaboration of Dr. Sturgis. I will never forget the stimulus and benefit I received from his critical attitude on one side and his enthusiasm for the whole book on the other. It was sheer pleasure to work with him. Similarly, as with the plates on testicular failure, the treatment of the physiology of menstruation was not easy, because too many unknowns still obscure the prospect of a clear-cut, invulnerable concept. My admiration for Dr. Sturgis's instructive contribution and for the way he mastered the difficulties are only surpassed by my gratitude to the fate that brought us together.

My reverence for Dr. Rubin goes back to my school days, and it made me very happy that I could obtain his and Dr. Novak's cooperation for the production of Section X. The major task and the tiresome working out of the details fell upon the shoulders of Dr. Novak, whose sound conservatism and astute wisdom provided the book and me with a vivid enlightenment. I am under special obligation to Dr. Novak for his handling of matter and text, because, more than in other sections, we felt, while preparing the chapter on diseases of the fallopian tubes, that the sectional arrangement according to organs had introduced some shortcomings. The congenital anomalies, and particularly the infections, could have been described in a more logical fashion in a discourse of these conditions affecting the entire female tract. Because division according to organ pathology was due to the chronologic development of the book and its parts, and because a change would have caused a number of other handicaps, a compromise became necessary, which, thanks to the discernment of the collaborators, was not too difficult.

Dr. Assali and Dr. Zeek have made the much-neglected pathology of the placenta and concurrent clinical phenomena their life's task. It was a thrilling experience for me to meet them, and I am deeply indebted to these two scientists for the interest they displayed and for the many hours they spent in acquainting me with the results of their own studies and the status of our knowledge in this sphere of science.

Last, because it concerns the most recent pictures I painted for this volume but assuredly not least, my thanks are tendered to Dr. Mitchell for his intelligent guidance in our selection of the conditions presented in Section VIII. His competent judgment was, furthermore, of great help in filling certain gaps in Section VI that had to be closed to make this section what I wanted it to be—an exhaustive survey of the anatomy of the female genital tract. Dr. Mitchell's illuminating texts that accompany my pictures in these two sections speak for themselves.

Finally, I must try to express my appreciation for the wonderful cooperation and encouragement I received from Dr. Oppenheimer. Officially, he was the editor of this volume, but actually he was far more—a friend, a counselor, a collaborator, and a ceaseless co-worker. His broad knowledge, his progressive point of view, and his flexible attitude helped tremendously in solving the most difficult problems.

Frank H. Netter, MD

CONTRIBUTORS

EDITORS

Roger P. Smith, MD
Adjunct Professor, Department of Obstetrics and Gynecology
Virginia Tech Carilion School of Medicine
Roanoke, Virginia
Sections 6–13

Paul J. Turek, MD
Director, The Turek Clinic
Former Professor and Endowed Chair
University of California, San Francisco
San Francisco, California
Sections 1–5, 14
Plate 11.9

CONTRIBUTOR

Mang L. Chen, MD
Reconstructive Urologist
G.U. Recon Clinic
San Francisco, California
Plates 14.1–14.7

CONTENTS

DEVELOPMENT OF THE GENITAL TRACTS AND FUNCTIONAL RELATIONSHIPS OF THE GONADS

Plate 1.1

Reproductive System: VOLUME 1

Indifferent (undifferentiated) stage

Labels: Paramesonephric (müllerian) duct; Mesonephros; Genital ridge; Hindgut; Mesonephric (wolffian) duct; Ureteric bud (metanephric duct); Metanephrogenic tissue; Cloaca; Cloacal membrane; Chromosome 11; WT1; SF1; Yolk sac stalk; Allantois; Transcriptional activation of SRY; Conversion of the genital ridge into the bipotential gonad; SRY; GATA4; FOG2; Chromosome Y; Chromosome 8; Chromosome 17; Chromosomes 10 and 13; Activation of SOX9; SOX9; FGF9; FGFR2; Genital tubercle; Bipotential gonads; Kidney (metanephros); Bladder; Urogenital sinus proper; Rectum; Perineum; DAX1; Chromosome X; WNT4 + RSPO1; Chromosome 1; Chromosome 3; FOXL2; Female gonadal development; Female; Male; Testis development; Kidney; Penis; Urethra; Gubernaculum; Testis migration; Wolffian duct differentiation; Masculinization of the genital anlage; Testis; Sertoli cells; Leydig cells; Insulin-like-3; Testosterone; Dihydrotestosterone (DHT); Antimüllerian hormone (AMH or MIF); Clitoris; Urethra; Vagina; Rectum; Uterus

C. Machado, M.D.

GENETICS AND BIOLOGY OF EARLY REPRODUCTIVE TRACT DEVELOPMENT

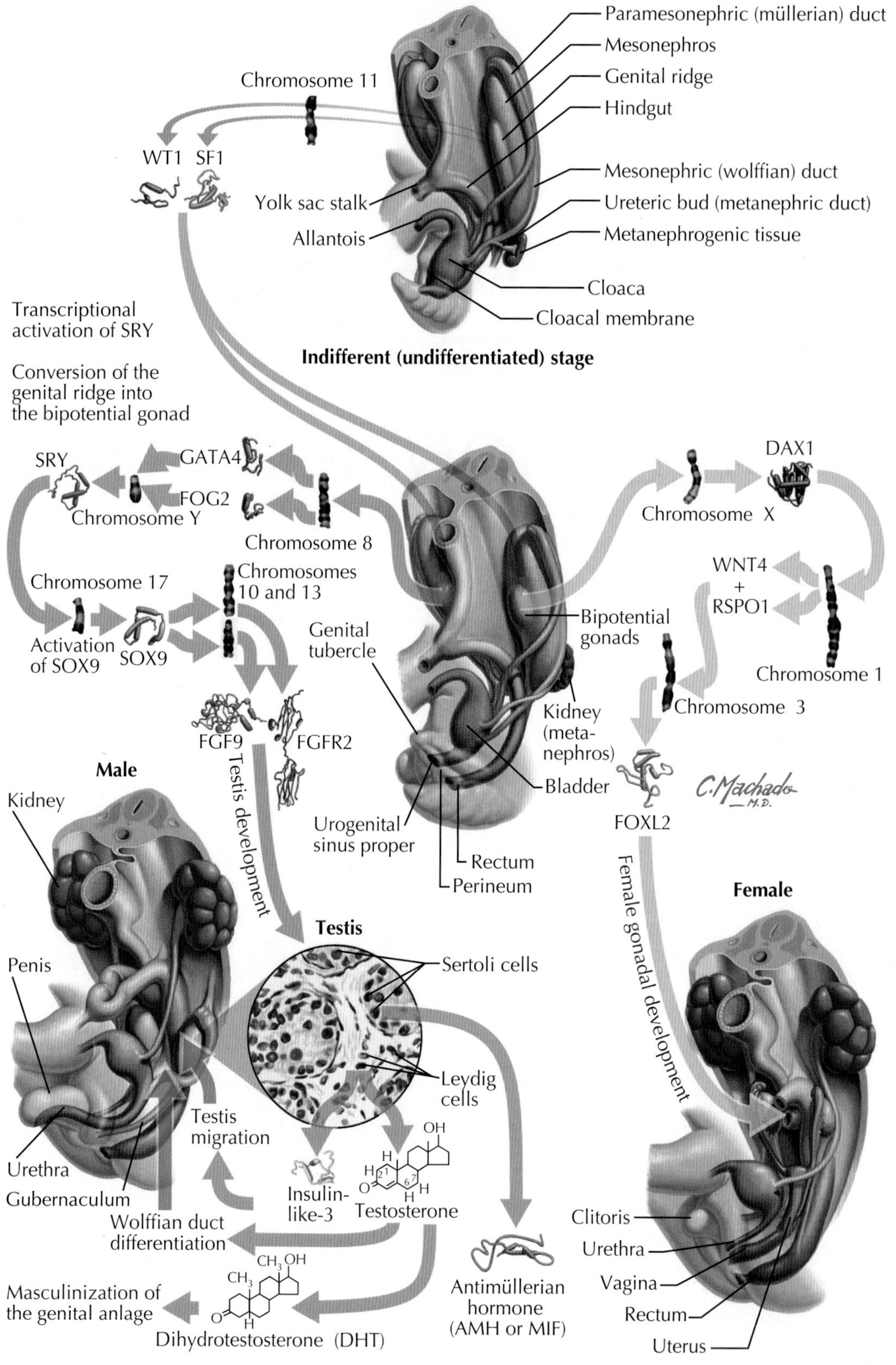

Most organisms have some form of sex-determination system that drives the development and expression of sexual characteristics. Sex determination can be genetic or can be a consequence of environmental or social variables. In humans, sex determination is genetic and is governed by specific genes and chromosomes. It is believed that the two human sex chromosomes (X and Y) evolved from other nonsex chromosomes (autosomes) 300 million years ago. Human females have two of the same kind of sex chromosome (XX), whereas males have two distinct sex chromosomes (XY). However, both male and female features can be found in an individual, and it is possible to have XY females and XX males. Analysis of such individuals has revealed the genes of sex determination, including SRY (sex-determining region Y gene) on the short arm of the Y chromosome, which is important for maleness. The *SRY* gene product is a protein that harbors a high-mobility group box sequence, a highly conserved DNA-binding motif that kinks DNA. This DNA-bending effect alters gene expression, leading to formation of a testis and subsequently to the male phenotype. Notably, individuals with XY chromosomes who lack the *SRY* gene on the Y chromosome are phenotypic females.

It is now clear that the *SRY* gene does not act in isolation to determine human sex. Other genes in other locations are also important for complete male sexual differentiation. DAX1, a nuclear hormone receptor, can alter *SRY* activity during development by suppressing genes downstream to *SRY* that would normally induce testis differentiation. A second gene, *WNT4*, largely confined to the adult ovary, may also serve as an "anti-testis" gene. Indeed, the discovery of these genes has significantly altered theories of sex determination. Previously, *SRY* gene presence was thought to determine male gonadal development from the bipotential gonad. The female genotype was considered the "default" developmental pathway for gonads. It is now clear that genes such as *WNT4* and *DAX1* can proactively induce female gonadal development, even in the presence of *SRY*.

Once gonadal sex is determined, several other events must occur for normal male sexual differentiation. Within the testis, Leydig cells make testosterone, a hormone that is critical for development of the internal genitalia, including the vas deferens, epididymis, and seminal vesicles through wolffian duct differentiation. Leydig cells also synthesize insulin-like-3 to promote transabdominal testis migration that begins testis descent into the scrotum. Dihydrotestosterone (DHT), a testosterone metabolite, masculinizes the genital anlage to form the external genitalia, including the penis and scrotum as well as the prostate. In addition, Sertoli cells within the developing testis synthesize *antimüllerian hormone* (AMH or MIF), which prevents the müllerian duct from developing into uterus and fallopian tubes and helps the early germ cells remain quiescent in the developing testis. Deficiencies in any of these developmental pathways generally result in either birth defects or intersex disorders. Such developmental variations, formerly termed *true* or *pseudohermaphroditism,* can include chromosomal abnormalities, ambiguous genitalia, phenotypic sex anomalies, or true intersex states.

HOMOLOGUES OF INTERNAL GENITALIA

Although sex is determined at the time of fertilization, phenotypic gender is determined by a complex tissue differentiation process that begins in the medial genital thickening or ridges on the posterior surface of the embryonic body cavity. During the fifth fetal week, primordial germ cells migrate from the yolk sac to the posterior body wall and induce the formation of genital ridges on either side of the midline. Here, these migrating cells induce the formation of undifferentiated primitive sex cords.

Signaled by the arrival of primordial germ cells, two sets of paired genital ducts, the mesonephric or nephric (wolffian) ducts and the paramesonephric (müllerian) ducts, also develop. The mesonephros is a prominent excretory structure that consists of a series of mesonephric tubules that connect with the elongating mesonephric (wolffian) ducts as the latter extend caudally until they terminate in the urogenital sinus on each side of the midline. The paramesonephric ducts develop lateral to each of the mesonephric ducts and are derived from the evagination of the coelomic epithelium. The upper ends open directly into the peritoneal cavity, whereas the distal ends grow caudally, fuse in the lower midline, form the uterovaginal primordium, and join the urogenital sinus as an elevation, the müllerian tubercle, which separates the urogenital area from the more posterior gut.

Under the influence of the *SRY* gene in the male primitive sex cord, the mesonephric (wolffian) ducts are maintained during development. As the developing male Sertoli cells begin to differentiate in response to SRY, they secrete a glycoprotein hormone, müllerian-inhibiting substance (MIS) or AMH, which causes the paramesonephric (müllerian) ducts to regress rapidly between the 8th and 10th fetal weeks. Müllerian duct remnants in the male include the appendix testis and the prostatic utricle. In females, MIS is not present, so müllerian ducts remain, and the mesonephric tubules and ducts degenerate in the absence of androgens, often resulting in remnant epoöphoron and paroöphoron cystic structures within the ovarian mesentery and Gartner duct cysts within the anterolateral vaginal wall. These structures are clinically important because they may develop into sizable and symptomatic cysts (see Plates 8.15 and 9.13).

In the male, under the influence of testosterone secreted by Leydig cells at 9 to 10 weeks, the majority of the mesonephric ducts develop into the vas deferens and body (corpus) and tail (cauda) of the epididymis. The mesonephric tubules nearest to presumptive testis form the globus major or caput of the epididymis and the efferent ductules that connect to the testis, forming ducts to transport sperm. The more cranial mesonephric tubules develop into the vestigial appendix epididymis, and the more caudal tubules may develop into remnants called *paradidymis*. The seminal vesicles sprout from the distal ends of the mesonephric ducts, whereas the prostate and bulbourethral glands develop from the urogenital sinus, thus revealing different embryologic origins. In the fully developed male embryo, the distal orifice of the mesonephric duct (ejaculatory duct) terminates in the verumontanum on the floor of the prostatic urethra.

During the 10th week of gestation in females, in the absence of MIS and androgens, the primordial müllerian ducts remain separate and form the fallopian tubes superiorly. At their caudal ends, the ducts join, fuse, and form

a common channel called the *uterovaginal canal,* which later develops into the uterus and proximal four-fifths of the vagina. The remainder of the distal vagina forms from paired thickenings on the posterior urogenital sinus, called *sinovaginal bulbs,* and the vaginal plate, which has an unclear origin.

Intersex disorders can result from failure of the müllerian or wolffian ducts to regress completely. An example of this is hernia uteri inguinale or persistent müllerian duct syndrome, in which MIS deficiency or receptor abnormalities cause persistence of müllerian

duct structures in an otherwise phenotypically normal male. This is commonly diagnosed during exploration for an infant hernia or undescended testicle because the müllerian structures can tether the testis in the abdomen and restrict normal scrotal descent. Vestigial remnants of the wolffian duct can also exist in fully developed females. Vestiges of the male prostate may appear as periurethral ducts in the female (see Plate 7.5). In addition, homologues of male Cowper glands are the major vestibular glands (Bartholin glands) in the female (see Plate 6.18).

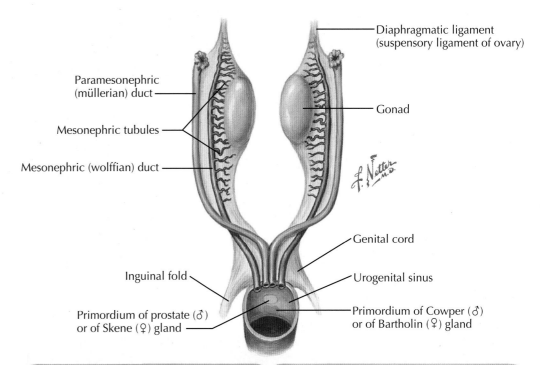

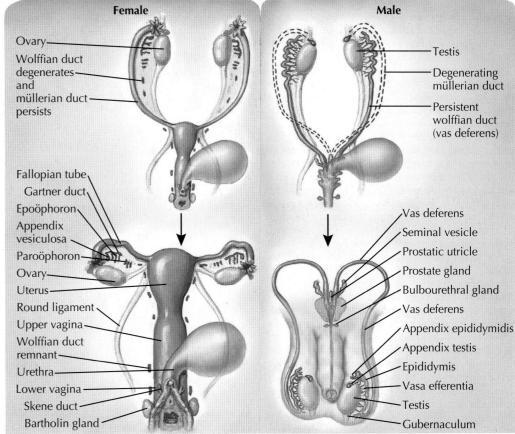

Plate 1.3

Reproductive System: VOLUME 1

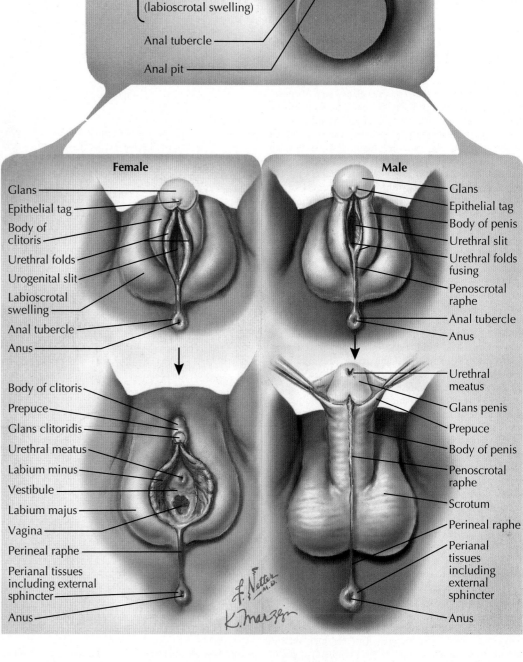

HOMOLOGUES OF EXTERNAL GENITALIA

Before 9 weeks of gestation, both sexes have identical external genitalia, characterized by a urogenital sinus. At this stage, the external genitalia consist of a genital tubercle above a urethral groove. Lateral to this are urethral or urogenital folds and even more lateral are the labioscrotal swellings or folds. The male and female derivatives from these structures are shown.

The bladder and genital ducts find a common opening in the urogenital sinus. This sinus is formed from the earlier urogenital slit, which is a consequence of the perineal membrane separating the urogenital ducts from the single cloacal opening.

In male development, the genital tubercle elongates, forming a long urethral groove. The distal portion of the groove terminates in a solid epithelial plate (urethral plate) that extends into the glans penis and later canalizes to form the urethra. The midline fusion of the lateral urethral folds is the key step in forming a penile urethra, but this fusion only occurs after the urethral plate canalizes distally. In the female, the primitive structures do not lengthen, and the urethral folds do not fuse in the midline. Instead, they become the labia majora.

The vagina develops as a diverticulum of the urogenital sinus near the müllerian tubercle. It becomes contiguous with the distal end of the müllerian ducts. Roughly four-fifths of the vagina originates from the urogenital sinus and one-fifth is of müllerian origin. In the male, the vaginal remnant is usually extremely small, as the müllerian structures atrophy before the vaginal diverticulum develops. In intersex disorders (formerly called *pseudohermaphroditism* and now termed *disorders of sexual development* [DSD]) such as androgen insensitivity syndrome (AIS), however, an anatomic remnant of the vaginal diverticulum may persist as a blind vaginal pouch.

In normal female development, the vagina is pushed posteriorly by a downgrowth of connective tissue. By the 12th week of gestation, it acquires its own separate opening. In female intersex disorders, the growth of this septum is incomplete, thus leading to persistence of the urogenital sinus.

Male and female external genitalia appear remarkably similar during the first trimester of development. The principal distinctions between them are the location and size of the vaginal diverticulum, the size of the phallus, and the degree of fusion of the urethral folds and the labioscrotal swellings.

FACTORS DETERMINING DIFFERENTIATION OF THE EXTERNAL GENITALIA

Similar to the genital ducts, there is a tendency for the external genitalia to develop along female lines. Masculinization of the genital ducts is induced by androgenic hormones, principally testosterone from Leydig cells in the fetal testis during the differentiation process. More important than the source of androgens, however, is the timing and amount of hormone. Examples of this include inappropriate androgen exposure from congenital adrenal hyperplasia (CAH) or from the maternal circulation, both of which can induce various degrees of masculinization of the female system characteristic of intersex disorders. By the 12th week, androgenic exposure will no longer cause fusion of the urethral and labioscrotal folds in the female, as the vagina has migrated fully posteriorly. Clitoral hypertrophy, however, may still result from such exposures at any time in fetal life or even after birth.

TESTOSTERONE AND ESTROGEN SYNTHESIS

Under the control of the anterior pituitary, three glands produce steroid hormones involved in reproduction: the adrenal cortex responding to adrenocorticotropic hormone (ACTH), and the ovary and testis, both under the influence of the gonadotropin luteinizing hormone (LH). For the majority of sex hormones that result from this stimulation, cholesterol is the precursor molecule.

In each of these organs, side chains are degraded from cholesterol to form pregnenolone and dehydroepiandrosterone (DHEA). In humans, DHEA is the dominant sex steroid and precursor or prohormone to all other steroid sex hormones, including testosterone and estrogens. In blood, most DHEA is found in its sulfate-bound form, DHEAS, and not in the free form. DHEA supplements are often used as muscle-building or performance-enhancing drugs by athletes. Pregnenolone is converted to progesterone, which by degradation of its side chain is converted to androstenedione and then to testosterone. These latter two hormones are the main products of testicular Leydig cells. Androstenedione, also termed "andro," is a dietary supplement banned by the US Food and Drug Administration that is also taken by athletes to improve performance. In the ovary, synthesis of androstenedione by theca interna cells and its subsequent conversion to estrone in follicular granulosa cells, along with conversion of testosterone to estradiol by aromatases, constitute the main secretory products. With polycystic ovary syndrome, enzymatic conversion of testosterone to estradiol in the ovary is impaired and DHEAS levels are elevated, leading to a characteristic androgenized phenotype in affected females. Estriol, a product of estrone metabolism in the placenta during pregnancy, is the third major estrogenic hormone in the female but is the least potent biologically.

About 5% of normal daily testosterone product is derived from the adrenal cortex, and the remainder is secreted by the testis into the systemic circulation. In the plasma, testosterone is virtually entirely bound (98%) by proteins such as sex hormone–binding globulin (SHBG) or albumin. The remainder of testosterone (2%) exists in a free or unbound form, which is the active fraction. Testosterone is conjugated in the liver and excreted by the kidney in this water-soluble form. Circulating estrogens have a similar bioavailability profile and are also carried on plasma proteins, notably albumin. Inactivation of estrogen occurs in the liver through conversion to less active metabolites (estrone, estriol), by conjugation to glucuronic acid, or by oxidation to inert compounds. There is also considerable

enterohepatic circulation of estrogens in the bile. Estrogen, testosterone, and their metabolites are ultimately excreted by the kidney, for the most part in the form of 17-ketosteroids in which a ketone group is present on the steroid ring. Examples of 17-ketosteroids include androstenedione, androsterone, estrone, and DHEA.

Although important for premenopausal females, the value of estrogen and progesterone supplementation in postmenopausal females is controversial. A randomized, controlled trial of 15,730 females in the Women's

Health Initiative was stopped early, after 5.6 years, because of the finding that risks (including stroke, blood clots, and breast cancer) outweighed benefits (lower risk of hip fractures and colon cancer) among subjects taking hormone supplements. Similarly, the value of testosterone supplements in older males who have reached andropause (androgen deficiency with age) is even more controversial, as large, randomized, placebo-controlled trials of sufficient duration to assess long-term clinical outcomes and events have not been undertaken.

Plate 1.5

Reproductive System: VOLUME 1

Hypothalamic-Pituitary-Gonadal Hormonal Axis

The hypothalamic-pituitary-gonadal (HPG) axis plays a fundamental role in phenotypic gender development during embryogenesis, sexual maturation during puberty, and endocrine (hormone) and exocrine (oocytes and sperm) function of the mature ovary and testis. Importantly, gonadal function throughout life, similar to the adrenal cortex and thyroid, is under the control of the adenohypophysis (anterior lobe of the pituitary) and hypothalamus.

HORMONE TYPES

Two kinds of hormones exist in the HPG axis: peptide and steroid. Peptide hormones are small secretory proteins that act via receptors on the cell surface membrane. Hormone signals are transduced by one of several second-messenger pathways involving either cAMP, calcium flux, or tyrosine kinase. Most peptide hormones induce the phosphorylation of various proteins that alter cell function. Examples of peptide hormones are LH and follicle-stimulating hormone (FSH). In contrast, steroid hormones are derived from cholesterol and are not stored in secretory granules; consequently, steroid secretion rates directly reflect production rates. In plasma, these hormones are usually bound to carrier proteins. Because they are lipophilic, steroid hormones are generally cell membrane permeable. After binding to an intracellular receptor, steroids are translocated to DNA recognition sites within the nucleus and regulate the transcription of target genes. Examples of reproductive steroid hormones are estradiol and testosterone.

HORMONAL FEEDBACK LOOPS

Normal reproduction depends on the cooperation of numerous hormones, and thus hormone signals must be well controlled. Feedback control is the principal mechanism through which this occurs. With feedback, a hormone can regulate the synthesis and action of itself or of another hormone. Further coordination is provided by hormone action at multiple sites and eliciting multiple responses. In the HPG axis, negative feedback is principally responsible for minimizing hormonal perturbations and maintaining homeostasis.

HORMONES OF THE HPG AXIS

As the integrative center of the HPG axis, the hypothalamus receives neuronal input from many brain centers, including the amygdala, thalamus, pons, retina, and cortex, and it is the pulse generator for the cyclical secretion of pituitary and gonadal hormones. It is anatomically linked to the pituitary gland by both a portal vascular system and neuronal pathways. By avoiding the systemic circulation, the portal vascular system provides a direct mechanism to deliver hypothalamic hormones to the anterior pituitary. Among the hypothalamic hormones, the most important for reproduction is gonadotropin-releasing hormone (GnRH) or LH-releasing hormone, a 10–amino acid peptide secreted from the neuronal cell bodies in the preoptic and arcuate nuclei. Currently, the only known function of GnRH is to stimulate the secretion of LH and FSH from the anterior pituitary. GnRH has a half-life of approximately 5 to 7 minutes. GnRH secretion is pulsatile in nature and results from integrated input from a variety of influences, including stress, exercise, diet, input from higher brain centers, pituitary gonadotropins, and circulating gonadal hormones.

The anterior pituitary gland, located within the bony sella turcica, is the site of action of GnRH. GnRH stimulates the production and release of FSH and LH by a calcium flux-dependent mechanism. These peptide hormones, named after their elucidation in the female, are equally important in the male. The sensitivity of the pituitary gonadotrophs to GnRH varies with patient age and hormonal status.

LH and FSH are the primary pituitary hormones that regulate ovarian and testis function. They are glycoproteins composed of two polypeptide chain subunits, termed a and b, each coded by a separate gene. The a subunits of each hormone are identical and similar to that of all other pituitary hormones; biologic and immunologic activity are conferred by the unique b subunit. Both subunits are required for endocrine activity. Oligosaccharide sugars with sialic acid residues are linked to these peptide subunits and may account for their differences in signal transduction and plasma clearance. Secretory pulses of LH vary in frequency from 8 to 16 pulses in 24 hours, generally reflecting GnRH release. Both androgens and estrogens regulate LH secretion through negative feedback. On average, FSH pulses occur approximately every 1.5 hours. The gonadal protein inhibin inhibits FSH secretion and accounts for the relative secretory independence of FSH from GnRH secretion. Activin, a structurally similar gonadal peptide, may act in a paracrine fashion to increase FSH binding in the ovary and stimulate spermatogenesis in the male, although serum levels of this substance are difficult to detect.

FSH and LH are known to act only in the gonads. In the testis, LH stimulates steroidogenesis within Leydig cells by inducing the mitochondrial conversion of cholesterol to pregnenolone and testosterone. FSH binds to Sertoli cells and spermatogonial membranes within the testis and is the major stimulator of seminiferous tubule growth during development and responds to inhibin secretion by Sertoli cells. Normal testosterone production in males is approximately 5 g/day, with secretion occurring in a damped, irregular, pulsatile manner. About 2% of testosterone is "free" or unbound and considered the biologically active fraction. The remainder is almost equally bound to albumin or SHBG within the blood. Testosterone is metabolized into two major active metabolites: DHT from the action of 5-alpha-reductase, and estradiol through the action of aromatases. DHT is a more potent androgen than testosterone. In most peripheral tissues, DHT is required for androgen action, but in the testis and skeletal muscle, conversion to DHT is not essential for hormonal activity. Testosterone stimulates the growth and maintenance of the secondary sex organs (prostate, seminal vesicles, penis, and accessory glands). In addition, testosterone is a potent anabolic steroid with various extragenital effects. In the brain, it influences libido, male aggression, mood, and aspects of cognition, including verbal memory and visual-spatial skills. It is responsible for an increase in muscle strength and growth and stimulates erythropoietin in the kidney. In bone marrow, testosterone causes accelerated linear growth and closure of epiphyses. It helps the liver to produce serum proteins and influences the male external appearance, including body hair growth and other secondary characteristics.

In the female, LH stimulates estrogen production from theca interna cells during the follicular phase of the menstrual cycle. The highest levels of estrogen during the menstrual cycle occur just before ovulation. FSH induces follicular development through a morphogenic effect on granulosa cells that line the graafian follicle. Eventually, this stimulation leads to the follicle's ripening and ovulation. With ovulation, the follicle is transformed into the corpus luteum, and the majority of granulosa and theca cells now become luteinized and produce progesterone simultaneously with estrogen. LH also influences preovulatory follicular enlargement, induces ovulation, stimulates the proliferation of the theca cells that secrete progesterone in the latter half of the menstrual cycle, and supports the development of the corpora lutea for 2 weeks after ovulation. Termed the *hormone of pregnancy,* progesterone supports endometrial development in early pregnancy, thickens the cervical mucus to prevent infection, decreases uterine contractility, and inhibits lactation during pregnancy. It is also necessary for the complete action of ovarian hormones on the fallopian tubes, uterus, vagina, external genitalia, and mammary glands. Interestingly, the ovarian estrogens and progesterone do not have the marked extragenital anabolic effects on muscle, kidney, blood, larynx, skin, and hair that are found with androgens.

A third anterior pituitary hormone, prolactin, can also influence the HPG axis. Prolactin is a large, globular protein that maintains the luteal phase of the menstrual cycle and induces milk synthesis during pregnancy and lactation in females. The role of prolactin in males is less clear, but it may promote sexual gratification after intercourse and induce the refractory period after ejaculation. It also increases concentration of LH receptors on Leydig cells and sustains normally high intratesticular testosterone levels. Although low prolactin levels are not usually pathologic, hyperprolactinemia in either sex abolishes gonadotropin pulsatility by interfering with GnRH release.

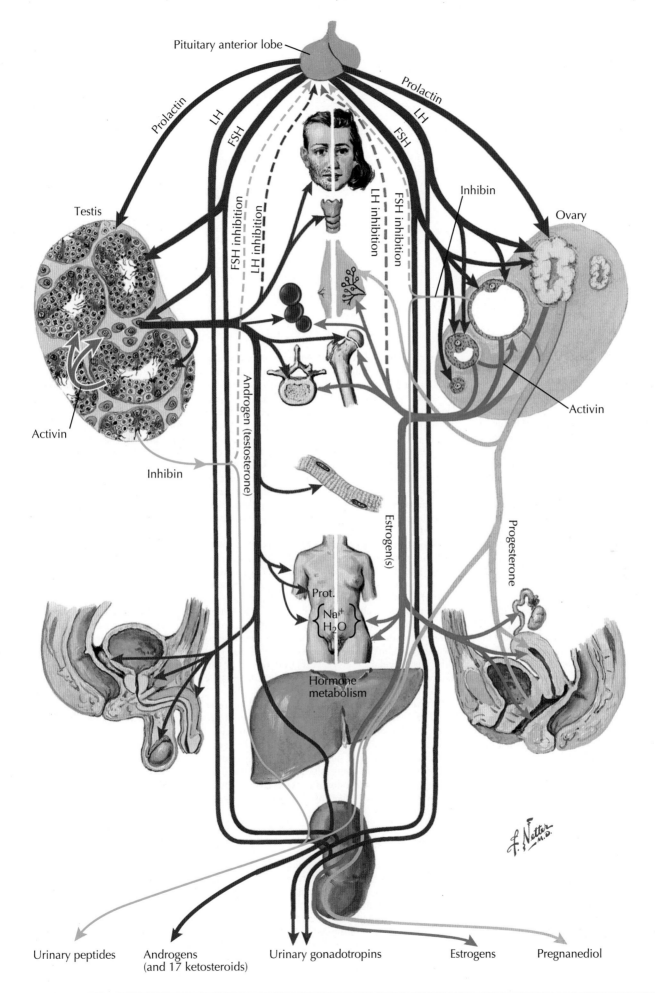

Plate 1.6   Reproductive System: VOLUME 1

PUBERTY: NORMAL SEQUENCE

The biggest differences between puberty in girls and boys are (1) the age at which it begins and (2) the major sex steroids involved. On average, girls begin puberty about 1 to 2 years earlier than boys (average age of 10.5 years in girls) and reach completion in a shorter time. Girls attain adult height and reproductive maturity about 4 years after the first changes of puberty. In contrast, boys accelerate more slowly but continue to grow for about 6 years after the first visible pubertal changes. Although boys are on average 2 cm shorter than girls before puberty begins, adult males are 13 cm taller than adult females. The hormone that dominates female development during puberty is estradiol, an estrogen. In males, testosterone, an androgen, is the principal sex steroid.

Puberty begins with GnRH pulsing, leading to a rise in gonadotropins, LH, and FSH and subsequently an increase in sex hormones. Indeed, exogenous GnRH pulses cause the onset of puberty, and brain tumors that increase GnRH may cause premature puberty. Puberty begins consistently at around 47 kg for girls and 55 kg for boys, and this correlation of pubertal onset with weight makes leptin the prime candidate for causing GnRH rise. Kisspeptin, a protein responsible for developmentally activating GnRH neurons and triggering GnRH release, is also involved in inducing pubertal onset. In addition, other genetic, environmental, and nutritional factors are thought to regulate pubertal timing.

PUBERTY: FEMALE

The first physical sign of puberty in females is usually a firm, tender lump under the areola(e) of the breasts, referred to as *thelarche*. In the Tanner staging of puberty, this is stage 2 of breast development (stage 1 is a flat, prepubertal breast). Within 6 to 12 months, the swelling is bilateral, softer, and extends beyond the areolae (stage 3). In another year (stage 4), the breasts are approaching mature size and shape, with areolae and papillae forming a secondary mound. This mound usually disappears into the contour of the mature breast (stage 5). Pubic hair is often the second change of puberty, usually within a few months of thelarche, and

is termed pubarche. The first few pubic hairs visible along the labia are Tanner stage 2. Stage 3 takes another 6 to 12 months, when hairs are too numerous to count and appear on the pubic mound. In stage 4, the hairs densely fill the pubic triangle. In stage 5, pubic hairs spread to the thighs and sometimes upward to the navel.

In response to estrogen, the vaginal mucosa also changes, becoming thicker and a dull pink in color. Whitish vaginal secretions (physiologic leukorrhea) can also be found. For 2 years after thelarche, the uterus and ovaries increase in size and follicles in the ovaries also enlarge. The ovaries contain small follicular cysts observable by ultrasound.

The first menstrual bleeding is referred to as *menarche* and typically occurs 2 years after thelarche. The average age of menarche in US girls is 11.7 years. Menses are not always regular for the first 2 years after menarche. Ovulation may or may not accompany the earliest menses, as about 80% of cycles are anovulatory in the first year after menarche. Although occurring more frequently with age after menarche, ovulation is not inevitably linked to the menstrual cycle, and girls with cycle irregularity several years from menarche can continue to have irregularity, anovulation, and possibly infertility.

Also in response to rising estrogen levels, the lower half of the pelvis and hips widen, creating a larger birth canal. The proportion of fat in body composition also increases, especially in the breasts, hips, buttocks, thighs, upper arms, and pubis. Rising androgen levels change the fatty acid composition of perspiration, resulting in an adult body odor and increased oil (sebum) secretions from the skin. This change increases the chances of acne.

PUBERTY: MALES

In males, testicular enlargement is the first physical sign of puberty and is termed gonadarche. Testes in prepubertal boys change little in size from 1 year of age until puberty, averaging about 2 to 3 mL in volume. Testicular size increases throughout puberty, reaching maximal adult size 6 years later. Although 18 to 20 mL is the average adult testis size, there is also wide ethnic variation.

The testis Leydig cells produce testosterone that induces most of the changes of sexual maturation and

maintains libido. Most of the increasing bulk of testicular tissue is due to growth of the seminiferous tubules, including Sertoli cells. The sequence of sperm production and the onset of fertility in males is not as well documented, largely because of the variable timing and onset of ejaculation. Sperm can be detected in the morning urine of most boys after the first year of puberty, and potential fertility can be reached as early as 13 years of age, with full fertility potential acquired at 14 to 16 years of age.

Pubic hair appears shortly after the genitalia start to grow. As in females, the first appearance of pubic hair is termed pubarche, and hairs are usually first visible at the base of the penis. The Tanner stages of hair growth are similarly classified in males and females, as described earlier. At about Tanner stage 3, the penis starts to grow. After the appearance of pubic hair, other body areas that respond to androgens develop heavier hair (androgenic hair) in the following sequence: axillary hair, perianal hair, upper lip hair, sideburn hair, periareolar hair, and facial beard. Arm, leg, chest, abdominal, and back hair become heavier more gradually. There is significant ethnic variation in the timing and quantity of hair growth.

Under the influence of androgens, the voice box, or larynx, grows in both sexes. Far more prominent in males, this growth causes the male voice to deepen about one octave, as the vocal cords lengthen and thicken. Voice change can be accompanied by unsteadiness of vocalization in the early stages. Most of the voice change occurs in stages 3 to 4 of male puberty, around the time of peak growth. Full adult voice pitch is attained at an average age of 15 years, usually preceding the development of facial hair by months to years.

By the end of puberty, adult males have heavier bones and nearly twice as much skeletal muscle as females. Some of the bone growth (e.g., shoulder width and jaw) is disproportionately greater, resulting in noticeably different male and female shapes. The average adult male has about 150% of the lean body mass of an average female and about 50% of the body fat. Muscle develops mainly during the later stages of puberty. The peak of the "strength spurt" is observed about 1 year after the peak growth rate. As with females, rising levels of androgens change the fatty acid composition of perspiration, resulting in adult body odor and acne. Acne typically resolves at the end of puberty.

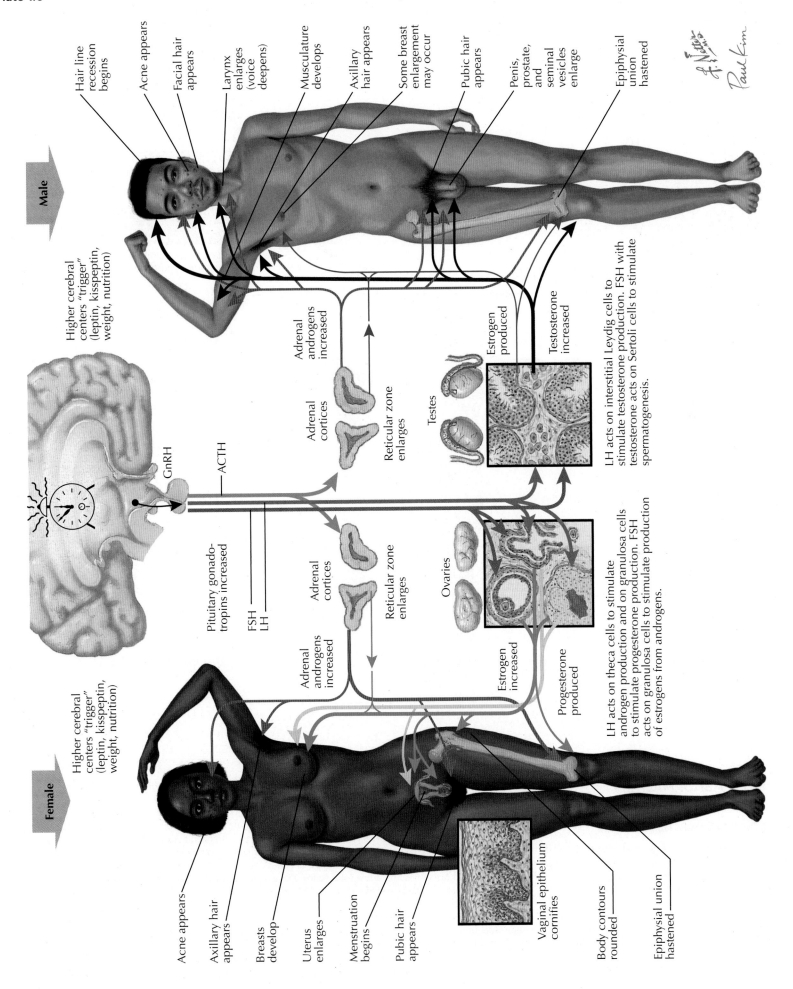

Male

Hair line recession begins

Acne appears

Facial hair appears

Larynx enlarges (voice deepens)

Musculature develops

Axillary hair appears

Some breast enlargement may occur

Pubic hair appears

Penis, prostate, and seminal vesicles enlarge

Epiphysial union hastened

Higher cerebral centers "trigger" (leptin, kisspeptin, weight, nutrition)

Adrenal androgens increased

Adrenal cortices

Reticular zone enlarges

Estrogen produced

Testosterone increased

Testes

LH acts on interstitial Leydig cells to stimulate testosterone production. FSH with testosterone acts on Sertoli cells to stimulate spermatogenesis.

GnRH

ACTH

Pituitary gonado-tropins increased

FSH
LH

Adrenal cortices

Adrenal androgens increased

Reticular zone enlarges

Ovaries

Estrogen increased

Progesterone produced

LH acts on theca cells to stimulate androgen production and on granulosa cells to stimulate progesterone production. FSH acts on granulosa cells to stimulate production of estrogens from androgens.

Higher cerebral centers "trigger" (leptin, kisspeptin, weight, nutrition)

Female

Acne appears

Axillary hair appears

Breasts develop

Uterus enlarges

Menstruation begins

Pubic hair appears

Vaginal epithelium cornifies

Body contours rounded

Epiphysial union hastened

Plate 1.7

Reproductive System: VOLUME 1

MALE GONADAL FAILURE

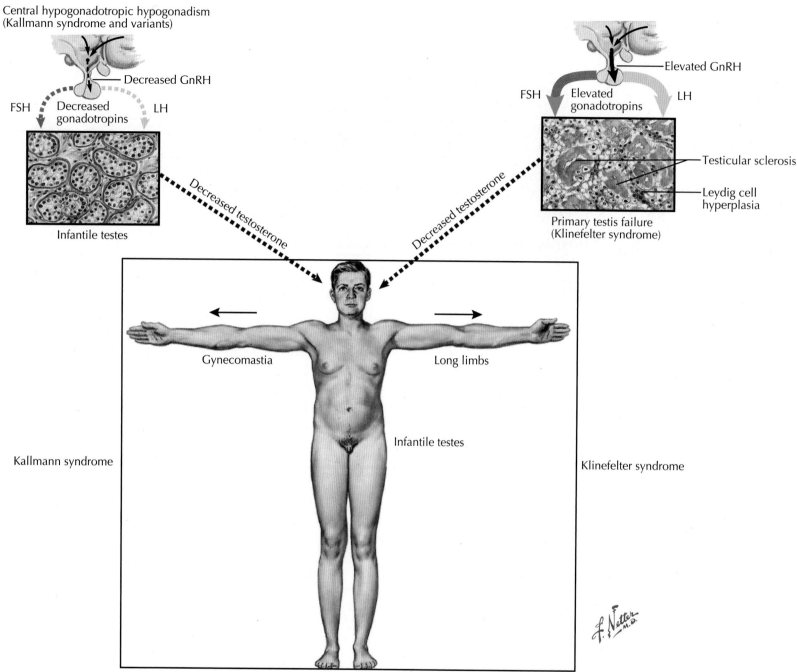

Central hypogonadotropic hypogonadism
(Kallmann syndrome and variants)

Decreased GnRH

FSH — Decreased gonadotropins — LH

Infantile testes

Decreased testosterone

Elevated GnRH

FSH — Elevated gonadotropins — LH

Testicular sclerosis

Leydig cell hyperplasia

Primary testis failure
(Klinefelter syndrome)

Decreased testosterone

Gynecomastia

Long limbs

Infantile testes

Kallmann syndrome

Klinefelter syndrome

PUBERTY: ABNORMALITIES

PUBERTY: ABNORMALITIES IN MALES

Abnormalities of puberty are generally due to issues of timing or dosage of sex steroids that normally govern phenotypic change. As discussed in Plate 1.5, androgens are converted to estrogens in the male by aromatase and because of this, male adolescence is frequently (80%) accompanied by gynecomastia. Issues of delayed puberty are a consequence of the lack of GnRH stimulation in patients with hypogonadotropic hypogonadism, as typified by Kallmann syndrome and its variants and Prader-Willi syndrome. Idiopathic hypogonadotropic

hypogonadism (IHH) or Kallmann syndrome is characterized by hypogonadism. Most patients experience a delay in puberty, although those with less severe defects may present with only infertility. Other findings include anosmia and midline abnormalities such as cleft palate and small testes. When anosmia is not present, the condition is termed IHH. The clinical diagnosis is confirmed by blood tests revealing a low total testosterone associated with low LH and low FSH levels in combination with normal prolactin. The condition is inherited as a familial disorder in one-third of cases. X-linked and autosomal inheritance patterns have been described. In the X-linked recessive form, deletions occur in *KAL1* (Kallmann-interval 1), a gene responsible for the migration of GnRH and olfactory neurons to the preoptic area

of the hypothalamus during development. As a consequence, there is failure of testicular stimulation by the anterior pituitary and hypothalamus and thus testis failure in addition to anosmia. Mutations in other genes have also been associated with IHH, including *Dax1* on the X chromosome (associated with CAH), the GnRH receptor, and *PC1* (associated with diabetes and obesity). Low testosterone is generally treated with testosterone replacement. Infertility due to azoospermia (no ejaculated sperm) can be treated with gonadotropin (LH and FSH) replacement over 12 to 18 months, which induces sperm in the ejaculate in 80% of males who are affected.

Primary testis failure, causing an inadequate testosterone surge at puberty and exemplified by Klinefelter

CAUSES OF MALE SEXUAL PRECOCITY

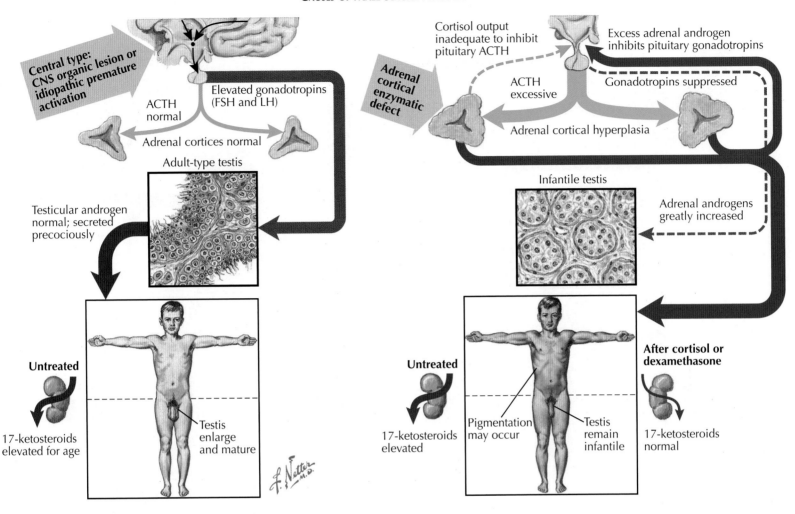

PUBERTY: ABNORMALITIES (Continued)

syndrome, may also produce a delay in the onset or sequence of pubertal events (Plate 1.7). Klinefelter syndrome is an abnormality of chromosomal number in which 90% of males carry an extra X chromosome (47,XXY) and 10% are mosaic with a combination of XXY/XY chromosomes. It is thought that approximately half of XXY cases are paternally derived, and recent evidence suggests that its occurrence may correlate with advanced paternal age. This syndrome may present with delayed puberty, increased height, decreased intelligence, varicosities, obesity, diabetes, leukemia, increased

likelihood of extragonadal germ cell tumors, and breast cancer (20-fold higher than normal males). Testis biopsies show sclerosis and hyalinization. In adults, hormones usually demonstrate a low testosterone and frankly elevated LH and FSH levels and generally require testosterone replacement. Natural paternity with this syndrome is possible, but almost exclusively with the mosaic or milder form of the disease. Biologic paternity in cases of pure XXY males is now possible with testicular sperm retrieval and assisted reproduction.

Sexual precocity, or the early onset of puberty, has a variety of causes in males (Plate 1.8). In idiopathic form (50% of cases), puberty proceeds in a normal pattern but begins earlier and is compressed into a shorter time frame. Although males who are affected are tall for their age during early puberty, the premature closure of

the epiphyses results in a markedly short stature in adulthood. Central causes of precocious puberty include brain tumors near the third ventricle, including astrocytoma, meningioma, or pinealoma, and are usually accompanied by diabetes insipidus and visual field defects. It can also be associated with congenital malformations such as hematomas of the brain.

Other causes of male precocious puberty are adrenal in origin and include CAH and benign or malignant virilizing adrenal cortical tumors (Plates 1.8 and 1.9). There are two major types of CAH: classic and nonclassic. The classic form is the more severe of the two and affects very young children and newborns. The nonclassic form is milder and usually develops in late childhood or early adulthood. Signs and symptoms of classic CAH in infants include an enlarged penis in

Plate 1.9

Reproductive System: VOLUME 1

CAUSES OF MALE SEXUAL PRECOCITY (CONTINUED)

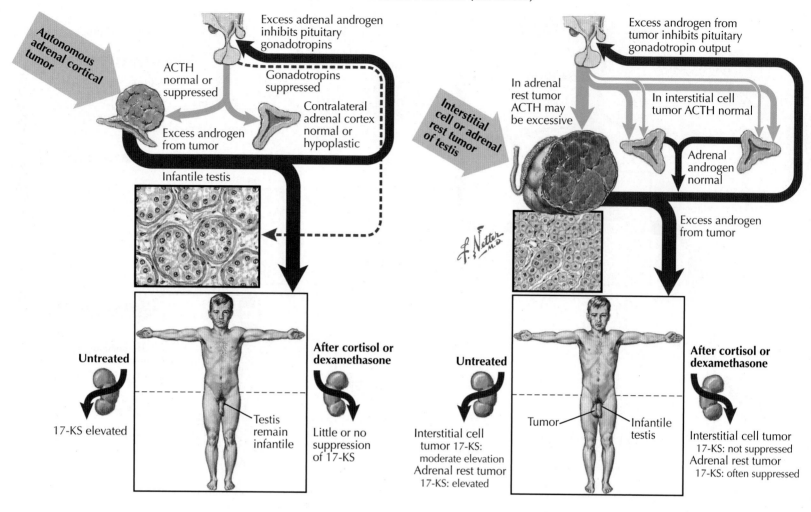

PUBERTY: ABNORMALITIES (Continued)

boys (macrogenitosomia), failure to regain birth weight, weight loss, acne, dehydration, vomiting, and pigmentation of the scrotum and perianal regions. Signs and symptoms of the classic condition in older children and adults include rapid growth during childhood, very early puberty with the development of pubic hair and deepening of the voice, shorter than average final height, and infertility. Nonclassic CAH generally presents with rapid growth during childhood and early puberty, severe acne, nausea, fatigue, low blood pressure, low bone density, high cholesterol, and obesity. Children can also often have slow recovery from infections and colds. Fundamentally, CAH results from a deficiency of one of the hydroxylase enzymes that are

required for cortisol synthesis from 17-hydroxyprogesterone. Impaired cortisol secretion activates pituitary gland secretion of excessive ACTH, and the adrenal gland undergoes compensatory hypertrophy as a result. In addition, large quantities of cortisol precursors are made that form the substrates for androgens. Excessive androgens contribute to the virilization and also downregulate pituitary gonadotropin secretion, so that the testes remain small and infantile despite other pubertal changes. The clinical signs of a virilizing adrenal adenoma or cortical carcinoma are similar to those induced by any other cause (Plate 1.8). These conditions can be differentiated from other causes by the lack of suppression of 17-ketosteroid secretion with exogenous glucocorticoids.

Primary testicular tumors can also cause precocious puberty (Plate 1.9). Based on proliferation of interstitial Leydig cells, these tumors can usually be palpated as nodular enlargement of one testis with a contralateral atrophic testis. Again, 17-ketosteroids are usually not

suppressed with glucocorticoids in this condition, and the adrenal glands are normal on imaging. Clumps of adrenal cells termed adrenal rests can also descend with the testis into the scrotum and be metabolically active and induce virilization. Adrenal rests are more likely to become active in cases of CAH in which there is excessive adrenal stimulation and can present as testis or peritestis enlargement. Even more rare are teratomatous rests in the scrotum that secrete excessive amounts of chorionic gonadotropin (hCG) that is similar to the gonadotropin LH and stimulates androgen production. These rests are highly malignant and are associated with growth of the contralateral testis as a result of gonadotropic-like stimulation.

PUBERTY: ABNORMALITIES IN FEMALES

Delayed puberty may occur for several years and then proceed normally in what is referred to as *constitutional*

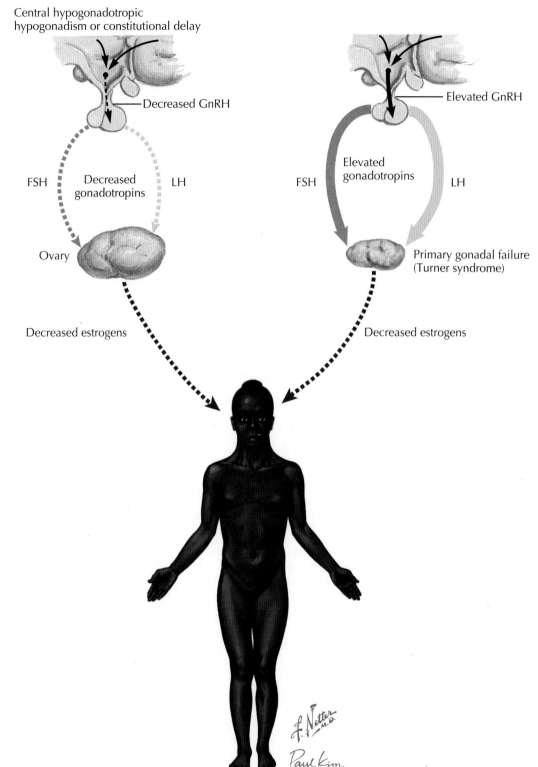

FEMALE GONADAL FAILURE

Central hypogonadotropic
hypogonadism or constitutional delay

Decreased GnRH

Elevated GnRH

FSH
Decreased
gonadotropins
LH

FSH
Elevated
gonadotropins
LH

Ovary

Primary gonadal failure
(Turner syndrome)

Decreased estrogens

Decreased estrogens

PUBERTY: ABNORMALITIES (Continued)

delay. It may also be due to poor nutrition from anorexia, extreme athleticism, and systemic disease such as chronic renal failure, hypothyroidism, and Cushing syndrome. Reproductive disorders such as Kallmann syndrome or Prader-Willi syndrome, gonadal defects characteristic of Turner syndrome, or a lack of response to sex steroids associated with androgen insensitivity disorders (in a genetic male) may also occur (Plate 1.10). Turner syndrome or Ullrich-Turner syndrome (a form of gonadal dysgenesis) occurs when one of the two female X chromosomes is constitutionally missing. When only a part of the X chromosome is missing, mosaic Turner syndrome may be present. Because this syndrome only affects the second X chromosome, the syndrome is only present in females. Occurring in 1 of every 2500 girls, the syndrome presents with characteristic physical abnormalities, such as short stature, broad chest, low hairline, low-set ears, and webbed neck. Girls with Turner syndrome typically have gonadal dysfunction (nonworking ovaries) that results in amenorrhea and sterility. Other health concerns include congenital heart disease, hypothyroidism, diabetes, vision and hearing problems, and autoimmune disease. Finally, there is also a characteristic pattern of cognitive deficits observed, with difficulties in visuospatial, mathematic, and memory areas. Rarely, cystic fibrosis and Frasier syndrome can result in delayed puberty.

There are two benign variants of sexual precocity in females: premature thelarche (benign mammoplasia) and premature pubarche. In the former, there is isolated premature development of breast tissue and in the latter, isolated pubic hair. Both may be associated with childhood obesity. True sexual precocity is usually due to central (nervous system) or ovarian causes (Plate 1.11). Adrenal tumors or hyperplasia in the female most commonly causes virilization and not true sexual precocity. Idiopathic sexual precocity is more common in girls than boys and presents with advanced stature and bone age, breast enlargement, vaginal wall

thickening, pubic hair, and acne. Axillary hair is rarely found but adult perspiration odors can be obvious. In addition, uterine enlargement can occur and irregular menstrual bleeding is possible. Central stimulation by gonadotropins can also result in large follicular cysts in the ovary, which may be difficult to distinguish from primary ovarian tumors. Spontaneous remission of idiopathic sexual precocity is not uncommon.

McCune-Albright syndrome, caused by a sporadic mutation in the *GNAS1* gene, is a special form of central

precocity that is associated with polyostotic fibrous dysplasia, a nonmetabolic skeletal disorder in which scar forms in bone that can lead to deformities and fractures (Plate 1.11). In this condition, sexual precocity is combined with lesions in the long bones and café-au-lait spots that stop at the midline. Thyroid enlargement is common, often with thyrotoxicosis. Girls who are affected may also have frontal bone and zygomatic arches, features characteristic of acromegaly, and polycystic ovaries and hirsutism. Primary hypothyroidism

Plate 1.11

Reproductive System: VOLUME 1

CAUSES OF FEMALE SEXUAL PRECOCITY

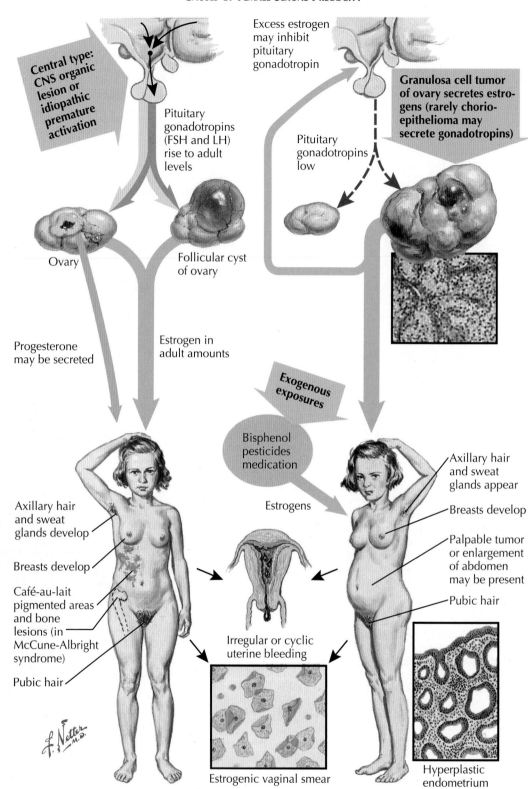

CNS, Central nervous system; FSH, follicle-stimulating hormone; LH, luteinizing hormone.

PUBERTY: ABNORMALITIES
(Continued)

can present with breast enlargement, early menstruation, and galactorrhea. These symptoms regress when thyroid replacement is given and suggest that pituitary gonadotropin hyperstimulation may be associated with excess thyroid-stimulating hormone stimulation.

Feminizing tumors of the ovary are a relatively common cause of sexual precocity in girls (Plate 1.11). Granulosa-theca cell tumors, more commonly known as *granulosa cell tumors,* belong to the sex cord–stromal group and include tumors made up of granulosa cells, theca cells, and fibroblasts in varying degrees. About 5% of these tumors occur in juveniles and the majority of the rest occur in postmenopausal females. Both types commonly produce estrogen, and estrogen production often is the reason for early diagnosis. Theca cell tumors are almost always benign and carry an excellent prognosis. The rare malignant thecoma likely represents a tumor with a small admixture of granulosa cells. It is not exactly known how these tumors arise, but it has been proposed that they are derived from either the mesenchyme of the developing genital ridge or precursors within the mesonephric and coelomic epithelium. Granulosa-theca cell tumors can be large, palpable, and can secrete large amounts of estrogen that causes heavy feminization. Some features of the syndrome, such as the growth of pubic and axillary hair, are attributed to associated pituitary stimulation. Complete tumor resection is mandatory for resolution of these symptoms. Rarer, but far more malignant, tumors of the ovary that can cause similar symptoms are progesterone-secreting luteomas and chorionepitheliomas. Exogenous estrogen intake through contaminated medications, foods, cosmetics, or exposure to endocrine disruptors such as bisphenol A and phthalates and estrogenic pesticides may underlie some cases of prior unexplained precocious puberty (Plate 1.11). Bisphenol A is an organic phenol compound that has been used primarily to make plastics for more than 50 years. It is used to make polyesters, plasticizers, polycarbonate, and epoxy resins, and is found in baby and water bottles, sports

equipment, medical and dental devices, dental fillings and sealants, eyeglass lenses, CDs and DVDs, and household electronics. Although good-quality human studies are currently lacking, animal studies have shown that excessive exposure to bisphenol A may be related to changes in anogenital distance, early puberty, changes in breast tissue that may predispose

to carcinogens, and decreased maternal behavior. Phthalates are a class of widely used industrial compounds known technically as alkyl aryl esters and are used as softeners of plastics, oily additives in perfumes, additives to hairsprays, lubricants, and wood finishers, and they have been linked to premature breast development in girls.

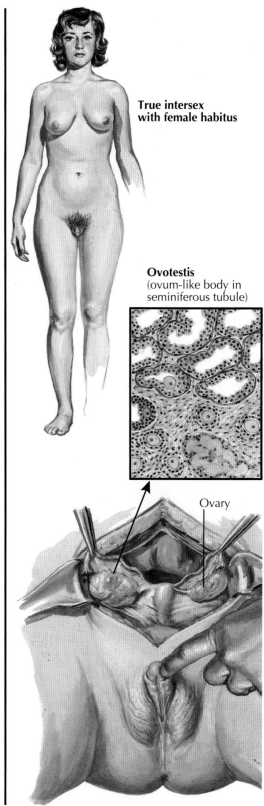

True intersex with male habitus

True intersex with female habitus

Ovotestis (ovum-like body in seminiferous tubule)

Ovary

Unicornuate uterus

Ovary

Testis

SEX DEVELOPMENT: TRUE INTERSEX

Intersexuality is that state in which sex chromosomes, genitalia, and/or secondary sex characteristics are neither exclusively male nor female. Patients who are intersex may have biologic characteristics of both the male and female sexes. Previously termed true hermaphroditism, a true intersex state is rare and exists when both testicular and ovarian tissue are present in the same individual, regardless of the karyotype. There may be an ovary on one side and a testis on the other, an ovotestis on each side, or a combination of these. These disorders have been alternatively designated as DSD.

The prevalence of intersex depends on the definition of the condition. Approximately 1% of live births exhibit some degree of sexual ambiguity. Between 0.1% and 0.2% of live births are ambiguous enough to consider surgical correction. When the definition is restricted to conditions in which chromosomal sex differs from phenotypic sex or in which the phenotype is not classifiable as either male or female, the prevalence is 0.018%.

True intersex is extremely rare, and it is even rarer that both types of gonadal tissue function. It has been described in patients with karyotypes 47,XXY; 46,XX/46,XY; or 46,XX/47,XXY. This condition is quite distinguishable histologically from mixed gonadal dysgenesis. It is caused by (1) the division of one unfertilized egg, followed by fertilization of each haploid egg and fusion of the two embryos early in development, or (2) an egg fertilized by two sperm followed by trisomic rescue such that a diploid embryo results, or (3) two eggs fertilized by two sperm cells, and these zygotes fuse to form a tetragametic chimera, or (4) abnormalities or mutations in the expression of the testis determining factor, the *SRY* gene.

In true intersex, the phenotype of the internal and external genitalia may be predicted from gonadal lateralization. In individuals with an ovary on one side and a testis on the other, müllerian structures persist on the side of the ovary, whereas atrophy of the fallopian tube and well-developed wolffian derivatives are found on the side of the testis. When ovarian and testis tissue occur on the same side, the development of wolffian structures is proportional to the degree of testicular maturation. With a well-developed testis, the gonads are found in the scrotum, and there is a proportional decrease in müllerian remnants. With a rudimentary testis, the gonad is usually located in a broad ligament adjacent to a normal uterus. External genitalia are often ambiguous, depending mainly on the amount of testosterone produced by testicular tissue during organogenesis from 8 to 16 weeks of gestation.

Adolescence and secondary sexual characteristics may be expected to mirror the degree of differentiation of gonadal structures. Usually, there is some degree of masculinization. However, coincidental signs of active estrogen secretion may include breast enlargement and menstruation. There is no absolute reason why the gonads may not develop to full spermatogenesis and oogenesis. However, spermatogenesis is unlikely if estrogens are secreted in significant quantities because of inhibition of FSH. Regardless of anatomy, the "true sex" of these individuals is the one to which they best adapt in society, and serious consideration of the need and role of gender reassignment surgery is widely accepted in the medical community.

Plate 1.13

Reproductive System: VOLUME 1

INTERSEX: MALE GONADAL

Gonadal intersex is an individual with the gonads of only one sex but with genitalia (internal and external) and secondary sex characters exhibiting sexual ambiguity. Such a simple classification of intersex is based purely on phenotype or morphology, without regard to genetic etiology. Factors that contribute to such disordered development include (1) gene mutations, (2) abnormal maternal hormonal influences, and (3) abnormal hormonal influences from the embryonic gonad, adrenal, or other endocrine organ. The type and degree of disordered development depend on the intensity and timing of these influences during embryonic life.

Male gonadal intersex exhibits varying degrees of female internal or external genitalia but have gonads that are testes. Although genetically male, they are often raised as female; the onset of puberty with growth of the penis, hair, and voice change usually precipitates medical evaluation for intersex. Simple penile hypospadias is a very elementary form of male gonadal intersex. In more severe forms, müllerian structures can develop to various degrees, and in most instances a bifid scrotum appearing as labial folds conceals a rudimentary blind pouch or well-developed vaginal cavity. The testes may lie intraabdominally, within the inguinal canal, or may have descended into a bifid scrotum. When the sex of the infant is unclear, exploratory surgery and gonadal biopsy to determine gonadal as well as genetic sex is considered during infancy. Most male gonadal intersex individuals develop emotionally as males during puberty, which has led to the performance of gender correction procedures, including release of penile chordee, construction of a penile urethra, orchiopexy, and, in some instances, excision of the vagina, uterus, and fallopian tubes.

Milder forms of male gonadal intersex include Klinefelter syndrome (47,XXY; 48,XXXY and mosaics), Kallmann syndrome (gonadotropin deficiency and anosmia), micropenis, and distal hypospadias. Aphallia is a birth defect in which the penis or clitoris is congenitally absent. It is a rare condition, with fewer than 100 cases reported. Its cause is not entirely clear, but it appears to be due to a failure of the fetal genital tubercle to form between 3 and 6 weeks after conception. Anatomically, the urethra opens on the perineum, and it can occur in both males and females.

There are several forms of gonadal dysgenesis that may also result in male gonadal intersex. The term *pure gonadal dysgenesis* describes conditions with normal sex chromosomes (e.g., 46,XX or 46,XY), as opposed to gonadal dysgenesis in which the genetic constitution involves missing or truncated sex chromosomes (e.g., Turner syndrome, 45,X). Mixed gonadal dysgenesis involves a genetic mixture of sex chromosomes (e.g., 46,XY/45,X). In this condition, there is a streak gonad that develops on one side, with a partially developed testis on the opposite side, and it can be associated with ambiguous genitalia. Importantly, streak gonads with

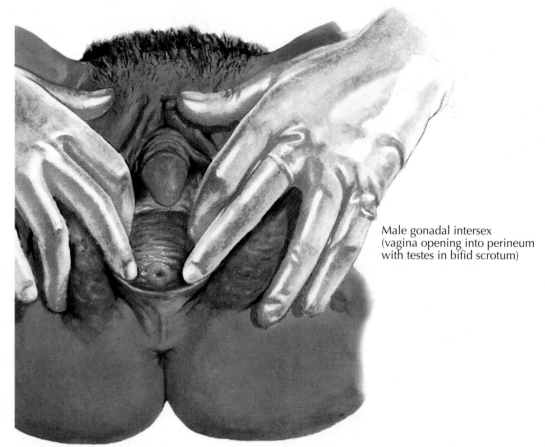

Male gonadal intersex
(vagina opening into perineum
with testes in bifid scrotum)

Abdominal testis

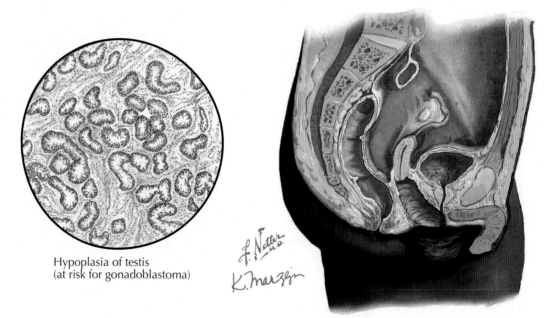

Hypoplasia of testis
(at risk for gonadoblastoma)

Y chromosome–containing cells have a high likelihood of developing cancer, especially gonadoblastoma. In Swyer syndrome, an example of 46,XY pure gonadal dysgenesis, there is atypical formation of both gonads early in gestation. In complete gonadal dysgenesis, the gonads do not function at all, resulting in a female appearance of the external genitalia. In partial gonadal dysgenesis, the testes function, but not at normal levels, resulting in a male with ambiguous genitalia. Because

the adrenal glands can make small amounts of androgens and are unaffected, pubic hair develops in most patients, although it often remains sparse. In complete forms such as Swyer syndrome, the diagnosis is often made due to delayed puberty. A karyotype reveals XY, and pelvic imaging demonstrates a uterus (no MIS present) but no ovaries (streak gonads are not usually seen). The absence of breasts and the presence of a uterus exclude the possibility of androgen insensitivity.

Normal female external genitalia (or slightly masculinized) vagina ends blindly

INTERSEX: MALE HORMONAL

There are several DSD that are accompanied by a normal karyotype (46,XY male) and are characterized by hormonal perturbations that induce sexual ambiguity. AIS, also referred to as *androgen resistance syndrome,* is a form of male disordered sex development caused by mutations of the gene encoding the androgen receptor (located on Xq11–12, X-linked recessive trait). More than 100 androgen receptor mutations causing AIS have been reported. Most forms of AIS involve variable degrees of undervirilization and/or infertility, termed partial AIS (PAIS), with the degree of ambiguity varying according to the structure and sensitivity of the abnormal receptor. Reifenstein syndrome is a form of AIS with obviously ambiguous genitalia, small testes in the abdomen or scrotum, sparse to normal androgenic hair, and gynecomastia at puberty. In more subtle cases, AIS due to a mild, partial androgen receptor defect can present simply as male infertility with a low ejaculated sperm concentration.

An individual with complete androgen insensitivity syndrome (CAIS, 1:20,000 births) has an entirely female external appearance, including undescended testes, despite the normal male karyotype. They are typically psychosexually female, in accordance with their external appearance and genitalia. The clitoris and vagina may be underdeveloped. Bimanual palpation reveals no evidence of internal genitalia (e.g., cervix, uterus), which can be confirmed laparoscopically. The testes may be found in inguinal hernias, in the canals, or intraabdominally. They appear as typical immature, undescended testes but are at higher risk for malignant degeneration (4%–9% chance) and should be removed. With CAIS, medical attention is sometimes sought because of the sudden appearance of testes within the inguinal canals during puberty, although the most common presentation is primary amenorrhea. It should be distinguished from another condition that presents with primary amenorrhea: vaginal underdevelopment and absence of female internal genitalia in 46,XX females due to inappropriate AMH production and termed *Mayer-Rokitansky-Küster-Hauser* (MRKH) syndrome.

Another condition, 5-alpha-reductase deficiency (5-ARD), can be observed in phenotypic females with a normal male karyotype. It is characterized by an absence of the enzyme 5-alpha-reductase, which converts testosterone to DHT. DHT is the primary androgen needed for the normal development of male external genitalia. Without DHT, prenatal genital development results in a female appearance. Individuals with 5-ARD can have normal male external genitalia, ambiguous

Relatively normal female habitus (inguinal herniae)

Testes operatively exposed in groins; laparotomy reveals complete absence of uterus, fallopian tubes, and ovaries

Section of testis typical of cryptorchidism (in situ neoplasia in upper left corner)

Urinary gonadotropins normal

17-KS normal or slightly elevated

Estrogen (normal levels for female)

genitalia, or normal female genitalia. They are born with testicles and wolffian structures but usually have female sex characteristics. Because of the normal action of AMH produced by the testis in utero, individuals with 5-ARD lack a uterus and fallopian tubes. Consequently, they are often raised as girls and often develop a female gender identity. Because male puberty depends more strongly on testosterone than on DHT, puberty will be virilizing unless the gonads are removed or a blocking medication is used. As a consequence of

virilization at puberty, gender identity issues may occur in adulthood. Phenotypic girls will also have primary amenorrhea.

Individuals with 5-ARD are generally capable of producing viable sperm. In those with feminized or ambiguous genitalia, there is a tendency toward a macroclitoris or microphallus. This structure may be capable of ejaculation as well as erection; however, assisted reproduction is necessary for fertility as intercourse may not be possible.

Plate 1.15

Reproductive System: VOLUME 1

INTERSEX: FEMALE

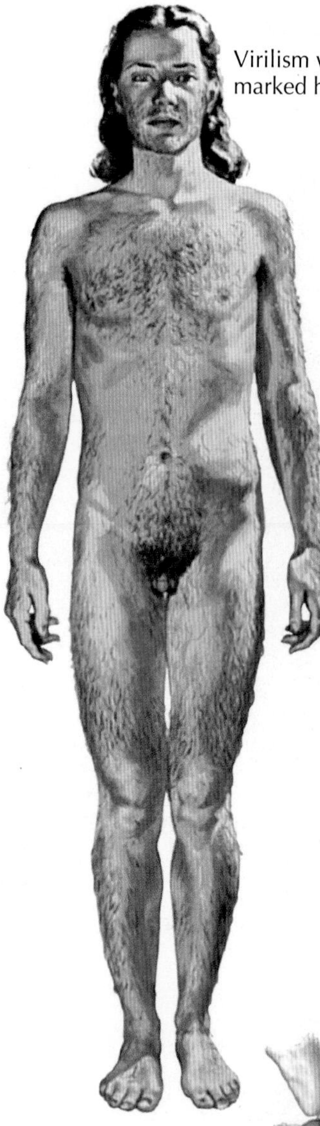

With female intersex an individual has ovaries but the external genitalia have a male appearance. This DSD usually results from hormonal disturbances. The maternal use of androgens or high doses of certain weakly androgenic synthetic progestogens (progestins) can masculinize or virilize the fetal female external genitalia during susceptible times in pregnancy. An example of a weakly androgenic substance is the sex steroid danazol, a derivative of ethisterone (17α-ethinyl-testosterone) that is used to treat severe endometriosis. Progestogens currently used for luteal support of pregnancy in in vitro fertilization (IVF) protocols or for prevention of preterm birth include progesterone, 17α-hydroxyprogesterone caproate, and dydrogesterone. Along with clitoral enlargement (clitoromegaly), some degree of fusion of the urogenital folds can occur with exposure from the 8th through the 12th week of gestation. This can present as ambiguous genitalia at birth. If exposure occurs after the 12th gestational week, then only clitoral enlargement occurs. Females with clitoral enlargement mature normally and have normal fertility, with almost total regression of the genital anomaly by adulthood. Surgical correction of labioscrotal fusion can be considered if desired. A much rarer cause of clitoromegaly is Fraser syndrome, characterized by defects including underdevelopment of the eyes (cryptophthalmos) and linked to the gene *FRAS1*, which may be involved in skin epithelial morphogenesis.

Müllerian agenesis (MRKH syndrome) is a congenital malformation characterized by a failure of the müllerian ducts to develop, resulting in a missing uterus and variable malformations of the vagina. Unlike other intersex conditions, MRKH is not associated with virilization but only absence of internal female genitalia. A female with this condition is hormonally normal, enters puberty, and develops typical secondary sexual characteristics. Usually, the vagina is shortened and intercourse may be difficult or painful. Medical examination demonstrates complete or partial absence of the cervix, uterus, and vagina. It is possible for females who are affected to have genetic offspring by IVF and surrogacy. Females with MRKH typically discover the condition when the menstrual cycle does not begin at puberty, as it is the second most common cause of primary amenorrhea.

The most common cause of female intersex is CAH, an endocrine disorder in which the adrenal glands produce abnormally high levels of virilizing hormones. In genetic females, this leads to an appearance that may be slightly masculinized (clitoromegaly) to very masculine. CAH refers to a constellation of autosomal recessive diseases that result from mutations in enzymes that mediate cortisol production from cholesterol (steroidogenesis). Most of these conditions involve excessive or deficient production of sex steroids, with 95% due to 21-hydroxylase deficiency. In addition to ambiguous genitalia, there can be vomiting due to salt-wasting, early pubic hair and rapid growth in childhood, precocious puberty or failure of puberty, virilization or menstrual irregularity in adolescence, infertility due to anovulation, and hypertension.

In its most common form, the vagina terminates in the posterior urethra; more rarely, it may open into the perineum, with the urethral orifice terminating in the anterior vaginal wall. The well-developed clitoris

Virilism with marked hirsutism

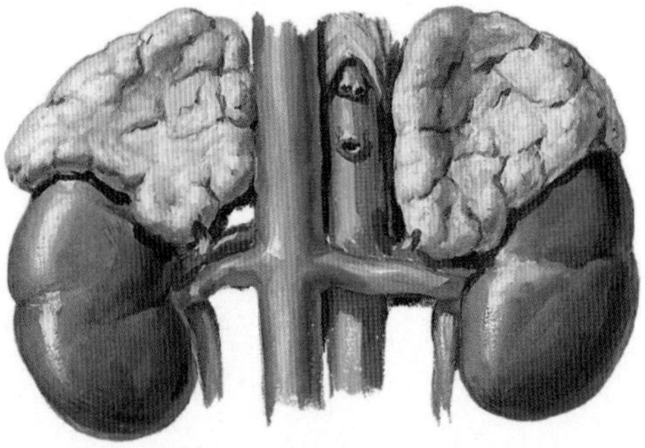

Adrenal cortical hyperplasia

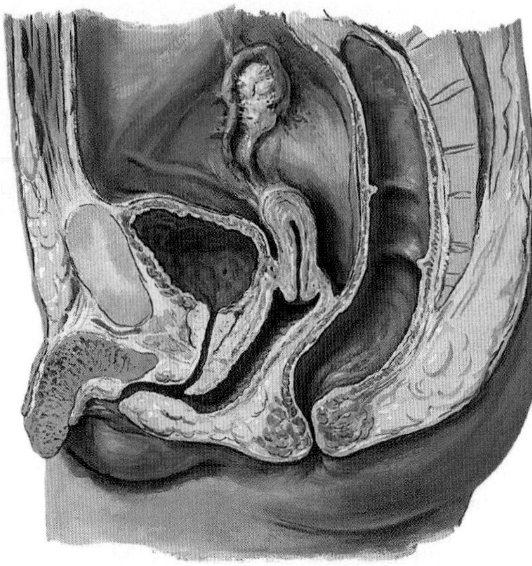

Genital configuration (vagina opening into urethra at base of hypertrophied clitoris; normally placed ovaries)

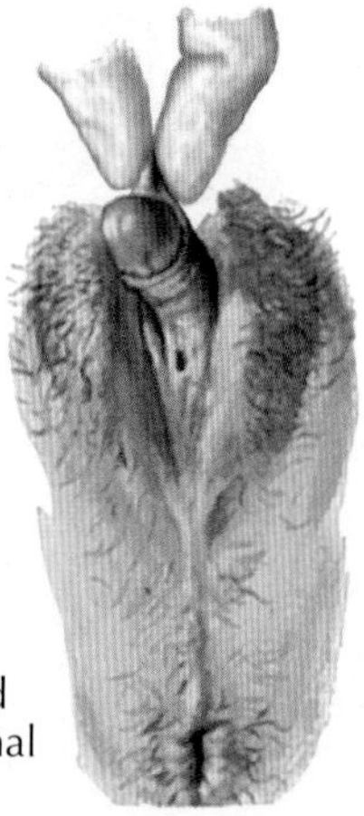

Genitalia: hypertrophied clitoris and urethrovaginal meatus

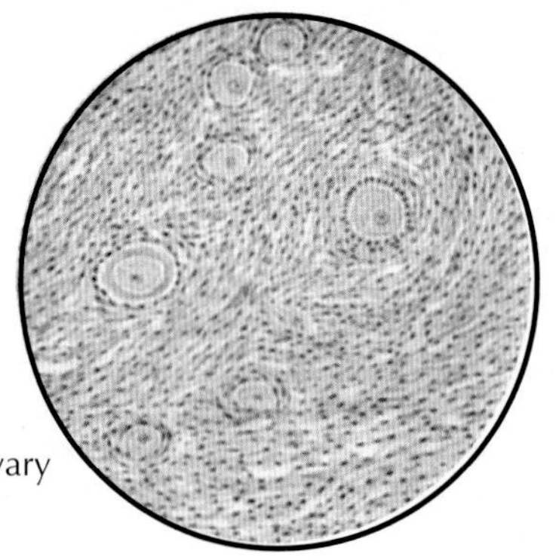

Hypoplastic ovary

resembles a hypospadiac penis with chordee, and the urethra is usually located in the penile base between two prominent labia majora, resembling a bifid scrotum. Palpation may reveal a small (hypoplastic) uterus and adnexa that result from androgenization.

In addition, there can be variations in secondary sex characteristics such as marked muscular growth, resulting in a short, stocky, or square body, and the general appearance of a well-developed male. Growth in stature is accelerated early, and the epiphyses close prematurely, resulting in an advanced bone age and a lower than average adult height. Other virilizing features, such as marked hirsutism of the face, torso, and extremities, are present. The voice becomes deep, with the thyroid

cartilage conspicuous. Breast development and menstruation are lacking. Signs of virilism are manifest usually at age 2 years and are characteristically progressive. The urine contains an abnormally large amount of 17-ketosteroids. Adrenal cortical tumors may also produce virilism, but they occur after birth when it is too late to cause ambiguous genitalia. Cortisol administration will suppress pituitary secretion of ACTH and reduce the activity of the hyperplastic adrenal cortex. This decrease fails to occur in patients with adrenocortical neoplasm and, thus, aids in the differential diagnosis. Treatment involves lifelong use of cortisol-like medications and gender-aligning surgery in some cases. Fertility is possible when the disease is well controlled.

PENIS AND MALE PERINEUM

Plate 2.1

Reproductive System: VOLUME 1

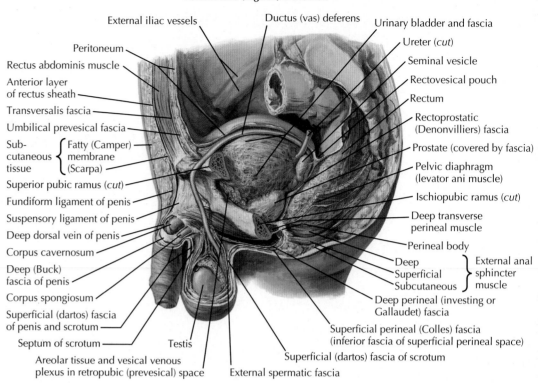

Paramedian (sagittal) dissection

External iliac vessels • Ductus (vas) deferens • Urinary bladder and fascia • Peritoneum • Rectus abdominis muscle • Anterior layer of rectus sheath • Transversalis fascia • Umbilical prevesical fascia • Subcutaneous tissue { Fatty (Camper) membrane (Scarpa) } • Superior pubic ramus (cut) • Fundiform ligament of penis • Suspensory ligament of penis • Deep dorsal vein of penis • Corpus cavernosum • Deep (Buck) fascia of penis • Corpus spongiosum • Superficial (dartos) fascia of penis and scrotum • Septum of scrotum • Areolar tissue and vesical venous plexus in retropubic (prevesical) space • Testis • External spermatic fascia • Ureter (cut) • Seminal vesicle • Rectovesical pouch • Rectum • Rectoprostatic (Denonvilliers) fascia • Prostate (covered by fascia) • Pelvic diaphragm (levator ani muscle) • Ischiopubic ramus (cut) • Deep transverse perineal muscle • Perineal body • Deep / Superficial / Subcutaneous } External anal sphincter muscle • Deep perineal (investing or Gallaudet) fascia • Superficial perineal (Colles) fascia (inferior fascia of superficial perineal space) • Superficial (dartos) fascia of scrotum

Median (sagittal) section

Urachus • Vesical fascia • Rectovesical pouch • Rectum • Urinary bladder { Apex / Fundus / Body / Trigone / Neck } • Pubic symphysis • Fundiform ligament of penis • Suspensory ligament of penis • Inferior (arcuate) pubic ligament • Transverse perineal ligament (anterior thickening of perineal membrane) • Perineal membrane • Corpus cavernosum • Corpus spongiosum • Superficial (dartos) fascia of penis and scrotum • Deep (Buck) fascia of penis • Superficial perineal space • Prepuce • Glans penis and external urethral meatus • Navicular fossa • Septum of scrotum • Buck fascia • Superficial perineal (Colles) fascia • Deep perineal (investing or Gallaudet) fascia • Bulbospongiosus muscle • Perineal body • Bulbourethral (Cowper) gland • Sphincter urethrae muscle • Rectoprostatic (Denonvilliers) fascia • Prostate • Seminal vesicle

PELVIC STRUCTURES

The relationships of male pelvic structures are illustrated in these complementary sagittal views—a paramedian and a median section. In the lower median view, the complete course of the *urethra* from the *bladder* to the *meatus* at the end of the *penis,* its passage through the *prostate gland* and the *urogenital diaphragm,* is shown. In the upper paramedian view, part of the pelvic bones (os ilium and ischium) have been removed, but both rami of the left *os pubis* and part of the inferior *ramus of the ischium* are present. The soft parts are sectioned laterally from the midline. This view allows visualization of the course of the *vas deferens* as it originates in the scrotum and ascends to pass over the superior ramus of the pubis and ultimately to the posterior surface of the bladder, passing over the ureter on each side ("water under the bridge"). Note too that the bladder, as a hollow smooth muscular organ, has muscle fibers that run in all directions, like a ball of yarn, to enable uniform concentric contractions during *micturition.* The paramedian view also illustrates the fact that all male urogenital organs exist in the extraabdominal, *retroperitoneal space* and are covered by the peritoneum superiorly. Both views outline the attachments and course of the ischiocavernosus and bulbocavernosus muscles and demonstrate the suspensory and fundiform ligaments.

Anatomic details of external and internal organs are discussed on Plates 2.2 and 3.1. However, well visualized here are the prostate gland below the bladder and paired *seminal vesicles* posterior to the bladder. The *preperitoneal space of Retzius* exists between the anterior surface of the prostate and bladder and the posterior surfaces of the symphysis and recti muscles. This retroperitoneal potential space contains veins, areolar tissue, nerves, and lymphatics and is bounded below by the superior surface of the urogenital diaphragm. The posterior surfaces of the prostate and the seminal vesicles are separated from the *anterior rectal wall* by a definite, fibrous layer of fascia termed the *rectovesical* or *Denonvilliers fascia* that covers the entire posterior surface of the prostate from its *apex,* over the surface of the seminal vesicles superiorly to the *rectovesical pouch.* Denonvilliers fascia is an important surgical landmark for operations that involve removal of the prostate or reflection of the rectal wall from the surface of the prostate.

The fascial planes of the urogenital region have considerable clinical significance because of their important function in supporting anatomic structures, their identification as surgical landmarks, and because their layered arrangement forms several interfascial spaces that control the spread of exudates, infections, malignancies, blood, or extravasated urine. In the plates that follow, these fascial layers will be shown in greater detail.

Plate 2.2

Penis and Male Perineum

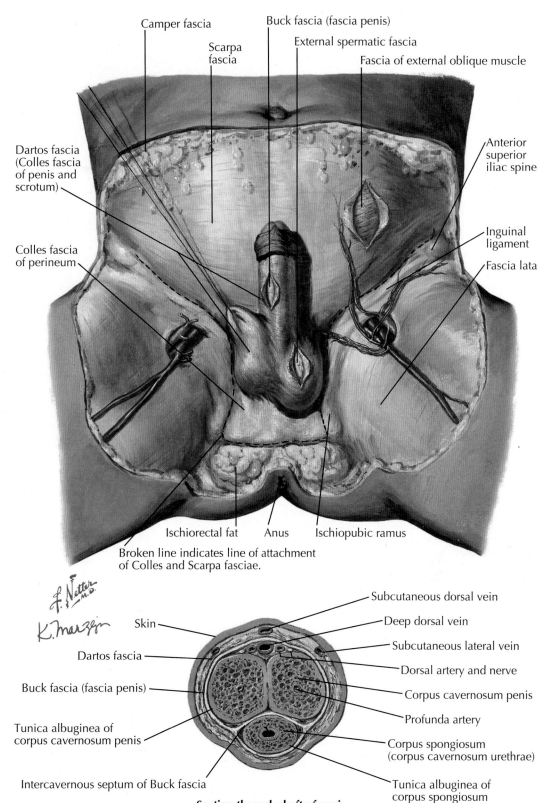

Camper fascia
Scarpa fascia
Buck fascia (fascia penis)
External spermatic fascia
Fascia of external oblique muscle
Dartos fascia (Colles fascia of penis and scrotum)
Anterior superior iliac spine
Colles fascia of perineum
Inguinal ligament
Fascia lata
Ischiorectal fat
Anus
Ischiopubic ramus
Broken line indicates line of attachment of Colles and Scarpa fasciae.

Skin
Subcutaneous dorsal vein
Deep dorsal vein
Dartos fascia
Subcutaneous lateral vein
Buck fascia (fascia penis)
Dorsal artery and nerve
Corpus cavernosum penis
Profunda artery
Tunica albuginea of corpus cavernosum penis
Corpus spongiosum (corpus cavernosum urethrae)
Intercavernous septum of Buck fascia
Tunica albuginea of corpus spongiosum

Section through shaft of penis

SUPERFICIAL FASCIAL LAYERS

The subcutaneous scrotal and perineal fasciae originate from the superficial fascia of the abdominal wall known as *Scarpa fascia*. This fascial layer is found deep to *Camper fascia* that backs the skin as a loose layer of fatty tissue. The abdominal Scarpa fascia is a true fascial layer that consists mainly of yellowy, elastic fibers that form a continuous membrane across the lower abdomen. In the upper abdomen, this fascia cannot be identified as a distinct membranous structure because it blends with the general superficial fascia of the upper abdomen. In the lower lateral abdominal region, Scarpa fascia is attached to the *Poupart ligament,* or to the *fascia lata* of the upper thigh just below this ligament. It passes over the external inguinal ring to continue inferiorly over the penis and scrotum into the perineum, where it fuses with the posterior inferior margin of the *urogenital diaphragm.* In the perineum, this fascia attaches laterally to the inferior rami of the pubis and the superior rami of the ischium and is called *Colles fascia.* As the fascia envelops the base of the penis, it is joined by additional fibers that extend from the dorsal penis to the symphysis, thus forming the *fundiform ligament.* Within the scrotum, this fascia is termed *dartos fascia* (dartos, meaning "flayed"), as it is reinforced by smooth muscle fibers.

Thus deep to the skin exists a continuous superficial fascial plane that begins in the lower abdomen and extends inferiorly to encompass the penis, scrotum, and anterior half of the perineum. Beneath it a potential space is formed in which fluids or exudates can accumulate and spread along well-defined planes. The points of fascial fixation, as described, lead to exudative, infectious, or extravasative processes taking on a characteristic "butterfly" shape of discoloration in this region. Although they can freely extend up the anterior abdominal wall to the clavicles, such processes do not normally extend beyond the inferior landmarks without penetrating this fascia.

In the scrotal midline, an inversion of the dartos fascia forms the *scrotal septum,* dividing the scrotal cavity into two halves. Anatomists differ as to whether a further inward extension of Colles fascia, termed the *major leaf* of Colles fascia, exists. It crosses the top of the scrotal cavity, thus forming a roof and separating it

from the superficial urogenital pouch superiorly. Urine extravasation from the *bulbar urethra* would not normally gain access to the scrotal cavity without rupture or penetration of this major leaf of fascia. However, this fascia may contain rows of transverse slitlike openings in some individuals, which would allow urine access to the scrotal cavity.

As the major leaf of Colles fascia nears the upper scrotal cavity, it divides near the anterior margin of

the scrotum, with a portion extending inward (see Plate 2.3). This so-called *deep layer* passes posteriorly, deep to the *bulbospongiosus muscles,* whereas the major leaf of Colles fascia in the perineal region is entirely superficial to the bulbospongiosus and *ischiocavernosus* muscles. The deep leaf of Colles fascia lying beneath the bulbospongiosus muscle, together with the superficial or major layer of fascia, forms a compartment for the bulbospongiosus muscle.

Plate 2.3

Reproductive System: VOLUME 1

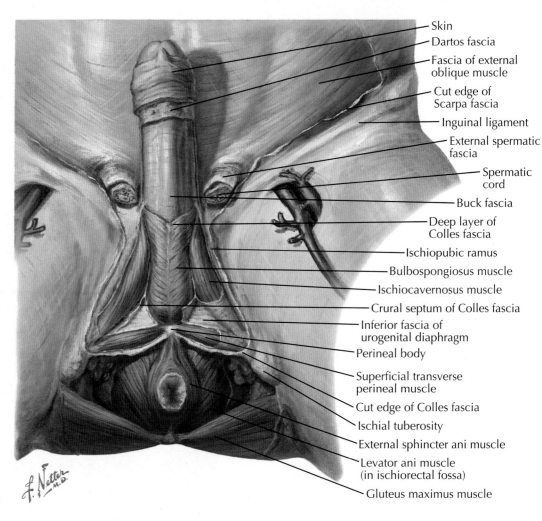

Skin
Dartos fascia
Fascia of external oblique muscle
Cut edge of Scarpa fascia
Inguinal ligament
External spermatic fascia
Spermatic cord
Buck fascia
Deep layer of Colles fascia
Ischiopubic ramus
Bulbospongiosus muscle
Ischiocavernosus muscle
Crural septum of Colles fascia
Inferior fascia of urogenital diaphragm
Perineal body
Superficial transverse perineal muscle
Cut edge of Colles fascia
Ischial tuberosity
External sphincter ani muscle
Levator ani muscle (in ischiorectal fossa)
Gluteus maximus muscle

Deep Fascial Layers

Beneath *Colles fascia,* within the urogenital triangle, is a potential space termed the *superficial perineal compartment.* Within this space, confined by the *inferior fascia of the urogenital diaphragm* on its deep aspect, lie the *bulbospongiosus,* ischiocavernosus, and *superficial transverse perineal* muscles. In addition, the bulb of the *corpus cavernosum urethrae* and the *crura of the corpora cavernosa penis* are found here. At the middle of the base of this triangle is the *perineal body,* a point of fusion between the muscles of the superficial perineal compartment and the adjacent *anal triangle* posteriorly.

The deep fascia *(Buck)* of the penis is a distinct structure lying beneath the *superficial dartos* or *Colles fascia. Buck fascia* is tenacious, dense, and whitish in appearance. It covers the penile corpora as a strong, fibrous, tubelike envelope and is adherent to the underlying *tunica albuginea* of the penis, which immediately covers the paired cavernous bodies (see Plate 2.2). Buck fascia is distinct from the tunica albuginea that covers the paired corporal cavernosa and the spongiosal bodies, though no demonstrable space exists between these adjacent fascial layers. Near the base of each crus, Buck fascia becomes less distinct as it merges with the tunica albuginea. At this point, it is continuous with the *deep suspensory ligament* of the penis, which is attached to the *symphysis pubis* (see Plate 2.1).

Buck fascia originates distally at the penile coronary sulcus and forms a transverse *intercavernous septum,* which separates the penis into two compartments: the paired corpora cavernosa dorsally and the single spongiosal body ventrally (see Plate 2.2, cross section). In the perineum, this fascia forms three compartments by covering each crus. Buck fascia covers the paired penile dorsal arteries and nerves and the deep dorsal vein (see Plate 2.2, cross section). In the perineum, Buck fascia lies beneath the reflected deep layer of Colles fascia that contains the bulbospongiosus and the ischiocavernosus muscles (see Plate 2.1).

Visualized in cross-sectional drawing on this page, a portion of *Colles fascia (crural septum)* spreads to cover the outer surfaces of the bulbospongiosus muscle and each ischiocavernosus muscle with the crura within. The cut margins of the crural septa, as they surround the ischiocavernosus muscles, are observed in the

Schematic view of fascial layers in a vertical section through perineum and urethral bulb

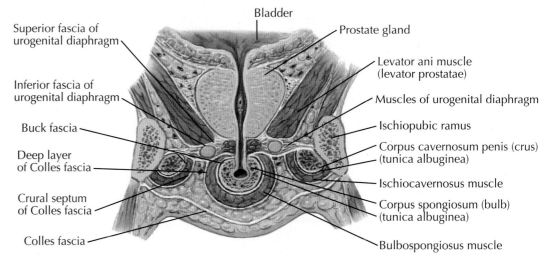

Superior fascia of urogenital diaphragm
Inferior fascia of urogenital diaphragm
Buck fascia
Deep layer of Colles fascia
Crural septum of Colles fascia
Colles fascia
Bladder
Prostate gland
Levator ani muscle (levator prostatae)
Muscles of urogenital diaphragm
Ischiopubic ramus
Corpus cavernosum penis (crus) (tunica albuginea)
Ischiocavernosus muscle
Corpus spongiosum (bulb) (tunica albuginea)
Bulbospongiosus muscle

upper drawing. The deep layer of Colles fascia, shown extending posteriorly under the distal aspect of the bulbocavernosus muscle, is also illustrated. At this point, the deep layer of Colles fascia also turns backward around each penile crus and around the corpus spongiosum. This reflected layer blends with Buck fascia surrounding the crura.

Thus in the urogenital triangle, four fascial layers cover the bulbous spongiosum and urethra. First is the

perineal layer of Colles fascia external to the bulbospongiosus muscle. Beneath this is the *deep extension of Colles fascia* below the bulbospongiosus muscle, followed by Buck fascia and, finally, the tunica albuginea. Only three fascial layers cover each crus of the penis: *Colles superficial fascia* overlying the ischiocavernosus muscles and Buck fascia beneath this muscle, which blends with the deep reflected layer of Colles fascia over the tunica albuginea.

Plate 2.4

Penis and Male Perineum

External urethral orifice (meatus)

Glans penis

Corona of glans

Frenulum

Neck of glans

Skin

Opening of preputial (Tyson) gland

Superficial (dartos) fascia of penis

Ischiopubic ramus

Deep (Buck) fascia of penis

External spermatic fascia investing spermatic cord (cut)

Anus

Superficial perineal (Colles) fascia (cut away to open superficial perineal space)

Deep perineal (investing or Gallaudet) fascia (cut away) over muscles of superficial perineal space

Ischiocavernosus muscle (cut away)

Superficial transverse perineal muscle

Ischial tuberosity

Deep layer of the superficial fascia

Ischial tuberosity

Perineal membrane

Gluteus maximus muscle

Perineal body

Levator ani muscle and inferior fascia of pelvic diaphragm roofing ischioanal fossa

Tip of coccyx

External anal sphincter muscle

Glans penis

Corpora cavernosa of penis

Intercavernous septum of deep (Buck) fascia

Corpus spongiosum

Pubic tubercle

Superior pubic ramus

Ischiopubic ramus

Bulb of penis

Crus of penis

Perineal membrane

Perineal body

External anal sphincter muscle

Ischial tuberosity

PENILE FASCIAE AND STRUCTURES

In this view, the distal end of the penis is shown intact to demonstrate the *glans* and the *frenulum* and the relationship to the *foreskin* or *prepuce*. In the sulcus between the *corona* of the glans and the internal surface of the foreskin are shown the openings of the *preputial glands (Tyson glands)* that excrete sebaceous material, a main constituent *of smegma*.

After removing the deep layer of *Colles fascia* and the overlying bulbospongiosus and ischiocavernosus muscles that cover the penile shaft and crura in Plate 2.3, the true extent of Buck fascia is revealed. In addition to covering the corpus spongiosum and both crura, Buck fascia anchors the bulbous portion of the urethra (corpus spongiosum) and each crus firmly to the pubis, to the inferior *rami* of the *ischium*, and to the *urogenital diaphragm*. The removal of Colles fascia at its posterior insertion in the urogenital diaphragm exposes the *superficial transverse perineal muscles* and the inferior surface of the *urogenital diaphragm*. Removing the urogenital diaphragm exposes the *deep transverse perineal muscle* as shown in Plate 2.5. The crural septum of Colles fascia, which extends between the bulbospongiosus and ischiocavernosus muscles, separates this portion of the perineum into three compartments. The *perineal body* is the focal point of attachment of the superficial transverse perineal muscles from each side and the anterior fibers of the external anal sphincter. Beneath the deep layer of the superficial fascia in the *anal triangle*, the greater part of the *pelvic diaphragm*, which includes the *levator ani muscle* as well as the *ischiorectal fossa*, is visible.

In the lower portion of Plate 2.4, Buck fascia has been removed from the penis, demonstrating the *corpus spongiosum*, which contains the urethra and also forms the spongiosal glans penis that forms a "cap" over the joined bodies of the *corpora cavernosa*. To allow for this, the paired corpora terminate distally in a pointed fashion, about 1 to 2 cm from the actual end of the penis. In the treatment of prolonged erections due to ischemic *priapism*, the blood within the corporal

bodies can be joined with that of the spongiosum to relieve this condition by surgically creating a hole between the spongiosal cap and the distal corporal bodies. The *intercavernous septum* of Buck fascia between the roof of the corpus spongiosum and the corpora cavernosa remains, as previously viewed in cross section in Plate 2.2.

Beneath Buck fascia, each corporal crus of the penis is firmly fixed to the rami of the pubis and *ischium*. The

cavernous spaces are surrounded by a thick, rigid fibrous capsule (*tunica albuginea*) consisting of both *deep* and *superficial* fibers. The latter course longitudinally and connect both corpora, but the deep fibers run in a circular manner and form a septum between the corpora after they become adjacent. Near the end of the penis, this septum becomes incomplete, allowing communication between the otherwise two distinct corpora cavernosa.

Plate 2.5   Reproductive System: VOLUME 1

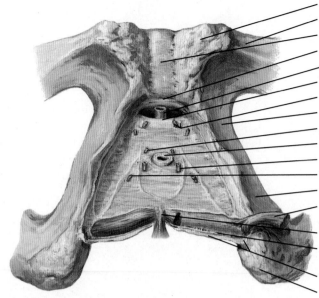

Pubic bone
Superior ramus of pubis
Symphysis pubis
Arcuate ligament of pubis
Deep dorsal vein of penis
Transverse ligament of pelvis
Dorsal artery and nerve of penis
Inferior ramus of pubis
Artery to urethral bulb
Urethra
Duct of Cowper (bulbourethral) gland
Cavernous (deep) artery of penis
Inferior ramus of ischium
Superficial transverse perineal muscle (*turned aside*)
Perineal body
Fusion of superficial and deep fascia of urogenital diaphragm
Cut edge of Colles fascia
Ischial tuberosity

UROGENITAL DIAPHRAGM

In the upper figure, the penis, bulbous spongiosum, and both crura have been removed, exposing the inferior surface of the *urogenital diaphragm*. This surface of the diaphragm is penetrated by the *membranous urethra* and the ducts of *Cowper (bulbourethral) glands* that lie within the confines of the inferior and superior fascial layers. Nerves, arteries, and veins that supply both the corpus spongiosum and corpora cavernosa also penetrate the inferior fascial layer of the urogenital diaphragm. The *deep dorsal vein* of the penis, which drains the glans penis and corpora cavernosa, passes through an aperture above the *transverse ligament* of the pelvis. This ligament is formed by the fusion of the superior and inferior fascial layers of the urogenital diaphragm. The urethra, after passing through the urogenital diaphragm, pierces the dorsal surface of the corpus spongiosum and is contained within it.

In the middle figure, the inferior fascial layer of the urogenital diaphragm has been removed. Note that the intramembranous Cowper (bulbourethral) glands and the *deep transverse perineal muscle* are now exposed. This muscle lies between the inferior and superior fascial layers of the urogenital diaphragm. Anteriorly, the fibers of this muscle surround the *membranous urethra* and are termed the *membranous urethral sphincter*. Injury to this muscle or its nerve supply, for example at the time of radical prostatectomy for prostate cancer, can result in urinary incontinence.

The bulbospongiosus, ischiocavernosus, and transverse perineal muscles lie within the *superficial perineal compartment* (see Plate 2.3). The bulbospongiosus muscle envelops the posterior part (bulb) of the corpus spongiosum, and its anterior fibers encircle both the corpus spongiosum and the paired corpora cavernosa (see Plate 2.3). It takes origin from the *perineal body* in the perineum as well as from a *median raphe* in the midline. It acts to expel the last drops of urine from the urethra during micturition and to aid in the penile erection.

The paired, fusiform-shaped ischiocavernosus muscles arise from the inner surfaces of the *ischial tuberosities* and *ischiopubic rami*. They cover and insert into the crura of the penis. They act to produce an erection by compressing the crura.

Dorsal artery and nerve of penis
Cowper (bulbourethral) gland
Cut edge of inferior fascia of urogenital diaphragm

Urethra
Membranous urethral sphincter
Deep transverse perineal muscle

Regions (triangles) of the perineum surface topography

Symphysis
Ischiopubic ramus
Urogenital triangle
Anal triangle
Ischial tuberosity
Tip of coccyx

The superficial transverse perineal muscles are slender slips that arise from the inner, anterior part of the ischial tuberosity and run transversely and insert into the central perineal body. Here, they blend with the *superficial external anal sphincter* (see Plate 2.4). The *perineal* branch of the *pudendal nerve* supplies all of these perineal muscles.

The bottom figure shows the relevant anatomic landmarks used to divide the perineum into two topographic regions: the *urogenital triangle* anteriorly and the *anal triangle* posteriorly. The bases of each triangle are shared and extend between the *bony ischial tuberosities,* roughly paralleling the course of the transverse perineal muscles. The apex of the urogenital triangle is the *pubic symphysis* anteriorly and that of the anal triangle is the tip of the *coccyx* posteriorly. Surgical procedures that traverse these anatomic regions, especially the anal triangle, are commonly performed in urology to remove the cancerous prostate (radical perineal prostatectomy).

Plate 2.6

Penis and Male Perineum

BLOOD SUPPLY OF PELVIS

The internal iliac (hypogastric) arteries supply the greater part of the pelvic wall and pelvic organs. Subject to variations, these arteries each divide into two major branches. The anterior branch gives off the following arteries: obturator, inferior gluteal, umbilical, superior vesical, middle vesical, inferior vesical, and internal pudendal, which supplies the external genitalia.

The blood supply of the bladder is derived from three arteries that enter it on each side and anastomose freely. The superior vesical artery, supplying the bladder dome, arises from the umbilical artery. The middle vesical artery, supplying the bladder fundus and seminal vesicles, may originate from either the internal iliac artery or a branch of the superior vesical artery. The inferior vesical artery, which usually arises as a major division of the middle hemorrhoidal artery, supplies the inferior portion of the bladder, the seminal vesicles, and the prostate. The arterial blood supply to the vas deferens (deferential artery) may rise from the superior vesical artery or from the inferior vesical artery.

The internal pudendal artery, which along with the gluteal artery stems from the internal iliac, or hypogastric, artery, supplies the external genitalia. The vessel courses downward and anteriorly to reach the lower portion of the greater sciatic foramen where, at the lower border of the piriformis muscle, it leaves the pelvis. In this region, the internal pudendal artery is adjacent to the ischial spine under the cover of the gluteus maximus muscle. The artery then passes through the sciatic foramen and enters the perineum, where it finally divides into the perineal artery and the deep (cavernous) and dorsal arteries of the penis. It is the internal pudendal-perineal segment of the artery that may be injured and result in vascular erectile dysfunction associated with long-term bicycle use. After the artery enters the perineum, it courses upward and anteriorly along the lateral wall of the ischiorectal fossa (Alcock canal), where it gives off the inferior rectal artery.

The prostatic blood supply is surgically relevant as "nerve-sparing" radical prostatectomy procedures attempt to identify and avoid cavernous nerves associated with these vessels to protect erectile function. The blood supply of the prostate comes from the inferior vesical artery (branch of internal iliac artery). The middle hemorrhoidal and internal pudendal arteries also send small branches to the apical prostate. Within the prostate, two groups of arteries are reliably observed. The internal or urethral groups supply approximately one-third of the prostatic mass and the urethra as far as the verumontanum. These vessels penetrate the prostatic capsule at the prostaticovesical junction and give off branches that enter and supply the lateral prostatic lobes (illustrated in a case of hyperplasia). Inside the gland they proceed in a perpendicular manner and reach the urethral lumen at the vesical orifice (neck) at a 7 to 11 o'clock position on the left and 1 to 5 o'clock position on the right of the orifice, as viewed cystoscopically. After the arteries pass these locations, they turn distally and course parallel to the urethral surface beneath the mucosa, supplying the prostatic urethra and also branching to the prostatic tissue.

The external or capsular arterial group supplies approximately two-thirds of the prostate. These vessels course along the posterolateral surface of the prostate, where they are identified during prostatectomy surgery and give off branches both ventrally and dorsally to

supply the outer surface of the gland. Many branches enter the prostatic capsule and anastomose to a moderate extent with vessels of the urethral group. At the apex of the prostate, the capsular arterial group penetrates inward to supply the urethra and that portion of the prostate in the region of the verumontanum.

Venous blood from the prostate drains through the puboprostatic and vesicoprostatic (pudendal) plexus

into the vesical and hypogastric veins. This plexus spreads between the lower part of the os pubis, the ventral surface of the bladder and the prostate, and receives major contributions from the deep dorsal vein of the penis and numerous prostatic veins to form the retropubic plexus of Santorini over the prostatic capsule. Control of this venous plexus is critical to reduce blood loss during radical prostatectomy procedures.

Left paramedian section: lateral view

- Abdominal aorta
- Common iliac arteries
- Ureter
- Right internal iliac artery and vein
- External iliac artery and vein
- Occluded part of umbilical artery
- Superior vesical artery
- Artery of ductus deferens
- Ductus deferens
- Inferior epigastric artery and vein
- Seminal gland
- Urinary bladder
- Vesical venous plexus (in retropubic space)
- Prostate
- Prostatic venous plexus
- Cavernous vein
- Superficial dorsal vein of penis
- Deep dorsal vein of penis
- Left dorsal artery of penis
- Deep external pudendal artery
- Anterior scrotal artery
- Testicular artery
- Ductus deferens
- Median sacral artery and vein
- Iliolumbar artery
- Left external iliac artery and vein
- Superior gluteal artery
- Patent part of umbilical artery
- Lateral sacral artery
- Obturator artery
- Inferior vesical artery
- Left piriformis muscle (cut)
- Coccygeus muscle (cut)
- Middle anorectal artery
- Inferior gluteal artery
- Internal pudendal artery
- Levator ani (cut)
- Inferior anorectal artery
- Prostatic branch of inferior vesical artery
- Internal pudendal vein
- Deep transverse perineal muscle (cut)
- Ischiocavernosus muscle (cut)
- Internal pudendal artery
- Perineal artery
- Posterior scrotal arteries

f. Netter M.D.
C. Machado M.D.

Arterial supply of prostate
(Frontal section, anterior view of specimen with benign hyperplasia)

- Inferior vesical artery
- Branch to prostate
- Urethral branches
- Capsular branches
- Hyperplastic middle lobe
- Hyperplastic lateral lobe
- Sphincter urethrae muscle

Plate 2.7   Reproductive System: VOLUME 1

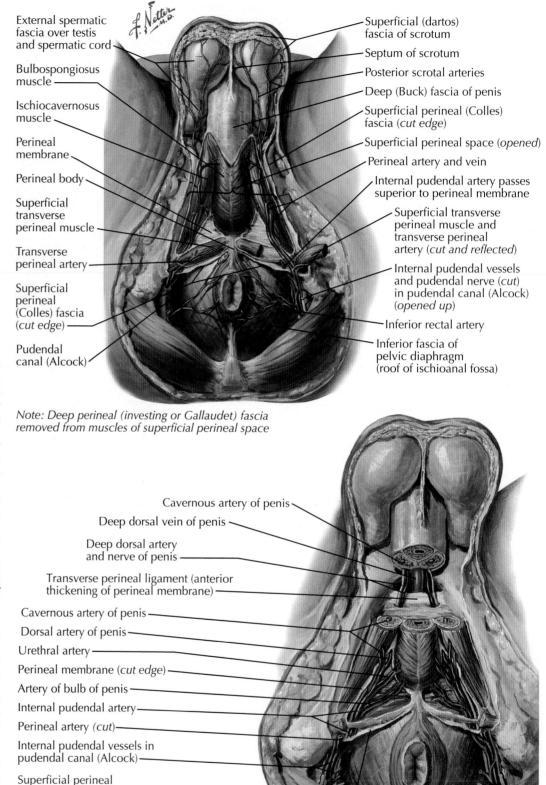

External spermatic fascia over testis and spermatic cord

Bulbospongiosus muscle

Ischiocavernosus muscle

Perineal membrane

Perineal body

Superficial transverse perineal muscle

Transverse perineal artery

Superficial perineal (Colles) fascia (cut edge)

Pudendal canal (Alcock)

Superficial (dartos) fascia of scrotum

Septum of scrotum

Posterior scrotal arteries

Deep (Buck) fascia of penis

Superficial perineal (Colles) fascia (cut edge)

Superficial perineal space (opened)

Perineal artery and vein

Internal pudendal artery passes superior to perineal membrane

Superficial transverse perineal muscle and transverse perineal artery (cut and reflected)

Internal pudendal vessels and pudendal nerve (cut) in pudendal canal (Alcock) (opened up)

Inferior rectal artery

Inferior fascia of pelvic diaphragm (roof of ischioanal fossa)

Note: Deep perineal (investing or Gallaudet) fascia removed from muscles of superficial perineal space

Cavernous artery of penis

Deep dorsal vein of penis

Deep dorsal artery and nerve of penis

Transverse perineal ligament (anterior thickening of perineal membrane)

Cavernous artery of penis

Dorsal artery of penis

Urethral artery

Perineal membrane (cut edge)

Artery of bulb of penis

Internal pudendal artery

Perineal artery (cut)

Internal pudendal vessels in pudendal canal (Alcock)

Superficial perineal (Colles) fascia (cut edge)

BLOOD SUPPLY OF PERINEUM

The internal pudendal artery, after emerging from the Alcock canal, gives off several branches. One, the perineal artery, passes beneath the Colles fascia in the perineum to course forward anteriorly, either under or over the superficial transverse perineal muscle. This vessel supplies the superficial structures of the urogenital diaphragm and sends a small branch, usually transversely, across the perineum (transverse perineal artery) that anastomoses with the artery from the opposite side. The perineal artery then continues anteriorly underneath the pubic arch and supplies both the ischiocavernosus and bulbospongiosus muscles. It also sends branches to the posterior scrotal surface.

The deep terminal branch of the internal pudendal artery pierces the inferior layers of the urogenital diaphragm and continues forward in the cleft between the ischiocavernosus and bulbospongiosus muscles, where it divides into the dorsal artery and the cavernous artery of the penis. As it courses between the inferior and superior layers of the fasciae of the urogenital diaphragm, it supplies the bulbous portion of the urethra and the corpus spongiosum. Distal to the bulbar urethra, a small branch passes downward through the inferior fascial layer of the urogenital diaphragm and enters the corpus spongiosum, where it continues to the glans penis (urethral artery).

The deep or cavernous artery of the penis pierces the inferior layer of the urogenital diaphragm, enters the crus penis obliquely on each side, and continues distally in the center of the corpus cavernosum of the penis. The blood flow within this artery is commonly measured by ultrasound in the evaluation of arterial erectile dysfunction. The dorsal artery of the penis pierces the inferior fascia of the urogenital diaphragm, just below the transverse ligament of the pelvis (see Plate 2.5), after which it traverses the suspensory ligament of the penis and courses forward on the dorsum of the penis beneath Buck fascia, where it terminates in the prepuce and glans penis. The paired dorsal arteries of the penis are situated between a single deep dorsal vein and paired dorsal nerves. The dorsal artery sends branches downward through the tunica albuginea of the penis into the corpus cavernosum, where they anastomose with the ramifications of the cavernous artery.

In general, the arteries supplying the internal and external genitalia are accompanied by similarly named

veins. The dorsal veins of the penis, however, pursue a different course. The subcutaneous dorsal (median and lateral) veins, which receive tributaries from preputial veins, pass proximal to the symphysis pubis, where they terminate in the superficial external pudendal veins that drain into the femoral veins. The single deep dorsal vein of the penis originates in the sulcus behind the glans penis and drains the glans and the corpus spongiosum. It courses posteriorly in a sulcus between the right and left corpora and passes between both of the

two layers of the suspensory ligament at the penile base (see Plate 2.6). It then passes through an aperture between the arcuate ligament of the pubis and the anterior border of the transverse pelvic ligament (see Plate 2.5). The deep dorsal vein then divides into branches that join the prostatic venous plexus. This plexus of thin-walled veins, with similar veins from the bladder and rectum, communicate freely with one another and with adjacent venous tributaries. Ultimately, they empty into the internal iliac veins.

Plate 2.8

Penis and Male Perineum •

BLOOD SUPPLY OF TESTIS

The internal spermatic artery originates from the abdominal aorta just below the renal artery. Embryologically, the testicles lie opposite the second lumbar vertebra and keep the blood supply that is acquired during the first weeks of life as they descend into the scrotum. The internal spermatic artery joins the spermatic cord above the internal inguinal ring and lies adjacent to the testicular veins (pampiniform plexus) to the testis mediastinum. Inferior to the scrotal pampiniform plexus, the spermatic artery is highly coiled and branches before entering the testis. Extensive interconnections, especially between the internal spermatic and deferential arteries, allow maintenance of testis viability even after division of the internal spermatic artery. A single artery enters the testis in 56% of cases; two branches enter in 31% of cases and three or more branches in 13% of testes. In males with a single testicular artery, its interruption can result in testicular atrophy. The testicular arteries penetrate the testis tunica albuginea and travel inferiorly along its posterior surface and penetrate into the parenchyma. Individual arteries to the seminiferous tubules, termed centrifugal arteries, travel within the septa between tubules. Centrifugal artery branches give rise to arterioles that become individual intertubular and peritubular capillaries.

The deferential artery (artery of the vas deferens) originates from either the inferior or superior vesical artery (see Plate 2.6) and supplies the vas deferens and the cauda of the epididymis. Near the testis, the internal spermatic artery and the deferential artery anastomose. A third artery, the external spermatic artery (cremasteric artery), arises from the inferior epigastric artery from within the internal inguinal ring, where it enters the spermatic cord. This artery forms a network over the tunica vaginalis and usually anastomoses at the testicular mediastinum with the internal spermatic and deferential arteries. The external spermatic artery also forms anastomotic patterns that supply the scrotal wall.

The veins of the spermatic cord emerge from the testis mediastinum to form the extensive pampiniform plexus. These veins gradually coalesce and, in 60% of cases, form a single trunk within the inguinal canal. The pampiniform plexus consists of three groups of freely anastomosing veins: (1) the internal spermatic vein group that emerges from the testicle and accompanies the spermatic artery to enter the vena cava; (2) the deferential group that accompanies the vas deferens to veins within the pelvis; and (3) the external spermatic (cremasteric) group that follows a course along the posterior spermatic cord. The latter group empties into branches of the superficial and deep inferior epigastric veins and into the superficial external and deep pudendal veins. These groups of veins afford routes of collateral circulation for blood return from the testicles.

The right internal spermatic vein enters the inferior vena cava obliquely below the right renal vein, whereas the left internal spermatic vein terminates in the left

Anterior view

Inferior vena cava
Abdominal aorta
Inferior mesenteric artery
Renal vessels
Internal spermatic vessels (part of spermatic cord)
Ureter
Common iliac vessels
Internal iliac vessels
External iliac vessels
Inferior vesical artery
Inferior epigastric vessels
Cremasteric vessels
Internal spermatic vessels in spermatic cord
Femoral vessels
Superficial external pudendal vessels (*cut*—pass superficial to spermatic cord)
Deep external pudendal vessels
Artery to ductus deferens
Pampiniform venous plexus
Deep dorsal vein and dorsal arteries of penis under deep (Buck) fascia of penis

renal vein at a right angle, apparently without natural valve formation. These differences in drainage patterns likely explain the fact that 95% of varicoceles occur on the left side, where natural resistance to increased abdominal pressure on retrograde flow through these veins is lower.

With varicocele formation, blood flow in the internal spermatic vein is reversed. With varicocelectomy, all veins except the deferential veins are ligated to reverse this process and improve pain or testis function. The

deferential vein affords a sufficient avenue for blood return. When performed in the retroperitoneum (Palomo or laparoscopic), varicocele recurrence rates after surgery are higher than when performed inguinally or subinguinally because of more complete ligation of all suspicious contributing veins observed more distally. Because of the increased number of pampiniform plexus veins subinguinally and the potential lack of a sufficiently collateralized arterial supply, varicocelectomy at this anatomic level is performed microscopically.

Plate 2.9

Reproductive System: VOLUME 1

LYMPHATIC DRAINAGE OF PELVIS AND GENITALIA

The scrotal skin contains a rich network of lymphatics that join the lymphatics of the penile skin and the prepuce. These channels, turning outward, terminate in the superficial inguinal nodes located in the subcutaneous tissue beneath the superficial fascia, inferior to the Poupart ligament and above the great saphenous vein. Penile and scrotal skin diseases can also progress to the deep inguinal lymph nodes beneath the fascia lata of the thigh, within the femoral triangle on the medial side of the femoral canal. Some lymphatics from the penile skin may also enter the subinguinal nodes that are deep inguinal lymph nodes located below the junction of the saphenous and femoral veins. Cloquet or Rosenmüller nodes in this nodal group are located in the external crural canal. Because of the communication between these nodes, it is important to inspect and remove all superficial and deep inguinal lymph nodes in penile cancer cases.

The lymphatics of the glans penis drain toward the frenulum. They then circle the corona, and the vessels from both sides unite on the dorsum to accompany the deep dorsal vein beneath Buck fascia. These lymph channels may pass through the inguinal and femoral canals without traversing nodes until they reach external iliac nodes that surround the external iliac artery and the anterior surface of the corresponding vein. Glans penis lymphatics may also terminate in the deep inguinal lymph nodes and the presymphyseal node located anterior to the symphysis pubis.

The lymphatic channels of the penile urethra, passing around the lateral surfaces of the corpora, accompany those of the glans penis outlined above or may pierce the rectus muscle to course directly to the external iliac nodes. The bulbous and membranous urethra drain through channels that accompany the internal pudendal artery and terminate in the internal iliac or hypogastric (obturator) nodes that are associated with the branches of the internal iliac (hypogastric) arteries or in the external iliac nodes.

The rich lymphatic network of the prostate, as well as the prostatic urethra, ends in the external iliac lymph nodes. Some lymphatics may accompany the inferior vesical artery to terminate in the internal iliac or hypogastric (obturator) nodes. These two nodal groups are most commonly surgically resected when regional spread of prostate cancer is suspected. Still others may cross the lateral surface of the rectum to terminate in the presacral and lateral sacral nodes within the concavity of the sacrum, near the upper sacral foramina and the middle and lateral sacral arteries. On the basis of this wide variation in lymphatic drainage of prostate cancer, lymph node dissection is performed for diagnostic but not therapeutic reasons.

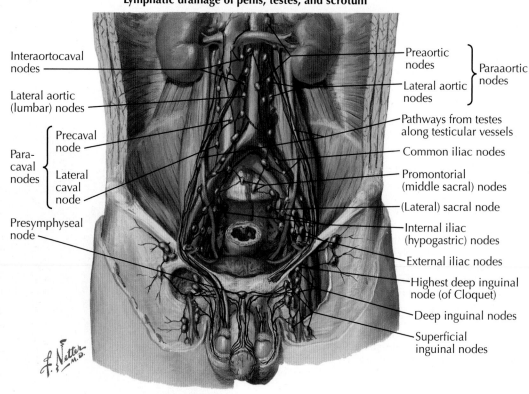

Lymphatic drainage of penis, testes, and scrotum

Interaortocaval nodes
Lateral aortic (lumbar) nodes
Para-caval nodes
Precaval node
Lateral caval node
Presymphyseal node
Preaortic nodes
Lateral aortic nodes
Paraaortic nodes
Pathways from testes along testicular vessels
Common iliac nodes
Promontorial (middle sacral) nodes
(Lateral) sacral node
Internal iliac (hypogastric) nodes
External iliac nodes
Highest deep inguinal node (of Cloquet)
Deep inguinal nodes
Superficial inguinal nodes

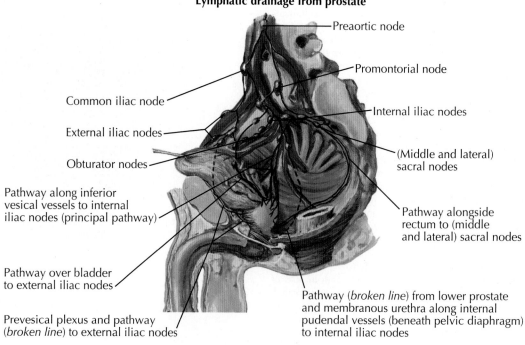

Lymphatic drainage from prostate

Preaortic node
Promontorial node
Common iliac node
Internal iliac nodes
External iliac nodes
Obturator nodes
(Middle and lateral) sacral nodes
Pathway along inferior vesical vessels to internal iliac nodes (principal pathway)
Pathway alongside rectum to (middle and lateral) sacral nodes
Pathway over bladder to external iliac nodes
Pathway (*broken line*) from lower prostate and membranous urethra along internal pudendal vessels (beneath pelvic diaphragm) to internal iliac nodes
Prevesical plexus and pathway (*broken line*) to external iliac nodes

The lymphatic vessels of the epididymis join those of the vas deferens and terminate in external iliac nodes. Nodal metastases from testicular tumors in these nodes indicate probable involvement of the epididymis because the lymphatic drainage of the testis follows the internal spermatic vein through the inguinal canal to the retroperitoneal space.

Depending on the side, testicular lymphatics, after angulating sharply toward the midline on crossing the ureter, terminate in defined groups of retroperitoneal nodes located along the vena cava and aorta from the bifurcation to the level of the renal artery. The lymphatics from the right testis drain mainly to the right paracaval nodes, including precaval, postcaval, lateral caval, and interaortocaval retroperitoneal lymph nodes. The lymphatics from the left testis drain mainly to the left paraaortic nodes, including the preaortic, lateral aortic, and postaortic lymph nodes. Lymphatic collaterals between the two testis sides exist, and contralateral metastases can occur when the ipsilateral nodes become obstructed.

Plate 2.10   Penis and Male Perineum

INNERVATION OF GENITALIA

Genitourinary organs receive a blend of autonomic and somatic nervous innervation. Autonomic nerves provide afferent and efferent innervation to organs, blood vessels, and smooth muscle and are characterized by the presence of peripheral synapses. Somatic nerves supply afferent and efferent innervation to skeletal muscle. Although these two nerve types leave the spinal cord within shared nerves, their course and function diverge widely.

The autonomic system is further divided into sympathetic and parasympathetic fibers. Sympathetic preganglionic fibers are found in the thoracic and lumbar spine, and parasympathetic preganglionic fibers originate in the cranial and sacral spinal cord. The pelvic organs receive a blend of these two autonomic nerve types through several pelvic ganglia. This autonomic innervation is demonstrated diagrammatically here, with a complete description of the anatomic and functional connections found elsewhere in this volume.

The parasympathetic fibers leave the spinal cord with the anterior spinal nerve roots from the sacral cord segments S2 through S4. After passing through the sacral foramen, they (nervi erigentes) enter the pelvic nerve plexus (inferior hypogastric) and follow blood vessels to visceral organs, including the descending and sigmoid colon, rectum, bladder, penis, and external genitalia.

The sympathetic fibers are derived from the thoracolumbar spinal cord segments (T10–L2). They descend through the preaortic plexus and abdominal chains to the presacral area and form a distinct midline nerve plexus usually located below the aortic bifurcation called the *superior hypogastric plexus*. Below this point, various ramifications of these nerves form the inferior hypogastric nerve plexus and branches from these two plexuses pass on to the pelvic organs. These adrenergic nerves terminate as postganglionic fibers and innervate the bladder neck, prostate, vasa deferentia, and seminal vesicles. They are primarily responsible for seminal emission (see table). Resection of this plexus or division of the abdominal sympathetic chain generally results in smooth muscle paralysis in these organs that is clinically manifest as either retrograde ejaculation or complete anejaculation, depending on the degree of injury.

The nerve supply of the penis is derived from the somatic pudendal nerve (S2–S4) and from the pelvic autonomic plexus. The pudendal nerve traverses the pelvis adjacent to the internal pudendal artery (see Plate 2.6) and is distributed to the same organs as the vessel supplies. The perineal branch supplies somatic motor function to the bulbospongiosus and ischiocavernosus muscles and also to the muscles of the urogenital diaphragm, including the sphincter urethrae (external sphincter). These muscles are important for somatic nervous system control of expulsion of the ejaculate that occurs with ejaculation. Sensory branches of this nerve are distributed to the skin of the penis (dorsal nerve of the penis), perineum, and posterior scrotum (see Plate 2.11).

Nerves emanating from the pelvic autonomic plexuses also distribute to the penis and through the cavernous

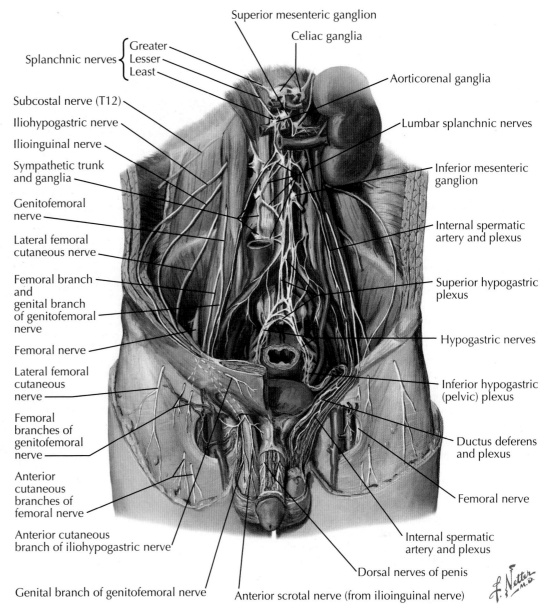

Splanchnic nerves { Greater / Lesser / Least

Superior mesenteric ganglion
Celiac ganglia
Aorticorenal ganglia
Subcostal nerve (T12)
Iliohypogastric nerve
Ilioinguinal nerve
Sympathetic trunk and ganglia
Genitofemoral nerve
Lateral femoral cutaneous nerve
Femoral branch and genital branch of genitofemoral nerve
Femoral nerve
Lateral femoral cutaneous nerve
Femoral branches of genitofemoral nerve
Anterior cutaneous branches of femoral nerve
Anterior cutaneous branch of iliohypogastric nerve
Genital branch of genitofemoral nerve
Lumbar splanchnic nerves
Inferior mesenteric ganglion
Internal spermatic artery and plexus
Superior hypogastric plexus
Hypogastric nerves
Inferior hypogastric (pelvic) plexus
Ductus deferens and plexus
Femoral nerve
Internal spermatic artery and plexus
Dorsal nerves of penis
Anterior scrotal nerve (from ilioinguinal nerve)

Effect of autonomic stimulation on genitourinary organs

Organ	Sympathetic stimulation	Parasympathetic stimulation
Urinary bladder		
Detrusor muscle	(β) Relaxation (usually)	Contraction
Trigone and sphincter	(α) Contraction	Relaxation
Ureter		
Motility and tone	Increase (usually)	Increase (?)
Male genitalia	Ejaculation	Erection

nerve innervate the smooth muscle of the paired cavernous spaces and the central cavernous artery and arterioles within the penis. Thus through the parasympathetic nervous system, they control cavernous vascular filling and erections.

Somatic nerves to the pelvic organs are derived from the lumbosacral plexus containing input from T12 to S4. They are demonstrated on the left side of the diagram. The iliohypogastric and ilioinguinal nerves are both derived from L1 and supply multiple

motor branches to the abdominal wall muscles and sensory innervation to the skin of the lower abdomen and genitalia. The lateral femoral cutaneous nerve and the genitofemoral nerve are derived from L1 to L3 and provide sensory input to the skin of the upper thigh and lateral genitalia. The genital branch of the genitofemoral nerve supplies the cremaster and dartos layers of the scrotum and is responsible for the cremasteric reflex that can be compromised with swelling of the spermatic cord as a consequence of testis torsion.

Plate 2.11

Reproductive System: VOLUME 1

INNERVATION OF GENITALIA AND OF PERINEUM

The nerves supplying the anterior scrotal wall are the ilioinguinal and the external spermatic branch of the genitofemoral branch of the lumbar nerves. The superficial perineal branches of the internal pudendal nerve, along with branches from the posterior cutaneous nerves of the thigh, innervate the posterior scrotal wall. The unstriated muscle in the dartos fascia is innervated by fine autonomic fibers that arise from the hypogastric plexus and reach the scrotum along with the blood vessels. Because of this complex innervation from various sources, the entire scrotum is difficult to anesthetize with local anesthesia, unlike the spermatic cord and testicles.

The nerves supplying the spermatic cord, epididymis, vas deferens, and testis track along the internal spermatic artery or the vas deferens to reach these organs (see Plate 2.10). Three nerves converge in the spermatic cord and innervate these organs. First, the superior spermatic nerve penetrates to the interior of the testicle and supplies it and associated structures. It accompanies the internal spermatic artery, originating from the 10th thoracic cord level, and passes through the preaortic and renal plexuses. Second, the middle spermatic nerve takes origin from the superior hypogastric plexus and joins the vas deferens at the internal inguinal ring and supplies mainly the vas deferens and epididymis. Third, the inferior spermatic nerve, derived from the inferior hypogastric nerve plexus and also coursing with the vas deferens, also supplies the vas deferens and epididymis.

In the lower figure, note that perineal nerve and dorsal nerve of the penis, both derived from the pudendal nerve (upper figure), course medial to the ischial tuberosity on each side of the perineum. Coursing parallel to these nerves are the perineal artery and the artery of the penis, both derived from the internal pudendal artery (see Plate 2.7). Recent research indicates that the pressure on the male perineum when sitting on a standard bicycle saddle is sevenfold higher than that observed sitting in a chair. It is thought that this increased pressure compresses either the perineal and dorsal nerves or the perineal and dorsal arteries, leading to perineal numbness and erectile dysfunction.

A spinal cord reflex termed the "bulbocavernosus reflex" (more appropriately, the bulbospongiosus reflex) refers to anal sphincter contraction in response to squeezing the glans penis. This reflex is mediated through the dorsal nerve of the penis (afferent) via the pudendal nerve to the inferior hemorrhoidal nerves (efferent) and tests the integrity of spinal cord levels S2–S4. In cases of spinal cord injury, the absence of this reflex documents continuation of spinal shock or spinal injury at the level of the reflex arc itself (cauda equina injury). Likewise, the return of the bulbospongiosus reflex signals the termination of spinal shock.

Referred pain to and from the scrotal region is of considerable clinical interest. In general, stimulation of the testis, epididymis, and tunica vaginalis can cause pain locally and also pain that projects to the lower abdomen, above the internal inguinal ring. Scrotal pain is likely perceived by the genital (external spermatic) branch of the genitofemoral nerve. Pain in the testis proper is referred to its point of origin in the retroperitoneum by referral through the superior spermatic nerve. Pain associated with renal stones may be perceived as arising from the testicle because both the testicle and kidney, including the renal pelvis, receive autonomic fibers from the same preaortic autonomic plexus near the renal arteries. Another source of this pain is radiating pain due to irritation of the genitofemoral nerve often adjacent to the upper ureter.

Sacral nerves
S1
S2
S3
S4
S5

Aortic plexus
Superior hypogastric plexus
Right and left inferior hypogastric nerves
Pelvic nerves (nervi erigentes)
Pelvic parasympathetics
Pelvic plexus
Rectal (hemorrhodial) plexus
Vesical plexus
Prostatic plexus
Small and large cavernous nerves
Posterior scrotal nerves (from perineal nerve)
Internal spermatic plexus on artery
External spermatic (genitofemoral) and anterior scrotal (ilioinguinal) nerves

Pudendal nerve
Inferior hemorrhoidal nerve
Perineal nerve
Dorsal nerve of penis

Posterior scrotal nerve
Perineal branch of lateral femoral cutaneous nerve
Posterior femoral cutaneous nerve
Ischial tuberosity
Perineal nerve
Dorsal nerve of penis
Inferior hemorrhoidal nerve

Plate 2.12

Penis and Male Perineum

Urethra and Penis

The figure shows the entire length of the male urethra as it traverses the prostate, pelvic diaphragm, and the penis. The natural curvature (see Plate 2.1) of the penis has been removed. The fascial relationships among tissues in the penis are not emphasized here but can be found in Plates 2.2 through 2.4. The pendulous, or penile, urethra and bulbous urethra extend through the center of the spongy tissue called the *corpus spongiosum* that joins with the paired corpora cavernosa to form the penile shaft. Each of the three spongy bodies is enclosed in a fibrous capsule, the tunica albuginea (see lower portion of Plate 2.3). The cavernosal and spongiosal bodies have a separate blood supply and there are normally no vascular anastomoses between them. Vascular shunts between these bodies may occur with trauma, however. The spongy tissue of the corpora cavernosa and spongiosum is composed of large venous sinuses that become widely dilated and engorged with blood during penile erection.

The urethral epithelium varies in different anatomic segments of the urethra. From the bladder neck to the triangular ligament (pars prostatica), the funnel-shaped coning of the trigone as it progresses distally into the prostatic urethra, the epithelium is transitional in character. In the membranous urethra (pars membranacea) that traverses the urogenital diaphragm, the epithelium assumes a stratified columnar form. The epithelium of the penile urethra (pars cavernosa) is composed of pseudostratified and columnar cells. Distally, in the fossa navicularis, the epithelial cells are stratified squamous in nature. The urethral mucosa is surrounded by the lamina propria that consists of areolar tissue with venous sinuses and bundles of smooth, unstriated muscle.

The floor of the prostatic urethra contains numerous orifices that represent the terminal ducts of the prostatic acini. Also on the prostatic urethral floor is an obvious elevation called the *verumontanum, colliculus seminalis,* or *prostatic utricle.* This mound of tissue contains a small pocket or utricle that represents the fused ends of each of the müllerian ducts (see Plate 1.2). In fact, the utricle is considered the male remnant of the female uterus. Just distal and lateral to the utricle are the slit-like orifices of the paired ejaculatory ducts, the obstruction of which is a well-defined cause of male infertility and male dyspareunia.

Within the penile periurethral tissue are many small, branched, tubular glands, the epithelia of which contain modified columnar, mucus-secreting cells. These glands of Littré are more numerous in the roof than the floor of the penile urethra. Also found in the roof of the penile urethra are many small recesses called the *lacunae of Morgagni,* into which the glands of Littré empty. These lacunae and glands may become chronically infected after urethritis, resulting in recurring symptoms and urethral discharge.

The pea-sized bulbourethral glands of Cowper lie laterally and posteriorly to the membranous urethra between the fasciae and the urethral sphincter within the urogenital diaphragm (see Plate 2.5). The ducts of these glands, about an inch long, pass obliquely forward and open on the floor of the bulbous urethra. The secretions from these glands form part of the seminal fluid during ejaculation.

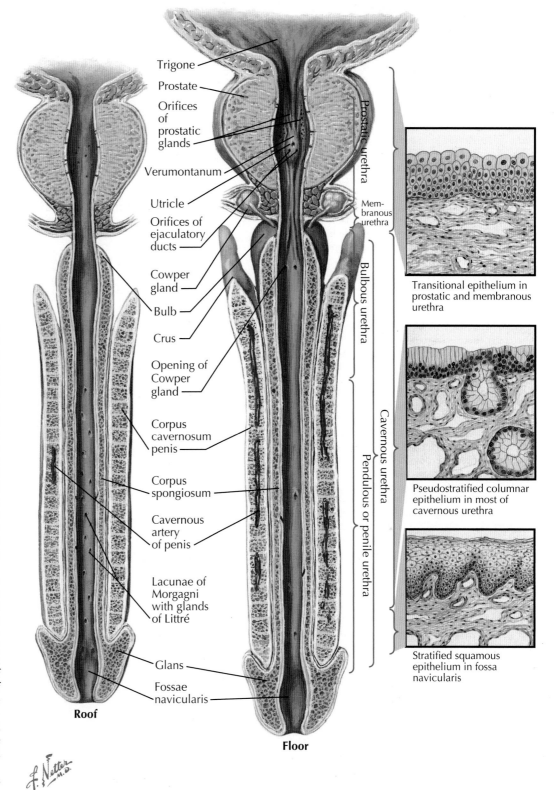

Trigone
Prostate
Orifices of prostatic glands
Verumontanum
Utricle
Orifices of ejaculatory ducts
Cowper gland
Bulb
Crus
Opening of Cowper gland
Corpus cavernosum penis
Corpus spongiosum
Cavernous artery of penis
Lacunae of Morgagni with glands of Littré
Glans
Fossae navicularis
Roof
Floor

Prostatic urethra
Membranous urethra
Bulbous urethra
Cavernous urethra
Pendulous or penile urethra

Transitional epithelium in prostatic and membranous urethra

Pseudostratified columnar epithelium in most of cavernous urethra

Stratified squamous epithelium in fossa navicularis

Plate 2.13

Reproductive System: VOLUME

ERECTION AND ERECTILE DYSFUNCTION

THE PENILE ERECTION

Penile erection is essentially a neurovascular event. Upon sexual stimulation, nerve impulses release neurotransmitters from the cavernous nerve terminals and relaxing factors from penile endothelial cells result in an erection. Nitric oxide released from parasympathetic nerve terminals is the principal neurotransmitter for penile erection. Within penile smooth muscle, nitric oxide activates a guanylyl cyclase that raises intracellular concentrations of cyclic guanosine monophosphate (GMP). Cyclic GMP in turn activates cGMP-dependent protein kinase, which results in the opening of the potassium channels, hyperpolarization, and sequestration of intracellular calcium. As a result of a drop in cytosolic calcium, smooth muscle relaxation occurs, leading to erection.

Subsequent to the activation of this signal pathway, three events are required for a normal erection. The first is relaxation of smooth muscle in the arteries and arterioles supplying erectile tissue, which results in a severalfold increase in blood flow. Second, and concomitantly, there is relaxation of the cavernous sinusoidal smooth muscle within the paired corporeal bodies, facilitating rapid filling and expansion of the sinusoids. And third, as a result, venous plexuses located between the cavernous sinusoidal spaces and the tunica albuginea covering the corporal bodies are compressed, resulting in almost total occlusion of venous outflow. These events effectively trap blood within the corpora cavernosa and raise the penis from a flaccid to an erect position (tumescence phase). Both masturbation and sexual intercourse trigger the bulbocavernosus reflex (see Plate 2.11) that causes the ischiocavernosus muscles to forcefully compress the blood-filled corpora cavernosa. During ejaculation, penile intracavernous pressures reach several hundred millimeters of mercury (rigid phase). During this phase, vascular inflow and outflow temporarily cease. Detumescence results when erectile neurotransmitter release stops, when phosphodiesterases break down second messengers, or as a result of sympathetic discharge during ejaculation. On return to the flaccid state, cyclic GMP is hydrolyzed to GMP by phosphodiesterase type 5. Currently, several oral agents prescribed for erectile dysfunction work by blocking phosphodiesterase enzyme activity.

ERECTILE DYSFUNCTION

Erectile dysfunction is traditionally classified as psychogenic or organic in nature. Among organic forms, there are neurogenic, hormonal, arterial, venous, or cavernosal and drug induced. It is now clear that cardiovascular risk factors suggestive of metabolic syndrome, such as hypertension, dyslipidemia, ischemic heart disease, obesity, and diabetes mellitus are associated with generalized penile arterial insufficiency. In fact, significant erectile dysfunction precedes heart attacks and stroke events by 5 to 7 years. Common causes of psychogenic erectile dysfunction include performance anxiety, strained relationship, lack of sexual arousability, and overt psychiatric disorders, such as depression and schizophrenia. Neurologic disorders such as Parkinson and Alzheimer diseases, stroke, and cerebral trauma can cause erectile dysfunction by decreasing libido or affecting the cerebral control of erection. In males with spinal cord injury, the degree of erectile function varies widely and depends on the lesion. Hormonally, androgen deficiency causes a decrease in nocturnal erections and

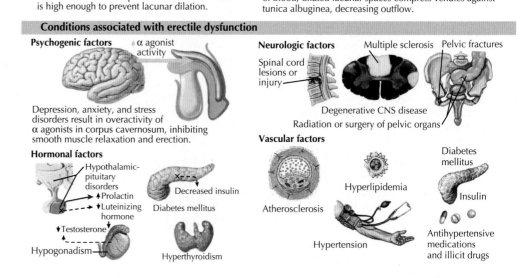

Chemical pathways of an erection

Nitrergic nerves
Endothelial cell

Sexual stimulation results in release of nitric oxide (NO) from nerve endings and endothelial cells in corpus cavernosum. This neurotransmitter acts through guanylyl cyclase to increase cGMP, resulting in increased Ca^{2+} efflux. The resultant decrease in intracellular Ca^{2+} produces smooth muscle relaxation. The cGMP is broken down by phosphodiesterase (PDE5). Drugs such as sildenafil act by blocking this enzymatic degradation and prolong cGMP action on corpus cavernosum.

Site of drug action
Linsidonine
Sodium
Nitroprusside

NO
Nitric oxide

Site of drug action
Prostaglandin

Prostaglandin E_1 (PGE$_1$)
Vasoactive intestinal polypeptide (VIP)

Corpus cavernosum smooth muscle cell

Guanylyl cyclase
G-protein G
Adenylyl cyclase

GTP
cGMP protein kinase
cAMP protein kinase
ATP

5'GMP
cGMP
cAMP
5'AMP

PDE5
K+
↓Intracellular Ca^{2+}

Site of drug action
Sildenafil
Vardenafil
Tadalafil

K+

↓Intracellular Ca^{2+} results in smooth muscle relaxation

Contracted trabecular smooth muscle
Relaxed trabecular smooth muscle
Compressed venule

Tunica albuginea
Tunica albuginea

Cavernosal artery
Cavernosal artery

Compressed lacunar space
Dilated lacunar space

Inflow
Outflow
Inflow
Compressed venule

Contracted helicine artery
Noncompressed venule
Helicine artery
Outflow

Flaccid state
Contracted trabecular smooth muscle limits inflow of blood into lacunar spaces while venous outflow is high enough to prevent lacunar dilation.

Erect state
Relaxed trabecular smooth muscle allows increased inflow of blood, dilated lacunar spaces compress venules against tunica albuginea, decreasing outflow.

Conditions associated with erectile dysfunction

Psychogenic factors
↑α agonist activity

Depression, anxiety, and stress disorders result in overactivity of α agonists in corpus cavernosum, inhibiting smooth muscle relaxation and erection.

Hormonal factors
Hypothalamic-pituitary disorders
↑Prolactin
↓Luteinizing hormone
↓Testosterone
Hypogonadism
Decreased insulin
Diabetes mellitus
Hyperthyroidism

Neurologic factors
Multiple sclerosis
Pelvic fractures
Spinal cord lesions or injury
Degenerative CNS disease
Radiation or surgery of pelvic organs

Vascular factors
Diabetes mellitus
Hyperlipidemia
Insulin
Atherosclerosis
Hypertension
Antihypertensive medications and illicit drugs

decreases libido. Hyperprolactinemia of any cause results in sexual dysfunction because of the inhibitory action of prolactin on gonadotropin-releasing hormone secretion, resulting in hypogonadotropic hypogonadism. Sexual function also progressively declines in "healthy" aging males. For example, with age the latent period between sexual stimulation and erection increases, erections are less turgid, ejaculation is less forceful, ejaculatory volume decreases, and the refractory period between erections lengthens.

ERECTILE DYSFUNCTION: EVALUATION

Erectile dysfunction can be the presenting symptom of various diseases. Therefore a thorough history (medical,

sexual, and psychosocial), physical examination, an appropriate laboratory tests aimed at detecting thes diseases should be performed. The physical examination should evaluate the breast, hair distribution, penis an testis, femoral and pedal pulses, and testing of genita and perineal sensation. Recommended laboratory test include urinalysis, complete blood count, fasting bloo glucose or hemoglobin A1c, lipid profiles, and testoster one. The provider should then assess the medical find ings, inquire about the goals and preferences of th patient (and partner), and discuss therapeutic options Cardiovascular risk factors should be determined an an appropriate referral made if these risks exist. In mos cases, erectile dysfunction can be treated with oral o local therapy.

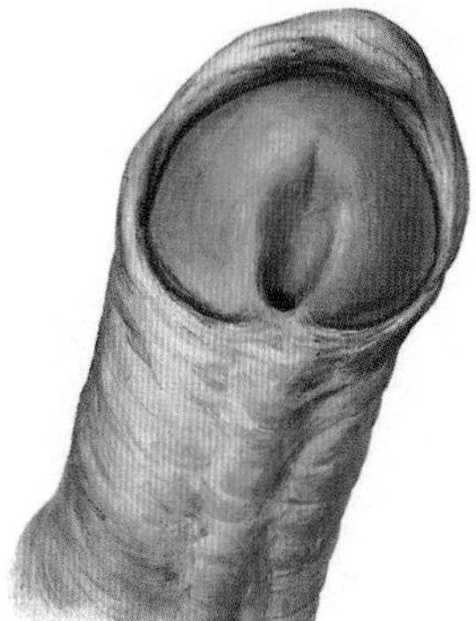

Plate 2.14

Penis and Male Perineum

HYPOSPADIAS AND EPISPADIAS

Hypospadias is a birth defect of the male urethra that involves an abnormally placed urethral meatus. Instead of opening at the tip of the glans penis, a hypospadiac urethra opens anywhere along a line (the urethral groove) from the penile tip along the ventral shaft to the junction of the penis and scrotum or perineum. This is among the most common birth defects of the male genitalia, second only to cryptorchidism, but the incidence varies widely from country to country, from as low as 1 in 4000 to as high as 1 in 125 boys. Hypospadias can occur as an isolated defect, or it can be observed in a complex syndrome of multiple malformations. The global incidence of hypospadias has increased since the 1980s, and this has been attributed to the wider application of assisted reproductive techniques and to endocrine disruptors. As it is considered to represent a degree of feminization or male pseudohermaphroditism (see Plate 1.13), hypospadias has also been associated with hypogonadism.

In hypospadias, the genital folds (see Plate 1.3) that normally unite over the urethral groove from the penoscrotal junction fail to close fully, thus creating a urethral meatus in a more proximal than normal location. The urethral meatus in one-half of cases is located just proximal to the normal meatus but still on the glans penis and is referred to as *glanular* or *first-degree hypospadias*. In penile or second-degree hypospadias, the urethral meatus is situated more proximally on the penile shaft. In perineal or third-degree hypospadias, the urethral opening is proximal to the penile shaft and is observed on the scrotal or perineal skin.

With hypospadias, the prepuce is usually redundant and forms a hood over the glans. In most cases, the urethra and corpus spongiosum fail to form normally, which results in a downward penile curvature (chordee) due to fibrous bands on the ventral undersurface. The scrotum may be bifid, with maldescended testes in some instances. Early correction of the chordee is important so that the penis and corporal bodies may grow straight. Androgens may be a valuable adjunct before surgery. Circumcision should not be performed because the hooded foreskin may be of use later as a source of flap tissue in urethral reconstruction.

Epispadias is a rare anomaly of the male urethra and is usually associated with exstrophy of the bladder (exstrophy-epispadias complex). It occurs in around 1 in 120,000 male and 1 in 500,000 female births. In this condition, the urethral orifice is observed on the dorsal penis just proximal to the glans (glanular epispadias) or is observed as an opening under the symphysis pubis in complete epispadias. Epispadias is a partial form of a spectrum of failures of abdominal and pelvic fusion in early embryogenesis. Although epispadias occurs in all cases of exstrophy, it can also appear in isolation as the least severe form of the complex. It occurs as a result of

Glanular hypospadias

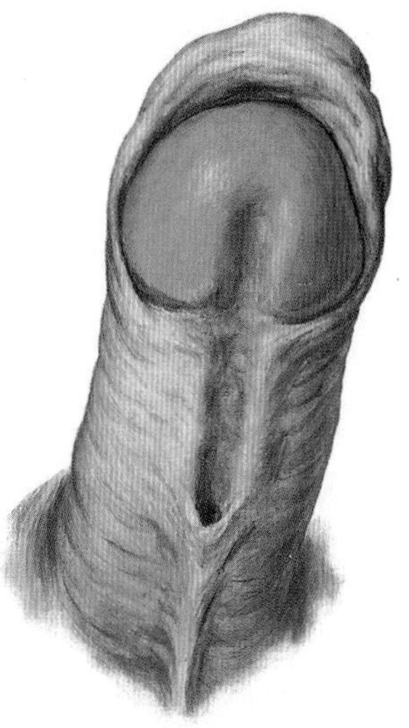

Penile hypospadias

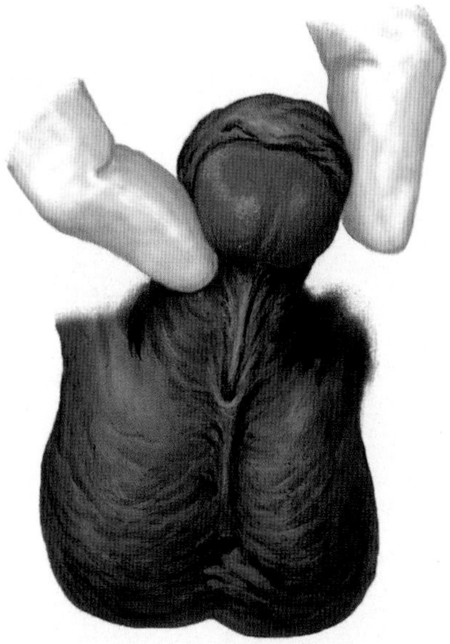

Penoscrotal hypospadias (with chordee)

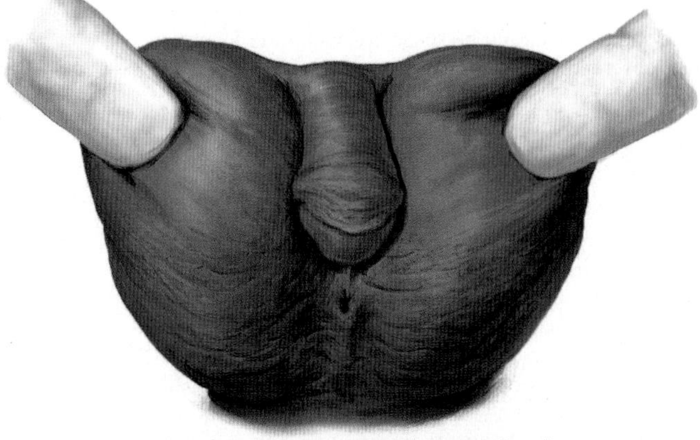

Scrotal hypospadias (bifid scrotum, chordee)

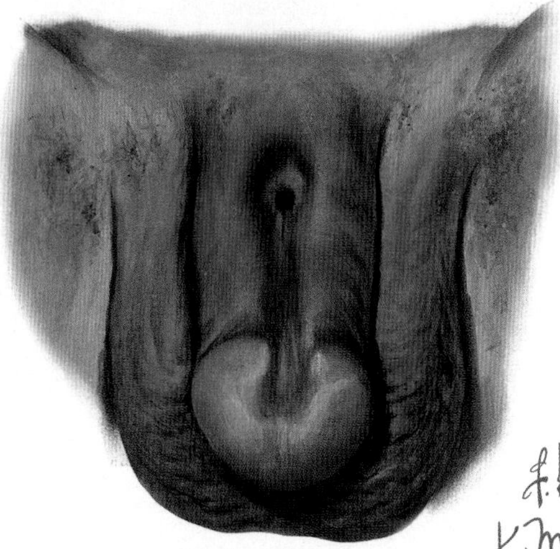

Penile epispadias

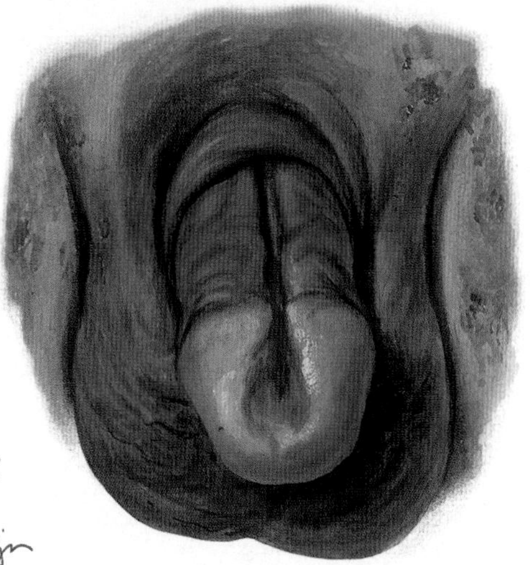

Complete epispadias

defective migration of the genital tubercle primordia to the cloacal membrane during the fifth week of gestation.

In this condition, the floor of the urethra is observed as a groove on the dorsum of the penis that is lined by mucosa and demonstrates openings of the periurethral glands (see Plate 2.12). The partial prepuce is located on the ventral penis. The epispadiac penis tends to curve upward and press against the mons pubis. The membranous and prostatic urethrae in most cases of complete epispadias are widely patent with incomplete development of the external sphincter muscle so that patients are commonly incontinent. The symphysis pubis may be well formed or may only be a fibrous band of tissue. Causes of epispadias are still unknown, but theories that postulate endocrine disruption, polygenetic predisposition, and viral infection have been put forth. Urinary tract reconstruction is necessary to restore continence and full penile function.

Plate 2.15

Reproductive System: VOLUME 1

CONGENITAL VALVE FORMATION AND CYST

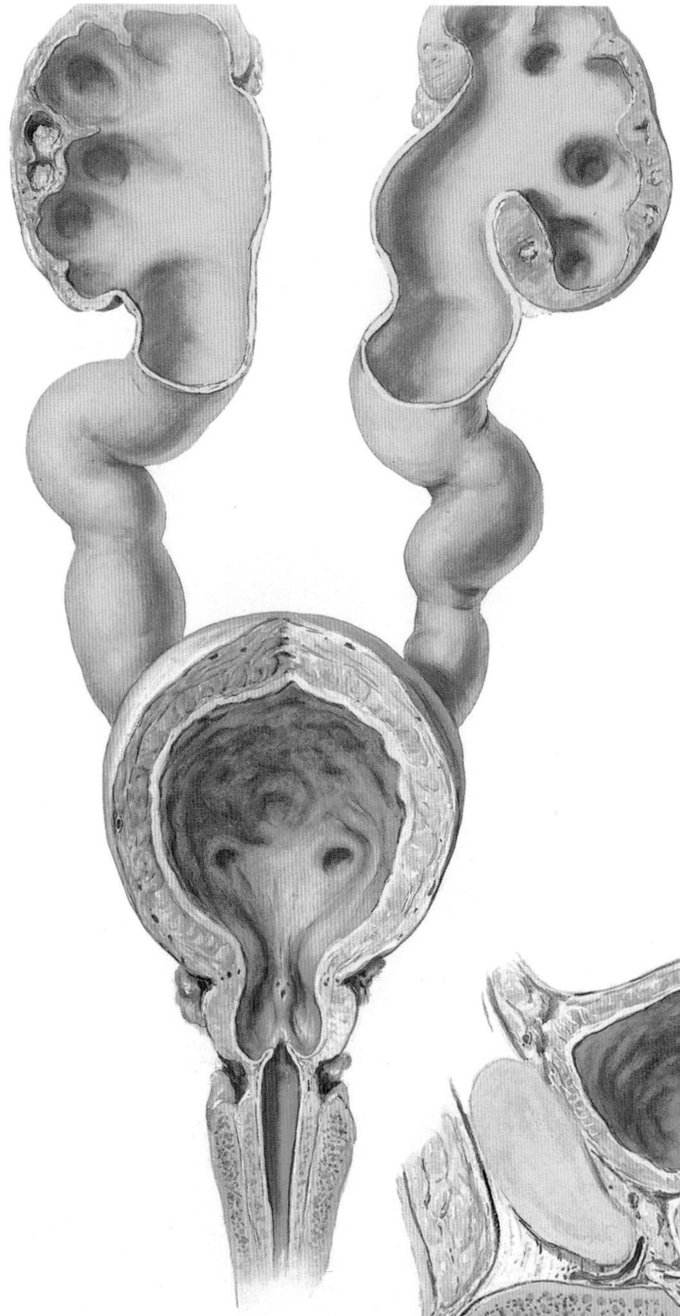

Congenital posterior urethral valves are serious anomalies of the posterior urethra. Thin folds of mucosa originate from the verumontanum and extend to the sides of the urethra and form a "wind sail" in the urethra. Urine flow fills the sails and results in chronic obstruction to urine flow, which then leads to compensatory bladder hypertrophy and eventually to bilateral hydronephrosis. The condition should be suspected when the following are observed: difficult urination, enuresis, intractable pyuria, recurrent urinary tract infection, or evidence of renal insufficiency. The diagnosis can be difficult to make, because the "valves" are difficult to see (the sails are floppy) when viewed in a retrograde fashion with cystoscopy. The diagnosis is best made with a voiding cystourethrogram. With transurethral approaches, the valve folds can be removed or fulgurated with complete relief of the urinary obstruction. Renal insufficiency, however, is usually irreversible.

Congenital cysts of the external genitalia are relatively rare. These cysts, simple or multiple, are usually situated along the median raphe of the penis at any point from the frenulum to the scrotum. On palpation they are freely movable, tense, rounded masses lying just beneath the skin.

Cysts of the internal genitalia may occur in the Cowper gland within the membranous urethra and also at the verumontanum (müllerian duct cysts). Cysts occurring in the verumontanum are vestigial ends of the müllerian ducts (see Plate 1.12) and can be large and project posteriorly to the prostate and seminal vesicles or occupy the space between the anterior rectal wall and the posterior bladder and prostate. Although usually small (a few centimeters), they can approximate the size of a large orange or present as an abdominal mass. There is usually communication by a small neck or channel to the utricle at the verumontanum. Wolffian or ejaculatory duct cysts are usually found laterally along either ejaculatory duct, unlike midline müllerian duct cysts. Either type of cyst can cause ejaculatory duct obstruction and present as a low ejaculate volume and azoospermia. They are treatable with transurethral cyst unroofing.

On occasion, wolffian and müllerian duct cysts may present with other symptoms beside infertility. A history of intermittent bloody urethral discharge, dysuria, a sensation of fullness in the rectum, or disturbances in sexual function that include hematospermia (blood in the semen) or dyspareunia (painful climax) are not uncommon. The diagnosis is confirmed with transrectal ultrasound, which may show the cyst in association with dilated seminal vesicles (>1.5 cm wide) or dilated ejaculatory ducts (>2.3 mm wide). Sophisticated adjunctive techniques such as vasodynamic pressure measurements, based on the same concept as urodynamic assessment of bladder function, can confirm physical

Urethral congenital valve with bladder hypertrophy and dilated ureters and renal pelves

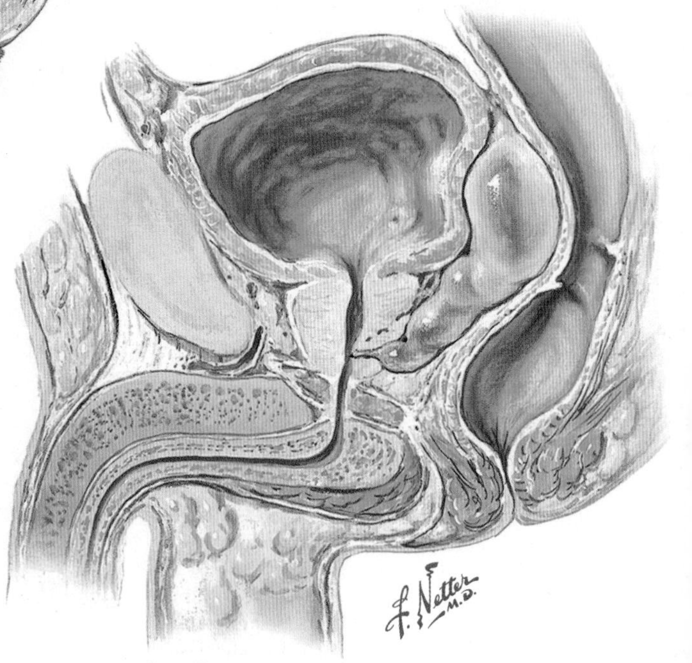

Congenital müllerian cyst

obstruction of the seminal vesicles in cases of partial ejaculatory duct obstruction.

Other congenital anomalies (not illustrated) are rare. Congenital urethral diverticula are located on the ventral urethra from the triangular ligament to the glans penis. These diverticula may, in rare instances, develop to a size that almost completely obstructs the urethra, similar to cases of acquired urethral diverticula resulting from strictures and tumors. Congenital stricture of the meatus causes dysuria and small ulcerations at the urethral meatus. Undiscovered meatal stenosis or strictures may lead to voiding dysfunction, cystitis, and pyelonephritis. Treatment requires antibiotics and urethral dilation or formal meatotomy. Absence or atresia of the urethra is very rare but may be associated with other anomalies in which the bladder urine drains through the urachus into the umbilicus or into the rectum. Congenital urethrorectal fistula, in which a communication exists between the membranous urethra and the rectum, is also very rare and is usually associated with imperforate anus.

Plate 2.16

Penis and Male Perineum

URETHRAL ANOMALIES, VERUMONTANUM DISORDERS

Diverticula are outpouchings of the urethral lumen that occur in both the anterior and posterior urethra. They may be congenital or acquired. The congenital variety, usually located in the penile urethra, is more frequent. Diverticula are further divided into true and false (pseudodiverticula) forms. The true diverticulum is generally congenital in origin and has a mucous membrane lining continuous with that of the urethra, whereas the wall of the false type is initially an unlined pouch as a result of a neoplastic or inflammatory process. Destruction of the mucosal lining of a true diverticulum by inflammation may render the two types indistinguishable. A false, acquired diverticulum may become epithelialized after surgical drainage of a periurethral abscess and may be interpreted as a true variety. Acquired diverticula are frequently observed in patients with spinal cord injuries who develop painless, undetected periurethral abscesses from chronic urethral catheters. These are "false" at the onset but appear "true" after epithelialization. Acquired pseudodiverticula are frequently found in the posterior urethra after instrumental trauma, whereas congenital diverticula are almost always located on the ventral wall of the anterior urethra.

Difficult urination (stranguria) or recurrent urinary tract infections are the most common presenting symptom. In addition, a common history is that during micturition, a mass appears in the perineum, scrotum, or under the penis that slowly disappears with dribbling of urine from the urethra. The condition is suspected by observation and palpation of the diverticular mass and the diagnosis is confirmed by urethroscopy and antegrade or retrograde urethrography. Diverticula are rarely asymptomatic and are best treated by complete excision and reconstruction of the urethral channel.

The accessory or duplicated urethra is very rare and has an unknown embryologic origin. They typically end blindly, generally at a depth of 3 to 10 mm (incomplete form, Effman type I), but can be much longer and connect with the urinary tract (complete form, Effman type II). They can communicate with the true, orthotopic urethra and for the most part are located ventral (hypospadiac) to the true urethral channel. When found dorsal to the true urethra, they are termed epispadiac duplicated urethrae. The most common type of urethral duplication is the Y type, in which a perineal meatus accompanies the usual orthotopic penile meatus. Retention of inflammatory exudates within these accessory structures can lead to recurrent abscess formation and intermittent purulent discharge. Infected anomalous tracts may require complete marsupialization or excision to eradicate the chronic inflammation.

Disorders of the verumontanum can be found in all age groups. The verumontanum represents the fusion of the terminal müllerian ducts (see Plate 2.12) and is located in the posterior urethral floor proximal to the external urethral sphincter. The only known function of this structure is to direct the semen during ejaculation. Congenital hypertrophy of the verumontanum is probably caused by maternal estrogens. It may be quite enlarged in young children and may nearly obstruct the prostatic urethra. Obstructive urinary symptoms such as stranguria and urinary frequency occur, until overflow incontinence develops. This form of incontinence in this age group can often be confused with benign enuresis. When severe, the back pressure induced by this obstruction on the upper urinary tract results in renal damage, especially if urinary tract infection is

present. Surgical removal of the histologically normal but enlarged verumontanum by transurethral resection is usually curative, but renal damage may persist.

Verumontanitis, or inflammation of the verumontanum, is usually due to underlying inflammation from chronic prostatitis, urethritis, or seminal vesiculitis. Visible changes include simple vascular engorgement or congestion, with or without edema. Chronic cases assume a granular and cystic appearance. Verumontanitis

in adults can provoke abnormal sexual symptoms, such as pain with ejaculation or hematospermia, and can cause urinary symptoms such as frequency and urgency. The ejaculatory ducts may be obstructed, leading to seminal vesicle dilation and pain radiating to the low back, perineum, scrotum, and rectum. The diagnosis is generally made by urethroscopy and treatment is directed at the underlying obstructive or inflammatory condition.

Diverticulum of urethra (other location indicated by *broken lines*)

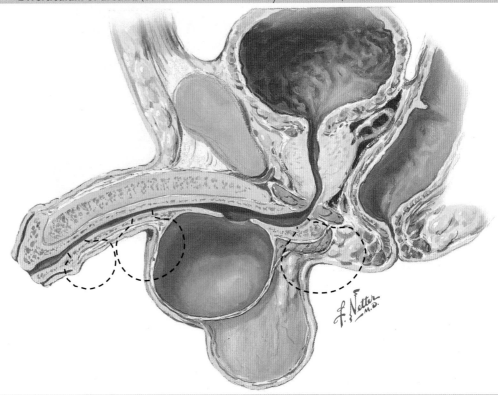

Accessory urethra

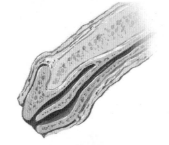
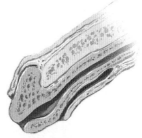
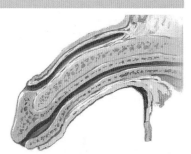

Disorders of the verumontanum: urethroscopic views

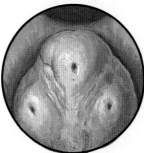
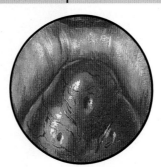
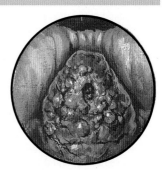

Hypertrophy

Intense congestion

Verumontanitis with granulations and small cysts

Plate 2.17

Reproductive System: VOLUME 1

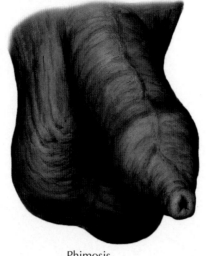

Phimosis

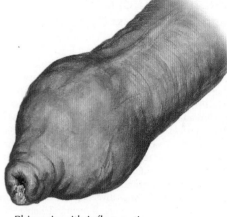

Phimosis with inflammation

PHIMOSIS, PARAPHIMOSIS, STRANGULATION

A redundant prepuce is normal in the newborn and during early childhood. *Phimosis* is diagnosed when the prepuce cannot be retracted behind the glans penis. If the foreskin is not retracted during early childhood and the congenital adhesions are not released, complete fibrous bands can develop between the prepuce and glans penis. When adhesions are present proximal to the glans corona, the preputial cavity or sulcus behind the glans near the fold of the inner preputial skin may be obliterated. These adhesions may be easily overlooked if the foreskin is partially retracted, exposing just the glans and not the entire preputial sulcus.

Phimosis may be so marked that the opening in the foreskin is pinhole sized. Urinary obstruction is rare but possible, with ballooning of the preputial cavity with urine upon micturition. When infected, the prepuce may become edematous, enlarged, and pendulous, with purulent discharge oozing from the red and tender preputial orifice. The retention of decomposing smegma, retained urine, and epithelium within this cavity may lead to ulcerative inflammatory conditions (see Plate 2.21), formation of calculi, and leukoplakia. A phimotic foreskin should be removed in any age group as the risk of acquiring penile cancer is greatly elevated in uncircumcised males demonstrating poor hygiene and retention of such carcinogenic decomposed secretions. Understand, however, that males who demonstrate excellent penile hygiene have no increased risk of contracting penile cancer compared with uncircumcised males. Circumcision has also been demonstrated to reduce the spread of HIV infection among heterosexual males and their partners in endemic areas.

Paraphimosis is the tight retraction of the foreskin behind or proximal to the coronary sulcus. It may result from the retraction of a congenitally phimotic prepuce or from the contraction of an essentially normal prepuce that has become swollen due to either edema or inflammation. In this condition, venous and lymphatic drainage is impaired resulting in marked edematous swelling of the prepuce and glans penis distal to the constricting ring. As swelling progresses, the impact of the constriction becomes more serious until the retracted preputial skin is impossible to manually reduce. Severe infection in the form of cellulitis, phlebitis, erysipelas, or gangrene of the paraphimotic foreskin may occur. Ulceration at the point of the constricting band may result in a release of the obstruction. In the

Adherent foreskin

Paraphimosis

Strangulation by metal ring

event of failure of manual reduction, incisions are made in the constricting band of retracted foreskin to relieve constriction (dorsal slit) and allow for swelling to reside before a formal circumcision is performed. Foreskin-preserving approaches to relieving paraphimosis have also been described.

Placing the penis into rigid devices such as bottles, pipes, and metal rings may result in strangulation similar to that observed with severe paraphimosis. Edema, thrombosis, inflammation, gangrene, and sloughing are

observed in neglected cases. With small constricting bands, the edema may become so excessive that the constricting object is not visible. Reduction of the device should be attempted before operation, as it may be possible to reduce the edema under anesthesia with constant manual pressure applied distal to the constricting ring. Metal objects, even hardened stainless steel, can be removed under anesthesia with the Gigli saw or jeweler's saws, making penile amputation from gangrene rarely necessary.

Plate 2.18

Penis and Male Perineum

PEYRONIE DISEASE AND PRIAPISM

PEYRONIE DISEASE

Peyronie disease (PD), also known as *induratio penis plastica,* is a benign condition that is associated with penile deformity. It occurs mainly in males 50 to 60 years of age, although it can occur at any age. The condition includes the triad of penile curvature, a plaque, and penile pain. Among these, penile curvature is the most obvious symptom and the one that leads to medical presentation. Interestingly, although generally thought be traumatic in origin, PD may also have an autoimmune etiology when associated with Dupuytren contracture of the palma fascia of the hand.

The penis may bend in any direction, although an upward bend is most common. Usually, the deformity is only evident during erection. Less commonly, a "waist" or "hourglass" defect may exist in which one segment of the penis is narrower than the surrounding areas. Even rarer are divots on one side of the penis. Importantly, PD is separate from chordee, which is a congenital penile curvature observed in newborns and is not associated with plaques or pain. A firm, flat, benign nodule or plaque may be felt on the penis and may contribute to curvature. The plaque is located within the tunica albuginea, the tough fibrous covering of the corpora cavernosal bodies. The plaque may accumulate calcium and become bone-like. Associated penile pain is most severe during erection but may be present at rest. Pain is often the first sign and occurs before noticeable bending. Bending occurs toward the side with the plaque. In most cases, the pain will resolve by 12 months although plaques and curvature may persist. About 50% of males who present with PD also have erectile dysfunction.

The principal finding is the deposition of scar within the penile tunica albuginea that forms the penile plaque. Pain occurs when active inflammation exists within the plaques. Erection dysfunction is typically a consequence of venoocclusive disease. PD has been linked to genetic connective tissue disorders. It is also thought to stem from minor trauma (often unnoticed) from penile buckling during sex, which shears layers of the tunica albuginea and disrupts small blood vessels. Bleeding and trauma induce the release of proinflammatory agents such as transforming growth factor-ß, fibroblast growth factor, interleukin-1, and fibrin. The inability to drain these inflammatory mediators away from the injury leads to prolonged inflammation and fibrosis. In 15% of patients, PD will resolve with time. In the remaining cases, the disease will stabilize or progress. In persistent cases, empirical medical treatments include antioxidants and antiinflammatory agents but are relatively ineffective. Penile "remodeling" or traction therapy with stretching devices is a valuable treatment for curvature less than 90 degrees. Collagenase *clostridium histolyticum,* an enzyme produced by the bacterium *Clostridium* that dismantles collagen, is an intralesional treatment approved by the US Food and Drug Administration that can dissolve the plaque. Surgical cures are routine with either penile plication (straightening) procedures or plaque excision and grafting procedures and may involve penile prosthesis implantation.

PRIAPISM

Priapism is a prolonged and often painful penile erection lasting more than 4 hours and not related to sexual desire or stimulation. The word is derived from the

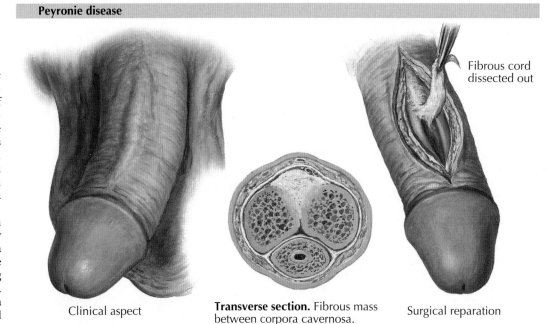

Peyronie disease

Clinical aspect

Transverse section. Fibrous mass between corpora cavernosa.

Fibrous cord dissected out

Surgical reparation

Ischemic priapism

Early: Thrombosis of corpora cavernosa (engorgement and priapism)

Late: Fibroid replacement (gristlelike)

Roman god Priapus, a deity renowned for his erect penis. Priapism can affect males at any age. There are two types of priapism, ischemic and nonischemic. Ischemic, low-flow, or venoocclusive priapism occurs when there is no penile blood flow and constitutes 95% of cases. With obstruction to flow, trapped blood increases pressure and the penile shaft becomes very hard and painful. Nonischemic priapism, also known as *high-flow priapism,* is rare (5%) and occurs with excessive blood flow through the penis as a result of arterial rupture or malformation within the erectile tissue, most commonly from blunt injury to the groin or pelvis. In nonischemic priapism, the penis is enlarged but not as rigid as a normal erection and there is usually less pain. It is critical to distinguish these two forms of priapism, as ischemic priapism is a medical emergency that can permanently injure the penis and lead to erectile dysfunction. This generally occurs after 48 hours of

unwanted erection as thrombosis within the cavernous spaces causes fibrosis and permanent loss of function.

Priapism can be idiopathic or secondary in nature. Drugs associated with priapism include papaverine, phentolamine, prostaglandin (when given for erectile dysfunction), trazodone, propranolol, hydralazine, thioridazine, antidepressants, and cocaine. Medical conditions associated with priapism include spinal cord injury, leukemia, gout, sickle cell anemia, and advanced pelvic and metastatic cancer. Treatment is directed at relieving the erection with corporal irrigation to remove blood clots, intracorporal injection of sympathomimetic drugs to contract arteries, surgical shunts to restore venous outflow and, as a last resort, penile prosthesis implantation. It is also important to find and treat the root cause of ischemic priapism with intravenous fluids, pain medication, oxygen, radiation, or chemotherapy.

Plate 2.19

Reproductive System: VOLUME 1

TRAUMA TO PENIS AND URETHRA

Beneath the deep layer of Colles fascia and Buck fascia (see Plate 2.4), the paired corpora cavernosal bodies of the penis are encased in a thick tunica albuginea layer. Rupture of the corpora cavernosa is rare but is encountered from direct trauma or penile fracture from vigorous intercourse or with the use of devices. Rupture of the tunica albuginea usually includes rupture of Buck fascia (see Plate 2.4), in which case the penis quickly swells as a result of extravasation of blood. Early surgical repair of the ruptured tunica albuginea may prevent thrombosis and subsequent fibrosis of the erectile tissue with consequent erectile dysfunction.

Isolated rupture of the urethra from trauma is not uncommon. It occurs as a result of three mechanisms: external or internal injury or obstructive disease. External blunt or penetrating injuries may involve the penile or bulbous urethra, more commonly the latter because of its immobility. Severe straddle injuries result from a blow to the perineum and bulbous urethra, usually after a fall astride a blunt or sharp object with the bulbous urethra crushed against the underside of the bony symphysis pubis. Pelvic fractures may physically separate the posterior (membranous) urethra from the bladder at the pelvic diaphragm or drive bone fragments into the urethra and corporal bodies where they attach to the pubic rami. The clinical presentation may include the inability to urinate and blood at the urethral meatus. Extensive injuries generally involve the corpus spongiosum surrounding the urethra and Buck fascia, with subcutaneous hematoma formation in the perineum and penis.

In cases of urethral tears limited to the mucosa, the only symptom may be blood at the urethral meatus. Abrasions and small tears generally cause blood at the meatus and hematuria, whereas more extensive lacerations result in periurethral and subcutaneous hematomas and urinary retention. With extensive injuries, passage of a Foley catheter may not be possible, and there may be the appearance of a rapidly developing subcutaneous hematoma. With meatal blood, before a catheter is attempted, an emergent retrograde urethrogram will demonstrate discontinuity or rupture of the urethra. Immediate surgical exploration is possible if the patient is hemodynamically stable, and the severed ends of the urethra can be anastomosed over a urethral catheter. Otherwise, urinary diversion with a suprapubic tube and delayed reconstruction are undertaken either sooner (within 5 days) or later (several months) after the injury with excellent results.

Urination with a urethral injury can result in extravasation of urine into the subcutaneous tissues outside of Buck fascia and beneath Colles fascia, where it spreads along known anatomic pathways (see Plate 2.20). In subtle, unrecognized injuries, urinary extravasation can lead to periurethral abscess and cellulitis and even fasciitis and gangrene of the genitalia (Fournier gangrene). Stricture formation, urinary incontinence, and erectile dysfunction are late sequelae of urethral trauma (see Plate 2.26).

Internal urethral injuries result from the passage of sounds, catheters, or foreign objects via the urethra. The urethral mucosa is easily penetrated by catheters, especially when used with a metal stylet or catheter guide. The penetration usually results in a false passage posterior to the urethra within the corpus spongiosum. The tunica albuginea and Buck fascia may also be penetrated, in which case blood and urine may pass to the subcutaneous tissues. Typically, this occurs

with attempts to dilate existing urethral strictures and is followed by a slowly developing periurethral abscess.

Spontaneous rupture of the urethra proximal to a preexisting urethral stricture may be due to increased intraurethral voiding pressure. Urethral rupture may be accompanied by chills and fever as urine and bacteria enter the circulation through the venous spaces of the corpus spongiosum ("urethral chill"). The most

devastating complication of this phenomenon is the occurrence of perineal and genital fasciitis (tracking along Colles fascia) due to gram-negative rods or anaerobic bacteria, otherwise known as *Fournier gangrene*. This life-threatening infection requires immediate, aggressive, and repeated tissue debridement and surgical drainage to avoid overwhelming sepsis and has measurable fatality rates in older patients or those who are immunocompromised or have diabetes.

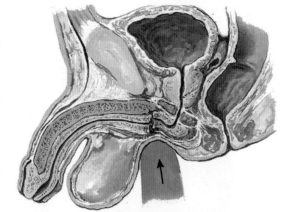

Straddle injury

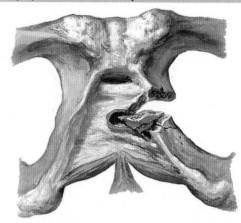

Injury due to fracture of pelvis

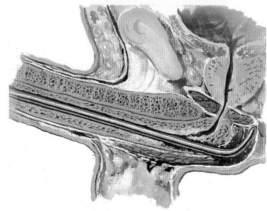

Injury from within (false passage)

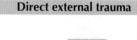

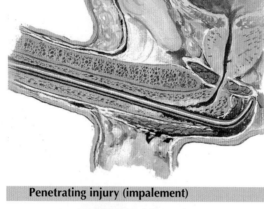

Direct external trauma

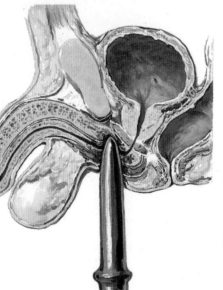

Penetrating injury (impalement)

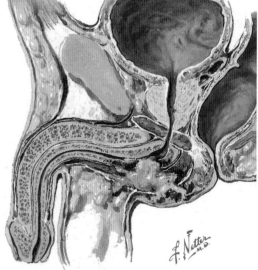

Perforation by periurethral abscess

Plate 2.20

Penis and Male Perineum

URINARY EXTRAVASATION

Urinary extravasation from the urinary tract will infiltrate specific anatomic spaces that are defined by well-described fascial planes (see Plate 2.2). Thus the degree and extent of urine extravasation depends not only on the type and severity of the injury but also on the involved fascial planes, making knowledge of these fasciae important in the treatment of this condition. Urine may extravasate from urethral perforation, resulting from periurethral abscess formation, instrumentation, external trauma (see Plate 2.19), or malignancy.

Most extravasation occurs in the bulbous urethra where the urine escapes into the well-vascularized corpus spongiosum that surrounds it. By this mechanism, infected urine enters the vascular system, often resulting in "urethral chill"—a sign of bacteremia. If the extravasation occurs gradually because of abscess formation in the bulbous urethra, it is at first limited by Buck fascia and appears as localized swelling deep in the perineum. If Buck fascia remains intact after penile urethral injury, extravasation causes swelling limited to the ventral penis. If the intercavernous or transverse septum of Buck fascia (see Plate 2.2) is penetrated, then the entire penis becomes symmetrically swollen.

Inflammatory processes eventually rupture through Buck fascia, and urine and exudate are then observed deep to Colles fascia in the perineum. Traumatic injury that extends through Buck fascia results in immediate spread of extravasate beneath Colles fascia. In the perineal region, extravasation may at first be restricted to the superficial urogenital pouch by the major leaf of Colles fascia. This fascial leaf is, however, easily penetrated, allowing fluid to descend into the superficial space of the scrotal wall, beneath the dartos fascia. The fascial arrangement also permits progression of extravasation superiorly from the superficial urogenital pouch to the space under Colles fascia of the penis. At the base of the penis, extravasated fluid will easily extend beneath the Scarpa fascia and track superiorly into the lower abdomen. This is termed the "butterfly" pattern of genital extravasation or bleeding. Extravasation can also extend to the lower abdominal wall from the scrotum by an additional route, along the spermatic cord canals.

Importantly, the posterior extension of extravasated fluid into the perineum beneath Colles fascia is restricted at the urogenital diaphragm to which Colles fascia is firmly attached (see Plates 2.2 and 2.3). Crush injuries to the perineum may rupture Colles fascia at this site of attachment, in which case urine will spread posteriorly and superiorly into the ischiorectal fossa space and perianal areas.

Anatomically, extravasated urine in the scrotum under Colles (dartos) fascia is still superficial to the external spermatic fascia (oblique muscle) of the scrotal wall. Thus extraperitoneal or retroperitoneal rupture of the urinary bladder can result in extravasation of urine into the scrotum through the inguinal canals. When this occurs, the scrotal fluid is located subcutaneously

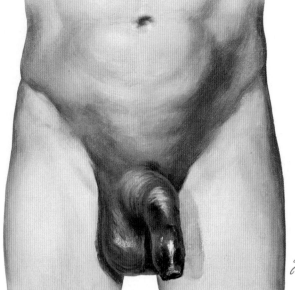

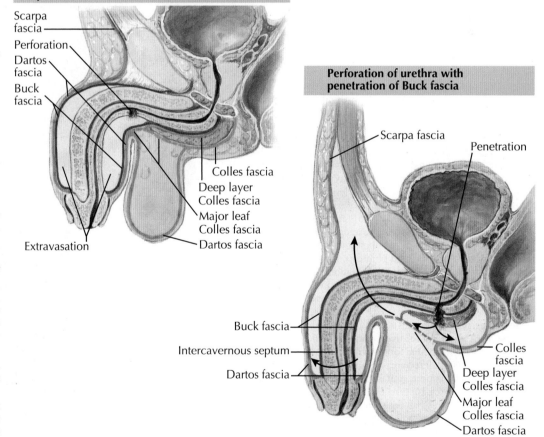

Perforation of urethra without penetration of Buck fascia

Scarpa fascia
Perforation
Dartos fascia
Buck fascia
Extravasation

Colles fascia
Deep layer Colles fascia
Major leaf Colles fascia
Dartos fascia

Perforation of urethra with penetration of Buck fascia

Scarpa fascia
Penetration
Buck fascia
Intercavernous septum
Dartos fascia

Colles fascia
Deep layer Colles fascia
Major leaf Colles fascia
Dartos fascia

beneath both the internal spermatic fascia and the external spermatic fascia, which are deep to the dartos fascia (see Plate 2.1).

A typical case of urinary extravasation from injury to the penile urethra is illustrated in the figure. Urine escapes through Buck fascia to beneath Colles fascia of the penis, where it extends inferiorly into the scrotum and superiorly under Scarpa fascia to the lower abdomen. Note the line of demarcation at the Poupart ligament, where Scarpa fascia is fixed to the fascia lata of the thigh,

limiting extension in this area (see Plate 2.2). Normal bacterial flora of the urethra include both aerobic and anaerobic organisms that are usually harmless saprophytes. However, they may become pathogenic when extravasated into remote tissues. In the presence of infected urine, intense cellulitis and gangrenous fasciitis may develop (Fournier gangrene) in these tissues that can progress quickly to necrosis and sloughing of the scrotum skin and is extremely lethal if not treated with antibiotics, the urine diverted, and the area surgically drained.

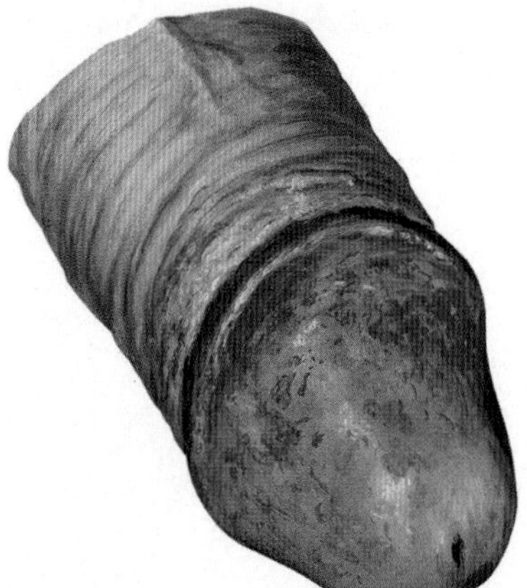

Plate 2.21

Reproductive System: VOLUME 1

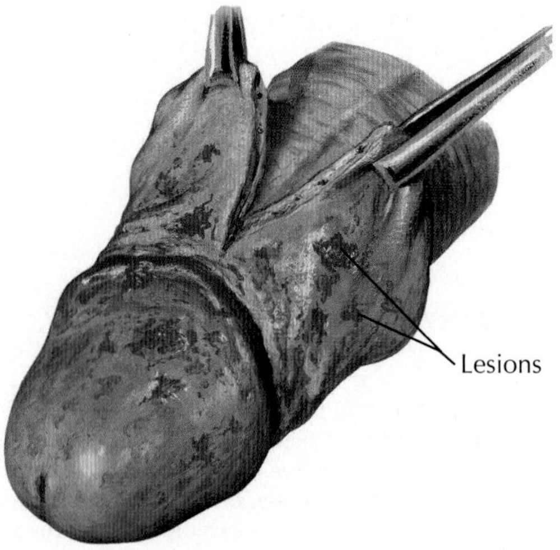

BALANITIS

Inflammation of the glans penis is termed balanitis. Inflammation of the preputial skin is referred to as *balanoposthitis*. Clinically, these conditions usually coexist, with the surface of the glans and prepuce both swollen, hyperemic, tender, and itchy. A yellow exudate and superficial ulcers or denudation of the glans surface are characteristic of balanoposthitis. In chronic balanitis, the glans epithelium becomes thickened and assumes a whitish appearance (leukoplakia).

By far the most frequent cause of simple balanitis is congenital or acquired phimosis (see Plate 2.17). In infants, balanoposthitis results from retained smegma, bacteria, and lack of hygiene associated with phimosis and dribbling urine or moist diapers. In adults, urinary incontinence may play an etiologic role. Seborrheic dermatitis, most commonly seen on the scalp, can also be found on the glans penis. Superficial fungal infections from *Candida albicans* are also common, especially in diabetics. Contact allergy from latex in condoms or ingredients in skin care products must also be considered. Balanitis circinata is a skin manifestation of reactive arthritis, characterized by arthritis, urethritis, and conjunctivitis. Generalized skin conditions such as lichen planus, psoriasis, erythema multiforme, erythrasma due to *Corynebacterium,* and erythema fixum are less common conditions that cause simple balanitis. Pemphigus, a group of autoimmune blistering diseases of the skin, and scabies usually produce distinctive lesions on the penile shaft rather than the glans penis. Rarely, phimosis secondary to obstruction of the inguinal lymph nodes from cancer, edema, or elephantiasis may also cause balanitis. Precancerous and cancerous lesions of the glans and prepuce are shown in Plate 2.27.

Balanitis xerotica obliterans, also termed lichen sclerosis, is a progressive form of balanoposthitis that primarily affects the foreskin, leading to whitening and loss of skin color, scarring, and phimosis. Involvement of the urethral meatus can lead to irritation, burning, and stenosis and may require a meatoplasty in cases of stricture. Long-term follow-up is needed to assess for recurrence.

Genital herpes simplex virus 2, caused by a double-stranded RNA virus, is a relatively common, venereally transmitted, painful, itching form of balanitis. Multiple lesions develop as small red areas upon which rounded translucent vesicles appear, containing clear, viral-rich, infectious fluid. After rupture of the vesicles, small round ulcers with a reddish base remain and heal. The infection usually recurs and is currently incurable, although the frequency and severity of infections can be reduced with antiviral therapy.

Erosive balanitis may be venereal, such as that due to syphilis or chancroid, or nonvenereal in origin, such as that due to histoplasmosis. Although unusual, anaerobic balanoposthitis is a classic form of nonvenereal, erosive balanitis caused by anaerobic gram-negative rods (genus *Bacteroides*). It is characterized by intense inflammation and edema of the prepuce, superficial glans ulcers, foul-smelling discharge, and bilateral inguinal lymphadenopathy. Infection tends to be locally destructive with severe tenderness and can result in tissue necrosis. The presence of phimosis and suboptimal

Simple balanitis

Erosive balanoposthitis
Lesions

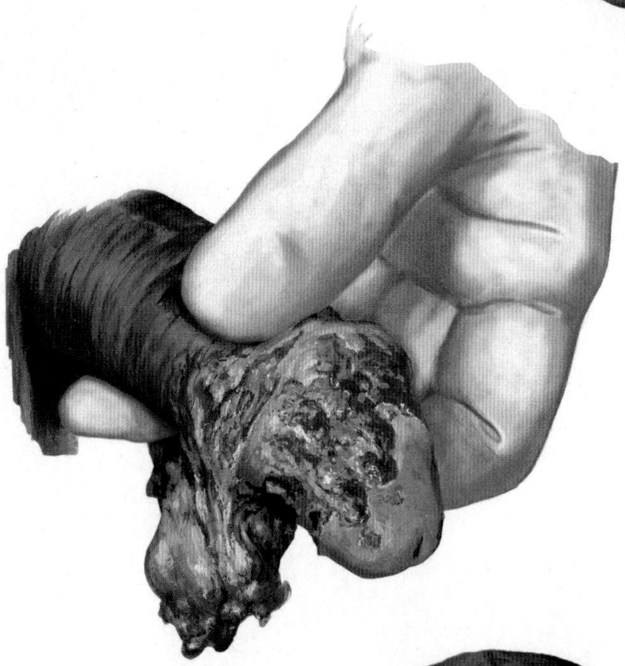

Gangrenous balanoposthitis

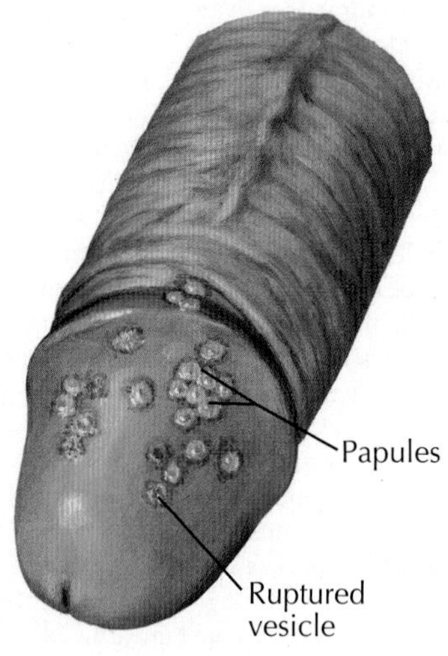

Herpes progenitalis
Papules
Ruptured vesicle

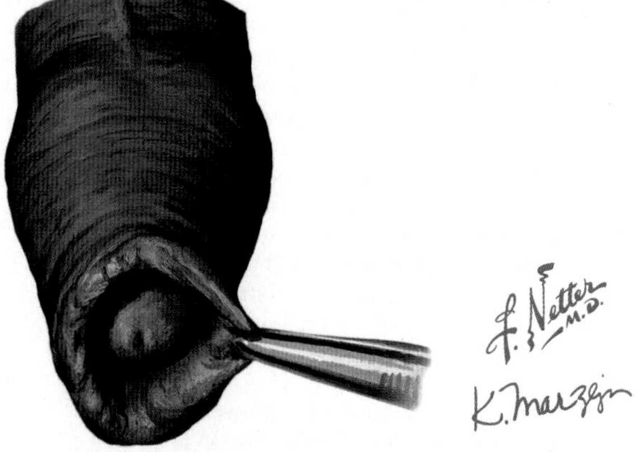

Atrophic balanoposthitis (leukoplakic)

hygiene appear to be prerequisites for this condition. The infection can be transmitted through sexual intercourse, contamination by colonized saliva, or extension from the perirectal area. It generally responds to the timely use of antibiotics and debridement if necessary.

Gangrenous balanitis, in some cases the evolution of erosive balanoposthitis, is generally caused by the same organisms. However, it progresses with such rapidity that an erosive stage may be entirely absent. The ulcers

are covered by gangrenous membranes that, when debrided, reveal deep extension of the process into the glans and preputial tissues. The ulcer bases are uneven yet have distinct borders surrounded by inflamed tissue. Within a day, the foreskin and even the entire glans and portions of the penile shaft can slough. Abscesses may also develop that involve the scrotum and extend superiorly to the abdominal wall and laterally to the thighs.

Plate 2.22

Penis and Male Perineum

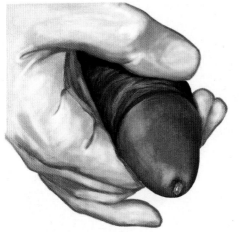

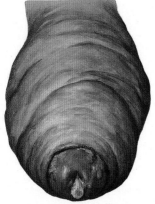

Severe gonorrhea

Mild gonorrhea or nonspecific urethritis

URETHRITIS

Gonorrheal urethritis *(Neisseria gonorrhoeae),* initially a sexually transmitted infection of the urethral mucosa, becomes symptomatic after the gonococci penetrate perimucosal tissues. Crypts and glands of the penile urethra fill with leukocytes and organisms. Chronic gonorrheal urethritis results from retention of gonococci in the urethral glands (Littré) and their intermittent discharge from these glands (carrier stage). The incubation period of gonorrhea is 3 to 5 days. In mild infections, the urethral discharge may be scant and often mistaken for nonspecific urethritis. Abundant purulent discharge and balanoposthitis (with preexisting phimosis) are typical of severe infections. In severe cases, the corpus spongiosum may become involved, resulting in painful erections. With extension of the infection into the posterior urethra, urinary frequency and dysuria occur. Infection of the prostate is usually asymptomatic unless a prostatic abscess is present. Gonorrhea may spread through the spermatic cord to the vas deferens (vasitis) and epididymis, resulting in epididymitis. Gonococcal endocarditis resulting from septicemia has been observed historically. The diagnosis is confirmed with bacterial cultures or urine or urethral swab DNA testing. If denudation of the epithelium in the urethra or vas deferens occurs from treatment, urethral strictures and infertility due to reproductive tract obstruction may develop. Risk factors for contracting the infection include having multiple sexual partners, a partner with a past history of any sexually transmitted diseases, and unprotected sex. Antibiotics are curative.

The term nongonorrheal urethritis or nonspecific urethritis refers to urethritis due to sexually transmitted diseases other than gonorrhea. This form of urethritis is more common than gonorrheal urethritis, with approximately 200 million new cases diagnosed annually worldwide versus 100 million new cases of gonorrhea. The clinical presentation can be identical to that of gonorrhea, and concurrent infections with several different organisms can occur. Responsible organisms are most commonly *Chlamydia trachomatis* (30%–40% of cases), the mycoplasma species *Ureaplasma urealyticum* and *Mycoplasma genitalium* (20% of cases), *Trichomonas vaginalis* (10%–15% of cases), and herpes simplex virus 2 (5% of cases). Nonspecific urethritis, when associated with conjunctivitis and arthritis, is

Sites of gonorrheal localization

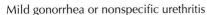

Posterior urethritis

Anterior urethritis

Lacunae of Morgagni and glands of Littré

Seminal vesiculitis

Vasitis

Prostatitis

Cowperitis

Epididymitis

Milky secretion in *Trichomonas* urethritis

Trichomonas vaginalis as seen in fresh specimen from urethral discharge

referred to as *reactive arthritis* and may be a consequence of sexually transmitted infections by nongonorrheal organisms. Urethral strictures can present with urethritis-like symptoms, and in rare instances the underlying cause may be a papilloma, polyp, or cyst of the urethra. Bacterial nongonorrheal urethritis is routinely cured with antibiotics in both partners.

Trichomonas vaginalis is a sexually transmitted, microscopic parasite that causes trichomoniasis. This is a relatively common form of nongonorrheal urethritis with an estimated 3 million new cases annually in the United States. Trichomonads are usually found in the urethral exudate or urethral urine and are recognized microscopically by their active motility and propelling flagella. Patients may be asymptomatic or have a slight thin, milky white urethral discharge in the morning. Itching, dysuria, and possibly urinary urgency may be present. It is curable with antibiotics.

Plate 2.23

Reproductive System: VOLUME 1

SYPHILIS

Syphilis is a sexually transmitted disease caused by the bacterium *Treponema pallidum*. It is often called "the great imitator" because many of its signs and symptoms are indistinguishable from those of other diseases. In the United States syphilis occurs mainly in females 20 to 24 years of age and in males 35 to 39 years of age. In the first decade of the 21st century, reported syphilis cases have increased 2% to 5% annually. More than half of the reported cases occur in men who have sex with men.

The primary syphilitic lesion, a chancre, appears at the primary site of inoculation without other symptoms after an incubation period of 6 to 90 days (mean, 21 days). In most cases, it occurs as a single lesion on the penis, but more than one chancre may be present. The chancre begins as a papule that later erodes. A grayish yellow and sometimes slightly hemorrhagic crust may be present on the surface of the erosion. The smooth base is usually moist, clean, and red. A serous exudate can be easily expressed. The classic chancre, uncomplicated by secondary infection, has a smooth, regular border that is neither rolled nor ragged. It represents an erosion of the skin surface rather than a deeper ulceration, and consequently the lesion heals without scar formation. The palpable induration is a result of vascular alterations and lymphocyte infiltration.

Chancres pursue a slow, indolent course that is characteristically pain free and accompanied in more than two-thirds of cases by inguinal lymphadenopathy. As spirochetes migrate into the body, the chancre heals gradually (and without treatment) over 3 to 6 weeks.

When syphilis occurs concurrently with other sexually transmitted diseases or infections, the chancre may lack characteristic features. In such cases, the primary penile lesion may be erroneously diagnosed as chancroid, superficial abscess, or simple abrasion. Chancres can also occur ventrally on the frenulum and appear as small atypical erosions. A presentation with phimosis with rubbery induration of the foreskin or as other atypical lesions should be investigated for syphilis. Intraurethral chancres, often manifesting as edema at the urethral meatus, can be misdiagnosed as mild nonspecific urethritis.

The definitive diagnosis rests on the dark-field demonstration of the spirochete *Treponema pallidum* in the serum exudate from the primary lesion or from aspirated fluid from an indurated lymph node. Serologic tests (rapid plasma reagin [RPR], Venereal Disease Research Laboratory [VDRL], fluorescent treponemal antibody–absorption test [FTA-ABS]) become positive only when antibodies are produced and become detectable several days or weeks from the appearance of the chancre. Worthy of its title as the "great imitator," syphilis may begin after direct inoculation into the vascular or lymphatic circulation without development of a primary skin lesion.

Syphilis is easily cured in the primary stage, but it is imperative to recognize and to properly treat syphilis early rather than to allow it to further evolve into its more refractory secondary and tertiary stages. Skin rash, mucous membrane lesions, and lymphadenopathy characterize the secondary stage of syphilis. The rash appears anywhere on the body and usually does not cause itching. Characteristically, it is rough, red, or reddish brown and occurs on the palms of the hands and the bottoms of the feet. Sometimes the rash is faint and barely noticeable. Additional symptoms may include fever, sore throat, patchy hair loss, headaches, weight loss, muscle aches, and fatigue. Secondary syphilis will also resolve without treatment. Tertiary or latent syphilis can last for years. The late stages of syphilis can appear 10 to 20 years after the infection was first acquired. In late syphilis, damage to internal organs, including the brain, nerves, eyes, heart, blood vessels, liver, bones, and joints is possible. Signs and symptoms include difficulty coordinating muscle movements, foot drop, paralysis, numbness, gradual blindness, dementia, and death.

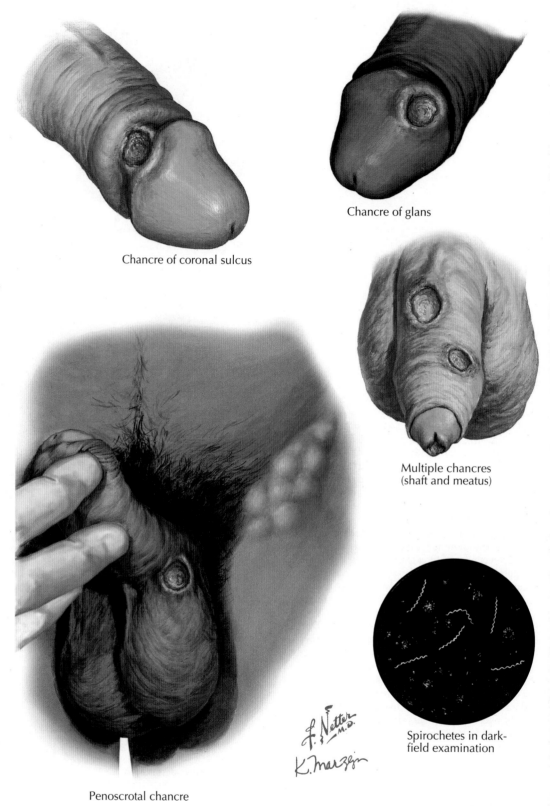

Chancre of coronal sulcus

Chancre of glans

Multiple chancres (shaft and meatus)

Penoscrotal chancre

Spirochetes in dark-field examination

Plate 2.24

Penis and Male Perineum

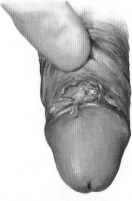

Soft chancre of chancroid

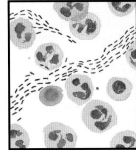

Ducrey bacillus

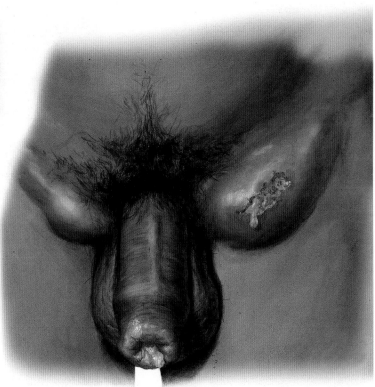

Chancroid under foreskin with marked adenitis

Chancroid, Lymphogranuloma Venereum

Chancroid, formerly called *soft chancre*, is a sexually transmitted disease characterized by painful ulcers and painful inguinal lymphadenopathy (buboes). The causative organism, *Haemophilus ducreyi*, was found by Ducrey in 1889. It is a gram-negative coccoid-bacillary rod that is found at the bottom of the initial ulcer, from which it spreads through lymphatic channels to the inguinal nodes, causing necrosis. *H. ducreyi* enters the skin through an epithelial break, usually after sexual intercourse. With a mean incubation period of 5 to 7 days, the bacteria secrete a cytolethal toxin that inhibits cell proliferation and induces cell death, causing the characteristic ulcer formation. The ulcer, very painful and often located around the sulcus of the glans, is characterized by a soft chancre with steep edges, irregular borders, undermined skin, and a ring of erythema. It begins as a small, congested area that develops into a macule and later a pustule surrounded by a hyperemic zone. A dirty floor due to the presence of exudate and sloughing tissue, and a profuse, purulent discharge are typical. Inguinal buboes may rupture after becoming an abscess and heal with scarring. This can result in chronic lymphatic obstruction and late elephantiasis-like changes to the penile and scrotal skin. The diagnosis is made from the clinical appearance of the lesions in the setting of negative *T. pallidum* by dark-field examination of exudate and negative herpes simplex virus 2 in exudate. The diagnosis can be confirmed by polymerase chain reaction (PCR) directed against one of two genomic segments (ribosomal RNA gene or the *GroEL* gene), or by Gram stain showing *H. ducreyi* appearing like "schools of fish," "railroad tracks," or "fingerprints." Organism culture is unreliable and insensitive. Immunochromatography is a more rapid but less available test that uses monoclonal antibodies to the hemoglobin receptor on the bacteria. Treatment involves incision and drainage of buboes and curative antibiotics.

Lymphogranuloma venereum (LGV) is a sexually transmitted disease caused by invasive *Chlamydia trachomatis (serovars L1, L2, L3)*. LGV may begin as a self-limited, painless genital ulcer that occurs at the contact site 3 to 12 days after inoculation. Most commonly it presents as proctocolitis in men who have sex with men. It usually heals rapidly unless secondary infection occurs. The secondary stage occurs from 10 to

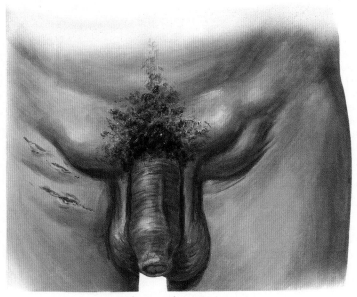

Lymphogranuloma venereum

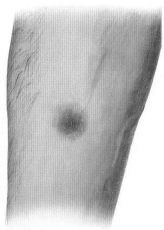

Positive Frei test

30 days later as the infection spreads to unilateral inguinal or femoral lymph nodes. Systemic signs of fever, decreased appetite, and malaise may occur as well. Buboes are typically painful at first and are associated with necrosis and abscess formation with chronic infection. There can be varying degrees of lymphatic obstruction and chronic edema caused by fibrosis as a result. The diagnosis is made by the appearance of the chronic ulcerative process in the inguinal area, and historically (before 1974) by a positive skin test (Frei

test) after intradermal injection of *Chlamydia* antigen. Ulcer biopsy histology is not pathognomonic. Complement fixation is more sensitive (80%) but it has cross reactivity with other *Chlamydia* species. Other blood tests such as microimmunofluorescence test for the L-type serovar of *C. trachomatis* and PCR of lesional swabs are very sensitive and specific, but test availability is limited. Bacterial culture from aspirated material is definitive but lacks sensitivity. Treatment with antibiotics is curative.

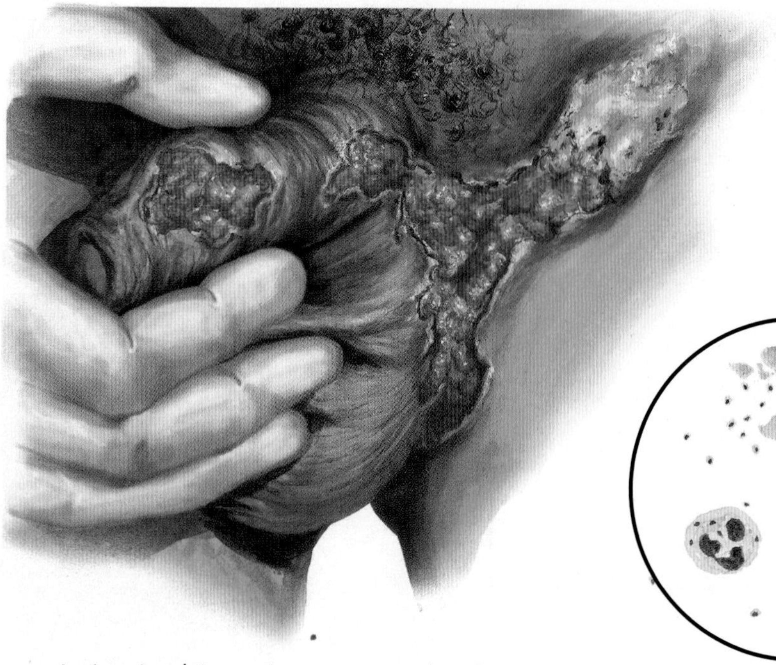

Plate 2.25

Reproductive System: VOLUME 1

Lesions involving groin, scrotum, and penis

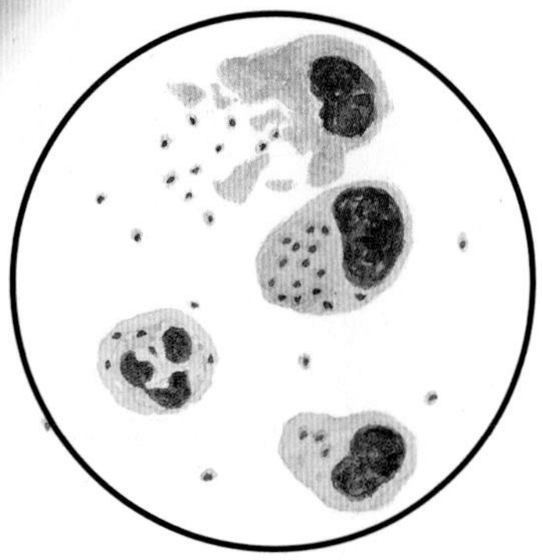

Donovan bodies

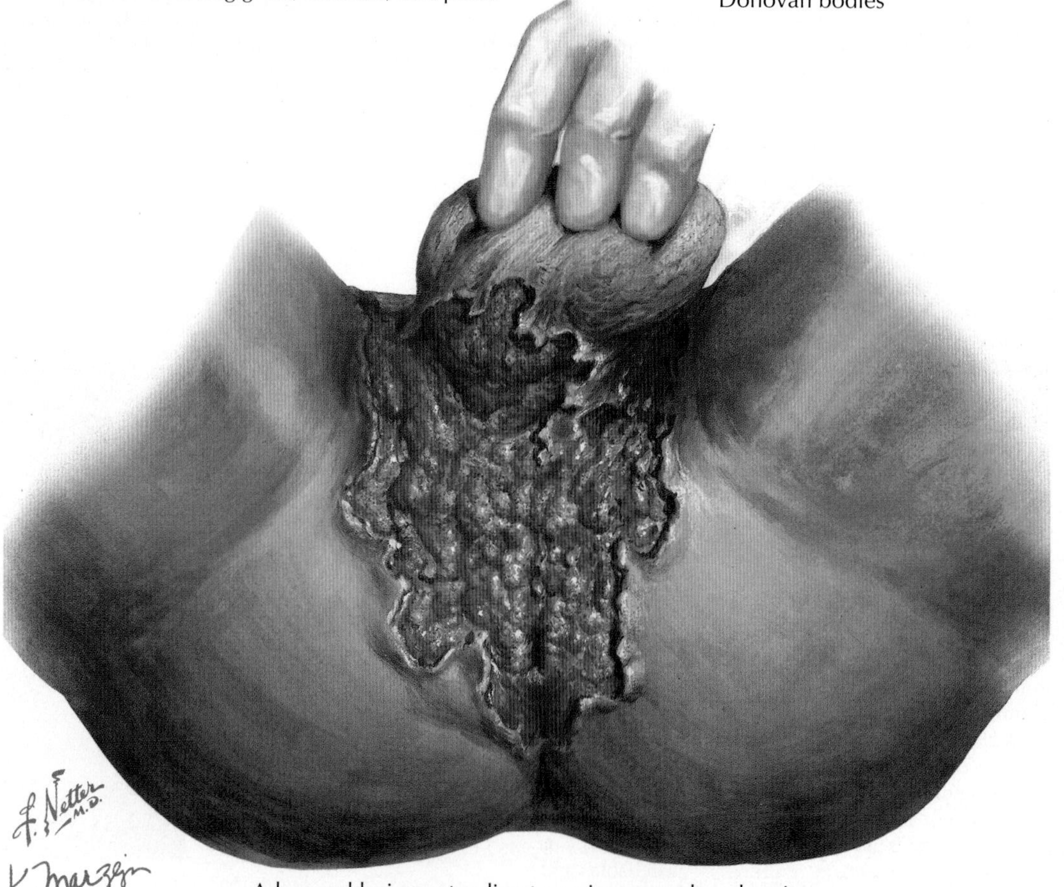

GRANULOMA INGUINALE

Granuloma inguinale (also known as *donovanosis*) is a sexually transmitted bacterial infection of endemic proportions in many underdeveloped countries. The pathognomic feature of the disease are Donovan bodies on Giemsa or Wright stain, intracellular inclusions representing the causative gram-negative *Klebsiella granulomatis* bacteria that have been engulfed by mononuclear phagocytes. Clinically, granuloma inguinale is characterized by painless genital ulcers that appear 10 to 40 days after contact and that can be mistaken for syphilis. There is typically no regional lymphadenopathy. Unlike syphilis, genital ulcers are highly vascular, can bleed and also progress to mutilate and destroy tissue as they are often superinfected with other pathogenic organisms. The lesions occur in the region of contact, which is typically the penile shaft or perineum, and contain Donovan bodies when the superficial layers of the ulcer are scraped or when stained granulation tissue is examined.

The earliest sign of the infection is a tiny macule that develops into a papule and finally a creeping, serpiginous, painless ulcer. Extensive and luxuriant granulations cover the ulcer base with considerable epithelial proliferation around the margin. No large abscesses develop, as in chancroid, but small necrotic areas are observed. Systemic symptoms and lymphadenopathy do not ordinarily accompany this infection. Granuloma inguinale must be differentiated from the other chronic ulcerative infections such as chancroid, chronic streptococcal infection, and syphilis. In later stages, granuloma inguinale may look like advanced genital cancers, LGV, and cutaneous amebiasis. In cases that do not

Advanced lesion extending to perineum and anal region

respond to curative antibiotics and surgical excision, carcinoma must be considered. The diagnosis is made by smears of scrapings from lesions, as the bacteria do not grow in ordinary culture media. No molecular tests are currently available to confirm the diagnosis. Although an infection may begin to reside after 7 days of treatment, a full 12 weeks of antibiotics is essential. Approximately 10% of healed lesions may relapse months later because the Donovan bodies persist beneath healed skin, mandating further treatment. Complications of granuloma inguinale infection include genital mutilation and scarring, loss of skin color in the genital area, and genital elephantiasis from scarring. Occasionally, bacteria spread hematogenously to the bones, joints, or liver; without treatment, anemia, wasting, and uncommonly death may occur. Concurrent testing for HIV is recommended for patients with granuloma inguinale.

Plate 2.26

Penis and Male Perineum

STRICTURES

Strictures of the male urethra may involve any segment, including the meatus, penile, bulbar, membranous, and prostatic urethra. The urethral narrowing may be mild, such that a stent or small cystoscope may pass, or severe, such that even a guidewire cannot be passed. Stricture length also varies from a short, simple narrowing to a long, complex stricture. Strictures may be single or multiple.

Strictures may develop after bacterial, viral, or sexually transmitted (*Chlamydia* and gonorrhea) infections or as a complication of indwelling catheters. Infections tend to lead to long, inflammatory strictures, with 50% occurring in the bulbar urethra, 30% in the penile urethra, and the rest elsewhere. Straddle injuries, penile trauma, punctures, and tears from improper use of sounds, catheters, stylets, and cystoscopes may also lead to severe, short strictures, generally in the bulbar urethra, with significant periurethral scar tissue that responds poorly to repeated dilation.

The degree and duration of urethral inflammation and individual propensity to form scar tissue all affect stricture onset and severity. Urethral strictures consist of poorly vascularized scar tissue that often responds to the trauma of repeated dilation with further inflammation and scar tissue. Scar tissue within the penile urethra usually occurs on the floor, whereas in the bulbar urethra, scar tissue is often located on the roof and may be palpable as an indurated mass that may invade the corpus spongiosum. Periurethral scar tissue can be extensive and of such long duration that the underlying urethral mucosa is completely denuded and appears stark white cystoscopically. The urethra proximal to a stricture may become dilated as a consequence of obstruction to urinary flow, resulting in bilateral hydronephrosis and renal insufficiency.

The most common symptoms are small caliber and weak or split urinary stream, urinary frequency, dysuria, and occasionally gross hematuria, pyuria, and urinary tract infection. Severe strictures may also lead to postvoid dribbling of urine. Acute urinary retention may also occur. Strictures are often complicated by infections that include prostatitis, epididymitis, cystitis, and, occasionally, pyelonephritis. Urethral abscess may develop with spontaneous extravasation of urine proximal to the blocked area, resulting in one or more urethrocutaneous fistulae often referred to as "watering pot perineum." Fistulae may heal spontaneously but then recanalize when abscesses recur. Granulation tissue usually lines the fistulous tracts. Extensive fistulae may open into the buttock and groin as well as the perineum. With chronic extravasation, virulent bacteria may lead to extensive penile, scrotal, and perineal cellulitis as well as gangrenous fasciitis (Fournier gangrene) (see Plate 2.20).

Urethral strictures are diagnosed in several ways. Often it is not possible to pass a urethral catheter. Or, the catheter may pass entirely, but as it enters the strictured area, it is held tightly and needs more force to pass. A nontraumatic retrograde urethrogram with a

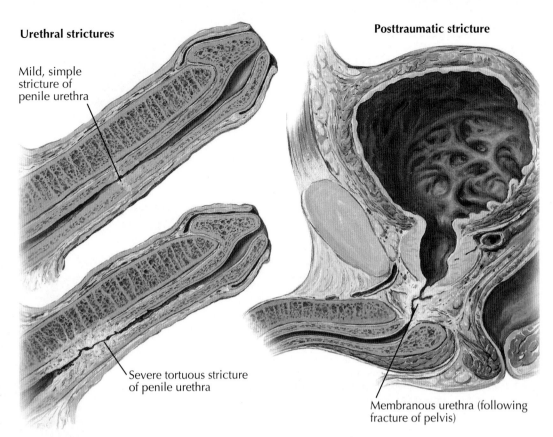

Urethral strictures

Mild, simple stricture of penile urethra

Severe tortuous stricture of penile urethra

Posttraumatic stricture

Membranous urethra (following fracture of pelvis)

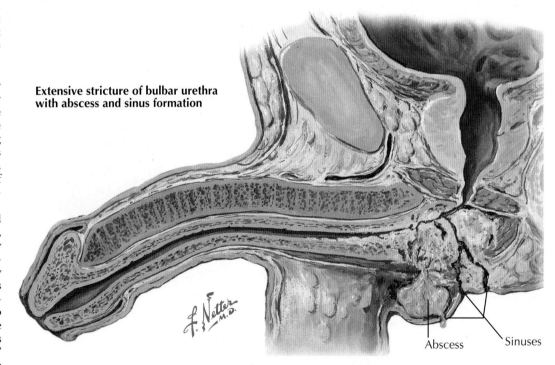

Extensive stricture of bulbar urethra with abscess and sinus formation

Abscess

Sinuses

plain film of the tilted pelvis can assess the severity and length of the strictured urethral lumen. High-frequency penile or perineal ultrasound is particularly good at assessing the extent of damage to associated corpus spongiosal tissue for surgical planning. Repeat dilation is usually only palliative treatment, as this may worsen scar tissue. For fine strictures of the bladder neck after radical prostatectomy, balloon dilation may often be sufficient. For other simple strictures, cystoscopy and

optical urethrotomy is effective in 80% of cases. If strictures recur after endoscopic treatment, formal urethroplasty in which all scarred tissue is excised and healthy urethra reanastomosed is often performed. The excision of long strictures may not allow end-to-end reconnection of the urethral tissue; in such cases, onlay or replacement tubular grafts with penile or preputial skin or bladder or buccal mucosa are routinely used with excellent and durable success.

Plate 2.27

Reproductive System: VOLUME 1

WARTS, PRECANCEROUS LESIONS, EARLY CANCER

The most frequent benign tumor of the penis, and the most frequent sexually transmitted disease, is condyloma acuminatum or verruca, commonly known as *venereal* (includes anal) *warts*. It is usually observed at the base of the glans and in the recess between the glans and a phimotic prepuce. Warts are made up of multiple villi projecting in a cauliflower-like appearance from a pedicled base. This highly contagious sexually transmitted viral infection is caused by over 200 subtypes of human papillomavirus (HPV) and is spread through skin-to-skin contact during oral, genital, or anal sex. Warts are caused by HPV strains 6, 11, 30, 42, 43, 44, 45, 51, 52, and 54; types 6 and 11 are responsible for 90% of genital warts cases. HPV also causes cervical and anal cancers; types 16 and 18 account for 70% of cancer cases.

There is no cure for HPV, but the treatment of visible warts is recommended, as it might reduce infectivity. Warts may disappear without treatment, but there is no way to predict whether they will grow or disappear. Topical solutions such as podophyllotoxin, imiquimod, sinecatechins, and trichloroacetic acid are routine, first-line treatments for small lesions. Surgical ablation with liquid nitrogen or lasers, and formal surgical excision are popular treatments for larger lesions. 5-Fluorouracil cream has been used to treat intraurethral lesions with mixed success.

Verrucae develop luxuriantly under moist conditions and if untreated, they progress to a large size with considerable ulceration and infection. Such giant condylomata are termed Buschke-Löwenstein tumors and can be grossly indistinguishable from carcinoma of the penis. At this stage, the lesion generally requires surgical excision. Verrucae should also be differentiated from the erosive, flat lesions of syphilis and those due to epitheliomas. Bowenoid papulosis is a term used to describe high-risk genital warts caused by HPV types 16 and 18. These lesions are often flatter and darker than verrucous lesions and are found in clusters. Bowenoid papulosis is of concern because although the appearance is similar to typical warts, histologically, they show early features of superficial squamous cell carcinoma.

Rarely lymphoma, myoma, and angiomyofibromas can involve the penile shaft. Angiokeratoma, or telangiectases, of small penile vessels can also appear as purple warts. Nevi and pigmented moles are uncommonly found on the penis. Fordyce spots, small (1–3 mm), white, raised bumps on the penile shaft skin, are naturally occurring sebaceous glands. Leukoplakia of the prepuce or glans, a common complication of chronic inflammation, occurs in solitary or grouped, discrete, white plaques; the skin becomes indurated, thickened, and leathery, with the surface assuming a bluish-white appearance. Within the plaque, hyperkeratosis, dermal edema, and lymphocytic infiltration are present, and this lesion is commonly associated with in situ squamous cell carcinoma and verrucous carcinoma of the penis. Complete surgical excision of leukoplakia is mandatory.

Balanitis xerotica obliterans is a progressive, sclerosing lesion of the preputial skin and meatus that presents with a finely wrinkled or puckered appearance of white parchment. Although not entirely clear, it may be related to lichen sclerosus et atrophicus, which has a similar appearance. These lesions may undergo periods of exacerbation and remission but only rarely resolve and may lead to precancerous leukoplakia.

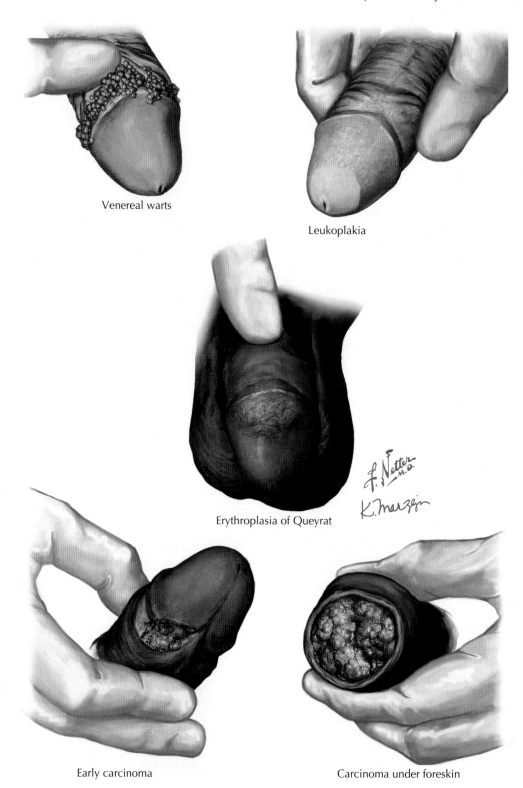

Venereal warts

Leukoplakia

Erythroplasia of Queyrat

Early carcinoma

Carcinoma under foreskin

Erythroplasia of Queyrat presents with characteristic solitary or multiple irregular erythematous plaques on the glans penis or preputial skin. When it occurs on the penile shaft, it is termed Bowen disease. The plaques can be smooth, velvety, scaly, or verrucous, and the edges are sharply marginated. Most commonly found in uncircumcised males, these lesions are synonymous with carcinoma in situ of the penis, therefore complete excision is necessary.

Squamous cell carcinoma of the penis often begins as a small excrescence in the coronal sulcus and near the frenulum in uncircumcised males. It may present with simple induration but later becomes ulcerated and develops into a large, fungating, often infected and foul-smelling mass. The entire glans penis may become involved, with extension into the corporal bodies and urethra. At presentation in 85% of cases, inguinal lymph nodes are indurated from either infection or metastasis. Disturbingly, more than half of patients who are affected have true lymph node metastases at the time of diagnosis. Partial phallectomy or total penectomy with perineal urethrostomy and radical lymph node excision is the treatment of choice.

Plate 2.28

Penis and Male Perineum

ADVANCED CARCINOMA OF THE PENIS

Practically all (95%) penile cancers are squamous carcinomas. Initially, there is thickening of the glans penis or preputial epithelium, with epithelial pearl formation, central degeneration, and keratinization. Penile cancers may be papillary and exophytic or flat and ulcerative. Cancer cells then penetrate the epithelial basal layers, extend to subcutaneous tissue, and subsequently to lymphatics. If untreated, penile autoamputation can occur.

Penile cancer is rare but deadly, with an estimated 2000 new US cases annually (<1% of cancers). One reason for the high mortality rate is that patients tend to delay seeking medical attention, with 15% to 50% delaying for more than 1 year from first awareness. Risk factors for penile cancer include lack of circumcision, poor penile hygiene, phimosis, age >60 years, multiple sexual partners, and tobacco use. In addition, HPV infection may increase the risk of penile cancer, because half of all penile cancers are associated with HPV types 16 and 18 viral infection. Premalignant lesions include erythroplasia of Queyrat, Bowen disease, and bowenoid papulosis and, based on their similar histologies, could be considered forms of intraepithelial neoplasia or carcinoma in situ for penile cancer. Retained, decomposing smegma, together with balanoposthitis, may contribute to the initiation of malignancy and explains why adult circumcision does not protect against cancer.

Penile cancer usually grows gradually and laterally along the surface of the penis. Buck fascia (see Plate 2.3) acts as a temporary barrier to corporeal invasion. Eventually, the cancer penetrates Buck fascia and the tunica albuginea, after which systemic spread is possible. Penile cancer metastasizes almost solely through the lymphatics, although occasionally hematogenous spread through the dorsal vein of the penis occurs with spread to the axial skeleton. Usually, the tumor metastasizes first to superficial inguinal lymph nodes (see Plate 2.9), but the central, presymphyseal lymph node and external iliac nodes may also be involved. Because the lymphatics of the penile shaft intercommunicate, metastases may occur bilaterally despite a unilaterally located primary lesion. The superficial inguinal nodes drain to the deep inguinal nodes beneath the fascia lata. From here, drainage is to the pelvic nodes. Inguinal lymph nodes extensively involved with tumor may erode through the skin and into the femoral artery and vein (see Plate 2.9). Although penile cancer can be suspected from its appearance, the diagnosis is established through biopsy of the primary lesion or lymph nodes.

Surgical excision constitutes definitive management of this condition. If the tumor is less than 2 cm in size and confined to the prepuce, circumcision may be sufficient. In small (<1.5 cm) glans lesions, Mohs micrographic surgery or laser ablation may spare the penis and eradicate tumor; however, local failure is far more common after organ-sparing procedures. Partial penile shaft amputation is appropriate when the cancer involves the glans and distal shaft. A 2-cm margin is necessary; attempts to limit the resection can result in recurrent tumor. If surgical resection with partial penectomy does not provide an adequate margin, a total penectomy is considered along with a perineal urethrostomy.

After treatment of the primary tumor, management of the inguinal lymph nodes follows. The decision to resect inguinal nodes in patients with no evidence of adenopathy, either clinically or after imaging studies, is

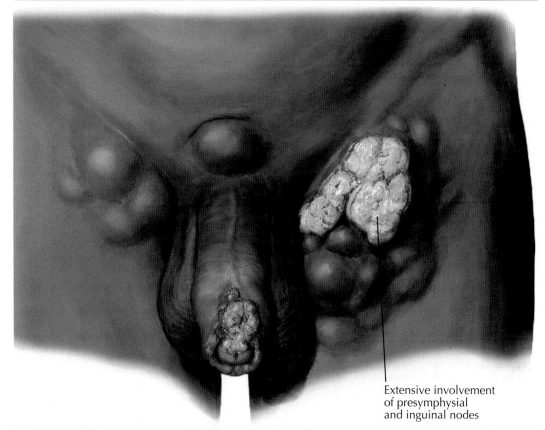

Advanced carcinoma of penis

Extensive involvement of presymphysial and inguinal nodes

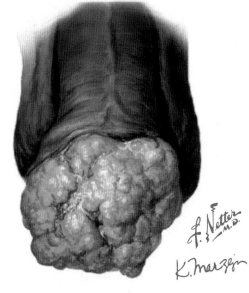

Extensive fungating carcinoma of penis

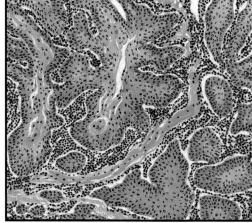

Squamous cell carcinoma of penis, histology

controversial. The incidence of occult metastases in patients without palpable adenopathy is 20% to 25%. In addition, radical inguinal lymphadenectomy has a high complication rate (80%–90%) that includes serous lymphocele formation, wound necrosis and infection, chronic leg edema, phlebitis, and pulmonary embolism. Therefore modifications to this procedure, including limited, superficial lymph node excision and sentinel lymph node biopsy (in which lymphoscintigraphy and intradermal blue dye is injected around the tumor and examined for its presence in the superficial inguinal lymph nodes to determine primary landing sites for cancer), have become popular to reduce the need for, and complications from, radical lymphadenectomy.

The indications for pelvic lymphadenectomy have not been clearly delineated without evidence of enlarged nodes on imaging. When two or more inguinal nodes contain cancer, the probability of pelvic node involvement is high and pelvic lymphadenectomy is indicated. Patients with negative inguinal lymph nodes rarely have pelvic node involvement. Regarding mortality, untreated patients with inguinal metastases rarely survive 2 years. Those with clinically palpable adenopathy and proven metastases have a 20% to 50% survival rate 5 years after definitive surgical treatment. The role of radiation and chemotherapy in penile cancer is palliative only.

Plate 2.29

Reproductive System: VOLUME 1

PAPILLOMA, CANCER OF URETHRA

Urethral warts (papillomas) are benign, sexually transmitted lesions that occur at the urethral meatus, in the fossa navicularis, along the penile urethra, and as far proximal as the prostatic urethra. However, 90% of lesions are observed in the distal urethra. Bladder involvement is rare. These are generally HPV-positive lesions, similar to condyloma acuminata (see Plate 2.27). Indeed, urethral papillomas are observed in 15% of males with condyloma of the external genitalia. The usual presentation is a mass protruding from the urethra, blood per urethra, hematuria, dysuria, or urethral discharge. Risk factors include multiple sexual partners and unprotected intercourse. Urethroscopy is important to determine the full extent of intraurethral lesions. Urethral meatal lesions can be treated by local excision, often accompanied by meatoplasty to improve access. The base of the lesion is generally fulgurated after excision. Deeper urethral lesions are treated cystoscopically with heat diathermy or CO_2 laser fulguration or cold cup excision. Recurrences are common after a single treatment, and therefore multiple treatments may be needed. The use of 5% 5-fluorouracil cream, although irritating, may help prevent recurrence.

True urethral polyps are rare, nonsexually transmitted, and occur almost exclusively in boys. They are characterized by benign urothelial-lined masses attached to a fibrovascular stalk and generally arise from the verumontanum. This location suggests that they may represent the embryologic persistence of müllerian structures. They may cause urinary urgency, dysuria, and frequency; hematuria; urinary tract infection; or occasionally urinary retention, especially if situated in the posterior urethra. They are visualized by cystoscopy and are removed by simple fulguration.

Primary urethral carcinoma of the urethra is rare but deadly. The most common type of urethral malignancy is squamous cell cancer (78% of cases) in the penile and bulbar urethra, but transitional cell carcinoma is also observed (15% of cases) in the prostatic urethra (see Plate 2.12). Occasionally, papillary adenocarcinoma of the urethra can originate from the glands of Littré or Cowper. Urethral cancer is more common in White individuals than in Black individuals, and it is the only urologic malignancy that is more common in females than in males. No formal risk factors have been identified, although cancer is thought to develop from chronic inflammation, infection, or irritation of the urethra. Patients with a history of bladder cancer have an increased risk of urethral cancer.

The onset of urethral cancer is insidious, and early symptoms are nonspecific. Because of this, the interval between symptom onset and formal diagnosis may be 3 years. Approximately one-half of patients give a history of urethral stricture and about 20% give a history of urethral discharge, often inviting treatment for a sexually transmitted disease. As the lesion progresses, urinary symptoms such as weak stream, post-void dribbling, and dysuria as well as sexual symptoms such as painful erections may occur. Some degree of urinary retention is observed in 25% of patients, and in 40% of patients a palpable indurated penile mass may be detected.

The diagnosis is made by cystoscopy, urethral biopsy, and cytologic washings. Tumors at the urethral meatus

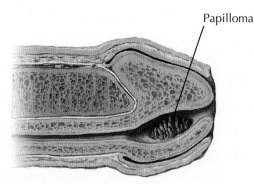

Papilloma of fossa navicularis

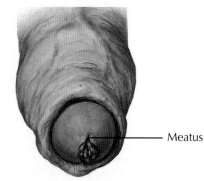

Papilloma protruding from meatus

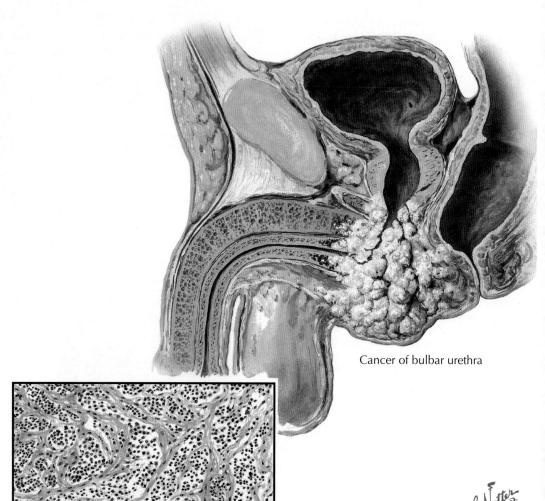

Cancer of bulbar urethra

Cuboidal cell cancer of bulbar urethra, histology

can simply be excised, although the entire urethra requires inspection. Noninvasive lesions may be managed expectantly, with repeat endoscopic incision for recurrences. Invasive lesions require more extensive surgery with wide urethral margins, often necessitating urethrectomy with penectomy. Depending on the location of the primary tumor in the urethra, metastases most commonly involve the inguinal lymph nodes, followed by lungs, liver, pleura, bones, and other distant organs. Surgery is the main curative treatment for urethral cancer, although multimodality treatment with chemotherapy and radiotherapy may also provide benefit. Four levels of surgical management are used for urethral cancer: (1) conservative therapy or local excision, (2) partial penectomy, (3) radical penectomy, and (4) pelvic lymphadenectomy and en bloc resection, including penectomy and cystoprostatectomy with removal of the anterior pubic bone (anterior exenteration) and urinary diversion. The 5-year survival rates are 60% for distal urethral tumors and less than 50% for proximal urethral cancers.

SCROTUM AND TESTIS

Plate 3.1

Reproductive System: VOLUME 1

SCROTAL WALL

The testicles are maintained in position within the scrotal cavity by the structures of the spermatic cord. Each testicle and spermatic cord is invested in six distinct tissue layers that are acquired as a result of the descent of the gonads from the retroperitoneum into the scrotum during fetal life.

From superficial to deep, the first layer is the scrotal skin, thin in texture, brownish in appearance, and highly distensible. It generally assumes a rugated pattern and is continuous with the skin of the mons pubis and penis superiorly, the perineum posteriorly, and the medial thighs laterally. Unlike these adjacent areas, the scrotal skin contains abundant sebaceous follicles, sweat glands, sparsely distributed hair, and a distinct median raphe that corresponds to the scrotal septum within the scrotum and is continuous with the median raphé of the perineum.

Beneath the scrotal epithelium is a thin, fibrous, net-like, and highly vascular tissue layer that contains elastic and smooth muscle fibers, and is termed the *tunica dartos* (*dartos,* meaning "flayed"). This is the superficial fascia of the scrotum (Colles fascia) that has been previously described (see Plate 2.2). It is a continuation of Scarpa fascia of the abdomen and Colles fascia of the urogenital triangle in the perineum (see Plates 2.2 and 2.3). The connective tissue from this layer extends inward to form the scrotal septum, which divides the scrotum into a compartment for each testicle.

Deep to the dartos fascia and separated from it by loose areolar tissue is the external spermatic fascia, a continuation of the external oblique fascia of the abdominal wall. Beneath the external spermatic fascia is the cremasteric fascia, which is composed of a double layer of areolar and elastic tissue that encloses a thin layer of striated muscle. The cremasteric fascia is a continuation of the internal oblique fascia and occasionally contains a few fibers from the transversus abdominus muscle. It is the cremasteric fascia that is responsible for the retraction of the testicles, protecting them from trauma and stimuli such as cold through the cremasteric reflex. This reflex is necessary for thermoregulatory control, as it maintains the testicles at the optimal temperature for spermatogenesis.

Deep to the cremasteric fascia is the internal spermatic fascia that closely invests the testicles and inner cord structures. This layer of loose connective tissue is a continuation of the transversalis fascia that lines the abdominal and pelvic cavities.

Beneath the internal spermatic fascia lies the tunica vaginalis. During development, the peritoneum forms two layers that cover each testis as it descends, one anteriorly and one posteriorly. The posterior peritoneum forms the visceral tunica vaginalis that surrounds the testicle where it is closely adherent to the tunica albuginea of the testicle. The outer, parietal layer of the tunica vaginalis is derived from the peritoneum of the anterior abdomen and is adherent to the overlying

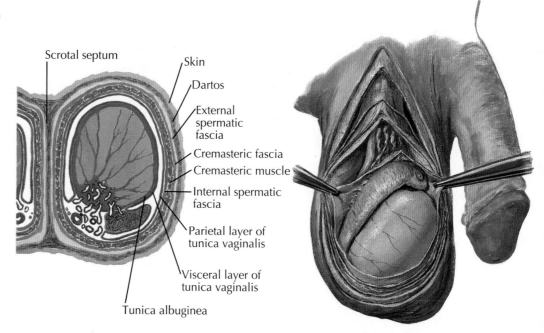

internal spermatic fascia. It is separated from the visceral layer by endothelial cells that form a small, fluid-filled space between it and the visceral layer. It is within this potential space that hydroceles form.

Within the spermatic cord, running along with the vas deferens, is the inferior spermatic nerve, derived from the pelvic plexus and carrying sympathetic and parasympathetic nerve fibers. It is believed that this nerve is the main neural regulator of testosterone secretion in the testis.

Two remnants from fetal development may be present in the adult scrotum and lie beneath the visceral layer of the tunica vaginalis: (1) the appendix testis (hydatid of Morgagni) on the upper pole of the testis and (2) the appendix epididymis (paradidymis), attached to the head (globus major) of the epididymis. The appendix testis represents remnants of the fallopian tube and is derived from the cranial end of the primitive müllerian duct, whereas the appendix epididymis is a vestige of the cranial end of the mesonephric duct (see Plate 1.2).

Plate 3.2

Scrotum and Testis

Anterior view

Inferior vena cava

Inferior mesenteric
artery

Abdominal aorta

Renal vessels

Internal spermatic vessels
(part of spermatic cord)

Ureter

Common iliac vessels

Internal iliac vessels

External iliac vessels

Inferior vesical
artery

Inferior epigastric
vessels

Artery to ductus
deferens

External spermatic
(cremasteric)
vessels

Internal spermatic
vessels in spermatic
cord

Femoral
vessels

Superficial
external
pudendal
vessels (*cut—
pass superficial
to spermatic
cord*)

Deep external
pudendal
vessels

Pampiniform
venous plexus

Deep dorsal vein and dorsal arteries
of penis under deep (Buck) fascia of penis

BLOOD SUPPLY OF THE TESTIS

The arterial supply to the testis is derived from three sources: the internal spermatic artery, the deferential (vasal) artery, and the external spermatic or cremasteric artery. The internal spermatic artery originates from the abdominal aorta just below the renal artery. Embryologically, the testicles lie opposite the second lumbar vertebra and keep the blood supply acquired during fetal life. The internal spermatic artery joins the spermatic cord above the internal inguinal ring and pursues a course adjacent to the pampiniform venous plexus to the mediastinum of the testicle. The vascular arrangement within the pampiniform plexus, with the counterflowing artery and veins, facilitates the exchange of heat and small molecules. For example, testosterone passively diffuses from the veins to the artery in a concentration-limited manner, and a loss of the temperature differential created by this system is associated with testicular dysfunction in males with varicocele and cryptorchidism.

Near the mediastinal testis, the internal spermatic artery is highly coiled and branches before entering the testis. Extensive interconnections between the internal spermatic and deferential arteries allow maintenance of testis viability even after division of the internal spermatic artery. The testicular arteries penetrate the tunica albuginea and travel inferiorly along the posterior surface of the testis within the parenchyma. Branching arteries pass anteriorly over the testicular parenchyma. Individual arteries to the seminiferous tubules, termed centrifugal arteries, travel within the septa that contain tubules. Centrifugal artery branches give rise to arterioles that supply individual intertubular and peritubular capillaries.

The deferential artery (artery of the vas) may originate from either the inferior or superior vesical artery (see Plate 2.6) and supplies the vas deferens and the cauda epididymis. A third artery, the external spermatic or cremasteric artery, arises from the inferior epigastric artery inside the internal inguinal ring, where it enters the spermatic cord. This artery forms a network over the tunica vaginalis and usually anastomoses with other arteries at the testicular mediastinum.

Veins within the testis are unusual in that they do not run with the corresponding intratesticular arteries. Small parenchymal veins empty into either the veins on the testis surface or into a group of veins near the mediastinum testis. These two sets of veins join with deferential veins to form the pampiniform plexus. The pampiniform plexus consists of branches of freely anastomosing veins from (1) the anterior (or internal) spermatic veins that emerge from the testicle and accompany the spermatic artery to enter the vena cava; (2) the middle deferential group that accompanies the vas deferens to pelvic veins; and (3) the posterior or external spermatic group that follows a course along the posterior spermatic cord. The latter group empties into branches of the superficial and deep inferior epigastric veins and the superficial and deep pudendal veins. The middle and posterior veins provide collateral venous return of blood from the testicles after internal spermatic vein ligation with varicocelectomy.

The right internal spermatic vein enters the inferior vena cava obliquely below the right renal vein forming a natural "valve" to reduce retrograde blood flow, whereas the left vein terminates in the left renal vein at right angles, without a natural valve. This anatomic relationship is thought to explain the fact that 90% of varicoceles are on the left side.

With varicocele formation, the blood flow in the internal spermatic vein is reversed, thus disturbing venous drainage from the testis and potentially elevating scrotal temperature. As a consequence, orchalgia and infertility can occur. In high-ligation varicocelectomy procedures (Palomo), the internal spermatic artery and vein are both ligated above where the deferential vessels and the external spermatic veins exit the spermatic cord, thus affording sufficient collateral circulation to maintain testis viability. During inguinal or subinguinal procedures, care is needed to spare the internal spermatic artery, as collateralization may be less extensive at this anatomic level.

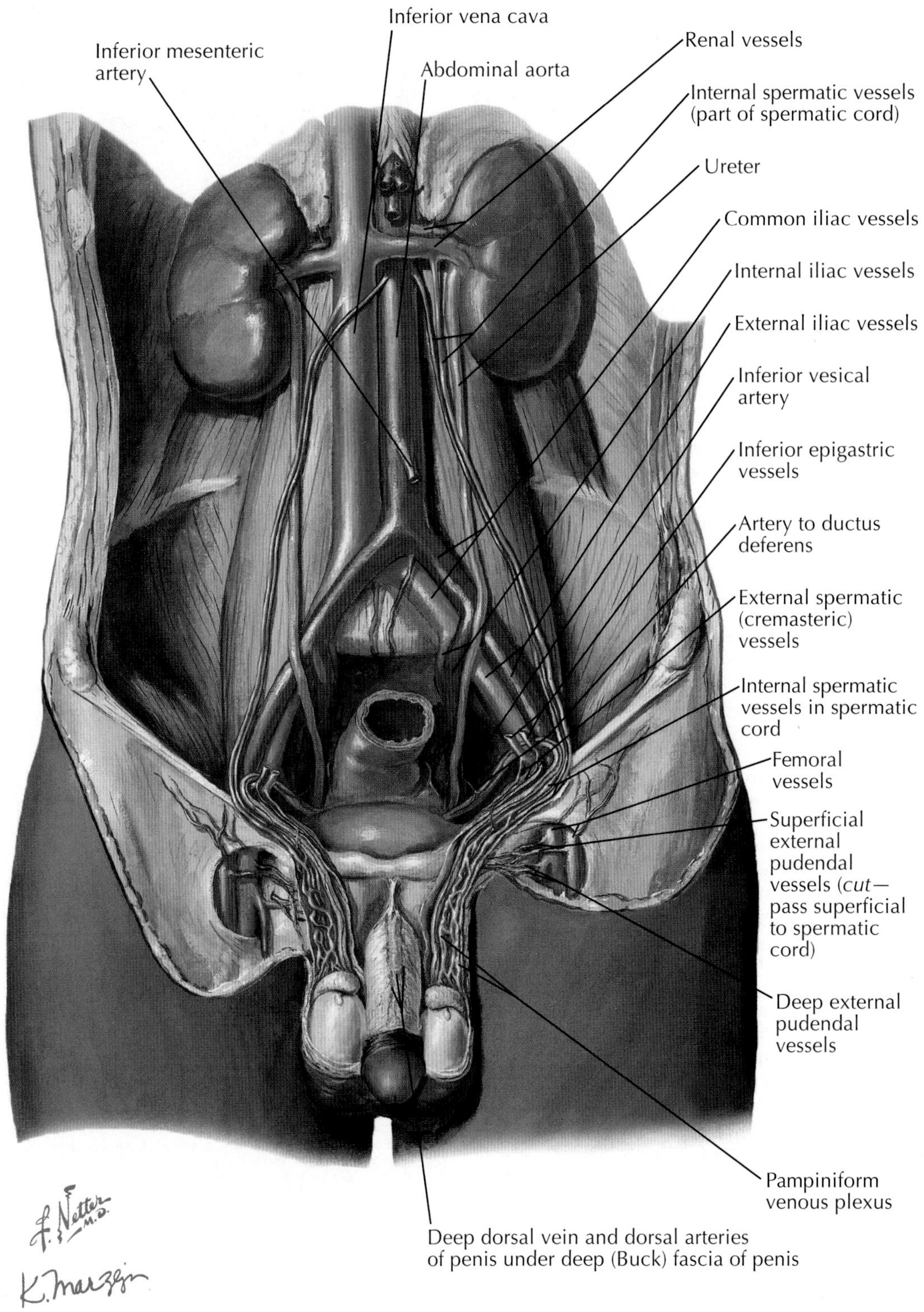

Plate 3.3

Reproductive System: VOLUME 1

Testis, Epididymis, and Vas Deferens

The testicle is encased within a thick, fibrous capsule known as the *tunica albuginea.* The tunica is covered by the closely adherent, glistening peritoneum (tunica vaginalis). Multiple septa from the capsule divide the interior of the testicle into several dozen pyramid-shaped lobules. The testis shows ethnic variations in size but is normally 4 cm in length and 3 cm in diameter (18–20 mL in volume).

Within each testicle, each lobule contains one or several tortuous seminiferous tubules that, when uncoiled, measure 0.3 to 0.6 m in length. These tubules converge at the testicular hilum (mediastinum testis), where they straighten and anastomose to form the rete testis. The rete testis tubules empty into 8 to 10 efferent ducts (ductuli efferentes) that carry sperm to the caput epididymis. Occasionally a blind-ending efferent duct is observed (vas aberrans). Spermatoceles are thought to be the result of pathologic dilation of the efferent ducts.

Testicular histology reveals evidence of both exocrine (sperm production) and endocrine (androgen production) functions within the organ. In the normal adult testis, seminiferous tubules are lined with a basement layer of laminated connective tissue containing elastic fibers and flattened myoid cells. On this layer rests the germinal epithelium and sustentacular cells known as *Sertoli cells.* The intertubular connective tissue contains groups of large polygonal cells termed *Leydig cells,* whose cytoplasm holds many lipid granules that contain testosterone and other androgens. Characteristics of maleness, including body hair, muscle mass, deepened voice, and sexual function, are several androgen-dependent functions.

The epididymis is a comma-shaped organ located along the posterolateral surface of the testis. It is a tightly coiled, tortuous duct 3 to 4 m in length, embedded in dense connective tissue. Passage through the epididymis induces many changes to newly formed sperm, including a gain in functional motility and alterations in surface charge, membrane proteins, immunoreactivity, phospholipids, fatty acid content, and adenylate cyclase activity. These changes improve cell membrane structural integrity, increase fertilization ability, and improve motility. Spermatozoa within the testis have very poor or no motility. They become progressively motile and functional only after traversing the epididymis. The transit time of sperm through the epididymis has been estimated at 12 days in humans.

Extensions from the tunical sheath that surrounds the epididymis enter interductal spaces and form septa that divide the duct into histologically characteristic regions: the caput or head, corpus or body, and cauda or tail. The 8 to 10 ductuli efferentes within the caput region coalesce to form a single epididymal duct within the corpus and cauda epididymis. The epididymis is distinguished histologically by its ciliated epithelium that consists of two main cell types: principal cells and basal cells. Principal cells vary in height along the length of the epididymis mainly because of the length of associated stereocilia. Principal cell nuclei are elongated and often possess large clefts and one or two nucleoli. Consistent with absorptive and secretory function, their cellular apices have numerous coated pits. There are far fewer basal cells than principal cells in the epididymis. Tear-shaped basal cells rest on the basal lamina and extend approximately toward the lumen, their apices forming threads between adjacent

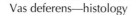

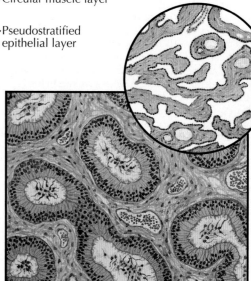

Vas deferens—histology

Epididymis—histology

principal cells. Thought to be derived from macrophages, they are likely the precursors of the principal cells.

The vas deferens originates as a continuation of the cauda epididymal duct. During this transition, the muscular coat of the tubule increases dramatically, the tortuosity of the duct decreases, and epithelial cells lose cilia. The vas continues for about 25 cm and becomes the ampulla of the vas before joining with the seminal vesicle and forming the proximal ejaculatory duct. In cross section, the vas

deferens has an outer adventitial connective tissue sheath containing blood vessels and small nerves, a muscular coat that consists of a middle circular layer surrounded by inner and outer longitudinal muscle layers, and an inner mucosal layer with a pseudostratified epithelial lining. The outer diameter of the vas deferens varies from 1.5 to 3 mm, and the lumen of the unobstructed vas deferens varies from 0.2 to 0.7 mm in diameter, dimensions easily handled using microsurgical approaches to surgical reconstruction after vasectomy or other blockage.

Plate 3.4

Scrotum and Testis

TESTICULAR DEVELOPMENT AND SPERMATOGENESIS

Histologically, newborn testes appear as "testis cords" that harbor mainly Sertoli cells and rarer early germ cells, called *gonocytes*, in layers without tubular lumina. Consistent with a brief surge in androgen levels during the first few months of life that is thought to hormonally imprint later androgen-dependent organs, large prominent interstitial Leydig cells occupy the spaces among the testis cords. In early childhood, little change occurs in the testis cords except for linear growth. At 5 to 7 years of age, lumina begin to appear in the cords and they gradually increase in diameter to become seminiferous tubules, characterized by primitive spermatogonial stem cells and marking the first stage of spermatogenesis. Mitotic activity of early spermatogonia begins at about 11 years of age; however, the age at which the germ cells begin to differentiate varies greatly, as does the onset of puberty. Primary spermatocytes appear soon thereafter, indicating the beginning of meiosis in the testis, and spermatids are noted at about 12 years of age. Once this germ cell maturation sequence (termed *spermarche*) begins, the testes enlarge rapidly, which constitutes the first sign of puberty (Tanner stage 1).

The interstitial Leydig cells mature concurrently with germ cells during early puberty, but androgen production lags slightly behind spermatogenesis. The pubertal surge in testosterone from mature Leydig cells is responsible for the remainder of pubertal development (Tanner stages 2 to 5). Spermatogenesis remains active throughout adult life but decreases during the seventh or eighth decade with the onset of andropause, as a response to decreased androgen production by Leydig cells.

Spermatogenesis is a continuous process in vertebrates (only seasonal in some moose species) and, in males, involves germ cell progression though 13 cell types over a period of 64 days. It consists of (1) a proliferative phase as spermatogonia divide to replace their number (self-renewal) or differentiate into daughter cells that become mature gametes; (2) a meiotic phase when germ cells undergo a reduction division, resulting in haploid (half the normal DNA complement) spermatids; and (3) a spermiogenesis phase in which spermatids undergo a profound metamorphosis to become mature sperm.

Spermatogenesis begins with type B spermatogonia dividing mitotically to form primary spermatocytes within the adluminal compartment. Primary spermatocytes are the first germ cells to undergo meiosis. As they move from the adluminal or basal to luminal or apical compartment of the Sertoli cell (as defined by intercellular tight junctions), they divide into secondary spermatocytes. The latter cleave immediately into spermatids, which metamorphose into mature sperm.

A cycle of spermatogenesis involves the division of spermatogonial stem cells into sperm. Several cycles of spermatogenesis coexist within the germinal epithelium at any one time and are described morphologically as stages. When viewed from a fixed point within a seminiferous tubule, six recognizable stages exist in humans. Superimposed on this, there is also a specific organization of spermatogenic cycles within the seminiferous

Testicular development

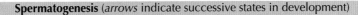

Neonatal testis

Infantile testis

Late prepubertal testis

Adult testis

Spermatogenesis (*arrows* indicate successive states in development)

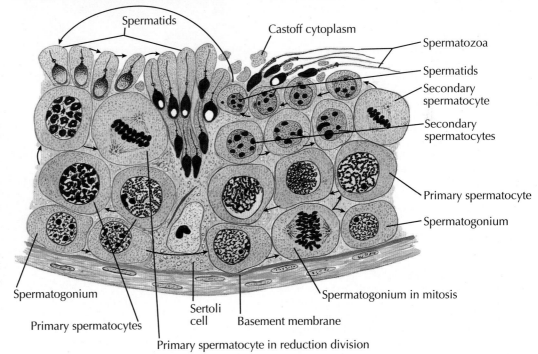

Spermatids

Castoff cytoplasm

Spermatozoa

Spermatids

Secondary spermatocyte

Secondary spermatocytes

Primary spermatocyte

Spermatogonium

Spermatogonium in mitosis

Spermatogonium

Primary spermatocytes

Sertoli cell

Basement membrane

Primary spermatocyte in reduction division

tubule space, termed spermatogenic waves. It is likely that human spermatogenesis occurs in a spiral or helical wave pattern that ensures constant and not pulsatile sperm production at 1200 sperms/heartbeat.

There are two important differences between mitosis and meiosis. During the phase of DNA synthesis in both mitosis and meiosis, reproducing cells have double the normal content of DNA ($4n$). In mitosis, DNA content is reduced to diploid ($2n$) after a single reduction division. However, in meiosis a second reduction

division (secondary spermatocytes to spermatids) occurs to generate daughter cells with haploid (n) DNA content consisting of 22 autosomes and either an X or a Y chromosome. The other difference is that mitosis produces identical daughter cells, whereas genetically different daughter cells result from meiosis. This occurs as a consequence of chromosomal synapse and recombination during meiosis, in which DNA is exchanged between sister chromatids and is the basis for genetic diversity in our species.

Plate 3.5

Reproductive System: VOLUME 1

DESCENT OF THE TESTIS

The early genital ridge on the posterior wall of the coelomic cavity contains the primordial testis and extends from the sixth thoracic to the second sacral segment. At 8 weeks' gestation, the testis, lying beneath the mesothelium (primitive peritoneum), becomes an elongated, spindle-shaped organ projecting into the coelomic cavity (future abdominal cavity). The mesothelium is thrown into two folds: the upper, diaphragmatic or cranial suspensory ligament extends to the diaphragm, whereas the lower, inguinal ligament or future gubernaculum terminates in the lower abdominal wall at a site where the inguinal bursa (future inguinal canal) is to develop. A pouch-like peritoneal evagination of the abdominal wall, termed the processus vaginalis, emerges during the sixth month. It grows to become the inguinal bursa, which, by the end of the seventh month is large enough to admit the testis. Concurrently, as a result of an involution of the cranial and adjacent mesonephros, the testis becomes mobile and is left suspended from the epididymis by the mesorchium, a fold of primitive peritoneum. By 7 months, the gonad is located several millimeters above the groin, with its long axis oriented obliquely or at right angles to the embryo.

At the end of the seventh month, the testes pass inferiorly through the inguinal canal. However, it is not uncommon to find them in the canal at birth, with final descent occurring postnatally. At the time of testis descent into the processus vaginalis within the inguinal bursa and scrotum, the portion of this processus vaginalis superior to the testis becomes obliterated sometimes weeks or months after birth. Persistence of the processus vaginalis after birth can result in what is called a *communicating hydrocele,* in which peritoneal fluid freely enters the tunical vaginalis space within the scrotum. This type of hydrocele is characterized by dramatic changes in size when assuming an upright or supine position.

The gubernaculum, originally discernible as a fibrous band in early fetal life, develops as the lower inguinal ligament and increases in size through the seventh month of gestation. It connects the upper end of the wolffian duct (epididymis), and with it the testis, to the lower abdominal wall. The distal attachment of the gubernaculum extends to the region of the inguinal bursa where the future external oblique layer of the abdominal wall develops.

The role of the gubernaculum in the descent of the testis is incompletely understood. What is known is that testis descent occurs in two stages: transabdominal migration and inguinoscrotal descent. Failure of either stage results in varying degrees in what is termed undescended testis or cryptorchidism. This is the most common urologic birth defect, occurring in 2% to 4% of full-term male births. It is also thought to be increasing in prevalence over the last few decades, possibly due to the influence of environmental factors acting as endocrine disruptors. Initially, the gubernaculum contracts and thickens to guide migration of the testis toward the

internal inguinal ring. In mice, this migration appears to be controlled by a testis-derived insulin-like/relaxin-like peptide (Insl-3). The human homologue of the mouse Insl-3 gene has been identified as an insulin- and relaxin-like molecule (*INSL3*) and is produced by Leydig cells. Mutations in the *INSL3* receptor, *RXFP2,* also known as *LGR8,* are also thought to be relevant for mammalian cryptorchidism. In studies of cryptorchid boys, mutations in the *INSL3* gene only occur in 1% to 2% of cases, suggesting that other factors must also play

a role in testis descent. The second phase of descent, transinguinal to scrotal, is thought to be androgen dependent. This is surmised from conditions such as androgen insensitivity (faulty androgen receptor activity) and Kallmann syndrome (defective androgen production) in which there is transabdominal but not inguinoscrotal descent observed. It also follows that endocrine disruptors that alter androgen balance in the third fetal trimester may also predispose male infants to cryptorchidism.

8 weeks (22.5 mm crown-rump)

Suprarenal gland
Suspensory (diaphragmatic) ligament
Gonads
Mesonephric (wolffian) duct
Gubernaculum
Urinary bladder

11 weeks (43 mm crown-rump)

Suprarenal gland
Kidney
Suspensory (diaphragmatic) ligament (atrophic)
Testes
Epididymis
Gubernaculum
Deep inguinal ring
Urinary bladder

4 lunar months (107 mm crown-rump)

Epididymis   Testis
Gubernaculum
Deep inguinal ring

8 lunar months (26 cm crown-rump)

Superficial inguinal ring
Ductus deferens
Scrotum (*cut open*)
Epididymis
Testis
Processus vaginalis
Gubernaculum
Cavity of tunica vaginalis (*cut open*)

Plate 3.6

Scrotum and Testis

SCROTAL SKIN DISEASES: CHEMICAL AND INFECTIOUS

Many skin diseases of infectious, allergic, or metabolic origin can involve the scrotum. Among many yeasts, molds, and fungi, only a few are infectious and are termed *dermatophytes* ("skin fungi"). Skin fungi live only on the dead layer of keratin protein on the skin surface. They rarely invade deeper and cannot live on mucous membranes. Infections by the fungus tinea cruris (ringworm) are very common in the groin and scrotum. It involves desquamation of the scrotal skin and contiguous surfaces of the inner thighs and itches ("jock itch"). Tinea begins with fused, superficial, reddish-brown, well-defined scaly patches that extend and coalesce into large, symmetric, inflamed areas. The margins of the lesions are characteristically distinct. The initial lesion may become macerated and infected and is painful and itches. Sweating, tight clothing, or obesity favor development and recurrence of this fungal infection, derived mainly from the genera *Trichophyton* and *Microsporum*. These same organisms cause tinea pedis or "athlete's foot."

Contact dermatitis (dermatitis venenata) is a localized rash or irritation of the skin caused by contact with a foreign substance. Only the superficial regions of the skin are affected, including the epidermis and the outer dermis. Unlike contact urticaria, in which a rash appears within minutes of exposure and fades away within minutes to hours, contact dermatitis takes days to fade away. The most common causes of allergic contact dermatitis are poison ivy, poison oak, and poison sumac. Common causes of irritant contact dermatitis are highly alkaline soaps, detergents, and cleaning products. Contact dermatitis of the scrotum may show a variety of lesions varying from erythema, to papules, to vesicles or pustules, but is always accompanied by itching. The scrotal skin is usually swollen, occasionally edematous, painful, and red. Treatment is directed toward discovery and elimination of the specific cause. Drug eruption is a form of contact dermatitis that may occur on the scrotum and elsewhere on the body after consumption of drugs to which the patient is allergic.

Allergic eczema or atopic dermatitis often occurs together with other atopic diseases like hay fever, asthma, and conjunctivitis. It is a familial and chronic disease and can appear or disappear over time. Atopic dermatitis can often be confused with psoriasis. It usually begins with superficial excoriation, localized edema, and exudation, after which the lesion progresses to dry, thickened skin with scale formation and a brownish hue. Marked pruritus or itching and pustule formation are characteristic. The underlying cause remains obscure. Herpes simplex virus 2 (see Plate 2.21) is a form of genital herpes located on the genitals that is more commonly observed on the penis than the scrotum.

Intertrigo or thrush is an erythematous, inflammatory condition occurring where contiguous skin surfaces are moist and warm. It is caused by the yeast *Candida albicans* that is normally found on the skin. It is usually symmetric on the scrotum and inner surfaces of the thighs, with frequent involvement of the penis and buttocks. Abrasions may lead to fissures and maceration, with the skin becoming secondarily infected with bacteria. If the diagnosis is in doubt, a KOH test can be performed to detect the candidal yeast. A bacterial culture can help

diagnose a secondary bacterial infection. Intertrigo is treated with antifungal creams such as clotrimazole and miconazole. Equally important is to keep the skin folds as dry as possible.

Other rare skin lesions (not illustrated) with a predilection for the scrotum are prurigo, which is a general term for itchy eruptions of the scrotal skin, and lichen planus, an inflammatory skin rash that forms scaly rings and plaques on the genitalia that are characteristically

violaceous, or purple colored. Erythrasma of the genital region, a chronic infection by the bacteria *Corynebacterium minutissimum*, appears as a brown, scaly, finely demarcated eruption that produces no symptoms. Tinea versicolor, caused by the fungus *Pityrosporum ovale*, is relatively common in adolescent and young adult males. It appears as enlarging brown macules without inflammation or other symptoms and is treated with typical antifungal creams.

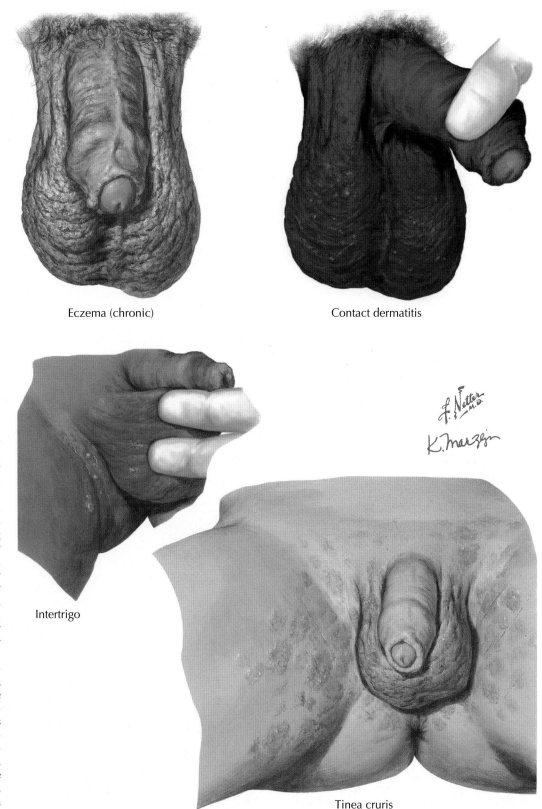

Eczema (chronic)

Contact dermatitis

Intertrigo

Tinea cruris

Plate 3.7

Reproductive System: VOLUME 1

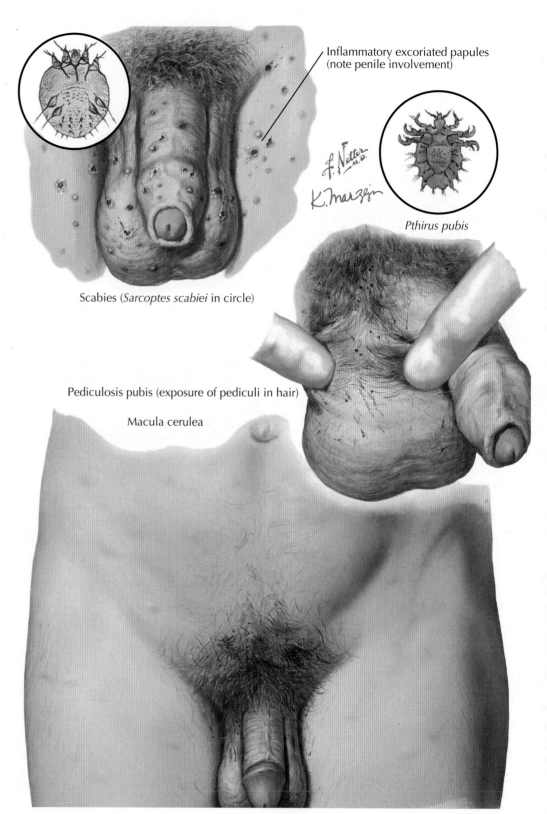

Inflammatory excoriated papules (note penile involvement)

Pthirus pubis

Scabies (*Sarcoptes scabiei* in circle)

Pediculosis pubis (exposure of pediculi in hair)

Macula cerulea

SCROTAL SKIN DISEASES: SCABIES AND LICE

Scabies is a contagious, parasitic skin disorder caused by the mite *Sarcoptes scabiei*. Mites are small, eight-legged parasites (in contrast to six-legged insects), 0.33 mm long, that burrow into the skin and that are especially active at night, producing intense nocturnal itching. Furrows are readily visible on the scrotum, and a tiny burrow can be detected at the point where the skin has been invaded. The furrows vary in length and coloration and are usually curved or arciform, resembling a small beaded or dotted thread. At the distal, closed end of the tortuous channel, a small vesicle develops where the mite is lodged. Scraping the vesicle usually produces the mite and eggs that can be visualized in 10% NaOH solution. The vesicles quickly transform into papules, pustules, incrustations, and excoriations that obscure the burrows. Once secondary excoriation and pustules develop, the original skin lesions are more difficult to recognize. In children, scabies is frequently complicated by impetigo of the buttocks. Skin-to-skin contact is the most common mode of spread, and human scabies is not obtained from animal contact. Scabies is curable with permethrin, crotamiton, or lindane creams.

Pediculosis pubis is a result of infestation by the crab louse *(Pthirus pubis)*. This ectoparasite feeds exclusively on blood and has an oral appendage that produces a skin lesion by suction. Unlike the body louse that lives in clothing, the crab louse resides on hairy body parts: in the genitalia, this louse attaches to pubic hair with its head buried in the hair follicle. Usually acquired during sexual contact, these lice rarely produce large skin lesions, and most commonly cause scratching. Because these organisms are most often spread through close or intimate contact, pediculosis is classified as a sexually transmitted disease (STD) that is not prevented with condom use. The skin may reveal a "bitten" appearance, showing small red points that may develop into papules. Scratching leads to excoriation, bleeding, and incrustation and a brownish discoloration of the skin. In addition, blue spots or macula cerulea up to 0.5 cm in diameter can occur on the skin as a result of the bite of the louse and is likely a consequence of a reaction between the louse saliva and the host blood. These blue spots do not disappear under pressure and are characteristic of pediculosis.

A careful search among the pubic hairs for nits, nymphs, and adults should be made in cases of pruritus. Lice and nits can be removed either with forceps or by cutting the infested hair with scissors and then examined with a microscope. Crab lice are also treated and killed with permethrin or lindane creams. A second treatment is recommended 10 days after the first. It is also crucial that all bed linens be changed and put into well-sealed plastic bags for 2 weeks before washing to destroy the lice eggs that may be a source of reinfestation.

Plate 3.8

Scrotum and Testis

Avulsion, Edema, Hematoma

Traumatic avulsion of the scrotum and penis is seen with animal attacks, motor vehicle accidents, assaults with sharp or high-velocity missiles, self-mutilation, and machinery-related (i.e., industrial, agricultural) accidents. It is most commonly observed in males aged 10 to 30 years. The entire scrotal tissue may be lost and complete sloughing of remaining skin may occur due to infection. Partial loss of the scrotum is managed by debridement, excision of islands of remnant full-thickness scrotal wall, and primary closure with absorbable sutures. If the complete scrotal skin has been avulsed, it may be necessary to transplant the uninjured testes into the subcutaneous tissues of the upper thigh or within the inguinal region. The ability of small fragments of remaining skin to regenerate a full-sized scrotum is remarkable, and transplantation of the testes can be avoided if some skin remains. The vascularity, compliance, and elasticity of the dartos layer allow scrotal flaps to cover substantial areas of loss. Clean granulation tissue usually coats the surface of the exposed testicles, followed by regeneration of the scrotum.

Complete scrotal loss requires skin grafting to expedite healing. Split-thickness grafting (0.20–0.36 mm) that is meshed to allow fluid to drain is ideal for scrotal coverage because it does not result in hair growth. With the penis, split-thickness skin grafts are needed for the denuded area, as the penile skin must be pliable to allow for erections. Healing by regeneration of skin from a nearby avulsed margin would result in a relatively inelastic covering. Testicles should be fixed together in a dependent position to minimize motion and maximize graft "take." The use of "thigh pouches" for the testes may be necessary with infected wounds until they are clean enough for grafting. Long-term success with skin grafting for scrotal injury is excellent. Only 20% of patients require significant revisions, and most of these can be managed in the office. Acute trauma without infection can be managed simply with wet-to-dry dressings until definitive graft placement.

Edema of the scrotum results from either localized or generalized pathology. The loose and elastic structure of the scrotum facilitates edema from even the slightest inflammatory reaction or vascular or lymphatic disturbance. Epididymo-orchitis is frequently accompanied by scrotal edema, as are allergic states or obstruction of the lymphatic or vascular system. Marked edema or anasarca that involves the scrotum can result from chronic cardiac insufficiency, liver cirrhosis, ascites, and renal failure. Malignancy affecting retroperitoneal and inguinal lymph nodes may, by obstructing the lymphatics, result in a nonpitting edema of the scrotum. Simple edema may also be the first sign of elephantiasis (lymphatic filariasis) and other tropical diseases. Trauma or surgery to the scrotum is usually followed by a considerable amount of edema. Notable edema may also result from spider bites or allergies (angioneurotic edema). When the edema is massive, the dependent portion of the scrotal skin may become moist, denude, and form ulcers. Patients with scrotal edema should elevate the scrotum to accelerate venous and lymphatic drainage.

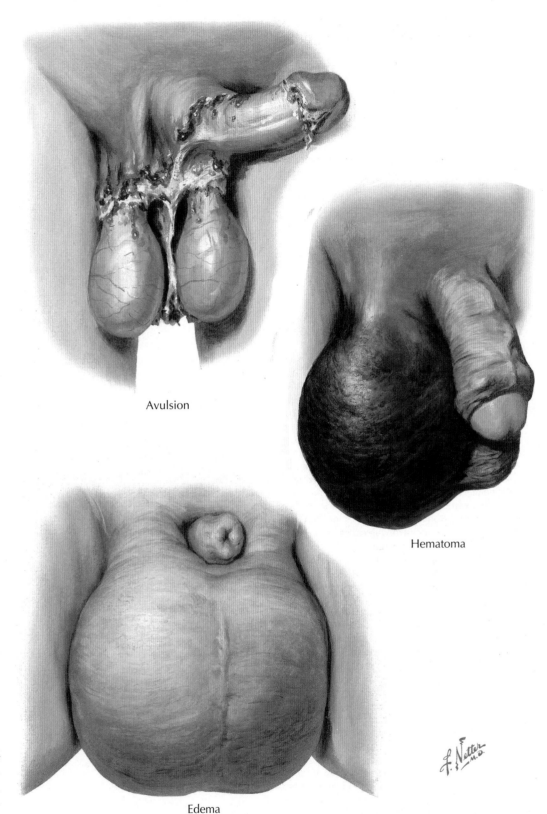

Avulsion

Hematoma

Edema

Scrotal hematoma or diffusion of blood through the subcutaneous scrotal tissue is most commonly observed after scrotal surgery or blunt trauma. The scrotum is an uncommon location for idiopathic bleeding, as its contracting smooth muscle layers efficiently compress blood vessels. With an acute bleed, the scrotum becomes dark and assumes a purple color. Over time, the coloration changes to yellow and then to normal color. However, it may take several weeks for blood pigments to be resorbed and for normal skin color to be completely restored. Hematoma is usually accompanied by variable degrees of edema and should be treated with moderate compression, suspension, and the application of ice or cold packs as early as possible. If bleeding is brisk, it may extend upward into the inguinal area and frequently over the penis under the continuity of the dartos and Scarpa and Colles fasciae (see Plate 2.20).

Plate 3.9

Reproductive System: VOLUME 1

HYDROCELE, SPERMATOCELE

A hydrocele is an accumulation of serous fluid greater in amount than that normally present between the parietal and visceral testis tunica vaginalis layers. As the testis descends (see Plate 3.5) from the retroperitoneum to the scrotum, it carries with it two layers of peritoneum. Abnormalities of these coverings and of the processus vaginalis communicating with the peritoneal cavity may lead to several kinds of hydrocele. The most common type is simple hydrocele, in which the normally formed tunica vaginalis is distended with fluid. In infantile hydrocele, the fingerlike processus vaginalis fails to close and extends upward to the upper scrotum or inguinal canal but does not communicate with the peritoneal cavity. In congenital or communicating hydrocele, with or without hernia, a lumen in the processus vaginalis permits communication with the abdominal cavity, so that bowel and peritoneal fluid may extend to the scrotum and hydrocele fluid may reach the peritoneal cavity. Congenital hydrocele may or may not be associated with descent of the bowel and inguinal hernia.

Hydrocele of the cord occurs as a localized collection of fluid in an encysted sac of peritoneum within the spermatic cord. It does not communicate with either the tunica vaginalis space below or the peritoneum above. Hernial hydrocele (not illustrated) is an accumulation of fluid within the tunica vaginalis as a result of a limited projection of the processus vaginalis from the peritoneal cavity inferiorly into the scrotum. However, the hernia pouch terminates before reaching the tunica vaginalis and does not communicate with it. Usually, neither bowel nor omentum is present in the sac, and the hydrocele fluid in the sac can be pressed back into the peritoneum. Rare types of localized hydroceles can also occur, involving either a portion of the epididymis or the testis.

Acute hydrocele is usually secondary to trauma, tumors, or underlying infection of the testicle or epididymis. Chronic hydrocele may be the end result of the acute form, but in many cases no history of an acute phase exists, nor are underlying diseases found, in which case it is termed *idiopathic* hydrocele. Hydroceles can follow trauma and occur after inguinal herniorrhaphy, varicocele ligation, or other retroperitoneal surgery that blocks lymphatic flow through the spermatic cord.

Hydrocele fluid is generally straw-colored and odorless and resembles serum. In acute cases, the fluid may be fibrinous, bloody, or even purulent. The parietal layer of the tunica vaginalis is usually thin, but it may become thickened and even calcified in chronic cases. Hydroceles are generally situated anterior to the testicle, which it displaces posteriorly in the scrotal cavity. Hydroceles should be differentiated from hernia, testicle tumors, hematocele, and spermatocele. Transillumination of the scrotum should reveal a "glowing" fluid sac with hydrocele. Aspiration of the hydrocele fluid for cytologic or chemical assessment should only be performed when coexistence of hernia has been excluded. The treatment is watchful waiting, repeated needle aspirations (as the fluid recurs quickly), or operative excision of the parietal tunica vaginalis. Aspiration followed by injection of sclerosing solutions is not as effective as tunica vaginalis excision. In long-standing hydroceles in which the tunica has become thick, some degree of testicular atrophy may result from chronic pressure.

A spermatocele is an intrascrotal cystic mass resulting from partial obstruction or diverticula of the efferent ductule system near the caput epididymis (see Plate 3.3).

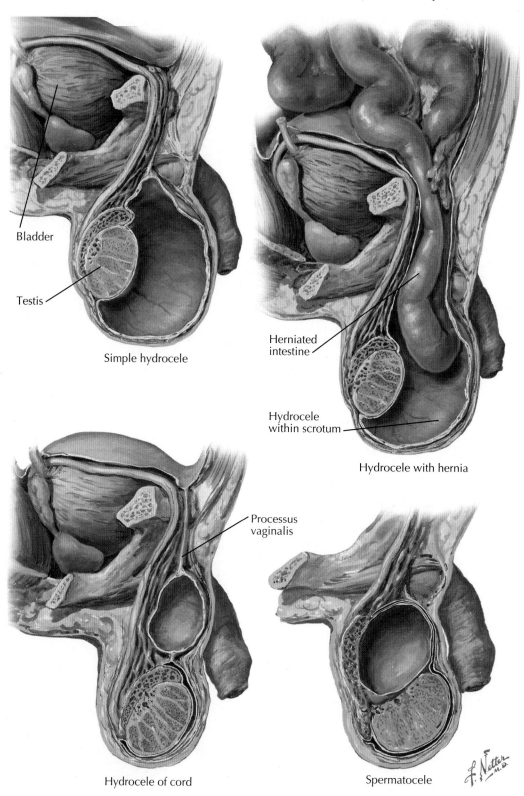

Bladder

Testis

Simple hydrocele

Herniated intestine

Hydrocele within scrotum

Hydrocele with hernia

Processus vaginalis

Hydrocele of cord

Spermatocele

When small, they can be confused with epididymal cysts (which generally remain small) and appendices of the testis and epididymis, but these latter structures do not contain sperm, unlike spermatoceles. The cyst is lined by pseudostratified epithelium and contains turbid, milky fluid, with immotile sperm and lipid granules. On palpation, spermatoceles appear as a round mass distinct from the testis, with a narrower "waist" between the testis and the cyst attached to it. Spermatoceles are located within the tunica vaginalis space, but an extravaginal variety can occur that lies posterior to the testis.

Spermatocele and hydrocele can occur concomitantly, in which case the former remains unrecognized unless the fluid is observed on aspiration. Most spermatoceles are asymptomatic, except for a slight dragging sensation in the scrotum due to a "mass effect." Spermatoceles tend to become symptomatic when they enlarge to the size of a normal 20-mL testis. Excision is the treatment of choice and should be only judiciously considered in reproductive-age males, as scarring in the epididymal bed of the excised lesion could obstruct the remaining efferent ducts and lead to duct obstruction and infertility.

Plate 3.10

Scrotum and Testis

VARICOCELE, HEMATOCELE, TORSION

Varicocele is defined as abnormal dilation and tortuosity of the pampiniform plexus of veins in the spermatic cord. Most varicoceles (90%) occur on the left side. The left internal spermatic vein terminates in the left renal vein at right angles, an insertion without a natural valve (see Plate 3.2). In contrast, the right internal spermatic vein enters the vena cava obliquely below the right renal vein. With varicocele, the blood flow in the internal spermatic veins is reversed, causing warm, corporeal blood to pool around the normally cooler testis. Varicoceles occur in about 15% of young males. The occurrence of an isolated right varicocele, or the sudden onset of a left varicocele after the age of 30 years, may indicate retroperitoneal disease, such as tumor, lymphadenopathy, hydronephrosis, or aberrant vessels. Most varicoceles develop as a consequence of the pubertal growth spurt. When symptomatic, they cause a pulling, dragging, or dull "congestive" discomfort in the testis and scrotum, a pain that promptly disappears in the supine position. Varicoceles are also the most common correctable cause of male factor infertility. The differential diagnosis on presentation includes epididymitis and inguinal hernia. Operative treatment is indicated (1) for ipsilateral orchalgia, (2) for male factor infertility in the presence of at least 1 year of adequate female fertility potential, and (3) when there is evidence of ipsilateral testicular atrophy in an adolescent.

Varicocele treatment consists of surgical ligation of the internal spermatic veins at the retroperitoneal (Palomo and modified Palomo procedure), inguinal (Ivanissevitch procedure), or subinguinal microscopic (Marmar procedure) approaches. In addition, laparoscopic ligation and radiographic embolization can also be attempted at the retroperitoneal level. The recurrence rate for ligation at the retroperitoneal level is approximately threefold higher than that for procedures at the inguinal or subinguinal level.

Hematocele is hemorrhage into the tunica vaginalis space, usually as a result of traumatic or surgical injury or testis tumor. Spontaneous hematocele is a known complication of arteriosclerosis, scurvy, diabetes, syphilis, neoplasia, and inflammatory conditions of the testis, epididymis, or tunica vaginalis. Hematocele may occur from birth injury and may also develop in various blood dyscrasias. After injury, hematocele is accompanied by scrotal edema, as the hematoma permeates the skin and subcutaneous tissues, lending the scrotal and penile skin a black appearance. A slowly developing hematocele may be indistinguishable from hydrocele except by its opacity to transillumination. Aspiration of bloody, rather than clear, fluid leads to a definitive diagnosis. If the diagnosis and etiology of hematocele are in doubt, surgical exploration is warranted to determine the underlying condition.

Axial rotation or torsion of the spermatic cord results in infarction and gangrene of the testicle. A 720-degree rotation is required for most cases of clinical torsion. Torsion occurs with equal frequency on either testis side, and also in the setting of cryptorchidism. The

main predisposing factor is abnormal mobility of the testis, usually due to a high insertion of the tunica on the spermatic cord, also termed the "bell clapper" deformity. The extent of the damage to the testicle depends on the degree and duration of the torsion. If uncorrected torsion persists for longer than 8 hours, complete testis infarction is likely. The success of surgical detorsion procedures is directly related to the duration of torsion. Although manual detorsion using palpation alone is possible, torsion is normally treated

by open surgery, at which time the testis is either removed if unviable or fixed to the scrotal wall or septum to preclude recurrence. At surgery, the contralateral, untorsed testicle also undergoes orchidopexy.

Torsion of the vestigial appendix testis or the appendix epididymis may also cause acute scrotal pain that must be differentiated from acute epididymitis and true testis torsion. Occurring most commonly in young boys, it can present with a "blue dot" sign as the necrotic appendix is viewed through the scrotal skin.

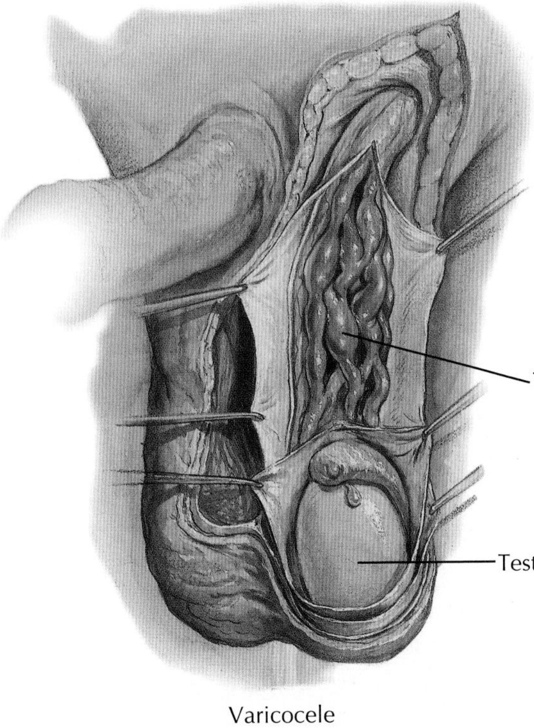

Varicocele

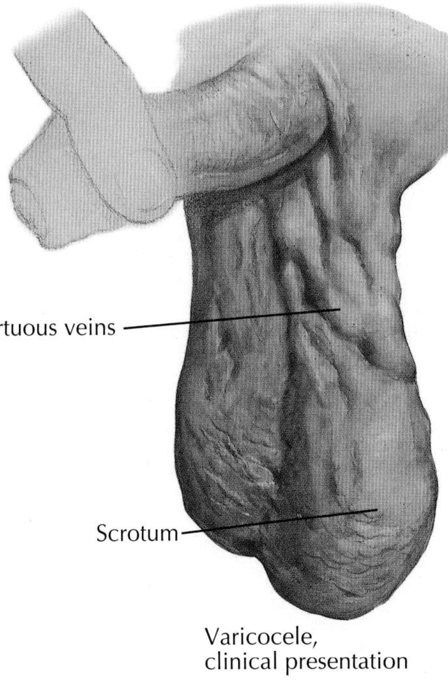

Tortuous veins

Testis

Varicocele, clinical presentation

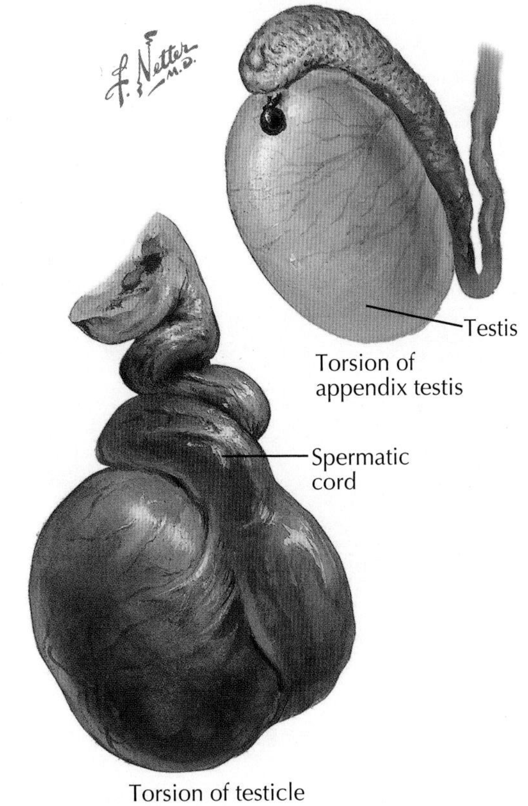

Tortuous veins

Scrotum

Torsion of appendix testis

Testis

Spermatic cord

Torsion of testicle

Hemorrhage in tunica vaginalis

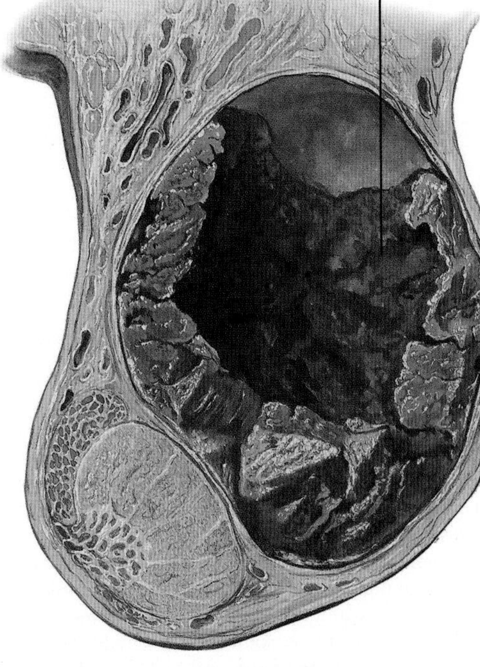

Hematocele

Plate 3.11

Reproductive System: VOLUME 1

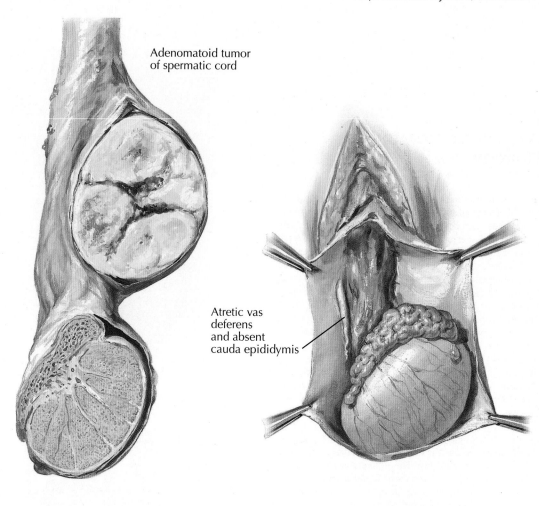

Adenomatoid tumor
of spermatic cord

Atretic vas
deferens
and absent
cauda epididymis

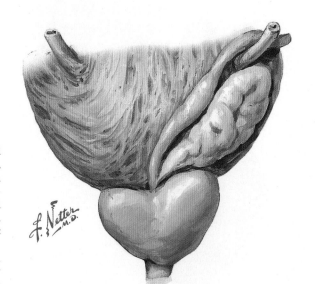

Absence of entire left seminal tract

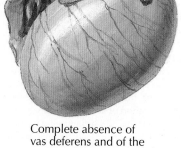

Complete absence of
vas deferens and of the
cauda and corpus epididymis

ANOMALIES OF THE SPERMATIC CORD

Tumors of the paratesticular tissues and spermatic cord are rare and can occur in all age groups. More often, paratesticular tissues are involved by extension from primary germ cell testis tumors. Benign tumors are observed in two of three cases and are usually mesodermal in origin and include adenomatoid tumors, lipomas, fibromas, occasionally myomas from the cremasteric muscle, hemangiomas, neurofibromas, and lymphangiomas. Adenomatoid tumors are the most common benign tumors, accounting for 30% of all paratesticular tumors. They present as solid, asymptomatic masses found on routine examination and are located in the epididymis, testis tunic, or, rarely, the spermatic cord. On sectioning, they appear uniformly white, yellow, or tan and exhibit a fibrous consistency. Histologically, epithelial cells with vacuoles and uniformly sized, round nuclei are observed. Occasionally, adenomatoid tumors are misclassified as mesotheliomas. *Dermoid cysts,* the term given to cysts lined by squamous epithelium, are also rare causes of scrotal masses. Mesotheliomas of the testis adnexa usually present as firm, painless scrotal masses in association with an enlarging hydrocele (see Plate 3.9) in older individuals. Grossly, they are poorly demarcated lesions with firm, shaggy, and friable areas

throughout. Microscopic examination reveals complex papillary structures and dense fibroconnective tissue containing scattered calcifications.

Malignant paratesticular tumors are also rare and include, in decreasing frequency, rhabdomyosarcoma (40%), leiomyosarcoma, fibrosarcoma, liposarcoma, and undifferentiated tumors. Patients generally present with a growing scrotal mass that is solid and nontransilluminating on palpation. These tumors must be differentiated from spermatic cord cysts, hydroceles, spermatoceles,

varicoceles (see Plate 3.10), and hernias. Most malignant tumors occur at the distal end of the cord near the scrotum, whereas benign tumors are more often encountered proximally toward the inguinal canal. Primary malignant tumors of the epididymis are exceedingly rare and mandate an evaluation for metastatic adenocarcinoma. The treatment of benign lesions is simple excision, whereas high inguinal orchiectomy, followed by radiotherapy and chemotherapy, is standard treatment for malignant lesions.

Plate 3.12

Scrotum and Testis

INFECTION, GANGRENE

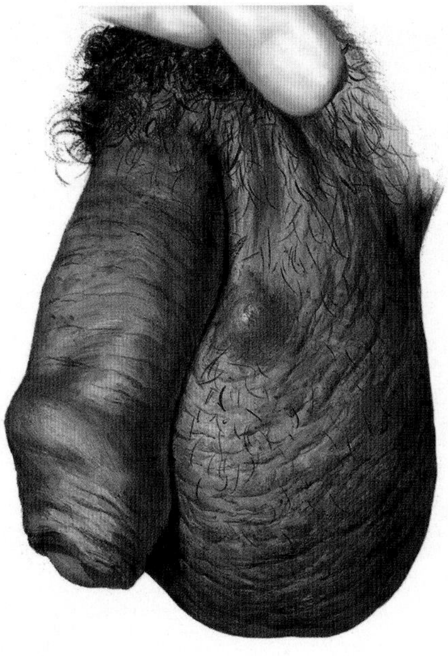

The scrotum is subject to infections, similar to skin elsewhere in the body. However, several anatomic issues predispose the scrotal skin to infection. Reduced ventilation and lack of sweat evaporation cause the scrotal skin to be moist. In addition, the proximity of the scrotum to the urethra and rectum can affect the bacterial type and load. Physical contact with the thighs favors skin maceration that can delay the healing process. Finally, the loose, fat-free, and contractile scrotal wall reacts to infection with considerable edema (see Plate 3.8), which can interfere with vascularity and prolong healing.

Primary abscess of the scrotal wall is rare. Abscesses secondary to underlying urethral, testicular, epididymal, perineal, or rectal pathology are more common. Scrotal boils or furuncles can occur from infection of hair follicles or sweat glands due to bacteria such as *Staphylococcus aureus*. They usually require incision and drainage along with antibiotics and are prone to recur if the sebaceous cyst is not entirely excised.

Scrotal erysipelas (Greek for "red skin") is a diffuse infection of the scrotal dermis and subcutaneous tissue. It is most commonly due to *Streptococcus pyogenes* (also known as *β-hemolytic group A streptococci*), although non–group A streptococci are also implicated. Erysipelas infections enter the skin through minor trauma, eczema, surgical incisions, abscesses, fistulae, and ulcers. People with immune deficiency, diabetes, alcoholism, skin ulceration, fungal infections, and impaired lymphatic drainage are at increased risk for this infection. Erysipelas is diagnosed by the appearance of well-demarcated rash and inflammation. Blood cultures are unreliable. It should be differentiated from herpes zoster and angioedema and be distinguished from cellulitis by its raised advancing edges and sharp borders. Erysipelas in the lower abdomen or adjacent skin areas may progress to the scrotum and can gradually invade the entire scrotum, with soft, loose tissues becoming markedly swollen, tense, smooth, and warm. Many blebs or vesicles form on the surface, and in some instances the infection is so intense that the scrotal skin becomes gangrenous. It is treated with penicillin, clindamycin, or erythromycin antibiotics.

Scrotal gangrene or necrotizing fasciitis of the scrotum is uncommon but lethal. It can occur after extravasation of infected urine into subcutaneous tissues secondary to urethral stricture (see Plate 2.20) or seeding from stool due to rectal fistula or fissure. It may also occur after mechanical, chemical, or thermal injury to the scrotum and is particularly prone to occur in individuals with underlying systemic immune disturbances, diabetes, or alcoholism. Scrotal gangrene has also been encountered as a complication of rare conditions such as embolism of the hypogastric arteries, *Entamoeba histolytica* infestation, and rickettsial diseases when accompanied by thrombosis of small blood vessels. Spread of the infection is usually limited by scrotal and pelvic fascial planes (see Plate 2.20).

Fulminating, spontaneous, or idiopathic gangrene (Fournier gangrene) of the scrotum is known for its dramatic, sudden onset. A combination of aerobic and anaerobic bacteria and fungi facilitate the rapid course of this infection. Staphylococcal bacteria clot the blood, depriving surrounding tissue of oxygen. Within this oxygen-depleted environment, anaerobic bacteria thrive and produce enzymes that digest tissue and further spread the infection. Males are 10 times more likely than females to develop Fournier gangrene, and those aged 60 to 80 years with a predisposing

condition are most susceptible. Alcoholism, diabetes mellitus, leukemia, morbid obesity, immune system disorders such as HIV and Crohn's disease, and intravenous drug users are at increased risk for developing gangrene. The condition also can develop as a complication of surgery.

With gangrenous infection, the scrotum becomes abruptly painful and reddened, usually limited to the demarcation of the scrotum. It may spread quickly under Scarpa fascia to the abdomen and even to the axilla, often

within hours. It can be differentiated from erysipelas, which begins in a localized area and spreads with a red, raised margin. Gangrene is typically accompanied by a "spongy" or "cracking" feel to the tissues in the scrotum, groin, and perineum on examination, which represents tissue crepitus from emphysema due to gas-producing anaerobic organisms. Treatment is emergent and involves making multiple incisions and wide debridement of affected tissues, irrigation with antibiotic solution, systemic broad-spectrum antibiotics, and fluid support.

Furuncle

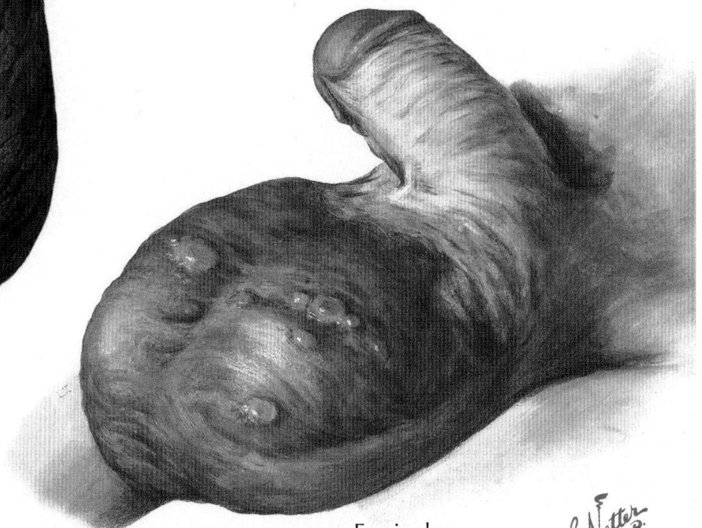

Erysipelas

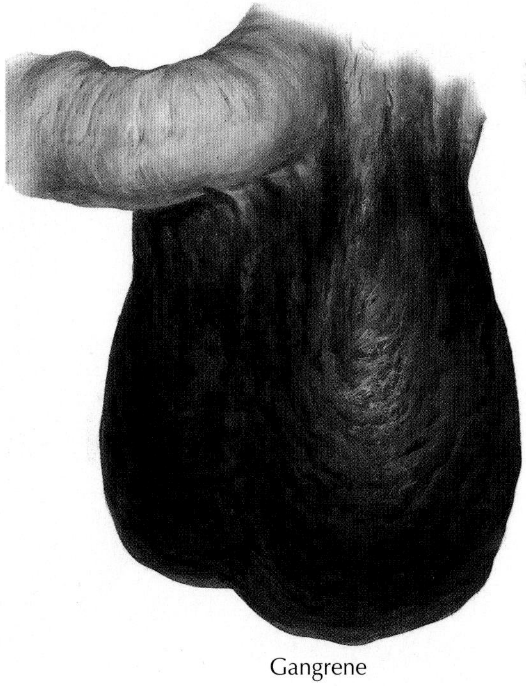

Gangrene

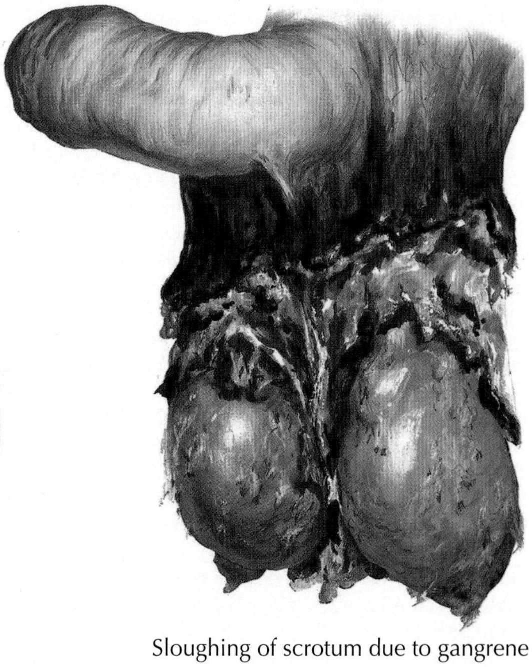

Sloughing of scrotum due to gangrene

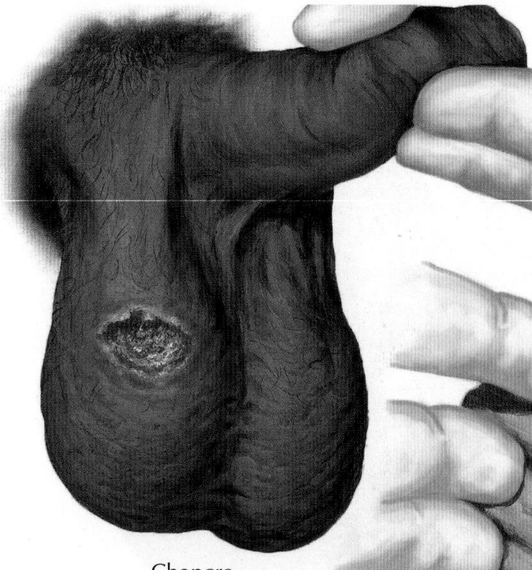

Plate 3.13

Reproductive System: VOLUME 1

Chancre

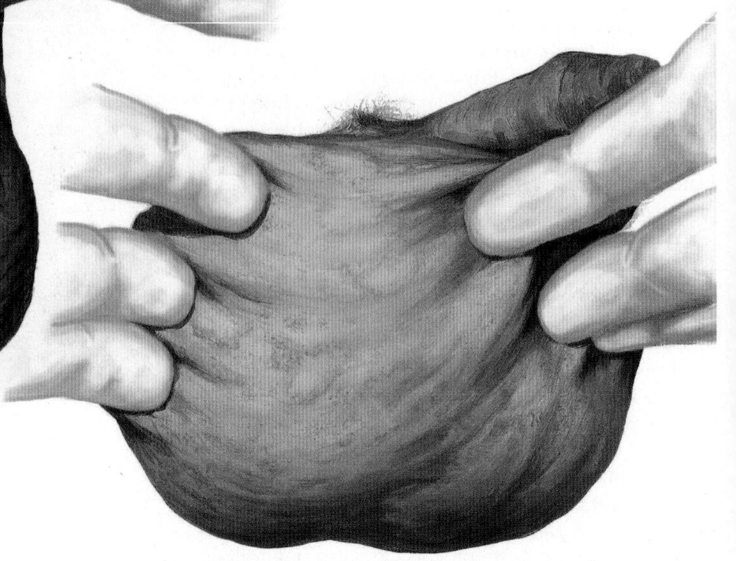

Very faint secondary lesions demonstrated by putting scrotal skin on stretch

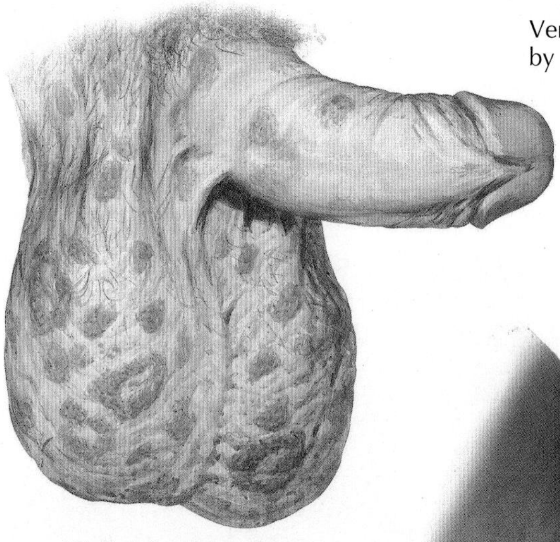

Well-defined annular and maculopapular syphilis (secondary)

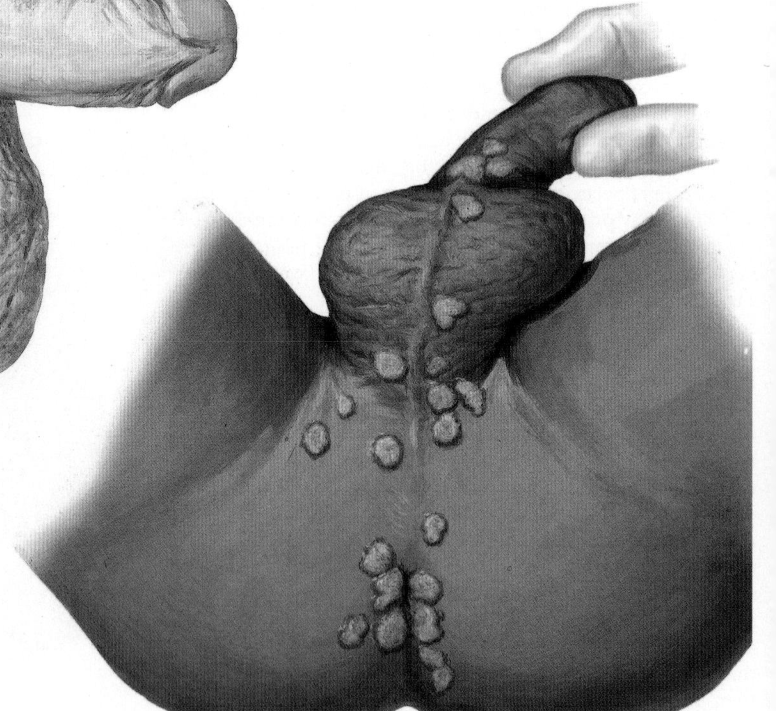

Condylomata lata

Syphilis

The scrotal skin is not an uncommon site for a primary syphilitic lesion. Syphilis infections reached an all-time low incidence in 2000, but have increased fourfold since. The primary stage of syphilis is marked by the appearance of a single sore (chancre), approximately 21 days after exposure. The chancre is usually firm, round, small, and painless, lasts 3 to 6 weeks, and heals without treatment. Regardless of location, the syphilitic chancre is grossly the same (see Plate 2.23). It may occur at the penoscrotal junction with barrier contraceptives. Lesions of the scrotum, however, are much more common in later forms of syphilis, especially during early and late relapses. They appear during relapse within the first 2 years but have been observed many years later as well. Anogenital cutaneous relapse occurs in 40% of untreated cases and scrotal lesions occur in 25% of relapsing cases.

In secondary syphilis, scrotal lesions may occur with a generalized cutaneous, nonpruritic rash and mucous membrane manifestation. This stage usually appears several weeks after the chancre has healed. Secondary syphilis may also mimic many other cutaneous diseases, but the generalized rash characteristically appears on the palms and on the undersides of the feet. On the scrotum, this rash may resemble tinea cruris, lichen planus (see Plate 3.6), or can appear as papules similar to urticaria pigmentosa. Follicular, nodular, and pustular lesions are relatively rarely observed on the scrotum, as secondary syphilitic rashes are more often papular or annular in character. The moist papule is the most common syphilitic lesion found on the scrotum. Annular recurrences are also observed in untreated and insufficiently treated patients. Annular lesions are actually moist papules with raised circular ridges that are elevated about 0.5 mm from the surrounding skin and may be covered by a light scale that exudes serum. Later the papillae appear as glistening or translucent elevated rings where the skin is stretched. The lesions can be hidden within the scrotal skin folds. If the scrotum is stretched, annular and papular lesions become obvious. Annular lesions may also occur in the tertiary stage. In addition to rashes, symptoms of secondary syphilis may include fever, swollen lymph glands, sore throat, patchy hair loss, headaches, weight loss, muscle aches, and fatigue. These symptoms will resolve without treatment but will progress to the latent and possibly late stages of disease. The annular and papular forms of cutaneous secondary syphilis are often misdiagnosed. Papular lesions sometimes develop into flat condylomata lata, with an eroded surface caused by nonspecific hypertrophy of the epidermis. They can be associated with condyloma acuminata near the rectum and can be found in similar individuals at risk for STDs. However, it is important to differentiate these two lesions: condyloma

acuminata are dry, cauliflower-like, and bulky, whereas condyloma lata are smooth, moist, and flat. It should be emphasized that scrotal lesions, even in relapsing syphilis, are infectious.

The latent stage of syphilis begins when primary and secondary symptoms disappear, and this stage can last for years. The late stages of syphilis develop in about 15% of untreated patients and can appear 10 to 20 years after infection was acquired. In late-stage syphilis, signs and symptoms include difficulty coordinating muscle

movements, paralysis, numbness, gradual blindness, and dementia. Ulceration on the scrotum in tertiary syphilis may occur from gummas of the testis and epididymis, which may become adherent to the overlying skin. Such chronic, indolent, and painless ulcers should not be confused with tuberculous ulcers, sarcoma, or necrotic teratoma, which cause similar manifestations. Lymphedema and mild pseudoelephantiasis of the scrotum can result from obstruction of syphilitic inguinal lymph nodes.

Plate 3.14

ELEPHANTIASIS

Lymphatic filariasis, or elephantiasis, of the scrotum presents as diffuse scrotal enlargement from hypertrophy and hyperplasia of the subcutaneous tissues and epidermis, which become leathery, coarse, and dry. Sebaceous glands are usually destroyed. The consistency of the leathery skin is that of nonpitting edema. The scrotum varies in size from slight enlargement to becoming monstrous in size, with the scrotum touching the ground and weighing as much as 200 pounds. The condition is indigenous to tropical areas. Filarial elephantiasis is caused by a nematode, *Wuchereria bancrofti* (90%), and is transmitted to humans by certain mosquito species (*Culex, Aedes,* and *Anopheles*). Other threadlike parasitic worms such as *Brugia malayi* (10%) and *Brugia timori* (<1%) may also cause elephantiasis. The adult worms in males are found in lymphatic channels and in subcutaneous tissues; the larval forms usually enter the bloodstream between the hours of midnight and 2 AM. These microfilariae produce no general symptoms except those associated with obstruction of lymphatics. Scrotal elephantiasis is a late sequela of filarial infection and results from lymphatic obstruction. Secondary bacterial infections can accentuate the process. Usually, a history of repeated episodes of lymphangitis and lymphadenitis associated with fever, malaise, rash, and tender lymph nodes after inoculation is obtained. With each episode of diffuse enlargement and swelling, the regression and healing is less complete. Superficial lymphatics may become dilated, rupture, and exude lymph.

Filariasis may begin as an insidious condition known as *lymph scrotum,* which is characterized by a mild enlargement of the scrotum along with cutaneous lymphatic ectasia. Three other presentations have been described with filariasis. The first is somewhat similar to lymph scrotum but involves the spermatic cord, which feels like soft, compressible vessels. In another presentation, the spermatic cord contains thick, rubbery masses, which represent a late fibrous reaction after lymphangitis. In this presentation, fibrous nodules, distinct from the vas deferens, are palpated throughout the spermatic cord. The third type of presentation, called "mumu," was observed during World War II as acute swelling and edema of the spermatic cord that gradually subsides after individuals leave an endemic area. This may represent an allergic reaction that develops after filarial inoculation.

Although positive skin tests and DNA polymerase chain reactions can detect filarial DNA and indicate disease, the definitive diagnosis is made by finding the microfilariae in the peripheral blood at night after filtration through micropore membrane filters. This can also quantify the load of microfilariae. However, once lymphedema develops, the microfilariae are absent in peripheral blood. Specific drug therapy involves diethylcarbamazine (microfilaria and adult worms), ivermectin (microfilaria), albendazole (adult filarial worms), and

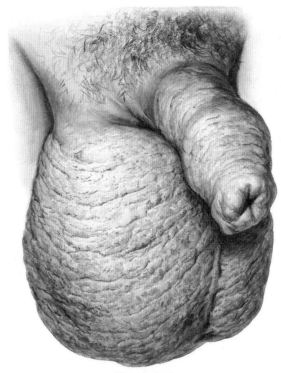

Nonfilarial elephantiasis

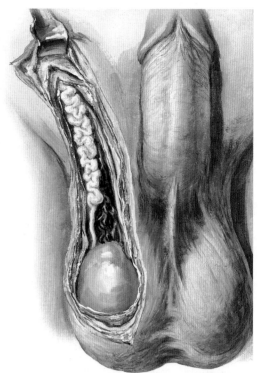

Asymptomatic lymphangiectasis

Male   Female

Wuchereria bancrofti (actual size)

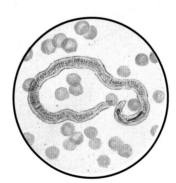

Wuchereria bancrofti (filaria) in blood

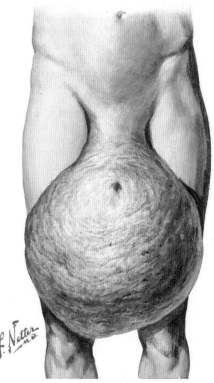

Giant filarial elephantiasis

possibly even doxycycline. Once lymphedema develops, there is no cure but reducing inflammation, and surgical removal of the elephantiasic genital tissue may help in selected cases.

Alternatively, elephantiasis may occur in the absence of parasitic infection. This nonparasitic form of elephantiasis is known as *nonfilarial elephantiasis* or *podoconiosis* and occurs in high frequency in northern Africa. Nonfilarial elephantiasis is thought to be caused by persistent

contact with irritant soils, or from lymphedema, lymph obstruction, or lymphangitis from a wide variety of causes, including infection. This elephantiasis may occur as a result of local disorders such as scrotal fistulae, or after inguinal lymphadenectomy, metastatic carcinoma, or inguinal lymphangitis from syphilis, lymphogranuloma venereum, tuberculosis, or granuloma inguinale. Treatment is aimed at eradication of infection and supportive care for the enlarged scrotum.

Plate 3.15

Reproductive System: VOLUME 1

CYSTS AND CANCER OF THE SCROTUM

Sebaceous cysts (epidermoid, epidermal cysts) of the scrotal wall are relatively common. Derived from sebaceous glands in the skin, cysts form either from overproduction of secretions or as a result of obstruction of the gland outlet. These cysts, usually scrotal, appear as smooth, round cystic tumors, varying in size from a few millimeters to, in rare instances, 8 to 12 cm. Although usually solitary or few in number, the occurrence of several hundred cysts has been described. The secretions contain cholesterol crystals and degenerated epithelial cells, and the fibrous cyst capsule is lined by stratified squamous epithelium with varying degrees of atrophy. Trichilemmal cysts (pilar cysts) are clinically indistinguishable from sebaceous cysts but contain keratinous rather than sebaceous material. Regarding the cyst type, inflammation is common in the obstructed duct and can lead to infection and pain. Sebaceous cysts are not precancerous but have been known to calcify. Definitive treatment is surgical excision, best performed after infection has been quelled with antibiotics. With excision, the entire epithelial sac that lines the cyst must be removed to avoid recurrence.

Angiokeratoma is a skin disorder characterized by the presence of multiple, small, punctate, violaceous (purple) lesions on the scrotal, and occasionally penile, skin. There can be hundreds of lesions present, but they are generally asymptomatic. They represent slightly elevated areas of venous ectasia and appear similar to punctate angiomas. As they are benign, treatment is usually unnecessary. However, if they bleed, local fulguration is effective.

Carcinoma of the scrotum is a rare cancer and for the most part an occupational disease confined to males exposed to petroleum and its products. It was the first cancer shown to be caused by an environmental carcinogen, and was named chimney-sweep's cancer in 1775 after its association with soot by Sir Percival Pott. It also occurs in males who are chronically exposed to tar, pitch, paraffin, shale, creosote, and crude wool. It has been observed in weavers who lean across machinery, and whose clothes become impregnated with oil, which then contacts the scrotum. It has also been described after x-ray therapy to the scrotum or after the chronic use of local treatments (psoralen and ultraviolet A) for scrotal psoriasis. An occasional case is observed without a history of occupational contact, and a recent rise in the incidence of scrotal cancers is thought to be associated with the HPV type 16 virus. The malignancy appears after two or three decades of exposure, usually between the ages of 45 and 70 years. The early lesion may be a small pimple or warty tumor that ulcerates, or the lesion may begin as an ulcer and develop into a large fungating mass.

Most carcinomas of the scrotum are squamous in type, but melanomas, basal cell carcinomas, and sarcomas have also been observed. Local remedies are usually applied without benefit before clinical presentation with pain. In about 50% of cases, metastases to inguinal lymph nodes are present when the patient is first seen. Metastatic spread occurs relatively quickly as the thin scrotal wall lacks natural barriers that tend to wall off neoplasia. Consistent with other squamous cancers, dissemination occurs chiefly by lymphatic rather than

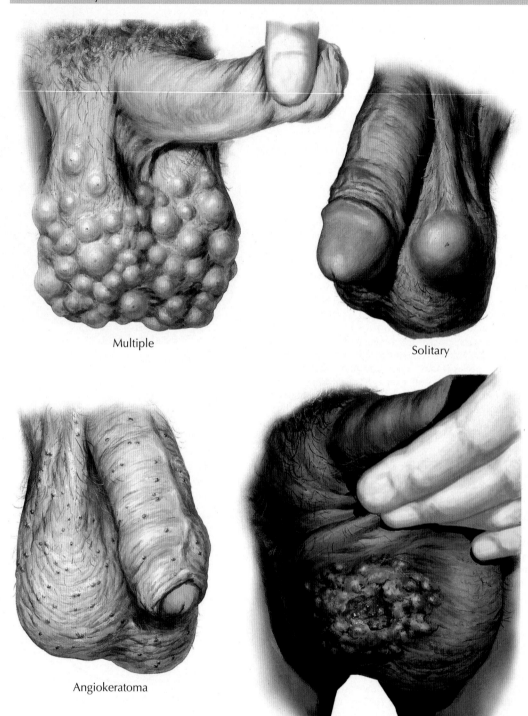

Sebaceous cysts

Multiple

Solitary

Angiokeratoma

Epithelioma (chimney sweep's or paraffin cancer)

hematogenous spread. If the malignancy has invaded the scrotal contents, metastases may spread directly to the periaortic nodes. Possibly due to its rarity or the nature of scrotal cancers, there is little relation between the duration of the cancer diagnosis, the grade of malignancy, and the prevalence of lymph node involvement. In very early, localized cases, a 75% cure rate is possible, with wide scrotal excision. Among those with lymph node involvement, 25% of patients are cured with bilateral inguinal and femoral lymphadenectomy.

Bilateral excision of draining lymph nodes is necessary, as the lymphatic channels in the scrotum are richly interconnected. The prognosis in metastatic cases is poor, and treatment can be quite morbid. Direct extension of tumor to deep femoral, external iliac, and hypogastric lymph nodes can occur, requiring dismemberment, lower limb removal, and hemipelvectomy. Chemotherapy and radiotherapy can be considered for downsizing tumors before resection but rarely result in cure when used as classic adjuvant therapy.

Plate 3.16

Scrotum and Testis

CRYPTORCHIDISM

Undescended testis (see also Plate 3.5) is the most common genital anomaly in males, observed in 2% to 4% of US boys at birth. Although most testis descent occurs prenatally, about 50% of undescended testes at birth subsequently descend during the first year of life. This condition may be an isolated birth defect (see Plate 3.5) due to failure of abdominal or inguinoscrotal testis descent, or it may be associated with conditions such as androgen insensitivity, Kallmann syndrome, spina bifida, Down syndrome, or endocrine disruption. Mechanical causes relate to adhesions, anatomic maldevelopments of the inguinal canal such as hernia uteri inguinalis, abnormalities of the inguinal ring, the mesorchium, the testis vascular supply, or gubernaculum. An actual congenital inguinal hernia is present in almost every case of true undescended testis, with the hernia sac below the testis in the scrotum. This leads to higher complications such as hydrocele formation and torsion in boys who are affected. Undescended testes are also at higher risk of malignant degeneration; this risk is related to the original location of the cryptorchid testis and is estimated to occur in 1 of 20 intraabdominal testes and 1 of 80 inguinal testes. Finally, it is also clear that both unilaterally and bilaterally cryptorchid males have higher rates of infertility (defined by paternity rates) compared with males with bilaterally descended testes.

In many prepubertal boys a condition termed "retractile testis" or pseudocryptorchidism can be confused with cryptorchidism. Unlike with true undescended testes, retractile testes can be pulled into the scrotum and will remain there for a finite period of time before drawing upward again. Retractile testes usually descend into normal position before or during puberty. It is controversial whether this condition harbors the same risks as truly cryptorchid testes in terms of infertility and malignant degeneration. In cases of obesity, the testes may be hidden under the mons pubic fat, and this can also be confused with cryptorchidism. A gentle examination, helped with moist heat, usually provides enough relaxation to permit manipulation of the testis into the scrotum. The cooling associated with undressing for an examination may prompt a cremaster reflex that elevates the scrotum superiorly. In as many as 25% of cases, the retractile testicle remains in the groin and is no longer movable. When this happens, the condition is called an *ascending testicle* or an *acquired undescended testicle* and is treated with orchidopexy.

The longer a testis remains undescended, the higher the risk of later malignant degeneration, testis hormonal failure, and infertility. In general, testes that undergo orchiopexy before puberty are less likely to become cancerous later in life compared with those that are repaired after puberty. Whether early orchiopexy reduces later infertility is unproven. Biopsies of cryptorchid testes at the time of postpubertal orchiopexy typically reveal tubular atrophy, germ cell aplasia (Sertoli cells only), and Leydig cell hyperplasia on histology. The time or critical age after which permanent damage occurs to the undescended testis is unknown. Degeneration within undescended testes is believed to begin as early as 5 to 6 years of age, and adults with childhood orchiopexy can show degenerating semen quality and progressive infertility with time. The optimum time for orchiopexy therapy is therefore unclear, but most clinicians recommend treatment before 1 year of age in a healthy infant.

Treatment for cryptorchidism includes watchful waiting, hormonal induction, or surgical repair. As a first-line treatment, clinicians may often try a short course of intramuscular human chorionic gonadotropin (hCG) to raise testosterone levels and encourage testis descent in inguinal cryptorchidism. hCG may be effective when cryptorchidism is due to hypopituitarism, but in most cases it likely stimulates descent of a testis that would otherwise normally descend. For definitive therapy, one- or two-stage orchiopexy procedures are performed to reduce the subsequent risk of torsion or inguinal hernia, to bring the at-risk testis into the scrotum for palpability of malignancy and for cosmesis.

Ectopic testis is a testis that descends but in a pathway that deviates from the usual scrotal end point. The most common landing sites for ectopic testes are (1) interstitial, on the oblique muscle; (2) pubopenile; (3) within the femoral triangle; and (4) perineal. Surgical replacement into the scrotum is indicated for proper testis function and to reduce pain or other complications.

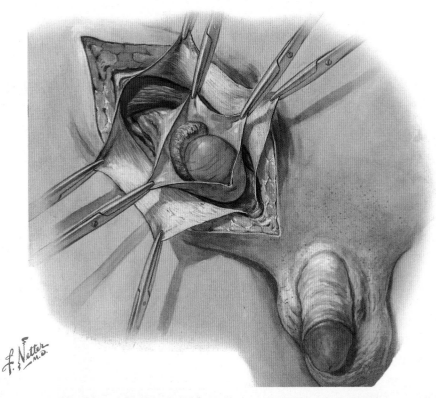

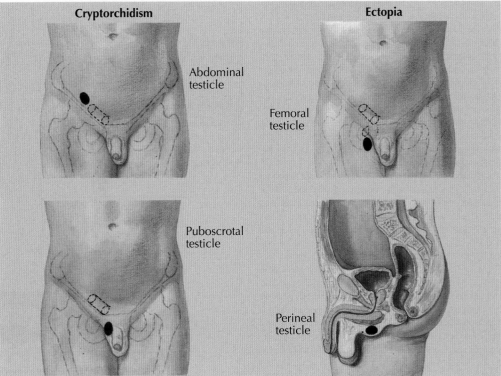

Cryptorchidism — Abdominal testicle, Puboscrotal testicle

Ectopia — Femoral testicle, Perineal testicle

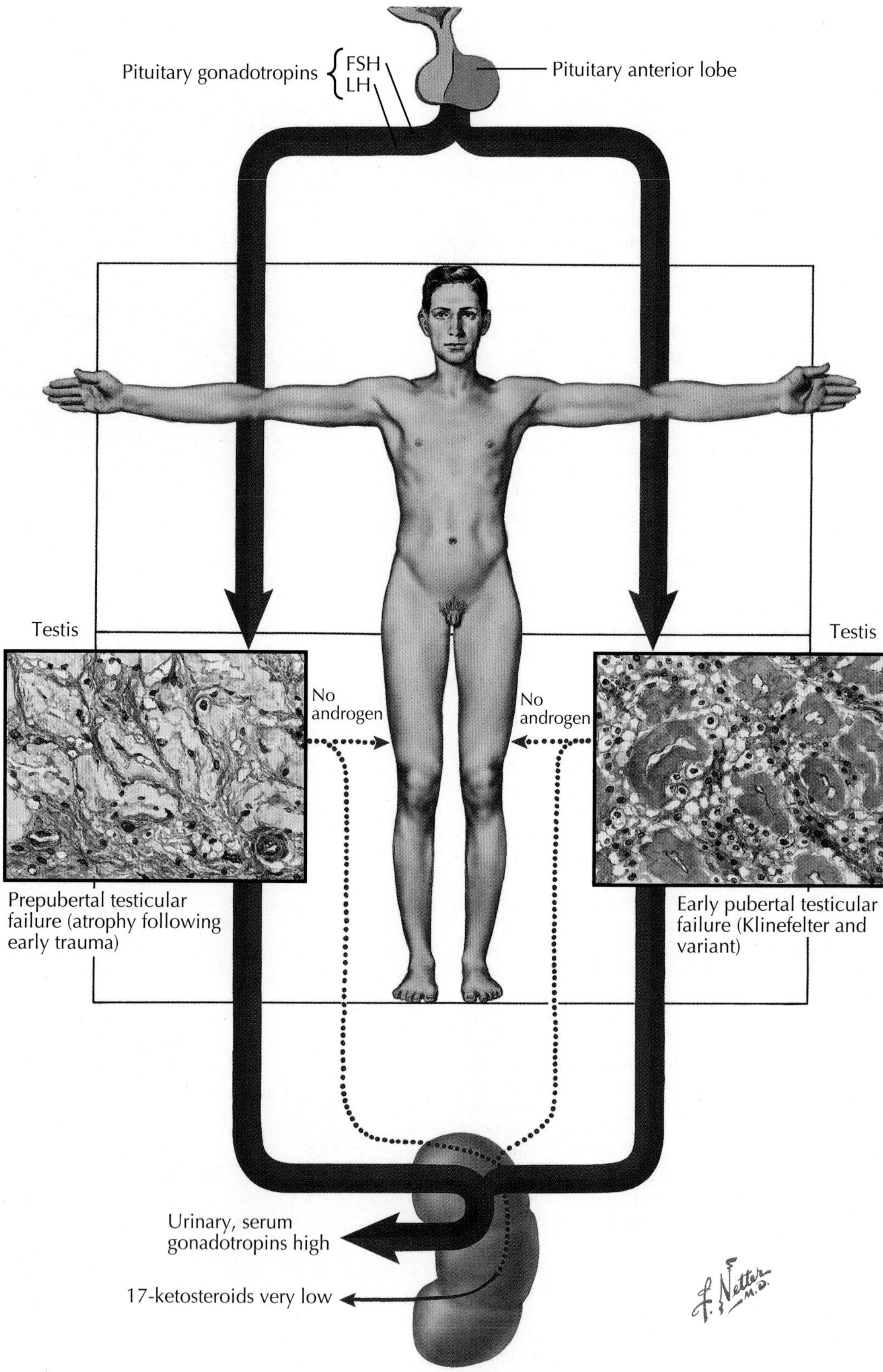

Plate 3.17

Reproductive System: VOLUME 1

Pituitary gonadotropins { FSH LH

Pituitary anterior lobe

Testis

Testis

No androgen

No androgen

Prepubertal testicular failure (atrophy following early trauma)

Early pubertal testicular failure (Klinefelter and variant)

Urinary, serum gonadotropins high

17-ketosteroids very low

TESTIS FAILURE: PRIMARY (HYPERGONADOTROPIC) HYPOGONADISM

Testicular failure may be unicompartmental and involve only exocrine function (spermatogenesis), or it may be bicompartmental and involve exocrine and endocrine (androgen) function. Endocrine deficiency due to interstitial or Leydig cell failure almost uniformly includes spermatogenic failure. *Hypogonadism* was originally used to delineate endocrine deficiency but customarily also refers to exocrine failure. Absence (e.g., castration, agenesis) of the testis is termed anorchia (formerly "eunuchism"). The term *eunuchoidal habitus* has been used to indicate a male body configuration that is characteristic of long-term androgenic deficiency, regardless of etiology.

Testicular deficiency is classified clinically as (1) primary (or intrinsic) testicular failure beginning prepubertally or very early in puberty, (2) primary testicular failure during puberty (see Plate 3.17), (3) secondary testicular failure from pituitary insufficiency or its variants (see Plates 3.18 and 3.19), and (4) predominantly germ cell failure and infertility (see Plate 3.22) without androgenic failure.

Primary testicular failure results from defects within the testis, usually occurring in the embryonic or prepubertal periods. Pituitary function is unimpaired, because there exists an appropriate, compensatory rise in gonadotropin production during and after puberty. It is also called *hypergonadotropic hypogonadism*. There is generally significant testicular atrophy, characterized histologically by sclerosis of the infantile (small) seminiferous tubules and a disappearance of Leydig cells in the interstitium and replacement with hyalinization. Genetic causes of testis atrophy include Klinefelter syndrome and its variants. Acquired causes are mumps with orchitis, bilateral trauma, neonatal or postnatal torsion, or cryptorchidism. Testis atrophy may also occur after chemotherapy or x-ray exposure from cancer therapy and as a consequence of bilateral inguinal herniorrhaphy.

The physical habitus of an affected male varies considerably, depending on whether the testis failure occurs before, during, or after puberty. Persistence of prepubertal physical features after puberty with failure of pubertal progression occurs with testis failure in childhood or during puberty. Patients may be tall and thin owing to marked overgrowth of the long bones. Bone age and maturation may be greatly delayed, and open epiphyses have been observed in affected 25-year-olds. Generally, the legs and forearms grow disproportionately long, resulting in a greater distance from the symphysis to the heel than from the symphysis to the top of the head. The arm span exceeds that of height by 2 cm or more. Genu valgum and kyphosis in later life and significant osteoporosis are also frequently encountered. The requirement for the development of these features is androgen deficiency during the period of rapid growth at puberty, regardless of the reason. As such, these physical characteristics are not restricted to patients with primary testicular failure but are common to all types of testis failure. Indeed, castration or estrogen administration after puberty during adult life does not cause regression of male secondary sex characteristics and only minimally alters physical features, except for gynecomastia, obesity, and skin changes.

Plate 3.18

Scrotum and Testis

TESTIS FAILURE: SECONDARY (HYPOGONADOTROPIC) HYPOGONADISM

Testicular deficiency due to failure of the anterior pituitary to secrete gonadotropins is termed secondary or hypogonadotropic hypogonadism. The hypothalamus is known to regulate anterior pituitary function, mainly through gonadotropin-releasing hormone (GnRH), a 10–amino acid peptide secreted from neuronal cells in the preoptic and arcuate nuclei. The only known function of GnRH is to stimulate gonadotropin secretion. GnRH has a plasma half-life of approximately 5 to 7 minutes, and it exhibits several types of rhythmicity: seasonal; circadian, resulting in higher testosterone levels during the early morning hours; and pulsatile, with GnRH peaks occurring every 90 to 120 minutes. The importance of the pulsatile GnRH secretory pattern in normal testicular function is aptly demonstrated by the ability of exogenously given GnRH agonists (leuprolide acetate) to stop testicular testosterone production by changing pituitary exposure to GnRH from a cyclic to a constant pattern.

In Kallmann syndrome, characterized by congenital hypogonadotropic hypogonadism, the GnRH precursor neurons fail to migrate normally, with a subsequent absence of hypothalamic GnRH. Individuals who are affected present with delayed puberty or infertility due to lack of testosterone production. Because the GnRH neurons comigrate with olfactory nerves, patients with Kallmann syndrome may also have anosmia. Causes of acquired pituitary hypofunction and secondary hypogonadism include severe stress, malnutrition, diabetes mellitus, chronic opiate use, sickle cell disease, hemochromatosis, and intracranial conditions such as prolactinomas, craniopharyngiomas, Rathke cleft cysts, and trauma. For this reason, pituitary imaging should be considered in cases of acquired secondary hypogonadism. Notably, not all brain or pituitary tumors necessarily disturb gonadotropin secretion and result in secondary hypogonadism.

The clinical picture of secondary hypogonadism is a similarly altered body morphology as that described for prepubertal or pubertal primary testicular failure (see Plate 3.17). In extreme cases, there is delayed growth of the external sexual organs, with the penis remaining small (micropenis) and the scrotum underdeveloped (hypoplastic). The prostate and seminal vesicles are small but present. The testes vary from infantile to small adult size, but testicular size does not correlate well with androgen function, because Leydig cells constitute only 10% to 15% of testicular volume. Testis biopsies generally reveal infantile seminiferous tubules containing undifferentiated spermatogonia, Sertoli cells, and Leydig cells. The histologic picture is essentially that of a prepubertal boy (see Plate 3.4).

There may be a complete absence of beard and bodily hair, with fine, sparse pubic hair characteristic of androgen deficiency. Baldness with advancing age is rare, unless the patient is treated with androgens. Skin may be smooth, pale, fine in texture, and dry, with little oiliness; acne rarely develops. The thyroid cartilage may be inconspicuous, and the voice high-pitched. There may also be a striking lack of muscular development and complaints of extreme fatigability. There may also be behavioral problems influenced by the adjustment needed due to sexual immaturity.

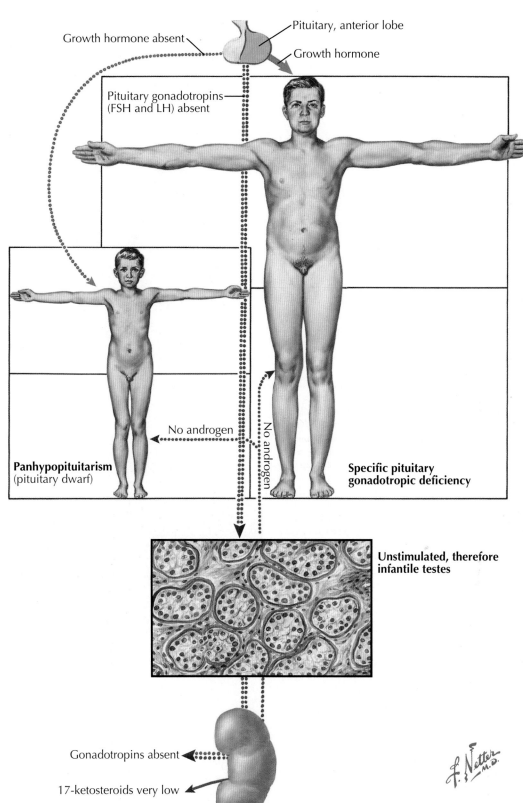

Growth hormone absent

Pituitary, anterior lobe

Growth hormone

Pituitary gonadotropins (FSH and LH) absent

No androgen

No androgen

Panhypopituitarism (pituitary dwarf)

Specific pituitary gonadotropic deficiency

Unstimulated, therefore infantile testes

Gonadotropins absent

17-ketosteroids very low

The anterior pituitary also secretes growth hormone in response to hypothalamic growth hormone–releasing hormone, thyroid-stimulating hormone, and adrenocorticotropic hormone (ACTH). Thus secondary hypogonadism can be associated with defective growth, hypothyroidism, and cortisol deficiency. When occurring together, this is referred to as *panhypopituitarism*. Boys with panhypopituitarism have greatly decreased height. However, they attain a mature skeletal ratio without disproportionate extremities

or eunuchoid features. They may also have infantile faces, acne-free skin, a lack of hair development owing to the deficient ACTH, and very low adrenal androgen levels.

With secondary hypogonadism, gonadotropin levels are undetectably low in conjunction with low androgens. This differentiates it from primary hypogonadism. In isolated cases, adrenal androgens may be sufficient to induce puberty, and so the presenting symptom may simply be infertility later in life.

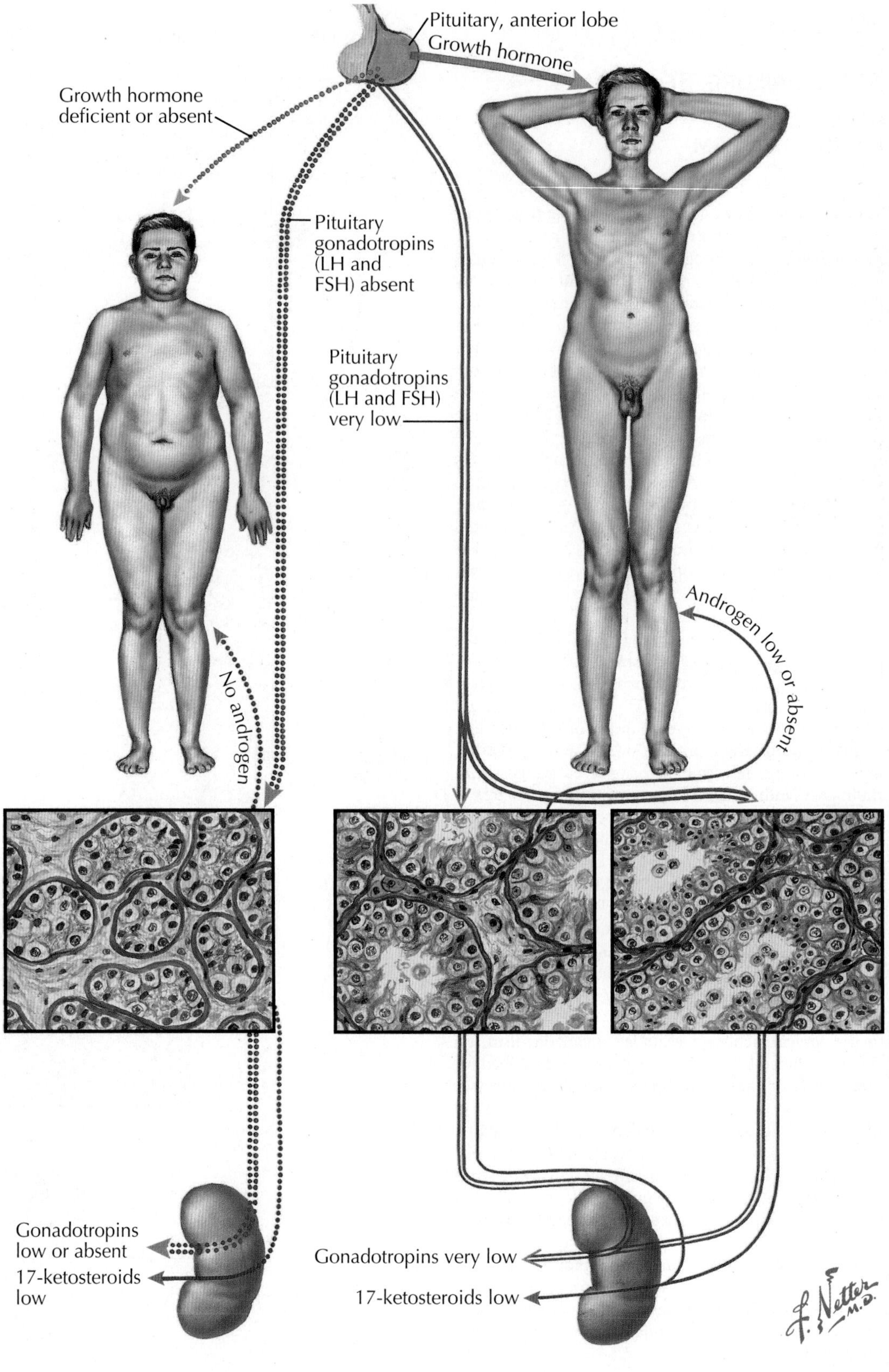

Plate 3.19

Reproductive System: VOLUME 1

Pituitary, anterior lobe

Growth hormone

Growth hormone deficient or absent

Pituitary gonadotropins (LH and FSH) absent

Pituitary gonadotropins (LH and FSH) very low

No androgen

Androgen low or absent

TESTIS FAILURE: SECONDARY HYPOGONADISM VARIANTS

Eunuchoid features common to primary (hypergonadotropic) and secondary (hypogonadotropic) hypogonadism are presented here in the classic physical phenotype (see Plates 3.17 and 3.18). However, most males with hypogonadism do not develop into exaggerated, tall, lean individuals. Most exhibit "in-between" morphogenetic types, as the onset of clinical hypogonadism occurs at various ages and has various degrees of influence. For example, many hypogonadal males are shorter than normal, although with skeletal proportions still characterized by long radial skeletal bones associated with delayed maturation of the epiphyses. Indeed, not all prepubertally hypogonadal males develop disproportionately long extremities, as additional factors are necessary for excess linear growth, including growth hormone status, nutritional and environmental factors, and thyroid balance.

Hypogonadal males with partial androgenic deficiency show all degrees of penile and testicular development. Many cases of secondary hypogonadism are not genetic but acquired and present after puberty as a result of extreme physical stress, anabolic steroids, chronic opiates, sickle cell disease, acquired pituitary cysts, diabetes mellitus, and hemochromatosis. These patients tend to have normal-volume testes and normal phallic length and may present only with symptoms of sexual dysfunction such as erectile dysfunction, low libido, or infertility.

Hair development in hypogonadal males varies with responsiveness to both testicular and adrenal cortical androgens. More hair can develop when testicular failure is incomplete and abundant; fine pubic hair may be present due to pituitary ACTH and resultant adrenocortical androgens. Hypogonadal males tend to be obese and have relatively undeveloped muscle and bone. In addition, fat tends to accumulate on the anterior abdominal wall, above the symphysis in the mons pubis area, around the mammary glands, and on the outer thighs and buttocks. However, such obesity can also be explained by dietary habits or other familial traits.

The treatment of primary hypogonadism is testosterone replacement. Testosterone can be given intramuscularly with weekly depot injections, by transdermally absorbed gels (daily), buccally absorbed tablets (daily), dermal patches (daily), implantable pellets (biannually), and oral pills (twice daily). Such replacement can be important to prevent the complications of long-term hypogonadism that include osteoporosis, anemia,

Gonadotropins low or absent

17-ketosteroids low

Gonadotropins very low

17-ketosteroids low

depression, heart disease, muscle wasting, memory loss, and possibly even higher rates of prostate cancer and metabolic syndrome. Cases of secondary hypogonadism may also respond to pituitary replacement with hCG that acts as luteinizing hormone (LH) and stimulates interstitial Leydig cell function and testosterone production. Many cases of acquired secondary hypogonadism are effectively treated with selective estrogen receptor modulators such as clomiphene citrate. In the

vast majority of hypogonadism cases, testosterone replacement will reduce pituitary follicle-stimulating hormone (FSH) and LH secretion by negative feedback homeostasis and induce sterility. The addition of injectable FSH therapy along with hCG can restore natural fertility to the majority of secondarily hypogonadal males. This is an important issue in secondary hypogonadism induced by anabolic steroid use by athletes and body builders.

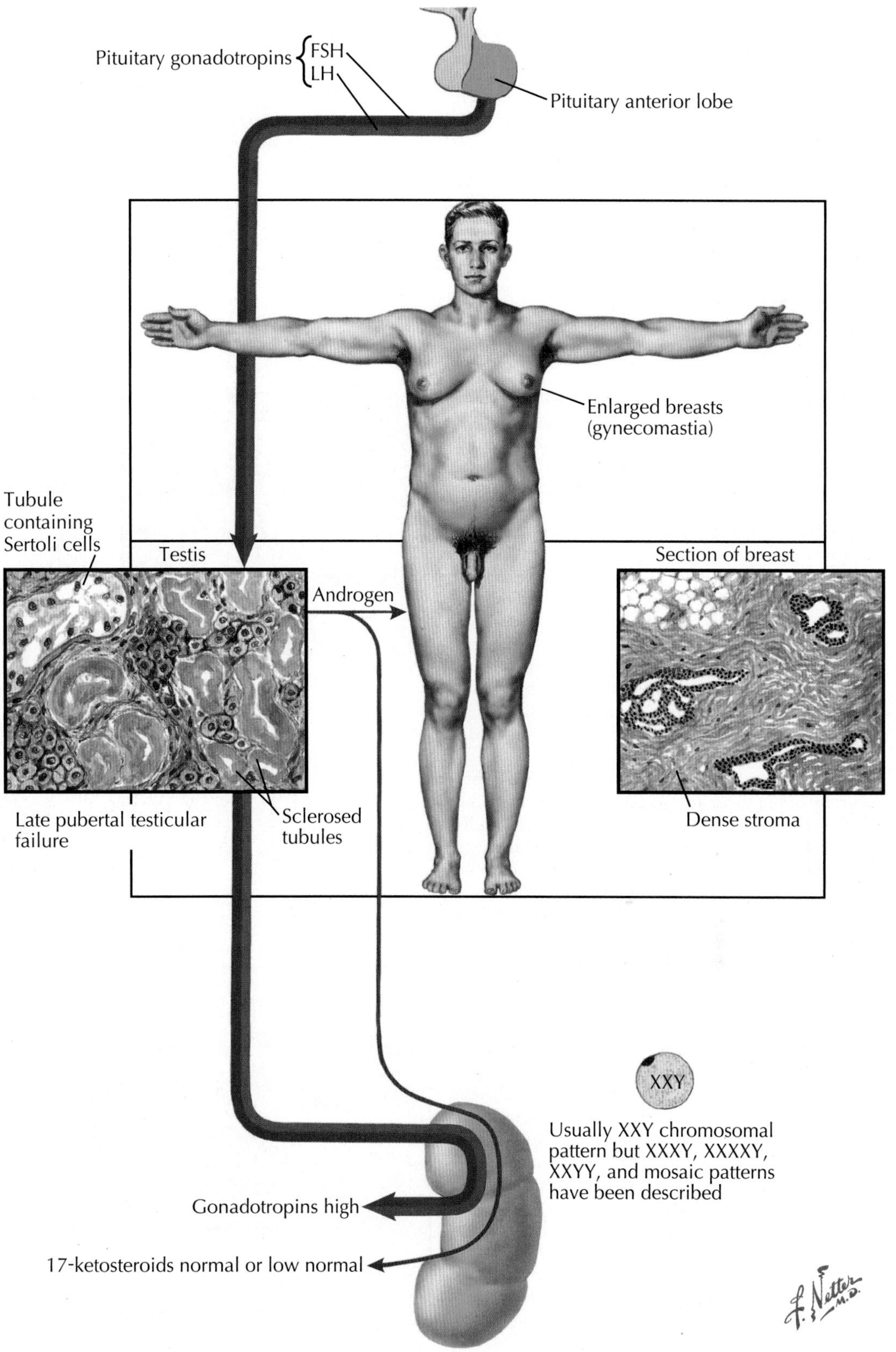

Plate 3.20

Scrotum and Testis

Pituitary gonadotropins { FSH, LH }

Pituitary anterior lobe

Enlarged breasts (gynecomastia)

Tubule containing Sertoli cells

Testis

Androgen

Section of breast

Late pubertal testicular failure

Sclerosed tubules

Dense stroma

Gonadotropins high

XXY

Usually XXY chromosomal pattern but XXXY, XXXXY, XXYY, and mosaic patterns have been described

17-ketosteroids normal or low normal

TESTIS FAILURE: KLINEFELTER SYNDROME

Klinefelter syndrome is the most common genetic cause of sterility due to primary gonadal failure; it is also a relatively common genetic anomaly in the general population, occurring in 1:500 boys. It is characterized by a male phenotype with a 47,XXY chromosomal constitution. Approximately 10% of patients with Klinefelter syndrome have mosaic 46,XY/47,XXY (or variants) patterns, and the remainder have a pure 47,XXY or variant constitution. Clinically, it is associated with a triad of findings: small, firm testes, azoospermia (no sperm count), and gynecomastia, although the latter is not necessarily a typical feature.

Approximately half of Klinefelter cases are paternally derived, and recent evidence suggests that its occurrence may correlate with advanced paternal age. This syndrome may also present with increased height, decreased intelligence, varicosities, obesity, diabetes, leukemia, and increased likelihood of extragonadal germ cell tumors and breast cancer (20-fold higher than 46,XY males). It usually presents as either delayed male puberty due to hypogonadism or with primary infertility later in life. Although nearly always associated with infertility in the pure chromosomal pattern, patients with Klinefelter syndrome often show a wide spectrum of masculinization ranging from a severe eunuchoid habitus to a normal male phenotype. The degree of gynecomastia is variable. Indeed, only 10% of patients with Klinefelter syndrome exhibit the classic attributes of this condition.

Reproductive hormones usually demonstrate a low testosterone and frankly elevated LH and FSH. Natural paternity with this syndrome is possible, but almost exclusively with the mosaic or milder form of the disease. Biologic paternity in cases of pure XXY males is now possible with assisted reproduction in conjunction with retrieval of testicular sperm.

Characteristically, the testes exhibit an irregular distribution of seminiferous tubules and tubular sclerosis separated by connective tissue and clumps of Leydig cells. Leydig cells are often increased in number and size and can form nests that appear as adenomas. Among seminiferous tubules, most contain only Sertoli cells, whereas in 60% of cases, other tubules will harbor pockets of spermatogenesis with sperm. The seminiferous tubule basement membrane is thickened and sclerosed, and there is significant intertubular hyalinization. Testicular abnormalities similar to those in Klinefelter syndrome can be brought about by radiation damage, mumps orchitis, or other testicular injury. Such a history is not typically elicited from patients with Klinefelter syndrome, however. Before adolescence, the testes are relatively normal in size but fail to develop normally in response to pubertal gonadotropin stimulation.

Interestingly, despite a uniformly abnormal somatic genotype, 75% to 100% of mature sperm from patients with 47,XXY harbor a normal haploid sex chromosome complement (X or Y), instead of XY or YY complements. The lack of significant gonosomal aneuploidy in the presence of somatic aneuploidy suggests that abnormal germ cell lines may arrest at a meiotic checkpoint within the testis or that somatic–germ line mosaicism is more common than previously thought.

Plate 3.21

Reproductive System: VOLUME 1

TESTIS FAILURE: DELAYED PUBERTY

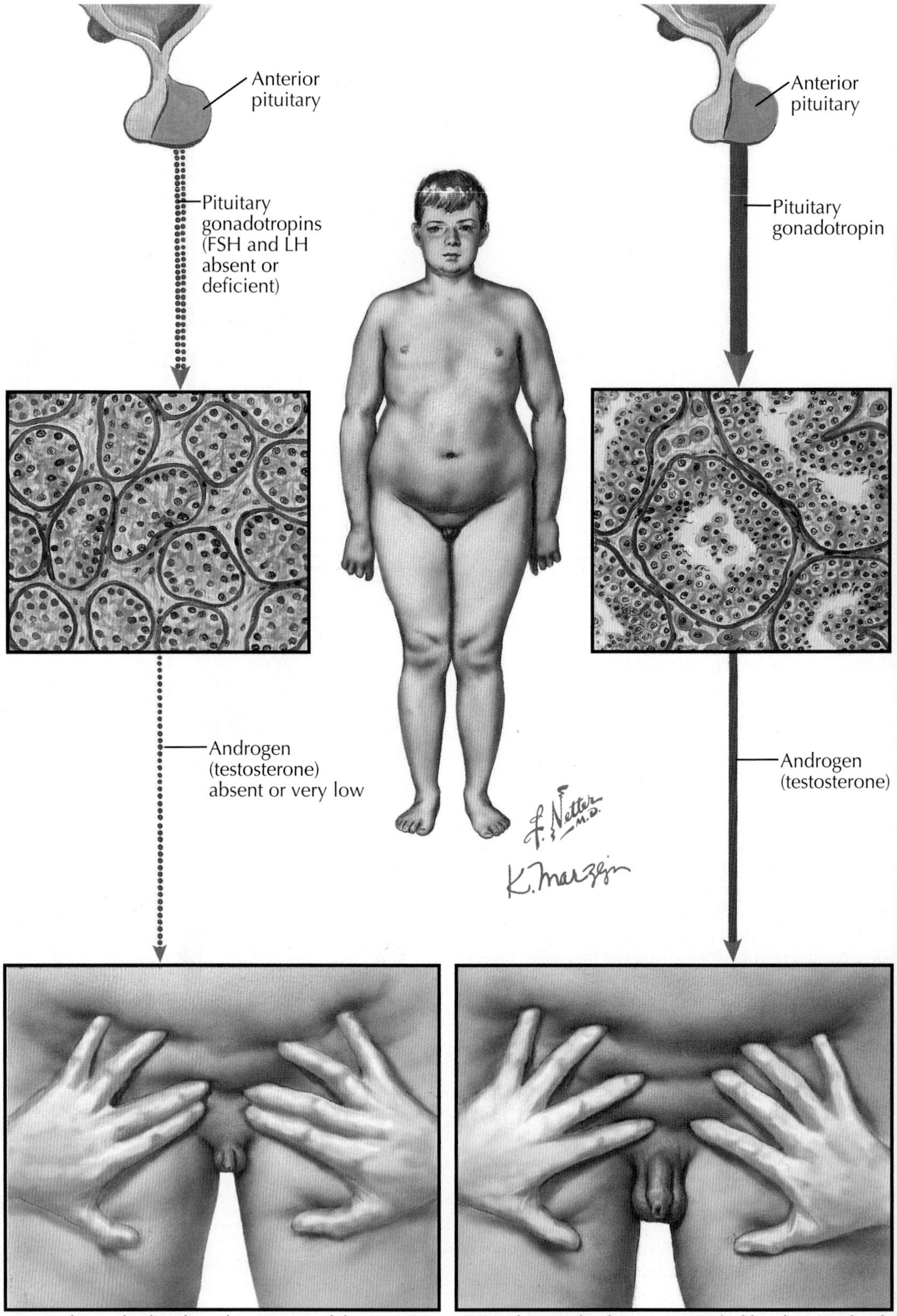

Puberty in the male occurs in progressive stages, most commonly identified by the classification into five stages by Tanner (see Plate 1.6). In addition to rapid development of sexual organs and other characteristics, during the later Tanner stages the testes produce sperm capable of fertility. Adolescence is the period of further development after puberty that ends when full maturity is reached. Before the onset of puberty (i.e., the prepubertal period), the testes are immature and quiescent as pituitary gonadotropins are released in only subthreshold amounts. As such, it is not possible to evaluate hypogonadism in prepubertal boys. It is also true that variations in male genitalia or stature during this period may not be due to absent or defective testes but may be ascribed to other factors, including those related to heredity, pituitary, thyroid, adrenal, growth hormone, or nutritional issues.

The real physical changes associated with puberty occur in response to the secretion of LH from the anterior pituitary gland. LH stimulates Leydig cells within the testis interstitium to produce androgens from cholesterol precursors. The age of onset and the rate at which it proceeds exhibit wide variation, lending tremendous variation in the length and degree of pubertal development in boys of any particular age.

Care providers are often called upon by parents to prognosticate regarding the sexual development of peripubertal boys, especially if the average age for pubertal onset has passed without genital growth. However, it is difficult to make an absolute diagnosis of hypogonadism during pubescence. A testicular biopsy is likely to reveal findings consistent with infantile testes, indicating only a lack of gonadotropic stimulation. Hormone assays for gonadotropins are more accurate but may change rapidly during this developmental period. The consistency of the testes, when soft and small, may possibly indicate true hypogonadism over time. Temporary breast development is normal during early male pubescence. Assessing linear growth or observing disproportionate bone growth can provide evidence of growth disorders such as genetic short stature.

If there is real concern about pubertal development, a diagnostic and therapeutic challenge with hCG (500–700 IU three times weekly for 3 weeks) can evaluate potential gonadal and pituitary factors. An increase in testis consistency or serum testosterone implies that the testis Leydig cells are normal. This in turn suggests that there may only be a delay in the onset of puberty, although the existence of a permanent pituitary defect is still a possibility.

Obesity and delayed genital development frequently coexist, but obesity in the vast majority of the cases is based on nonendocrine causes (see Plate 3.19). Careful examination of most obese boys with alleged genital underdevelopment reveals no evidence of delayed

Anterior pituitary

Pituitary gonadotropins (FSH and LH absent or deficient)

Androgen (testosterone) absent or very low

Anterior pituitary

Pituitary gonadotropin

Androgen (testosterone)

Genitalia underdeveloped (majority of these cases later become normal)

Normal genitalia for age (revealed by drawing back obese abdomen and thighs)

puberty. A thorough examination of suspected micropenis that involves retraction of the pendulous abdomen and excessive mons pubic fat most commonly exposes a "hidden" penis and testes that are within the normal limits for age.

The management of most boys with delayed puberty and persistently infantile genitalia remains watchful waiting. Although the onset of puberty may be delayed, full genital and linear growth usually ensues with time.

Indeed, weight loss from diet management in cases of obesity may hasten the onset of puberty. Regular medical follow-up with anthropometric measurements can help with the early detection of true pubertal abnormalities resulting from hypogonadism or dwarfism. Treatment with gonadotropins or androgens may be considered when the lack of sexual development affects other quality-of-life issues such as school performance, athletic development, or concerns regarding socialization.

Plate 3.22

Scrotum and Testis

SPERMATOGENIC FAILURE

Infertility is defined as the inability to conceive after 1 year of unprotected intercourse. It occurs in approximately 10% to 15% of reproductive-age couples worldwide. In 30% to 40% of cases, male factor infertility is involved. Among male factors, spermatogenic failure leading to oligospermia (low sperm count) or azoospermia (no sperm count) is very common. Unlike with clinical hypogonadism, there is usually no evidence of androgenic failure in most infertile males. Indeed, most infertile males are otherwise healthy and have no evidence of hypopituitarism or other endocrine or metabolic disturbances. However, the diagnosis of infertility may place males at higher risk of subsequently developing cancer, including testis and prostate cancer. In addition, it is now clear that infertile males have a higher comorbidity burden than do fertile males. In this way, infertility may be viewed as a biomarker of both current and future health issues in affected males.

The evaluation of male infertility involves a thorough history and physical examination, an assessment of testosterone and FSH levels and, ideally, two semen analyses. Reproductive toxins such as tobacco, wet heat exposure (hot baths), ionizing radiation, heavy metal exposure, and antiandrogen medications should be eliminated, and ideal body weight (body mass index = 19–25) should be sought. The physical examination should investigate for testis cancer, varicoceles, and abnormalities of the excurrent ducts, such as congenital absence of the vas deferens. Hormone assessment can evaluate the integrity of both the exocrine (sperm) and endocrine (androgen) hormonal axes critical for testis function. It is clear that normal sperm production requires normal levels of both FSH and testosterone. Two semen analyses are helpful for reducing the technical variability and better understanding the inherent biologic issues with semen quality. Adjunctive testing is possible but predicated mainly on the findings from this initial evaluation and the decision whether testing will (1) reveal a general health issue or (2) alter management of the fertility issue.

In cases of severe spermatogenic failure, termed *nonobstructive azoospermia,* there may be microfoci of sperm production in the testis, despite the lack of any sperm in the ejaculate. This is even true in cases of iatrogenic spermatogenic failure due to chemotherapy for cancer treatment. Procedures such as the testis biopsy, fine-needle aspiration "mapping," and microdissection testis sperm extraction are strategies used to determine whether sperm are present in the testis of azoospermic males. If present, testis sperm is routinely used to achieve pregnancies with in vitro fertilization and intracytoplasmic sperm injection. The most common histologic patterns obtained from the diagnostic testis biopsy (see Plate 5.6) in nonobstructive azoospermic males are as follows:

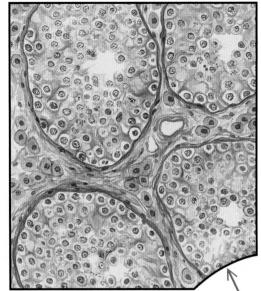

Maturation arrest

Pituitary gonadotropins normal (but may be elevated)

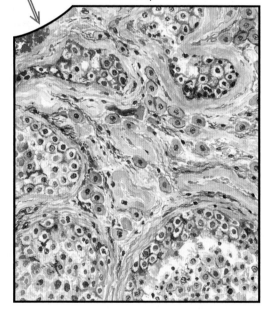

Germinal cell aplasia (Del Castillo or Sertoli cell only syndrome)

Pituitary gonadotropins (elevated)

Pituitary gonadotropins (elevated)

Hypospermatogenesis

Pituitary gonadotropins normal (but may be elevated)

Incomplete fibrosis

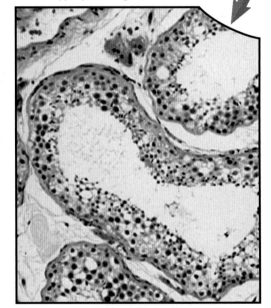

Maturation arrest of spermatogenesis. This tubular morphology describes spermatogenesis that abruptly ceases during meiotic prophase such that germ cells beyond primary spermatocytes are absent (early maturation arrest). The arrest may also be incomplete (not in all tubules) or occur at other stages, most commonly at the spermatogonial stage or the spermatid stage (late arrest). Gonadotropins are usually normal. This condition can be transitory after febrile illnesses and testosterone deficiency, but in 50% of cases it is a consequence of errors in meiotic recombination.

Germ cell aplasia (Sertoli cell–only syndrome). Often called *Del Castillo syndrome,* this histology is characterized by tubules devoid of germinal epithelium and containing only Sertoli cells. Normal Leydig cells appear to be increased in number. Causes may be acquired or congenital and may represent the failure of primordial germ cell migration to the somatic testis during early development (see Plate 1.2). FSH levels are usually high in this condition.

Hypospermatogenesis represents a thinning of the normal germinal epithelium such that mature sperm production declines to a point below the threshold required for ejaculation. Unlike maturation arrest, all stages of spermatogenesis are present in this condition. It is commonly observed after cancer chemotherapy, with varicocele, cryptorchidism, and tobacco use. FSH levels are generally elevated.

Tubular sclerosis consists of replacement of the seminiferous tubule lumen with acellular fibrosis. Interstitial Leydig cells are present in normal or decreased numbers. It is a consequence of noxious agents, viral (mumps) and bacterial orchitis, and vascular injury from torsion and may lead to progressive peritubular fibrosis. In severe cases, FSH and LH levels are usually elevated.

Patients with azoospermia caused by obstruction (see Plate 5.5) show normal spermatogenesis on biopsy.

Plate 3.23

Reproductive System: VOLUME 1

INFECTION AND ABSCESS OF TESTIS AND EPIDIDYMIS

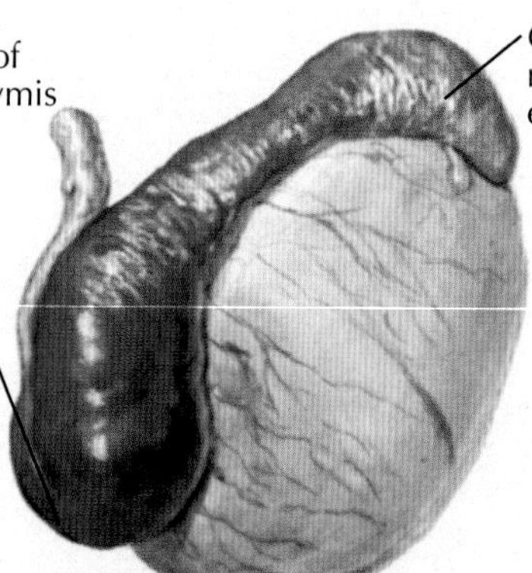

Acute testicular infections are rare. More commonly, orchitis develops secondary to suppurative epididymitis and is termed *epididymo-orchitis*. Orchitis occurs through three possible routes: via lymphatics, via the bloodstream, and ascending through the vas deferens. The most common setting for bacterial orchitis in males older than 35 years is age-related prostatism or urethral strictures resulting in urinary tract obstruction and gram-negative urinary tract infections. In males younger than 35 years, STDs such as chlamydia and nongonorrheal urethritis (NGU) are the most common culprits. Inflammatory orchitis may occur in response to bacterial toxins; autoimmune responses; trauma; torsion; chemicals such as iodine, thallium, lead, and alcohol; and medications (amiodarone). In such cases, pathogenic organisms may not be cultured from the urine or from inflamed or necrotic tissue.

Acute bacterial orchitis is usually accompanied by high fevers and sudden scrotal pain and swelling. The onset is so acute that it may be confused with testicular torsion, except that the latter has no associated fever or bacteriuria. A reactive hydrocele is common, and the overlying scrotal skin shows redness and edema. These associated features often make it clinically difficult to distinguish among isolated orchitis, epididymitis, or epididymo-orchitis. The inflamed testicle is tense and bluish in appearance, with many punctate hemorrhages on the surface. There may be considerable edema of the testis within the fixed, noncompliant tunica albuginea, which can result in ischemia and seminiferous tubule loss and atrophy. The process may progress to suppuration, abscess formation, and in rare cases, testicular autoamputation.

Mumps orchitis complicates approximately 20% of mumps cases and rarely occurs before puberty. As a viral glandular infection, mumps can affect the parotid glands, the pancreas, and the testis. Epididymis involvement in this process is rare. Orchitis usually develops 4 to 6 days after parotitis and generally subsides in 7 to 14 days. The signs and symptoms of this virus infection are similar to those of other interstitial orchitides. Scrotal pain and testicular swelling are the prominent features. Early testicular histologic findings include transitory edema that quickly progresses to marked interstitial inflammation. Seminiferous tubule sclerosis, gross testicular atrophy, and infertility are serious sequelae. About 70% of mumps orchitis cases are unilateral, and in 50% demonstrable testicular atrophy occurs. Treatments have included wide incision of the testis tunical albuginea and systematic corticosteroids or interferons to reduce the effects of inflammation and edema.

Epididymitis is by far the most common type of intrascrotal infection or inflammation. It may be classified as sexually transmitted (i.e., gonorrheal, chlamydial, NGU), bacterial (gram-negative, tuberculous), inflammatory, posttraumatic, and idiopathic. Infecting organisms reach the epididymis through the vas deferens from infected urine, prostate, or seminal vesicles. Infection may also spread retrograde through lymphatics and, rarely, through hematogenous routes.

Gonorrheal epididymitis, now rare, was historically a common complication of gonorrheal urethritis (see Plate 2.21). It rarely involves the testicle, appearing first in the globus minor or cauda epididymis, which becomes swollen, tense, and tender. Although small abscesses may develop, suppuration is rare, and resolution

Globus minor of epididymis — Globus major of epididymis

Acute epididymo-orchitis

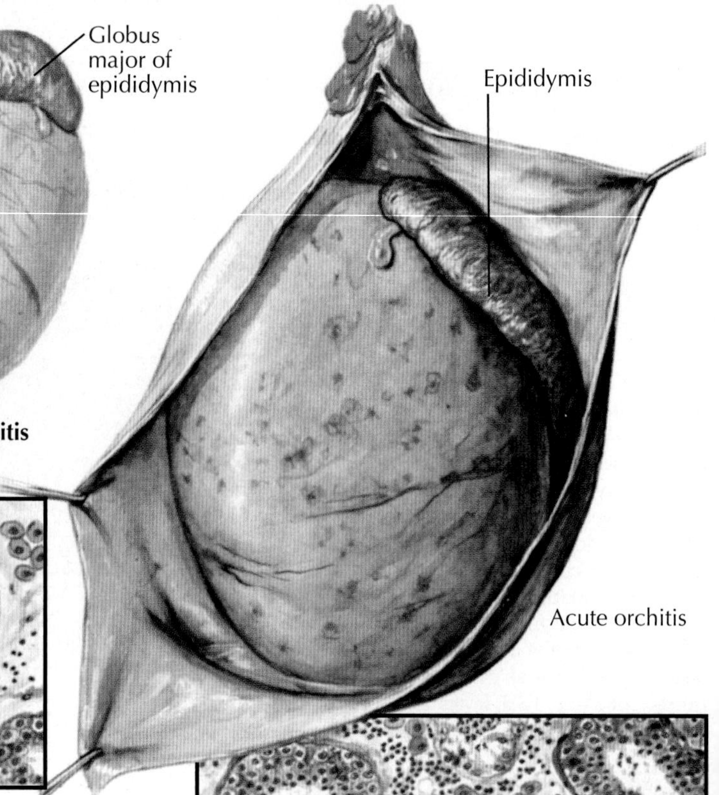

Epididymis

Acute orchitis

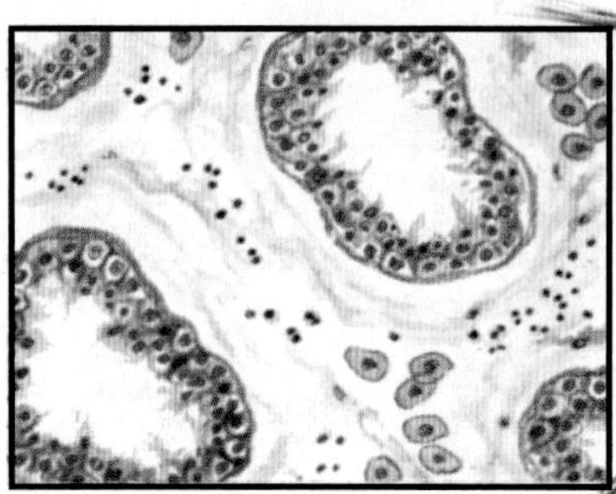

Mumps orchitis. Early stage; edema.

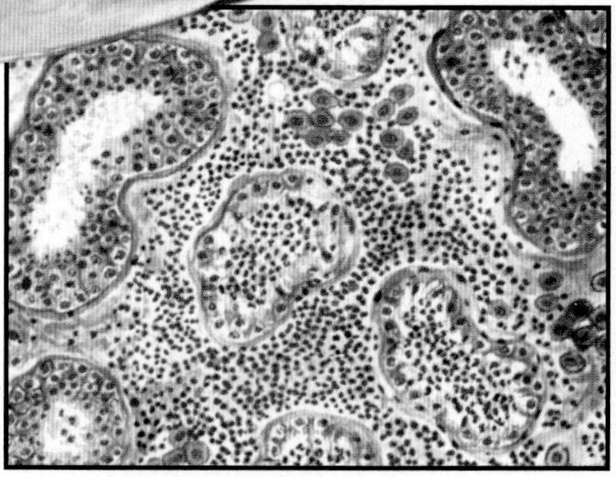

Mumps orchitis. Advanced stage.

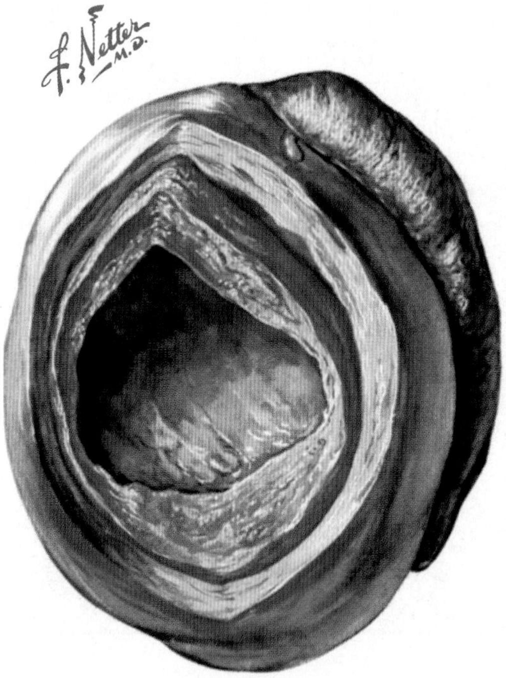

Abscess of testis

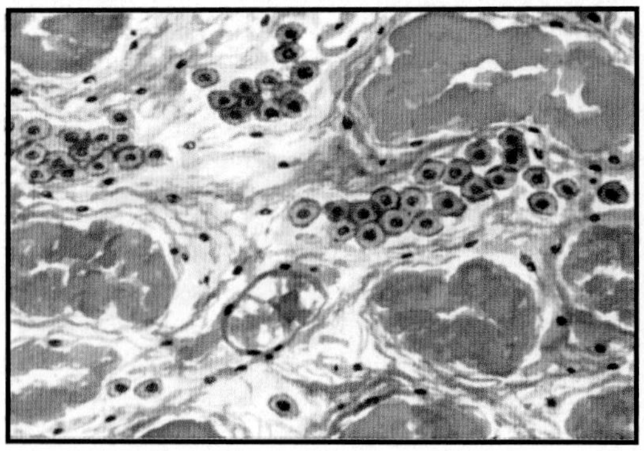

Mumps orchitis. Sequelae.

is common, accompanied by sterility due to excurrent ductal obstruction from scar tissue if bilateral.

Posttraumatic epididymitis due to urethral catheterization, cystoscopy, and other surgical procedures is also relatively uncommon with widespread antibiotic use. Epididymitis may become chronic and be a source of recurrent pain and swelling due to ejaculatory duct reflux of urine through the vas deferens with strenuous physical activity or after organ congestion due to vasectomy. If epididymitis does not respond to rest, scrotal elevation, and antibiotics, antiinflammatories may be added. Antibiotic-refractory epididymitis should raise clinical suspicion for tuberculous epididymitis (see Plate 3.24) and warrants examination of first morning urine or tissue for acid-fast bacillus. Epididymectomy is a rarely used treatment option but can be effective after vasectomy.

Plate 3.24

Scrotum and Testis

SYPHILIS AND TUBERCULOSIS OF THE TESTIS

Syphilis of the testicle was once a common sequela of untreated primary syphilis but is now very unusual. Historically, syphilitic orchitis occurred as an interstitial infection or caused necrosis or gumma formation. The interstitial infection is insidious and indolent, unilateral or bilateral, and usually painless. An accompanying hydrocele is the rule. The testicle is usually hard and smooth (like a billiard ball) as a result of infiltration of plasma cells and fibrous tissue, which eventually leads to testicular fibrosis. Gummas or syphilitic granulomas are characterized by areas of necrotic nodules in the testicle. The fibrous tissue surrounding the coalesced gummatous nodules also results in considerable hardness to palpation. The epididymis is rarely involved during the initial stage of testis infection, although syphilitic epididymitis may be a primary presentation of syphilis. As the tunica vaginalis and epididymis become involved, there is adherence and extension to the scrotal skin, which may slough and ulcerate. Although patients do not experience significant pain, there may also be enlargement of the inguinal nodes. Despite the dramatic presentation of a hard testis, it was frequently unnoticed by both patient and physician.

Tuberculosis of the testicle is almost always preceded by epididymal infection; primary involvement of the testicle alone is rare. Once uncommon, there has been a resurgence of tuberculous epididymitis in inner-city areas and in males who are HIV positive. Because 15% of tuberculosis occurs as an isolated genitourinary infection without systemic miliary signs or symptoms, this presentation of tuberculosis appears identical to other forms of bacterial epididymitis but is suspected when the infection is refractory to common bacterial antibiotics. The disease is frequently bilateral and will not heal without specific antituberculous therapy. Extension of tuberculous epididymitis to the testicle is a common but later development in untreated cases. More often, epididymo-orchitis occurs from constitutional disease. Systemic tuberculous infection proceeds in a descending fashion down the genitourinary tract from renal tuberculosis to the bladder, prostate, vas deferens, and epididymis. The affected vas deferens often feels like a "string of pearls" with intermittent, skip areas of scarring and atrophy between areas of normal vas deferens.

Genital tuberculosis begins with classic tubercle formation, either localized or diffuse. Destruction of tissue

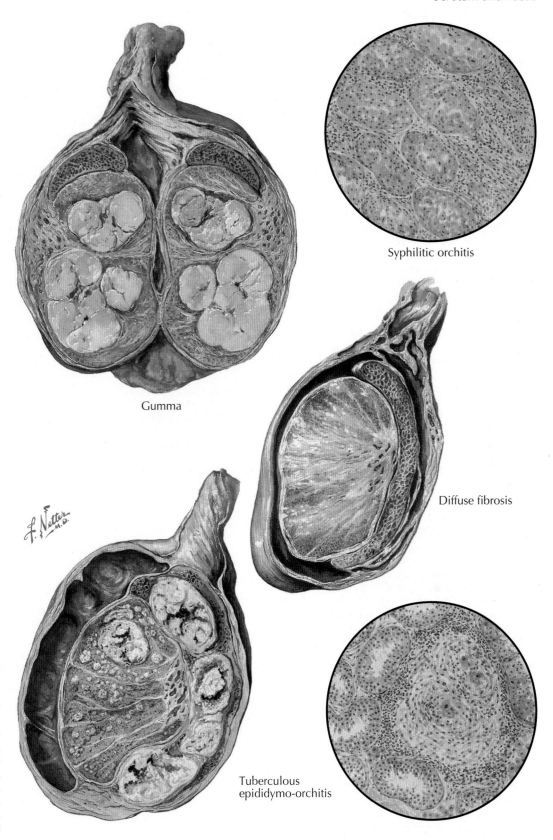

Gumma

Syphilitic orchitis

Diffuse fibrosis

Tuberculous epididymo-orchitis

by caseation follows, often accompanied by fibrosis and calcification. Not uncommonly, there may be involvement of the scrotal skin through cutaneous sinuses or the development of a rigid, thick tunica vaginalis containing clear or purulent fluid. When untreated, there is a great tendency for the infection to become chronic and stagnant. The process may remain dormant for long periods of time and then become acute or subacute.

Left untreated, tuberculosis is lethal to two of every three infected persons. The mainstay of treatment for the last 50 years has involved multidrug therapy with isoniazid, rifampicin, pyrazinamide, and ethambutol. Although this therapy is considered curative, multidrug-resistant strains are increasing. With healing, scar tissue is common and surgical procedures may be necessary to restore function in the genital tract.

Plate 3.25

Reproductive System: VOLUME 1

TESTICULAR TUMORS: SEMINOMA, EMBRYONAL CARCINOMA, YOLK SAC TUMORS

Testicular cancer is the most common cancer in males 15 to 35 years old. It most commonly affects White males and is rare among males of African descent. Worldwide incidence has doubled over the past 40 years, with the highest prevalence rates in Scandinavia, Germany, and New Zealand. A major risk factor for its development is cryptorchidism (undescended testicle). Other risk factors include infertility and a family history of testis cancer and possibly intersex conditions, inguinal hernia, mumps orchitis, sedentary lifestyle, and environmental exposures. Testicular tumors most commonly present as lumps in or hardening of the testis or as an enlargement within the scrotum due to a mass or hydrocele. They are generally painless but can be associated with increased testicular sensitivity.

Although testis cancer can be derived from any cell type found in the testicles, more than 95% of testis cancers are germ cell tumors. Most of the remaining 5% are sex cord–gonadal stromal tumors derived from Leydig cells or Sertoli cells. Other tumors such as lipomas, fibromas, adenomatoids, and sarcomas are rare. Secondary tumors from metastatic cancer, lymphoma, or leukemia are also rare. Adult germ cell tumors are grouped into five general types, according to fundamental histologic and biologic behavior patterns.

Seminomas constitute 40% of germ cell tumors. They are classified as typical (90%) or spermatocytic (10%) and are homogeneous, lobulated, yellow, orange, or pinkish tumors that are well circumscribed but not encapsulated. Histology reveals large, round or polygonal, uniform cells with clear cytoplasm, distinct cell membranes, and septated architecture. Tumor cells contain a prominent, centrally placed nucleus usually occupying about half of the cellular volume and may be arranged in disordered masses resembling tubules without lumen, similar to ovarian dysgerminomas (see Plate 10.22). The stroma may contain plasma cells and lymphocytes. Eighty percent of tumors occurring in undescended testes are seminomas. They are likely to be derived from spermatogonial stem cells within the testis.

Seminomas have little tendency to invade the spermatic cord; they metastasize mainly through lymphatics to retroperitoneal lymph nodes. In 10% of cases, serum hCG levels are elevated. They are very radio- and chemosensitive. When small (<1 cm) and solitary, they may be amenable to enucleation and partial orchiectomy; however, radical orchiectomy is needed for most tumors because of their size or number. When treated early, active surveillance or adjuvant treatment with retroperitoneal radiation or two cycles of cisplatin-based chemotherapy is usually recommended, with extremely high cure rates.

Embryonal carcinomas are the most common type of nonseminomatous germ cell tumor, accounting for about 20% of testis malignancies. These tumors resemble the tissues of early embryos and are likely to be derived from a multipotent primordial stem cell. This type of tumor can grow rapidly and metastasize. Grossly, they have the appearance of soft tissue, with areas of hemorrhage and necrosis. Histologically, embryonal carcinomas are composed of large masses of pleomorphic, embryonic epithelial cells that may simulate glandular structures with papillary organization or trabecular cells. These tumors stain with keratin, OCT-4, and CD30, are associated with an abnormal isochromosome 12 karyotype, and may be

Seminoma

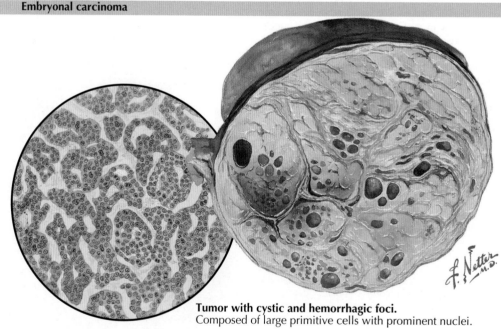

Solid yellow tumor. Composed of uniform cells with single, central nuclei arranged in solid clusters.

Embryonal carcinoma

Tumor with cystic and hemorrhagic foci.
Composed of large primitive cells with prominent nuclei.

associated with elevated serum lactate dehydrogenase and placental alkaline phosphatase (PLAP) levels. Cells may be arranged in lobules or into papillary, cystic, and other patterns of either differentiated or poorly differentiated structures, including cytotrophoblast and syncytiotrophoblast. Treatment is by radical orchiectomy and with either cisplatin-based chemotherapy or retroperitoneal lymph node dissection for early-stage disease. Cure rates higher than 90% are possible in most cases.

Endodermal sinus tumors (yolk sac tumors) are unusual, very aggressive, malignant testis cancers. These tumors recapitulate embryonal yolk sac tissue and uniformly secrete α-fetoprotein that is measurable in serum. In pure form, they are most commonly found in young boys; in adults, they usually occur as a component of mixed germ cell tumors. Grossly, the cut surface is heterogeneous because of extensive hemorrhage, necrosis, and cystic degeneration. Histologically, they are characterized by a pleomorphic intermingling of epithelial and mesenchymal elements (Schiller-Duval bodies) in an attempt to form yolk sac tissue. Treatment is radical orchiectomy and cisplatin-based chemotherapy.

Plate 3.26

Scrotum and Testis

TESTICULAR TUMORS: TERATOMA, CHORIOCARCINOMA, IN SITU NEOPLASIA

Teratomas (Greek for "monstrous tumor") are encapsulated tumors with tissue or organ components resembling normal derivatives of all three germ layers but foreign to the location in which they are found. Teratomas have been reported to contain hair, teeth, bone, and very rarely more complex organs such as eye, torso, and hands and feet. Teratomas constitute about 5% of testicular tumors and are generally classified as malignant. They occur in several forms, including mature and immature teratomas and dermoid cysts, the latter of which contains developmentally mature skin, (ectoderm) and are considered benign.

Teratomas show a remarkably wide variation in gross and microscopic appearance. Histological components of the tumors tend to represent tissues of the embryonic ectoderm, mesoderm, and endoderm: glandular tissue, cysts, cartilage, joints, skin, teeth, neuroepithelium, epidermoid cysts, enteric glands, smooth muscle, salivary glands, respiratory epithelium, lymphoid tissue, transitional epithelium, and even cardiac muscle and bone. Teratomas may be so poorly differentiated that only unrecognizable structures are present. Pure teratomas do not increase α-fetoprotein or hCG levels. The prognosis for a teratoma, if it contains no malignant focus of leukemia, sarcoma, or carcinoma, is favorable because of the infrequent occurrence of metastases. In the testis, teratomas are most commonly found in association with other nonseminomatous germ cell tumor types and are malignant. When found in association with embryonal carcinoma or choriocarcinoma, they are called *teratocarcinomas*. Pure teratomas are relatively chemo- and radioresistant and are treated by radical orchiectomy and surgical extirpation in general.

Especially in mixed germ cell tumors, the histology of the primary tumor may not conform to that of metastases, which may contain any combination of the primary tumor cell types. For example, adult teratomas may metastasize as teratomas or as embryonal carcinomas. It may be that relatively undifferentiated malignant primary tumor cells undergo a maturation process during metastasis.

Choriocarcinomas are among the most highly malignant tumors in the body. This fast-growing tumor develops from trophoblastic cells that form the placenta and help embryos attach to the uterus. They are rare (<2% of testis tumors) and most commonly observed in conjunction with embryonal carcinomas and teratocarcinomas. They uniformly secrete hCG into the serum. Grossly, they appear remarkably hemorrhagic and necrotic. Histologically, they consist of giant syncytiotrophoblastic cells with large, atypical nuclei intermingled with cytotrophoblasts, surrounding blood spaces, similar in structure to placental chorionic villi. Aggressive treatment with surgical resection and cisplatin-based chemotherapy has resulted in high cure rates.

Testicular germ cell cancers may begin in a noninvasive form called *carcinoma in situ* (CIS) or intratubular germ cell neoplasia. CIS may not always progress to invasive cancer, and it is estimated that it takes 5 years for CIS to progress to an invasive form of germ cell cancer. It is found in the contralateral testis in 5% of testis cancer cases. In addition, it is currently thought that CIS is the common precursor to all testis germ cell tumor types (except for juvenile yolk sac and teratoma tumors and

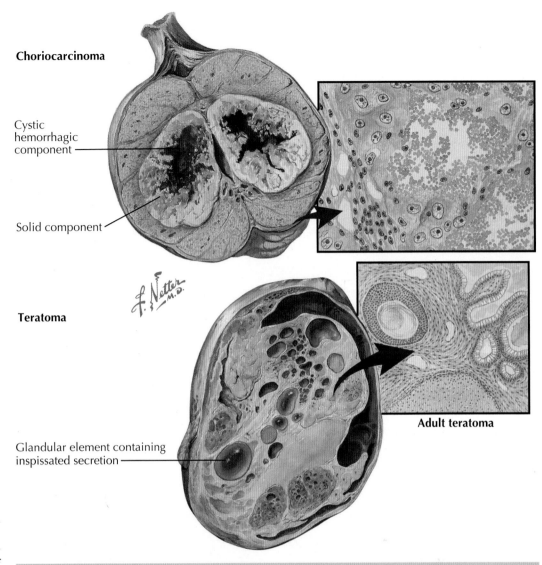

Choriocarcinoma

Cystic hemorrhagic component

Solid component

Teratoma

Glandular element containing inspissated secretion

Adult teratoma

In situ neoplasia of testis

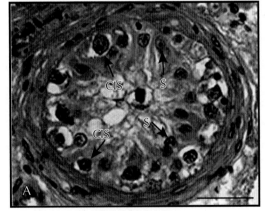

A. High power

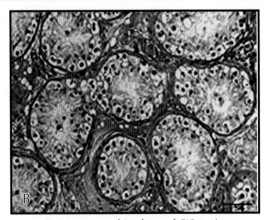

B. Low-power histology of CIS testis

spermatocytic seminomas). The assumption that CIS is the precursor of germ cell tumors is supported by the frequent observation of CIS in testis tissue surrounding invasive cancer and the development of invasive germ cell cancers in patients in whom CIS has been diagnosed. CIS causes no symptoms and has few findings, as it is generally found on testis biopsy. CIS cells are large with distinct nucleoli and are located in a single row at the usually thickened basement membrane of seminiferous tubules. Testicular tissue with CIS is frequently atrophic

and may be dysgenetic, with poorly differentiated tubules, poor spermatogenesis, and microcalcifications. The most common marker for CIS is PLAP, a tissue-specific alkaline phosphatase. The best treatment for CIS is controversial, because CIS does not always become invasive cancer. However, if treatment is chosen, localized low-dose radiotherapy (14–16 Gy) to the testis eradicates CIS and germ cells (and therefore fertility) while maintaining Leydig cell function and androgen balance in most males.

SEMINAL VESICLES AND PROSTATE

Plate 4.1   Reproductive System: VOLUME 1

PROSTATE AND SEMINAL VESICLES

The prostate, seminal vesicles, and bulbourethral glands of Cowper are the accessory glands of male reproduction and contribute to the makeup of seminal fluid. Prostatic secretions are acidic and constitute the first portion (10%–20%) of the ejaculate. The seminal vesicles contribute fluid of basic pH and account for the majority of seminal fluid (80%). Vasal fluid containing sperm constitutes the remainder of the ejaculate (10%). The adult prostate, a firm, rubbery organ weighing 20 g, is located inferior to the bladder neck and surrounds the posterior urethra. It is posterior and inferior to the symphysis pubis, superior to the urogenital diaphragm, and anterior to the rectal ampulla. The prostatic base abuts the bladder wall; posteriorly, a fascial sheath called *Denonvilliers fascia* (see Plate 2.1) separates the prostate from the rectal wall. The space of Retzius between the symphysis pubis and the anterior surface of the prostate and bladder is a potential space filled with connective tissue, fat, and a rich venous plexus. The cavernous nerves that control penile erection travel between the prostate and rectum at the 5 and 7 o'clock positions posteriorly and can be injured during prostate resection for cancer. The puboprostatic ligaments attach the lateral and anterior surfaces of the prostate to the symphysis pubis.

The current concept of prostate anatomy suggests that there are four basic anatomic regions or zones, including the anterior prostate, central gland, transition zone, and peripheral gland. The anterior prostate is entirely fibromuscular and nonglandular, and it appears to have little significance in prostatic function or pathology. This zone makes up approximately one-third of the bulk of prostatic tissue. The central gland is composed of the proximal urethra, the prostate tissue around the urethra and ejaculatory ducts, and the smooth muscle of the internal sphincter. It forms the central portion of the prostate and extends from the base of the prostate to the verumontanum. Although this zone accounts for only 5% to 10% of the glandular tissue in young males, it can exhibit significant growth with age. The transition zone immediately surrounds the urethra and is where benign prostatic hyperplasia (BPH) develops. The peripheral zone is composed entirely of acinar tissue of alveoli lined with columnar epithelium embedded in the relatively thick fibromuscular stroma and makes up 20% of the glandular volume. It constitutes the posterior surface of the prostate, including the apical, lateral, posterolateral, and anterolateral portions of the prostate. The prostatic alveoli drain through a system of branching ducts that empty into the floor and lateral surfaces of the posterior urethra. Prostatic acini may also contain soft bodies known as *corpora amylacea,* composed of prostatic secretions and epithelial cells. The peripheral zone represents approximately 75% of glandular volume in the adult prostate. The vast majority of prostatic carcinomas arise in the peripheral zone of the prostate. Normal prostatic secretions discharged with the ejaculate are milky and contain citric acid, choline, cholesterol, various enzymes, prostatic acid phosphatase, and prostate-specific antigen (PSA), a serine protease that liquefies

Ureteral orifice

Prostate
Utricle
Ejaculatory duct orifice
Cowper gland
Urogenital diaphragm
Membranous urethra
Openings of Cowper gland ducts

Colliculus
Urethral crest
Cavernous urethra

Frontal section

Sagittal section

Posterior view

Seminal vesicle
Ureter
Vas deferens

Superior fascia of urogenital diaphragm
Muscles of urogenital diaphragm
Ampulla of vas
Prostate
Cowper glands
Ischio-pubic ramus

Histology of prostate

Prostate superior view
Fibromuscular stroma
Transitional zone
Central zone
Urethra
Peripheral zone
Ampulla vas deferens
Seminal vesicle

Prostate transverse section
Fibromuscular stroma
Transitional zone
Urethra
Central zone
Peripheral zone

the seminal fluid 15 to 30 minutes after it is ejaculated as a coagulum.

The paired seminal vesicles, derived from the wolffian duct, are pouch-like structures 8 to 10 cm long that lie posterior to the bladder and anterior to the rectum. The distal end of the vas deferens (ampullary vas) and seminal vesicles fuse to form the paired ejaculatory ducts that enter the prostate posteriorly and terminate within the utricle in the posterior urethra (see Plate 2.12).

The seminal vesicles consist of tubular alveoli, separated by thin connective tissue, surrounded by a thick smooth muscle wall. The seminal vesicles serve as the "bladder" of the reproductive tract, contracting in response to hypogastric nerve stimulation and emptying fructose-rich fluid into the sperm-filled ejaculatory ducts during ejaculation. Hypogonadism results in a reduction in prostate and seminal vesicle glandular activity and decreased ejaculate volume.

Plate 4.2

Seminal Vesicles and Prostate

DEVELOPMENT OF PROSTATE

The glandular prostate originates from the epithelium of a narrow tube of cloacal mesoderm (primitive posterior, or prostatic urethra). Glandular tissue does not become evident until fetal week 10, when epithelial evaginations or buds extend posteriorly from the floor of the primitive urethra into the surrounding mesenchymal tissue. By the 11th week, lumina form within the epithelial cords and cellular buds form primitive acini. Mesenchymal cells differentiate into smooth muscle, fibroblasts, and blood vessels. During the 12th week, the epithelium continues to proliferate while connective tissue septae extend into the acini, and the stroma of the gland thins as the ducts and acini expand. By 13 to 15 weeks, testosterone concentrations have reached peak embryonic levels. Androgen-mediated epithelial-mesenchyme interactions cause simple cuboidal epithelial cells to differentiate. By the end of the 15th week, the secretory cells are functional, the basal cell population has developed, and scattered neuroendocrine cells are present. Maturation of the gland continues while embryonic testosterone levels are high; however, as testosterone levels fall during the third trimester, the gland enters a quiescent state that persists until puberty. At puberty, when testosterone levels again increase, the epithelium proliferates, giving rise to the complex folding seen in the mature gland. The prostate doubles in size during this phase of development, and as androgen receptors are expressed by epithelial cells, the full secretory phenotype is established.

During early prostate development, five groups of epithelial buds, tubules, or lobes develop and are termed (1) middle, (2) right lateral, (3) left lateral, (4) posterior, and (5) anterior. The term *lobes* used here should not be confused with the same term used to describe the cystoscopic view of prostatic enlargement later in life (see Plate 4.9). The lateral tubules, 37 to 40 in number, evaginate from the right and left lateral walls of the primitive urethra. Their orifices are located between the primitive bladder neck and the verumontanum ("mountain ridge"). As they grow posteriorly and outward, they eventually form the greater part of the gland, the peripheral zone, in the adult prostate. As they branch laterally, they extend superiorly to meet and form a commissure of glandular tissue in the ventral aspect of the adult prostate anterior to the urethra (the anterior zone).

The middle or median lobe develops from 7 to 12 tubules located in the floor of the urethra proximal to the ejaculatory ducts. They are separated from the lateral tubules by connective tissue and eventually become the central and transition zones.

The posterior lobe arises from 4 to 11 tubules that appear in the third month of development and arise from the floor of the urethra distal to the seminal colliculus. They eventually contribute, along with the lateral lobes, to the posterior zone of the prostate. The acini and ducts of the posterior lobe grow posteriorly behind the ejaculatory ducts, where they are separated from other prostatic zones by a layer of fibromuscular tissue in the adult. These tubules are large and are also separated by fibrous tissue from the ejaculatory ducts. Carcinoma of the prostate (see Plate 4.10) develops

more commonly in the posterior zone than in other prostatic regions, whereas benign hypertrophy (see Plates 4.7–4.9) originates mainly in the transition zone.

The anterior or ventral lobe consists at first of rather large and numerously branched tubules, averaging nine in number. At fetal age 16 weeks, these tubules begin to atrophy and in the newborn are reduced to a just few acini.

The 8 to 19 small tubules composing the subcervical glands of Albarrán develop under the floor of the prostatic urethra just distal to the bladder neck. These branching tubules are short and consist of fine and cylindrical epithelia. Other small tubules may also develop under the mucosa of the trigone (glands of Home). Neither set of tubules is a common source of hypertrophy or cancer in the adult.

Bladder

Albarrán subcervical glands
Urethra
Anterior lobe
Colliculus
Lateral lobe
Median lobe
Ejaculatory duct
Posterior lobe
Utricle
Lateral lobe

Schematic cross section above the level of the utricle

Anterior lobe
Urethra
Lateral lobe
Median lobe
Ejaculatory duct
Posterior lobe

Plate 4.3

Reproductive System: VOLUME 1

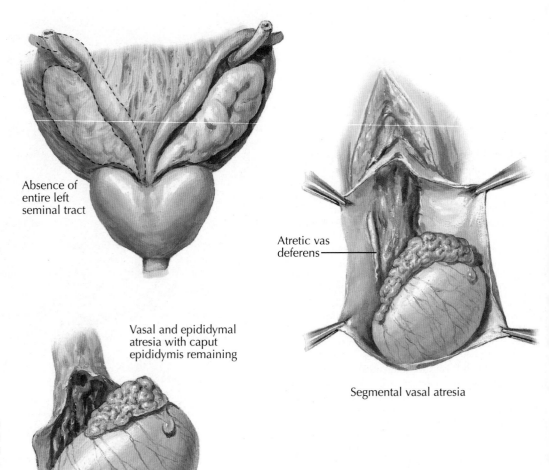

Absence of entire left seminal tract

Atretic vas deferens

Vasal and epididymal atresia with caput epididymis remaining

Segmental vasal atresia

2000 possible mutations in CFTR gene on chromosome 7 leads to faulty NaCl channels and buildup of mucus with cystic fibrosis.

Extracellular

Mucus buildup

Chloride ions

Intracellular

Normal NaCl channel

Faulty NaCl channel

J. Perkins
MS, MFA, CMI

SEMINAL VESICLE AGENESIS

The congenital absence of one or both seminal vesicles is part of a syndrome termed congenital absence of the vas deferens (CAVD). In the vast majority of cases CAVD is due to mutations in the cystic fibrosis transmembrane regulator gene *(CFTR)*. Mutations in *CFTR* occur in 1:2500 births and constitute the most common autosomal recessive disease in humans. *CFTR,* which encodes the cyclic adenosine monophosphate (cAMP)-regulated chloride channel, was initially cloned in 1989 from patients with cystic fibrosis. Currently, over 2000 different *CFTR* mutations have been described. Clinical features of cystic fibrosis include chronic pulmonary obstruction and infection, exocrine pancreatic insufficiency, neonatal meconium ileus, and male infertility.

Virtually all patients with cystic fibrosis have bilateral CAVD characterized by various defects in wolffian or mesonephric duct development (see Plate 1.2). Anatomically, the body and tail of the epididymis, vas deferens, seminal vesicles, and ejaculatory ducts are affected or absent, but the testis, and its efferent ducts, and a remnant of the caput epididymis are always present as they have divergent developmental origins.

As expected, seminal vesicle absence causes male infertility associated with low-volume, sterile semen. Interestingly, 1% to 2% of males who are infertile have CAVD without cystic fibrosis. These patients exhibit the same spectrum of wolffian duct defects as those with cystic fibrosis, but generally lack the severe pulmonary, pancreatic, and intestinal problems. Soon after *CFTR* was cloned in patients with cystic fibrosis, the same *CFTR* mutations were discovered in healthy males who are infertile with CAVD. Predictably, *CFTR* mutations are found very frequently in males who are infertile with CAVD and consist mainly of compound heterozygotes in which a different mutation exists in each of two *CFTR* copies on chromosome 7. In addition to formal *CFTR* mutations, another genetic abnormality found with CAVD consists of variations in the polythymidine tract in the splicing region of intron 8 (IVS8; 5T, 7T, and 9T regions), a noncoding sequence of DNA within *CFTR*. A reduction in the polythymidine tract decreases the efficiency of exon splicing, leading to a reduction in

CFTR mRNA and presumably a decrease in mature, functional CFTR protein, thus contributing to the CAVD phenotype. Isolated CAVD is now considered a genital form of cystic fibrosis. Infertility due to CAVD is generally treated by using sperm retrieval and assisted reproduction.

Although most patients with CAVD have bilaterally absent seminal vesicles, unilateral absence also occurs (CUAVD). Males who are affected are also clinically healthy except that they have a palpable vas deferens on

one side and can be naturally fertile. Importantly, generalized wolffian duct anomalies leading to seminal vesicle absence can occur from cystic fibrosis–unrelated gene mutations. Such patients, constituting roughly 10% of CAVD cases, have associated ipsilateral renal hypoplasia or agenesis and do not harbor known *CFTR* mutations. Finally, female partners of males affected with CAVD should be genetically screened and counseled for *CFTR* mutations to fully inform the couple of the residual risk of having offspring with cystic fibrosis.

Plate 4.4

Seminal Vesicles and Prostate

PELVIC AND PROSTATIC TRAUMA

Penetrating trauma to the prostate gland is rare as it is protected from penetrating objects by the surrounding bony pelvis. However, penetrating injury to the prostate is possible from broken pelvic bones as a consequence of pelvic fracture. The real concern with prostatic trauma, however, involves injury to the posterior and prostatomembranous urethra that lie superior to the urogenital diaphragm. This is most commonly a consequence of forceful blunt trauma to the pelvis.

Posterior urethral injuries may occur in three ways: (1) Internal trauma with perforation of the membranous and prostatic urethra during unskilled use of rigid endoscopy instruments such as sounds or cystoscopes. This usually results in only temporary injury to the prostatic parenchyma but can lead to more long-term "acquired" diverticula, prostatic abscess, or prostatorectal fistula. (2) External trauma with direct injury to the prostatic capsule by either missiles or sharp objects through the perineum. Although rare, these usually involve injury to Colles fascia and to the urogenital diaphragm as well (see Plate 2.19). (3) The most common and clinically important injuries involve damage to the prostatomembranous urethra from fractures of the bony pelvis. The prostate is firmly held in a relatively fixed position by the dense puboprostatic ligaments that attach its anterior surface to the undersurface of the os pubis (see Plate 4.1) and by its attachment by the urethra to the pelvic diaphragm inferiorly. However, the prostatomembranous urethra, measuring 1 cm long between the apex of the prostate and the urogenital diaphragm, is very fragile and easily subjected to disruption from shear force. Pelvic fracture and particularly separation of the symphysis pubis often dislocates the prostate and severs the prostatomembranous urethra from the urogenital diaphragm. Alternatively, bony os pubis fragments from the rami and ischium may sever the prostatomembranous urethra. Finally, any injury violent enough to disrupt the puboprostatic ligaments usually also injures the prostatomembranous urethra, even with minimal bony fractures.

Prostatomembranous urethral rupture should be considered in all cases of trauma to the pelvic girdle. The inability to urinate and blood at the urethral meatus are particularly important symptoms and signs. A rectal examination may reveal superior displacement of the prostate from its normal position, often to the point of impalpability. A retroperitoneal hematoma or urine extravasation may also accumulate and, when significant, may be palpated as a soft mass on rectal examination. Urethral catheterization should not be attempted in cases of pelvic injury and blood at the meatal tip unless retrograde urethrogram imaging reveals an intact urethra, as this procedure could convert a partial to complete urethral disruption.

The majority of posterior urethral injuries usually require urgent treatment of shock, bleeding, and fracture management. With urethral bleeding, the possibility of a coexistent intra- or extraperitoneal bladder rupture must also be considered. With an intact urethra and a small extraperitoneal bladder rupture, the simple insertion and maintenance of catheter drainage may be sufficient for early management. For intraperitoneal bladder rupture, surgical exploration and repair is generally needed.

With complete prostatomembranous urethral disruption, primary surgical reanastomosis of the urethra or primary realignment of the urethral ends over a catheter, performed immediately or in a delayed fashion, are necessary. Primary surgical repair is performed through perineal, transpubic, or suprapubic exposure and is partly determined by the limitations of patient positioning resulting from pelvic fracture and stability. Evacuation or drainage of extravasated urine is also advised. Failure to anastomose or accurately approximate the severed urethral ends leaves a mucosal defect that results in extensive cicatrix and stricture formation in the urethral gap. A significant delay in urethral realignment because of other life-threatening conditions allows a displaced prostate to become fixed by fibrous tissue and complicates alignment surgery. In addition to urethral stricture formation, erectile dysfunction is a common complication of this form of urethral injury.

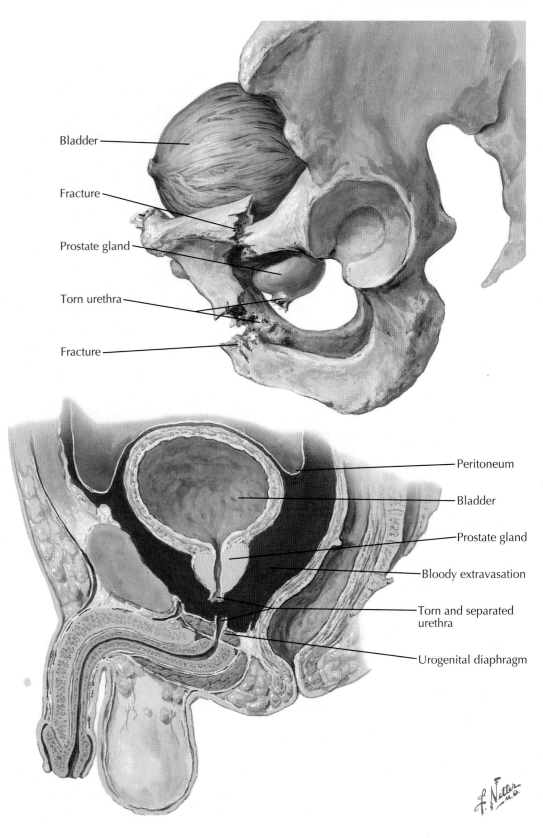

Bladder

Fracture

Prostate gland

Torn urethra

Fracture

Peritoneum

Bladder

Prostate gland

Bloody extravasation

Torn and separated urethra

Urogenital diaphragm

Plate 4.5

Reproductive System: VOLUME 1

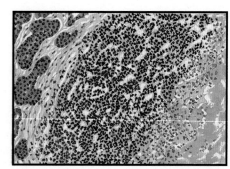

Section through edge of infarct. Leukocytic and round cell infiltration about zone of necrosis. Metaplasia of epithelium in adjacent acini.

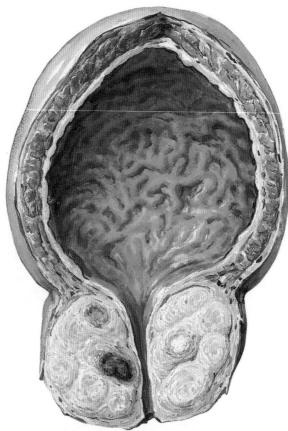

Infarcts in hypertrophic prostate (recent and healing infarcts on right side, old fibrosed infarct on left)

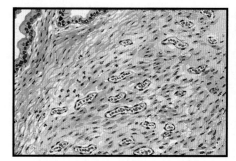

Section of healing infarct. Fibroblasts and new blood vessels growing in.

PROSTATIC INFARCT AND CYSTS

Prostatic infarction, recent or healed, is found in up to 25% of cases of benign hypertrophy when the excised glandular tissue is carefully studied. They generally produce few, if any, clinical symptoms but if large enough can mimic acute prostatitis or cause hematuria and urinary retention. The infarcted areas may be single, multiple, and up to several centimeters in size and are usually located around the periphery of an area of prostatic hyperplasia within the transition zone. They occur more often with significant hyperplasia and in instrumented patients, although they can occur without obvious cause or infection. Prostatic infarcts are thought to be due to arterial obstruction from enlarging hyperplastic nodules, infection, or inflammation on the urethral branches of the prostatic artery (see Plate 2.6).

Grossly, prostatic infarcts show mottled yellowish areas surrounded by a hemorrhagic margin. Within the area of infarction, the tissue loses its normal structure and becomes necrotic. Acutely, swelling and edema compress the surrounding acini. Interestingly, with infarction the epithelium of the immediately surrounding acini may be altered, in which normal cells are replaced by polygonal and sometimes squamous cells. This multiplication of cell layers often fills and obliterates the lumen of the adjacent acinus. Histologically, these cells lack characteristics of metaplasia, including keratinization and intercellular bridges, and therefore more closely resemble regenerative dysplastic cells than squamous epithelium. These marginal changes are not malignant or precancerous and should not be considered squamous cell carcinoma.

Prostatic cysts occur in 10% of adult males and generally have little clinical significance. They can be congenital due to müllerian or wolffian duct remnants. Other cysts may be of parasitic origin from schistosomiasis or *Echinococcus* infection. Hemorrhagic cysts can occur within degenerating areas of advanced prostatic carcinoma. The

Retention cysts of prostate

Sagittal section

Microscopic section showing compressed, flattened epithelial lining

Frontal view

common prostatic cyst is a simple retention cyst that arises from prostatic acini, generally beneath the trigone. It is likely a consequence of obstructed acini and can be multilobular from rupture of the thin walls between adjacent obstructed acini. Such cysts may project into the urethra or into the bladder neck. When located near the gland periphery, they may be palpable on rectal exam as soft, fluctuant masses. Prostatic retention cysts of 6 to 8 mm diameter are not uncommon, but larger cysts up to

several centimeters in size are relatively rare and can be symptomatic.

Prostatic cysts are lined by thin, flattened, columnar epithelia. When they project into the bladder or urethra, they are covered with the mucous epithelium of the surrounding structure. Cyst contents on aspiration appear thin and milky. Symptomatic cysts that project into the prostatic urethra or the bladder neck are easily removed by transurethral resection.

Plate 4.6

Seminal Vesicles and Prostate

PROSTATITIS

Prostatitis is the term given to a complex constellation of symptoms and findings related to the prostate. Currently, there are four general categories of clinically defined prostatitis. They are differentiated based on symptoms and the urinalysis findings of bacteruria and pyuria. The categories are acute bacterial (NIH class I), chronic bacterial (NIH class II), inflammatory (NIH class IIIA) or noninflammatory (NIH class IIIB), and asymptomatic inflammatory prostatitis (NIH class IV). Class III prostatitis is also termed chronic nonbacterial prostatitis/chronic prostatitis and pelvic pain syndrome (CPPS).

Acute bacterial prostatitis typically presents with acute urinary tract infection (UTI) symptoms and infected urine, typically with gram-negative organisms. It is unusual but may be related to urologic instrumentation and chronic catheter use. Clinically, it involves the acute onset of irritative voiding symptoms, dysuria, pelvic and perineal pain, fever, and hematuria. Not uncommonly, a rectal exam reveals a tender, "boggy" prostate. Cloudy, infected urine is a feature that differentiates it from prostatic infarction. Histologically, prostatic acini are filled with exudate, and the stroma is infiltrated with leukocytes. When severe, urinary retention may result, which is treated with urethral or suprapubic catheter drainage. The infection requires broad-spectrum, gram-negative antibiotics that are later adjusted to bacterial sensitivity.

Chronic bacterial prostatitis can occur with or without an antecedent acute form and is characterized by acute or chronic symptoms and infected urine. Patients experience recurrent episodes of bacterial UTI caused by the same organism, usually *Escherichia coli,* another gram-negative organism, or enterococcus. Between symptomatic episodes, lower urinary tract cultures can document an infected prostate gland as the focus of recurrent infections. Indwelling catheters, instrumentation, recurrent UTIs, bladder stones, or spread from distant infections such as abscessed teeth, bronchitis, pneumonia, or sinusitis may underlie this diagnosis. Chronic prostatitis can be asymptomatic but is usually associated with complaints of scrotal, penile, low back, inguinal, or perineal pain; sexual dysfunction; and irritative or obstructive urinary symptoms. The finding of a boggy or fluctuant prostate on rectal examination is unusual. Histologically, prostatic acini contain increased leukocytes and the stroma is infiltrated with plasma cells and varying degrees of fibrosis. Prostatic ducts can also be chronically inflamed and dilated, indicating an infection that extends from the urethra.

Class III inflammatory or noninflammatory prostatitis is not primarily a disease of the prostate or the result of an inflammatory process but is a moniker for a symptom complex suggestive of bacterial prostatitis but in the absence of bacteruria. More than 90% of patients who are symptomatic fall into this category of prostatitis. Symptom duration and intensity can be significant and can be associated with profound effects on patient quality of life. Pyuria can be present (IIIA) or absent (IIIB) in the urine, semen, or in the urethral fluid obtained after expressed prostatic massage. Urologic pain complaints are the primary component of this syndrome, and exclusion criteria include the presence of active urethritis, urogenital cancer, urinary tract disease, functionally significant urethral stricture, or neurologic disease affecting the bladder. This prostatitis category recognizes the limited understanding of the causes of this syndrome and the possibility that organs other than the prostate gland may be causally important.

Acute prostatitis

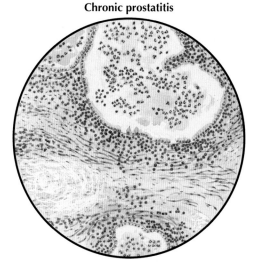

Histology. Polymorphonucleur leukocytes infiltrate the prostatic acini and the stroma.

Chronic prostatitis

Histology. A mixed infiltrate of neutrophils and lymphocytes is present, and the acini are separated by an increase in fibrotic stroma.

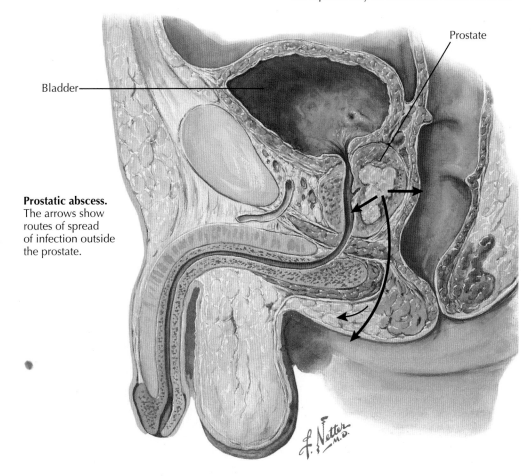

Bladder

Prostate

Prostatic abscess. The arrows show routes of spread of infection outside the prostate.

Asymptomatic inflammatory prostatitis is diagnosed in patients without a history of genitourinary tract pain complaints. The diagnosis is made during evaluation of other genitourinary tract issues, including (1) the finding of inflammation on a prostate biopsy for possible prostate cancer because of an elevated serum PSA level and (2) elevated leukocytes in the seminal fluid of patients who are infertile (pyospermia). Treatment is aimed at decreasing PSA levels or restoring normal semen quality, as pain is not a component of this diagnosis.

Prostatic abscess as a consequence of acute prostatitis is unusual with modern antibiotic therapy. Abscess can occur with metastasis from distant infectious foci or as a complication of immunosuppressive disease. Symptoms are similar to those of acute prostatitis, but stranguria and tenesmus are more common, along with acute urinary retention. Prostatic abscess can sometimes be detected on rectal examination with the finding of a boggy and tender gland. If untreated, the abscess usually spares rectal involvement due to Denonvilliers fascia posteriorly, but rupture and drainage into the posterior urethra is possible. Treatment with incision and drainage through endoscopic unroofing or transrectal or perineal drainage may be required along with appropriate antibiotics.

Plate 4.7

Reproductive System: VOLUME 1

PROSTATIC TUBERCULOSIS AND CALCULI

Tuberculous prostatitis is rare, but the gland is infected in about one of eight patients who die of tuberculosis. Tuberculous prostatitis is observed in 75% to 90% of tuberculosis involving the genitourinary tract. If the infection is confined to the genitourinary tract, the prostate and seminal vesicles are involved in 100% of cases, whereas epididymitis occurs in about 60% of cases. Most males who are affected (80%) are younger than 50 years. It is generally assumed that tuberculous prostatitis develops secondary to active tuberculosis elsewhere in the body and through a hematogenous route.

Of males with prostatic tuberculosis, 50% have dysuria and 40% have perineal pain. Patients may also present with male infertility, a well-described complication of prostatic tuberculosis. Sterile urethral discharge or pyuria and terminal hematuria may also be associated with this condition. Rarely, perineal swelling, drainage, and urinary fistula constitute the most overt presentation. Tuberculous prostatitis may also be painless and may remain undiscovered except when palpated by rectal examination in cases of urinary tract or epididymal tuberculosis. When the prostate is involved, its palpation may reveal a normal or enlarged gland that is irregular or nodular in contour, and firm or granular in consistency. Soft areas can be palpated when caseation is present. Tuberculosis in the prostate does not differ from that encountered elsewhere in the body. Histologically, there is destruction of normal glandular tissue and replacement by a crumbly, yellow mass of caseous material surrounded by fibrous capsules. Healing proceeds with fibrosis and calcification. After antibiotic treatment, the prostate may become fibrotic.

Prostatic calculi may be found with or without glandular hyperplasia. They contain protein, cholesterol, citrates, and inorganic salts, mostly calcium and magnesium phosphate. Most cases are encountered in patients older than 40 years. Calculi are located diffusely within dilated acini and this distribution can, although not necessarily, be associated with other pathologic findings, such as prostatitis. It is difficult to establish whether conditions

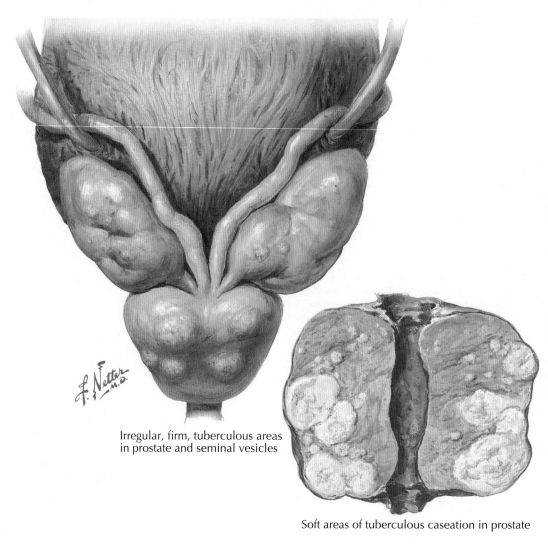

Irregular, firm, tuberculous areas in prostate and seminal vesicles

Soft areas of tuberculous caseation in prostate

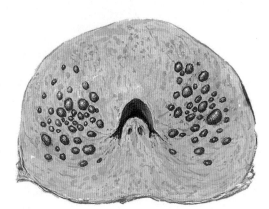

Calculi (diffuse) in chronic prostatitis

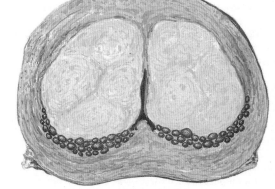

Calculi associated with benign prostatic hyperplasia

precede the formation of calculi or vice versa. The symptoms and urinary findings in cases of calculi are characteristic of chronic prostatitis and not usually due to the presence of calculi alone. However, calculi may be the source of recurrent prostatitis if bacterial infection cannot be cleared in their presence.

Calculi that occur at the junction of the transition and posterior zones of the prostate are called *corpora amylacea* and are common in patients with benign enlargement of the prostate. They are thought to occur

because as prostatic secretions become "inspissated" from the disarray of the duct architecture from benign prostatic hyperplasia they eventually calcify. The diagnosis is usually made when calcifications are visualized on transrectal ultrasound imaging. On rare occasions, calculi protrude into the posterior urethra from the orifice of a prostatic duct and grow into a urethral calculus. In most cases, prostatic calculi are not specifically treated as they are incidental findings from prostatic imaging.

Plate 4.8

Seminal Vesicles and Prostate

HEMATOSPERMIA

Hematospermia or hemospermia is defined as the macroscopic presence of blood in the semen. It has been documented in medicine since the time of Hippocrates. Generally considered a benign condition, the true incidence of hemospermia is unclear, but it likely occurs in less than 0.5% of males younger than 50 years. It is most prevalent in younger males, with a mean age of 37 years at presentation. It is typically painless. The time from symptom onset to medical presentation is short due to the visually alarming nature of the disorder. Most (75%) affected patients present for care after only one or two episodes of bloody semen. The disorder can be acute or chronic and ranges in duration from 1 to 24 months.

The etiology of hemospermia is multifactorial. Anatomic sources of blood in semen include the seminal vesicles, prostate, epididymides, vasa deferentia, and urethra. Inflammation and infection in any of these constituent organs constitute the largest root causes (40%). Traumatic mucosal irritation occurs with prostatic and seminal vesicle calculi and seminal vesicle cysts. Infections with bacteria, viruses, mycobacteria, and parasites have been described, the most common of which are *Enterococcus faecalis*, herpes simplex, *Chlamydia trachomatis*, tuberculosis, and *Ureaplasma urealyticum*. Iatrogenic causes due to urethral instrumentation, transrectal ultrasound prostate biopsies, and external beam and brachytherapy radiation therapy for prostate cancer are becoming increasingly common. Ejaculatory duct obstruction from utricular (müllerian) and wolffian cysts or ectopic calcification within the utricle is another common cause of hemospermia. Benign urethral polyps and proliferative urethritis are more uncommon obstructive causes of bloody semen. Prostate, testicular, and seminal vesicle malignancies have been reported in 3% of cases. Arteriovenous and congenital malformations of the seminal vesicles and verumontanum are much rarer causes of hemospermia. Bleeding diatheses from anticoagulant therapy and metabolic disorders such as von Willebrand disease, hemophilias, and liver disease have also been associated with hemospermia. Despite this wide variety of underlying causes, a significant number of hemospermia cases remain idiopathic.

The medical evaluation of hemospermia is performed with the goal of identifying treatable and life-threatening conditions. The amount, color, frequency, and duration of hemospermia is ascertained. Persistent or recurrent episodes of bloody semen in an older male (>50 years) typically merit a more thorough evaluation. The sexual partner should be excluded as an underlying cause and can be verified by the finding of bloody semen with condom use. A thorough medical history should identify significant risk factors as previously outlined. The physical examination should include vital signs to identify fevers or hypertension, an abdominal examination to identify hepatomegaly or splenomegaly, and a thorough genital and rectal exam that includes inspection of the urethral meatus, spermatic cords, testes, and epididymides for masses or tenderness. With single episodes of hemospermia in young patients, no further evaluation is needed. With recurrent hemospermia or its occurrence in older males, the evaluation should include a sexually transmitted disease panel (chlamydia, gonorrhea, ureaplasma) and herpes viral titers, a midstream urinalysis for culture and sensitivity, and acid-fast or parasitic evaluation if the history is suggestive of exposures. A semen analysis can be very valuable in distinguishing

Congenital variations in ejaculatory duct anatomy

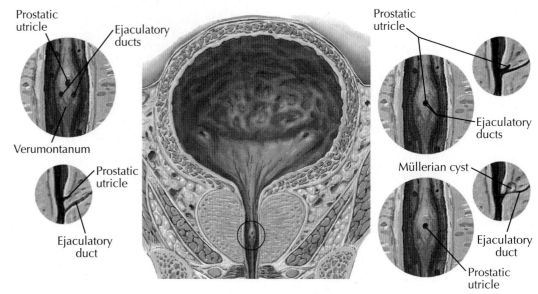

Possible causes of hematospermia

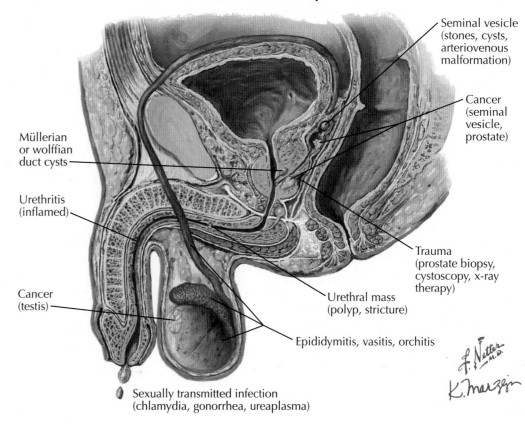

true hemospermia from other causes of ejaculate discoloration. Likewise, a serum PSA is indicated in males older than 50 years to screen for prostate cancer or prostatitis. The best imaging technology for delineating anatomic causes of bloody semen is transrectal ultrasound (TRUS), which detects lesions in 75% of recurrent cases that have failed conservative management. T2-weighted magnetic resonance imaging of the pelvis is another excellent imaging technology for seminal vesicle and accessory sex gland anatomy, and its ability to localize blood is especially relevant for hemospermia. Cystoscopy and seminal vesicle aspiration are last-resort options for this condition.

Treatment for hemospermia is directed at root causes. In the majority of cases, bleeding is self-limited and is managed expectantly. Infectious causes are treated specifically. Empirical antibiotic treatment is considered when infection is suspected but not confirmed on diagnostic testing. Anatomic lesions such as ejaculatory duct stones, cysts, or urethral polyps are generally transurethrally incised or excised. Seminal vesicle cysts or malformations can be excised laparoscopically. There is anecdotal evidence that finasteride may help resolve symptoms in cases of chronic idiopathic hemospermia.

Plate 4.9

Reproductive System: VOLUME 1

EJACULATORY DUCT OBSTRUCTION

Ejaculatory duct obstruction (EDO) underlies 1% to 5% of male infertility. Although originally described in males with azoospermia with complete blockage, it is now clear that EDO is a more complex anatomic condition that can take several forms.

The ejaculatory ducts are paired, collagenous tubes that commence at the junction of the ampullary vas deferens and seminal vesicle, course through the prostate, and empty into the prostatic urethra at the verumontanum. The duct has three regions: an extraprostatic portion, a middle intraprostatic segment, and a distal segment within the verumontanum. Ejaculatory continence is maintained and urinary reflux prevented by the acute angle of duct insertion into the urethra.

Physiologically, the relationship between the seminal vesicle and ejaculatory duct is similar to that of bladder and urethra. Just as bladder outlet obstruction can result from prostatic blockage, so too can physical blockage of the ejaculatory ducts cause EDO. By similar reasoning, "functional" or neurologic dysfunction of the seminal vesicle may be similar to voiding dysfunction due to bladder myopathy. At times, a "functional" issue can be mistaken for "physical" ejaculatory duct blockage, thus adding further complexity to the diagnosis of EDO.

Ejaculatory duct obstruction presents with infertility, postejaculatory pain, or hemospermia. Low-volume azoospermia defines complete or classic EDO and represents the physical blockage of both ducts. Unilateral complete or bilateral partial physical obstruction results in incomplete or partial EDO. Both are associated with either one or more of low ejaculate volume, postejaculatory pain, or hemospermia. However, partial EDO is uniquely associated with oligoasthenospermia.

EDO can result from seminal vesicle calculi, müllerian duct (utricular) or wolffian duct (diverticular) cysts, postinflammatory scar tissue, medications or medical conditions, calcification, or congenital ductal atresia. With congenital blockage, genetic evaluation for cystic fibrosis gene mutations is indicated (see Plate 4.3). Transrectal ultrasound may reveal dilated seminal vesicles, ejaculatory duct cysts, calculi, absence of the vas, or müllerian duct remnants. Associated risk factors for EDO include prior urinary tract infection, epididymitis, perineal trauma, orchalgia, and perineal pain. It is important to discontinue medications that may impair ejaculation. Although rare, a digital rectal examination revealing enlarged, palpable seminal vesicles may suggest EDO.

Procedures used to confirm the diagnosis of EDO include seminal vesicle sperm aspiration (a normal seminal vesicle should not have sperm in it, unlike a blocked one), contrast seminovesiculography (injection of contrast in a manner similar to vasography to locate the obstruction), and seminal vesicle chromotubation (a variant of vesiculography in which colored dye is injected and ejaculatory duct patency assessed visually). A prospective study of these three techniques deemed patency with chromotubation the most accurate way to diagnosis ejaculatory duct obstruction.

Because of the complexity of diagnosing partial EDO, testing has been developed that can differentiate physical from functional forms of EDO. Similar to the concept of urodynamics for bladder outlet obstruction, ejaculatory duct manometry measures the "opening pressures" of the ejaculatory duct, defined as the pressure above which fluid from the seminal vesicle that passes through the ejaculatory duct enters the prostatic urethra. Patients who are fertile have remarkably consistent and low opening

pressures, defined as <45 cm H_2O, and males who are infertile with EDO have significantly higher ED pressures. Based on the well-established pressure-flow concept used to evaluate bladder outlet obstruction, diagnostic ED manometry can differentiate complete from partial, and physical from functional forms of EDO.

Once EDO is confirmed diagnostically, the treatment is transurethral incision or resection of the ejaculatory ducts (TURED), performed in an outpatient setting under anesthesia. Similar to transurethral

resection of the prostate for BPH, the technique combines cystourethroscopy with resection of the verumontanum in the midline (for complete obstruction) or laterally (for unilateral obstruction) with cutting current. When performed correctly, cloudy, milky fluid is usually seen refluxing from the opened ducts. Postoperatively, a small Foley catheter is placed for 24 hours. Impressive and durable increases in semen quality and fertility are common after the procedure.

Ejaculatory duct anatomy

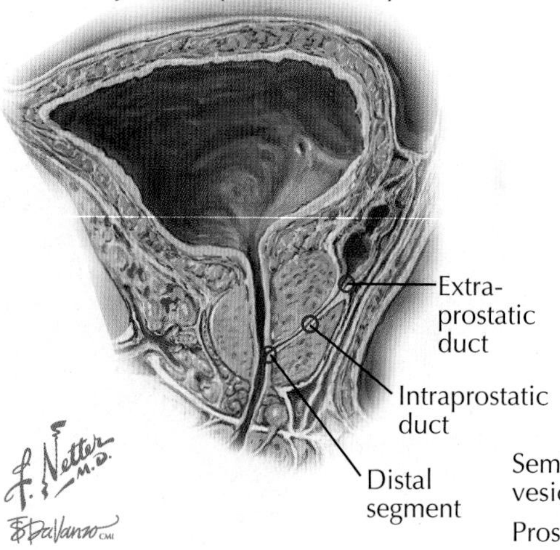

Extra-prostatic duct
Intraprostatic duct
Distal segment

Diagnosis of EDO by ejaculatory duct manometry

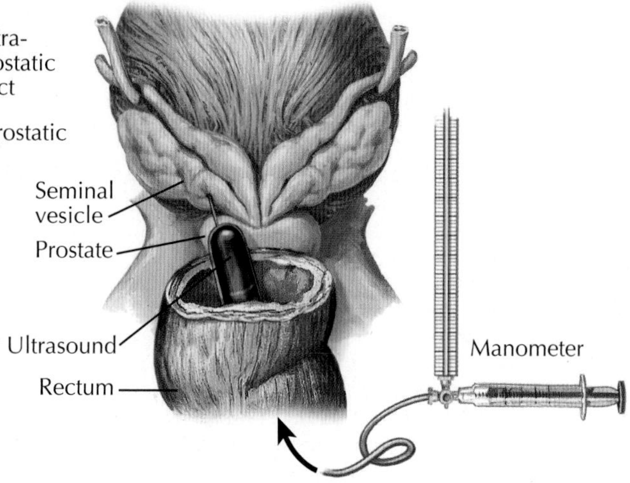

Seminal vesicle
Prostate
Ultrasound
Rectum
Manometer

TURED procedure

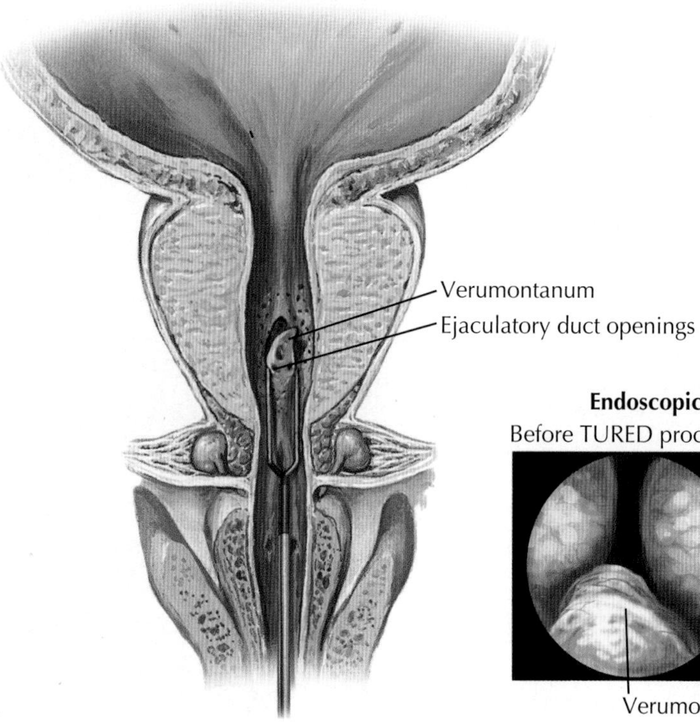

Verumontanum
Ejaculatory duct openings

Endoscopic view of TURED for EDO

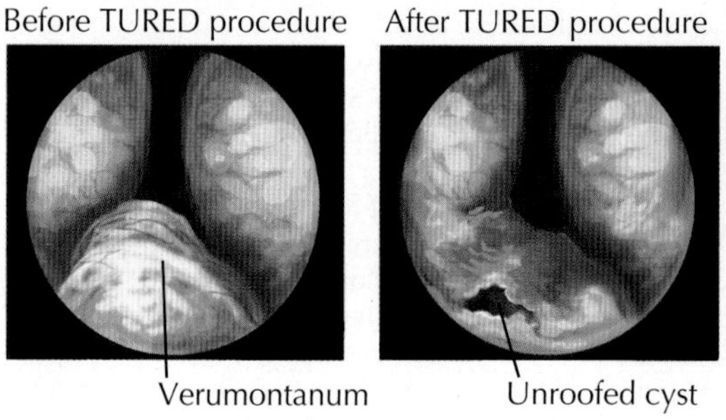

Before TURED procedure   After TURED procedure

Verumontanum   Unroofed cyst

Plate 4.10

Seminal Vesicles and Prostate

SEMINAL VESICLE SURGICAL APPROACHES

The seminal vesicle is a uniquely male organ, derived from the mesonephric duct (see Plate 1.2) beginning at 13 fetal weeks. The normal adult seminal vesicle is 5 to 8 cm in length, less than 1.5 cm in width, and has a volume of 10 mL. The blood supply is derived from the deferential artery or, occasionally, from branches of the inferior vesical artery. The seminal vesicles receive innervation from adrenergic fibers via the hypogastric nerve.

Primary pathologic states of the organ are rare. Congenital lesions include ureteral ectopy, cysts, and aplasia, many of which can be managed expectantly. Infections of the seminal vesicles are uncommon, but tuberculosis and schistosomiasis can cause masses, abscesses, and calcifications. Primary benign tumors include papillary adenoma, cystadenoma, fibroma, and leiomyoma. Malignant neoplasms are extremely rare and include papillary adenocarcinoma and sarcoma. Radical excision of the organ is the standard treatment for malignancy. Far more common than primary malignancy is secondary involvement from adenocarcinoma of the bladder, prostate, or rectum, and lymphoma. Few established alternatives to surgery exist for seminal vesicle tumors.

A variety of open surgical approaches to the seminal vesicles have been described, including transvesical, transperineal, paravesical, retrovesical, and transcoccygeal methods. In addition, a laparoscopic retrovesical approach has gained popularity. The chosen approach depends on the nature of the lesion to be excised and surgeon experience.

TRANSVESICAL APPROACH

With the patient supine, an infraumbilical, extraperitoneal incision is made, the rectus muscles separated, and the space of Retzius entered. A Balfour retractor exposes the anterior bladder wall, which is then opened with a vertical incision. The retractor is repositioned within the bladder to expose the trigone and posterior bladder wall. With a cutting Bovie, a vertical incision is made through the trigone near the bladder neck and the ampullae of the vasa deferentia are visualized posteriorly. The seminal vesicles are identified lateral to the ampullae, dissected free, ligated, and divided. A metal clip placed across the cut end of the seminal vesicle minimizes organ spillage. The distal vascular pedicle is identified and controlled with clips or ties, and the organ is removed. Too deep a dissection risks violating Denonvilliers fascia and entering the rectum.

TRANSPERINEAL APPROACH

This approach to seminal vesiculectomy is virtually identical to that described for radical perineal prostatectomy (see Plate 4.18). To adequately expose the seminal vesicle, the rectum should be dissected off the posterior prostate to a point higher than that needed for perineal prostatectomy. The vasal ampullae can be spared for the excision of a simple seminal vesicle cyst or small tumor but may need resection in the setting of cancer or infection.

PARAVESICAL AND RETROVESICAL APPROACHES

The paravesical approach commences with an infraumbilical incision to expose the space of Retzius, and the

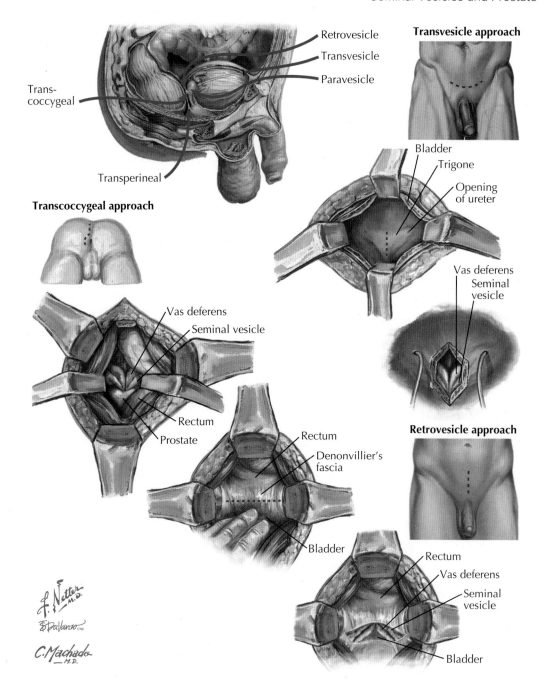

bladder is bluntly dissected away from the pelvic side wall. The vas deferens is tracked medially toward the bladder base to help locate the seminal vesicle. The plane between the bladder and seminal vesicle is developed laterally to medially. As the seminal vesicle is dissected, the awareness that the vas deferens crosses over the ureter helps avoid ureteral injury. The bladder is rolled medially for better exposure. The neck of the seminal vesicle is defined at the prostate base and the organ ligated with absorbable suture.

The retrovesical approach is appropriate for bilateral seminal vesicle excision of small cysts or tumors. A midline, infraumbilical, intraperitoneal incision is made to gain access to the bladder dome and the cul-de-sac between bladder and rectum. The small and large bowel are packed superiorly, and the peritoneal reflection near the posterior bladder is incised over the rectum. With sharp dissection, the bladder is peeled forward off the rectum until the ampullae and the seminal vesicle apices are visualized. In a manner similar to the paravesical approach, the seminal vesicles are dissected to the

prostatic base and the organ ligated. The retrovesical approach is currently most commonly performed laparoscopically (see Plate 4.20).

TRANSCOCCYGEAL APPROACH

Less commonly used, this dissection is appropriate for individuals in whom the perineum or lower abdomen is not accessible because of limitations in patient positioning or due to multiple prior surgeries. With the patient in the prone, jackknife position, an incision is made along the coccyx and angled into a gluteal cleft. The coccyx is removed and the gluteus maximus muscle retracted laterally to expose the rectosigmoid colon. After Denonvilliers fascia is incised deep to the rectum, it is dissected off the prostate with exposure of the seminal vesicles. Injury to the neurovascular bundle is more likely with this approach because it is directly in the path of dissection. After the seminal vesicles are removed, the rectum is carefully inspected for injury. The wound is closed in anatomic layers, and a drain is placed.

SPERM AND EJACULATION

Plate 5.1

Reproductive System: VOLUME 1

ANATOMY OF A SPERM

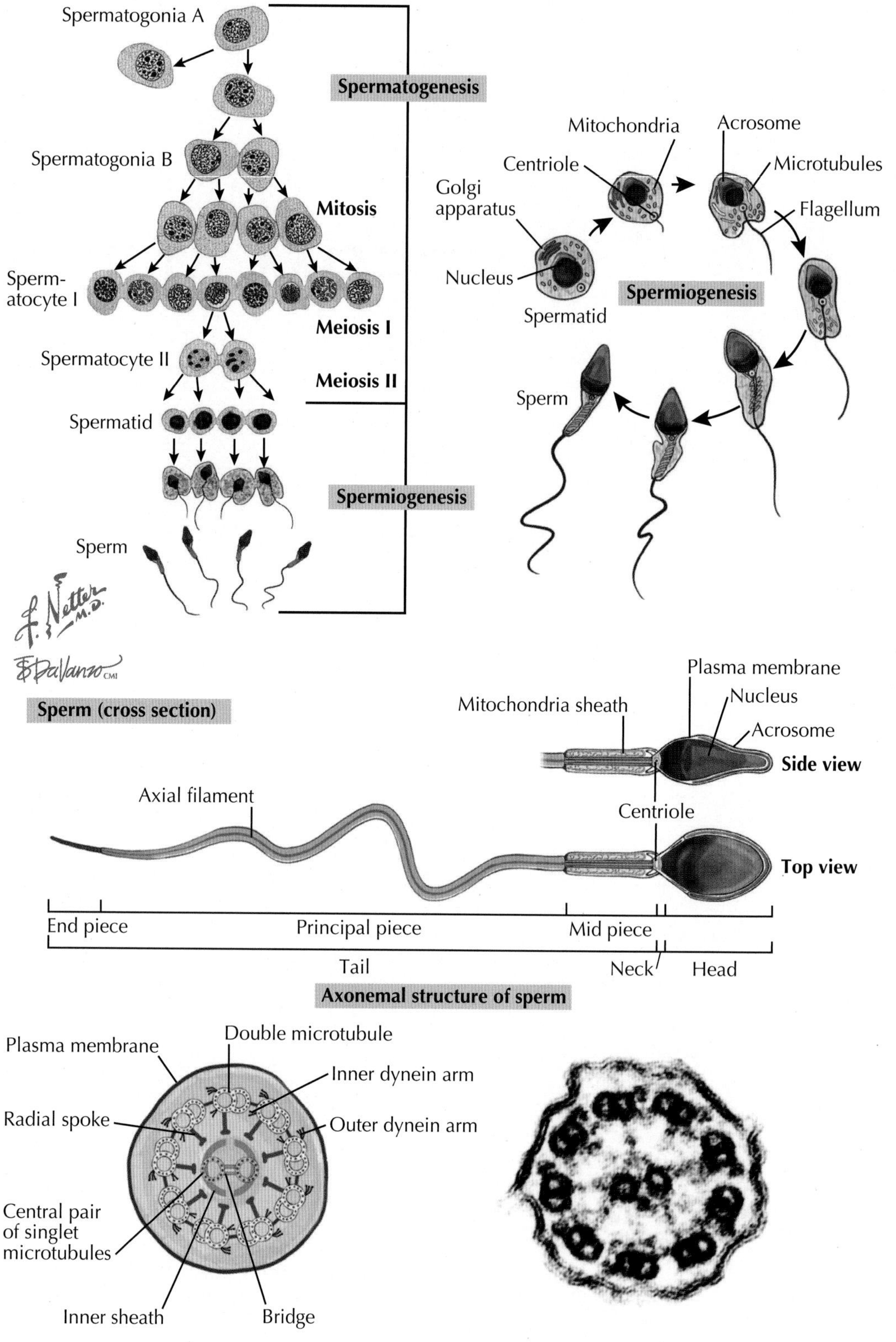

The mature spermatozoon is an elaborate, specialized cell produced in massive quantity, up to 1200 per second. Spermatogenesis begins when type B spermatogonia divide mitotically to produce diploid primary spermatocytes ($2n$), which then duplicate their DNA during interphase. After a meiotic division, each daughter cell contains one partner of the homologous chromosome pair, and they are called *secondary spermatocytes* ($2n$). These cells rapidly enter a second meiotic division in which the chromatids then separate at the centromere to yield haploid early-round spermatids (n). Thus theoretically, each primary spermatocyte yields four spermatids, although fewer actually result, as the complexity of meiosis is associated with germ cell loss.

The process by which spermatids become mature spermatozoa within the Sertoli cell takes several weeks and consists of several events: the acrosome is formed from the Golgi apparatus; a flagellum is constructed from the centriole; mitochondria reorganize around the midpiece; the nucleus is compacted to about 10% of its former size; and residual cell cytoplasm is eliminated. With completion of spermatid elongation, the Sertoli cell cytoplasm retracts around the developing sperm, stripping it of unnecessary cytoplasm and extruding the sperm into the tubule lumen. The mature sperm has remarkably little cytoplasm.

The human spermatozoon is approximately 60 μm in length and is divided into three anatomic sections: head, neck, and tail. The oval sperm head, about 4.5 μm long and 3 μm wide, consists of a nucleus containing highly compacted chromatin, and an acrosome, a membrane-bound organelle harboring the enzymes required for penetration of the outer vestments of the egg before fertilization. The sperm neck maintains the connection between the sperm head and tail. It consists of the connecting piece and proximal centriole. The axonemal complex extends from the proximal centriole through the sperm tail. The tail harbors the midpiece, principal piece, and endpiece. The midpiece is 7 to 8 μm long and is the most proximal segment of the tail, terminating in the annulus. It contains the axoneme, which is the 9 + 2 microtubule arrangement, and surrounding outer dense fibers. It also contains the mitochondrial sheath helically arranged around the outer dense fibers. The outer dense fibers, rich in disulfide bonds, are not contractile proteins but are thought to provide the sperm tail with the elastic rigidity necessary for progressive motility. Similar in structure to the midpiece, the principal piece has several columns of outer dense fibers that are replaced by the fibrous sheath. The fibrous sheath consists of longitudinal columns and transverse ribs. The sperm terminates in the endpiece, the most distal segment of sperm tail, which contains axonemal structures and the fibrous sheath. Except for the end-piece region, the spermatozoon is enveloped by a highly specialized plasma membrane that regulates the transmembrane movement of ions and other molecules.

The spermatozoon is a remarkably complex metabolic and genetic machine. The 75 mitochondria that surround the axoneme contain enzymes required for oxidative metabolism and produce adenosine triphosphate (ATP), the primary energy molecule for the cell. Mitochondria are semiautonomous organelles that produce cellular energy and can also cause apoptotic cell death through the release of cytochrome c. Mitochondria are composed of double (outer and inner) membranes. Five distinct respiratory chain complexes span

Spermatogonia A

Spermatogenesis

Spermatogonia B

Mitosis

Sperm-atocyte I

Meiosis I

Spermatocyte II

Meiosis II

Spermatid

Spermiogenesis

Sperm

Golgi apparatus

Centriole

Mitochondria

Acrosome

Microtubules

Flagellum

Nucleus

Spermatid

Spermiogenesis

Sperm

Sperm (cross section)

Plasma membrane

Nucleus

Acrosome

Mitochondria sheath

Side view

Axial filament

Centriole

Top view

End piece

Principal piece

Mid piece

Tail

Neck

Head

Axonemal structure of sperm

Double microtubule

Plasma membrane

Inner dynein arm

Radial spoke

Outer dynein arm

Central pair of singlet microtubules

Inner sheath

Bridge

the width of the inner membrane and are necessary for oxidative phosphorylation: the NADPH dehydrogenase, succinate dehydrogenase, cytochrome $bc1$, cytochrome c oxidase, and ATP synthase complexes. The sperm axoneme contains enzymes and structural proteins necessary for the chemical transduction of ATP into mechanical movement. The plasma membrane covering the sperm-head region harbors specialized proteins that participate in sperm-egg interaction.

The axoneme is the true motor assembly and requires 200 to 300 proteins to function. Among these, the microtubules are the best-understood components. Sperm microtubules are arranged in the classic 9 + 2 pattern of nine outer doublets encircling an inner central doublet. The protein dynein extends from one microtubule doublet to the adjacent doublet and forms both the inner and outer "arms" of the axoneme. Sperm with outer arm mutants have reduced motility and those with inner arm mutants have no motility. Radial links or spokes connect a microtubule of each doublet to the central inner doublet and consist of a complex of proteins. Tektins are proteins associated with the outer microtubular doublets, and nexin links are proteins that connect the outer doublets to each other and maintain the cylindrical axonemal shape.

Plate 5.2

Sperm and Ejaculation

SEMEN ANALYSIS AND SPERM MORPHOLOGY

Although not an accurate measure of fertility, the semen analysis, if abnormal, suggests that the probability of achieving fertility is lower than normal. For a male infertility evaluation, two semen analyses, performed with 2 to 3 days of sexual abstinence, are sought due to the large biologic variability in semen quality. Lubricants should be avoided and the specimen kept at body temperature during transport.

Normal values have been defined for the human semen analysis by evidence-based criteria (World Health Organization). Fresh semen is a coagulum that liquefies from 5 to 30 minutes after ejaculation. After liquefaction, semen viscosity is measured and should not show any stranding. Ejaculate volume should be at least 1.5 mL, as smaller volumes may not sufficiently buffer against vaginal acidity. Although most commonly a consequence of collection error, low ejaculate volume may also indicate retrograde ejaculation, ejaculatory duct obstruction, or androgen deficiency. Sperm concentration should be >15 million sperm/mL. Reasons for low sperm concentrations can include medications, exposures, systemic disease, hormonal disorders, varicocele, unilateral blockage, and genetic syndromes. Sperm motility is assessed in two ways: the proportion of all sperm that are moving and the quality of sperm movement. A normal value for sperm motility is 43% motile along with an average quality or progression score. The causes of low sperm motility, the most common abnormal semen analysis finding, are myriad and often reversible.

There has been debate recently concerning precisely which semen analysis values should be considered "normal," as controlled studies of fertile and infertile couples suggested other thresholds may be more appropriate, and sperm production is known to be susceptible to wide individual, geographic, and seasonal variation. When assessing semen quality, it is important to realize that spermatogenesis takes 60 to 80 days to complete, so that an individual semen analysis reflects biologic influences occurring 2 to 3 months prior. Likewise, medical or surgical therapy directed at improving semen quality will take several months to become manifest in improved semen quality.

Although seasonal variation exists, sperm production is a rapid and relatively constant process in humans. This is in part due to the anatomy of sperm production within the seminiferous tubules. A cycle of spermatogenesis involves the division of primitive germ cells into later germ cells. Many cycles of spermatogenesis coexist within the germinal epithelium at any one time, and they are described morphologically as stages. In addition, there is also a specific organization of spermatogenic cycles within the tubular space, termed spermatogenic waves. Although well described in other mammals, the exact configuration of spermatogenic waves in humans has been debated. The best evidence suggests that human spermatogenesis exists in a spiral or helical cellular arrangement that ensures that sperm production is a continuous and not a pulsatile process.

The formal evaluation of sperm shape is termed morphologic assessment. Several descriptive systems exist to evaluate morphology and within each system sperm are designated normal or abnormal based on specific size criteria. Although it is essentially judging a book by its cover, since the late 1980s it has been believed that sperm morphology may correlate with fertility potential as reflected by in vitro fertilization (IVF). In general, the percentage of sperm with normal morphology has the

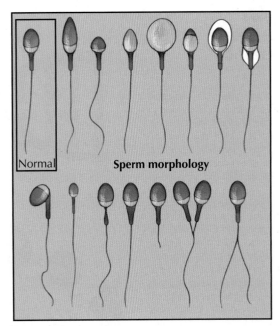

Normal | Sperm morphology

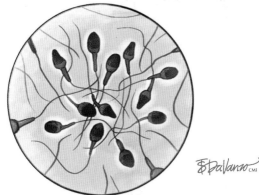

Sperm viewed under microscope

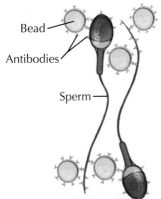

Bead

Antibodies

Sperm

Sperm antisperm antibody test (Immunobead method)

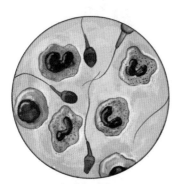

Seminal leukocytes

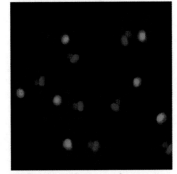

Evaluation of sperm chromosomes (FISH method)

greatest discriminatory power among all descriptors of semen quality in distinguishing fertile from infertile semen, although no particular value is diagnostic of fertility. Sperm morphology can be altered by toxic and occupational exposures, varicocele, fevers, medications, and systemic disease. It appears that sperm morphology is a sensitive indicator of overall testicular health, because the sperm morphologic characteristics are determined during spermatogenesis.

Other fertility assays can evaluate whether the seminal environment is abnormal, which may contribute to male infertility. Two such tests include an evaluation for excessive semen leukocytes (leukocytospermia) and testing for antisperm antibodies that can inhibit sperm

transport through the female reproductive tract and impair sperm–egg interaction at fertilization. Sperm genetics can also be directly assessed for chromosomal normalcy with in situ hybridization techniques. More recently, sperm DNA fragmentation testing in which tightly wound sperm DNA is unraveled in vitro in neutral, acidic, or basic environments to examine the integrity of the double-stranded DNA helix, has shown to correlate with natural fertility and embryo development. It also appears that sperm epigenetic patterns of both repressed and expressed genes show similar correlations to fertility. These tests can complement the routine semen analysis in the male evaluation and better estimate the chances of fertility.

Plate 5.3

Reproductive System: VOLUME 1

OLIGOSPERMIA: SPERM PRODUCTION PROBLEMS—GENETIC AND EPIGENETIC

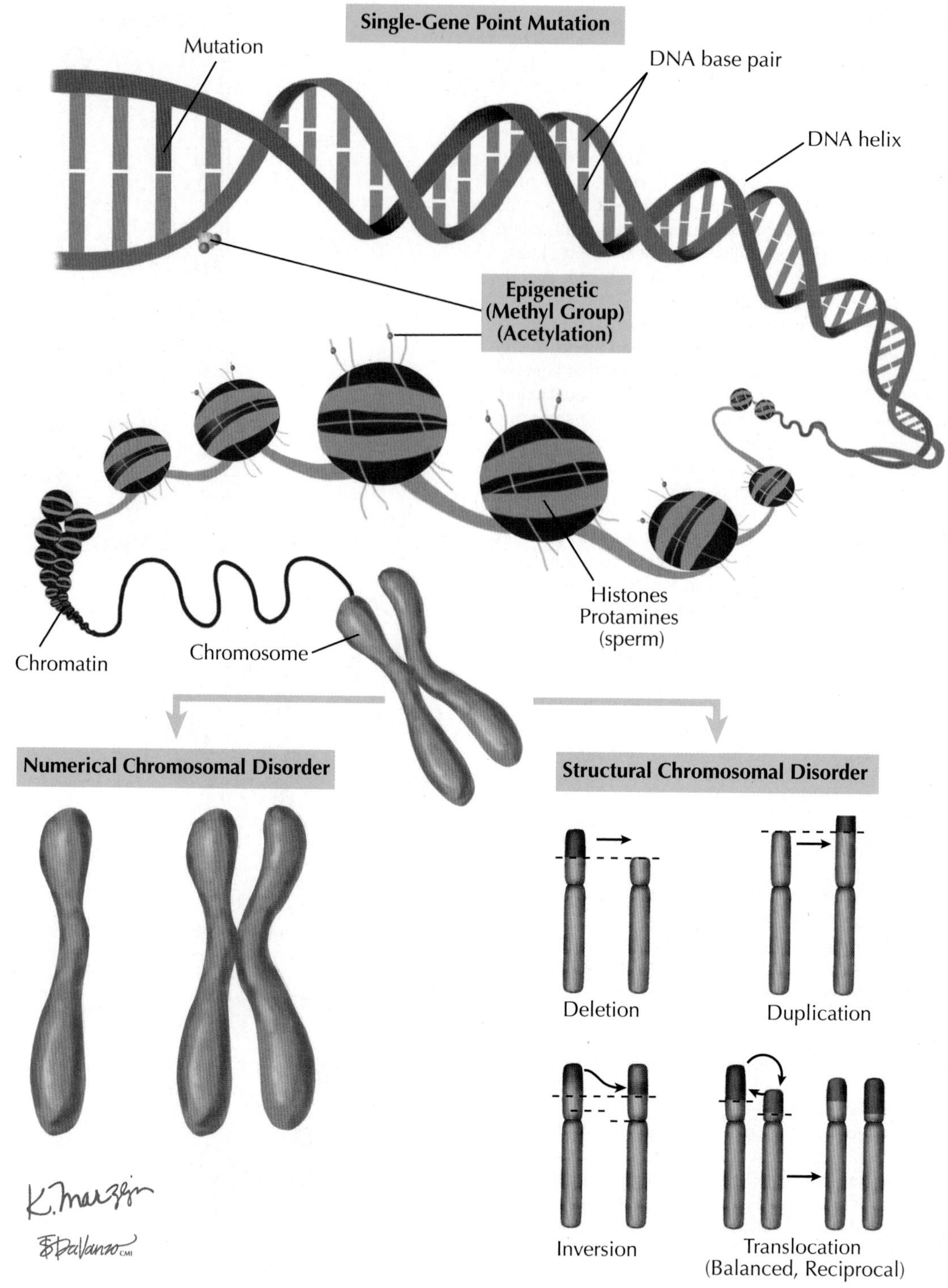

Defined as a low sperm concentration in semen, a significant proportion of oligospermia is likely due to underlying genetic causes. Genetic defects are generally divided into three categories: (1) point mutations in single genes that follow the rules of mendelian genetics; (2) chromosomal disorders in which changes in whole segments of chromosomes occur that are classified as either structural or numerical in type with loss (deletion), gain (duplication), or exchange (balanced defect) of genetic material, or numerical chromosomal defects with extra or missing chromosomes, and (3) polygenic or multifactorial genetic defects. These three genetic categories explain most disorders of human biology. Another recently elucidated mechanism for low sperm production is epigenetic, in which the pattern of genes expressed and repressed within the genome are altered, without affecting the DNA sequence itself. A fifth, rarer category of mutations, termed mitochondrial disorders, consists of mutations in nonchromosomal DNA within these subcellular organelles.

A blood test for cytogenetic analysis (karyotype) can determine whether such a genetic anomaly is present. Patients at risk for abnormal cytogenetic findings include men with oligospermia and atrophic testes, elevated follicle-stimulating hormone (FSH; see Plate 1.4) values, and no other attributable causes based on lifestyle or medical history. A classic genetic cause of low sperm concentrations is XYY syndrome typically associated with tall stature, hypotrophic testes, and higher risk of leukemia. Chromosomal translocations or inversions are also an infrequent cause of male infertility and low sperm counts. When segments of chromosomes are exchanged, a translocation results. When a chromosome breaks in two places and the material between the breakpoints reverses orientation, an inversion results. Such exchanges may either interrupt important genes at the breakpoint or interfere with normal chromosome pairing during meiosis because of imbalances in chromosomal mass. Many translocations have been associated with male infertility. The most common among these are the Robertsonian translocations that occur in chromosomes 13, 14, 15, 21, and 22, as these five autosomal chromosomes have arms that are particularly discordant in length. This type of translocation is eightfold more common in men who are infertile than in normal males.

Interestingly, in humans it is clear that 10% of known genes are involved with spermatogenesis or fertility. Therefore it is not surprising to find that single-gene mutations constitute a significant proportion of genetic oligospermia. Some occur as part of genetic syndromes such as myotonic dystrophy, Noonan syndrome, mixed gonadal dysgenesis, sickle cell anemia, congenital adrenal hyperplasia, congenital unilateral absence of the vas deferens (CUAVD), Kallmann syndrome (see Plate 3.18), Prader-Willi syndrome, and Kennedy disease. Other single-gene mutations appear to be specific for spermatogenesis and include autosomal genes such as the acrosin gene, *BAX, BCL16, c-kit, ATM, HSP70.2, RAD6B, MDHC7, CREM,* and *DNA11* and *12.* But by far the most common genetic causes of oligospermia are mutations in Y chromosome genes. Before its firm association with male fertility, the Y chromosome was widely considered a genetic black hole, an evolved, broken remnant of the X chromosome. It was apparent that the Y harbored the male sex-determining region (testis-determining region, *SRY*), but it was also home to gene regions that govern

stature, tooth enamel, and hairy ears as well as "junk" genes. In 1992 three gene regions were identified on the long arm (Yq) of the Y chromosome, labeled AZFa (azoospermia factor a), AZFb, and AZFc, that harbored important male fertility genes. Although men with AZFa and b deletions are most commonly sterile or azoospermic (see Plate 5.6), those with AZFc deletions can present with low sperm counts, typically below 5 million sperm/mL in ejaculated semen.

Epigenetic alterations to DNA are natural and common occurrences and are influenced by age, environment, lifestyle, and illness. Epigenetic modifications underlie normal development and also pathologic diseases such as cancer, autoimmunity, and now infertility. All four known types of epigenetic modifications are known to occur in

sperm and include DNA methylation, chromatin remodeling, histone modification, and noncoding RNAs. Early research revealed that the *H19* locus was 100-fold more often abnormally imprinted in men with oligospermia compared with those with normal sperm counts. Recently it has become clear that "banks" or "arrays" of many more imprinted genes are correlated with low sperm counts. In addition, abnormal sperm epigenetic profiles appear to correlate not only with semen analysis parameters but also with reproductive competence as defined by embryo quality and miscarriage rates. As sperm epigenetic patterns are heritable, there is the potential for both intergenerational transmission of infertility and other epigenetic disease to offspring as well as transgenerational implications for grandchildren.

Single-Gene Point Mutation

Mutation

DNA base pair

DNA helix

Epigenetic (Methyl Group) (Acetylation)

Histones Protamines (sperm)

Chromatin

Chromosome

Numerical Chromosomal Disorder

Structural Chromosomal Disorder

Deletion

Duplication

Inversion

Translocation (Balanced, Reciprocal)

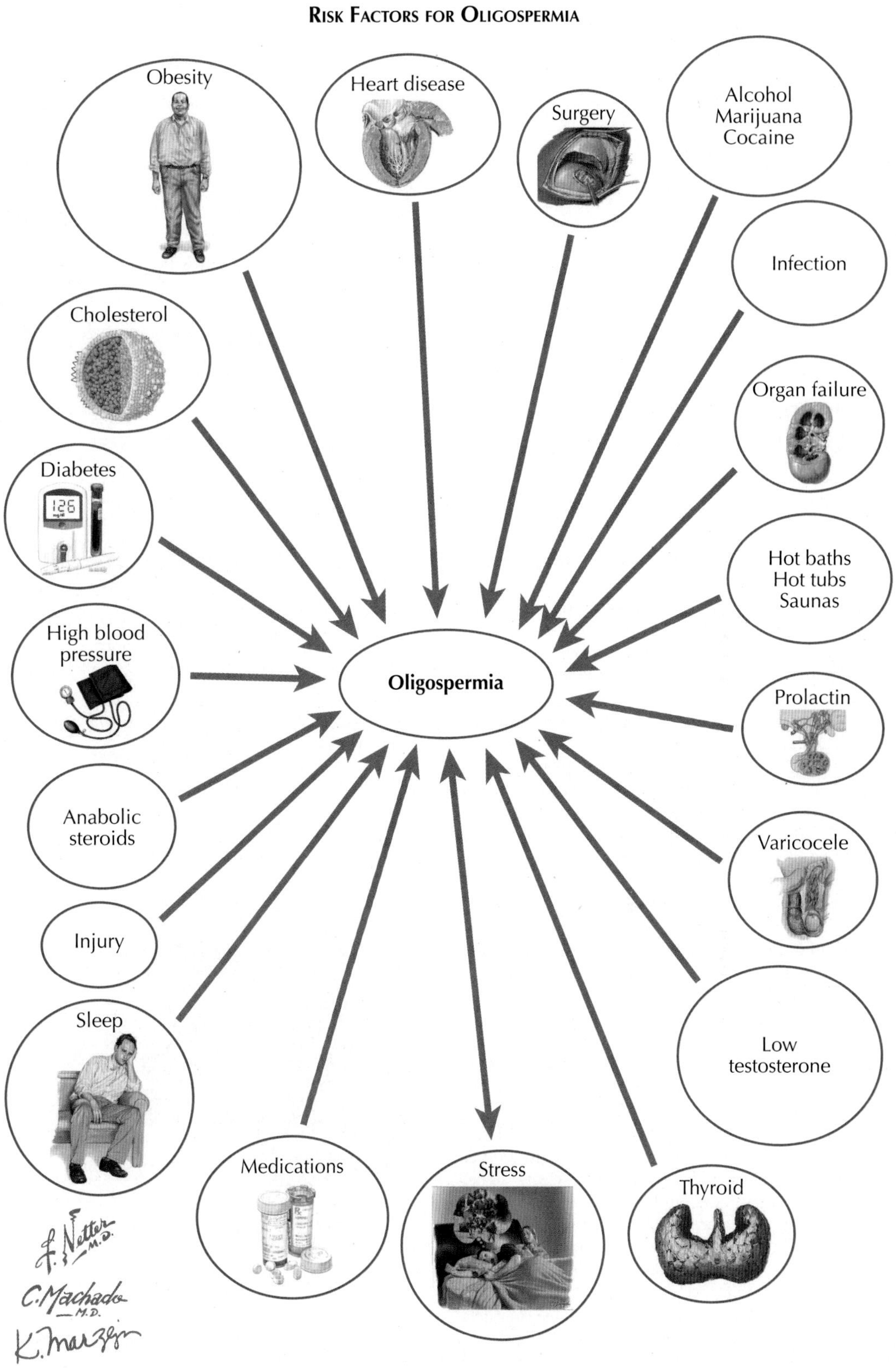

Plate 5.4

Sperm and Ejaculation

RISK FACTORS FOR OLIGOSPERMIA

Obesity

Heart disease

Surgery

Alcohol Marijuana Cocaine

Infection

Cholesterol

Organ failure

Diabetes

Hot baths Hot tubs Saunas

High blood pressure

Oligospermia

Prolactin

Anabolic steroids

Varicocele

Injury

Sleep

Low testosterone

Medications

Stress

Thyroid

OLIGOSPERMIA: SPERM PRODUCTION PROBLEMS— HORMONAL AND ACQUIRED

The medical history and physical examination are valuable in determining the root causes of low sperm counts and male infertility. This is because sperm production in the testicles runs at peak capacity in the setting of good overall health, at approximately 1000 sperm per heartbeat. Therefore lifestyle choices and disorders that impair health can significantly reduce sperm production and fertility. A thorough history can elucidate factors such as fevers, systemic illnesses such as diabetes, obesity, thyroid imbalance, cancer, and infections. Medications that are known to impair spermatogenesis include finasteride, cimetidine, diethylstilbestrol, spironolactone, sulfasalazine, and testosterone and its associated esters. It is also well recognized that severe stress, be it emotional, physical, travel or sleep-related, or financial, can induce impressive secondary hypogonadism and impair spermatogenesis.

A social history may detect the habitual use of the gonadotoxins alcohol, tobacco, marijuana, and other recreational drugs. Exogenous or anabolic steroids are the most commonly detected hormonal cause of oligospermia in men of reproductive age. Frequent use of hot baths, tubs, saunas or steam rooms is known to lower sperm counts. There is debate about whether radiation from cell phones or Wi-Fi alters sperm production. An occupational history determines exposure to ionizing radiation, chronic heat, benzene-based solvents, dyes, pesticides, herbicides, and heavy metals, all of which can impair sperm production.

The physical examination can also reveal root causes of oligospermia. The presence of undescended testes, either unilateral or bilateral, either corrected or uncorrected, is associated with lower sperm counts. A past history of testicular torsion, mumps orchitis, or bacterial epididymo-orchitis is also linked to impaired semen quality and infertility. The long-term effects of Zika, Ebola, or COVID-19 viral infections on spermatogenesis do not appear to be significant as these viruses do not easily cross the blood-testis barrier and infect the testicular parenchyma. By far the most common acquired cause of oligospermia is the presence of a clinical varicocele on exam. This dilation of veins within the pampiniform plexus is a consequence of humans assuming an upright posture and results in the retrograde flow of corporal venous blood into the peritesticular region. Spermatogenic impairment with varicoceles is thought to be due to either reflux of metabolites or elevated temperature in the peritesticular region.

It is now recognized that male fertility potential is a true "biomarker" of overall health. This concept was first brought to light with the finding that the male infertility evaluation detects significant medical illnesses in 1% to 5% of cases. Further research demonstrated that men who are infertile develop higher rates of testicular and prostate cancer later in life than do men who are fertile. Most recently, men who are infertile have been shown to have a higher comorbidity burden (e.g., diabetes, obesity), higher rates of cardiovascular disease, and possibly shorter lift expectancies than men who are fertile. Notably, the vast bulk of this body of research is based on semen analyses demonstrating oligospermia, emphasizing the true biologic significance of this finding.

Plate 5.5

Reproductive System: VOLUME 1

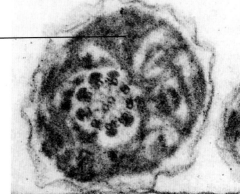

ASTHENOSPERMIA: GENETIC AND ACQUIRED CAUSES

The movement of sperm is termed motility. Asthenospermia is reduced or absent sperm motility. Among the descriptive features of sperm observed on a semen analysis, sperm motility correlates best with fertility, because sperm must travel from the cervix, where they are deposited, to the fallopian tube to fertilize the egg. This journey is equivalent to a human swimming hard and fast for 5 miles. Sperm are generally immotile within the testicle and acquire their characteristic motility during their passage through the epididymis before ejaculation.

It is thought that 200 to 300 genes govern sperm motility, many of which are involved with the sperm axoneme, the motor assembly within the sperm tail (see Plate 5.1). The best described of these are the ciliary gene mutations known to be causative for Kartagener syndrome, a form of primary ciliary dyskinesia characterized by (1) immotile or dyskinetic beating of cilia in respiratory epithelial cells that impairs mucus clearance, leading to recurrent lung infections, sinusitis, and bronchiectasis; (2) male infertility due to subtotal or complete lack of motility in ejaculated sperm, and (3) mirror reversal of body organ positioning (situs inversus) due to faulty cilia within cells of the embryonic node. The four causative ciliary genes in this syndrome include *DNAH5* coding for the outer dynein arms; *DNAI1,* coding for intermediate dynein chain 1; *DNAH11,* coding for dynein heavy chain, and *TXNDC3,* coding for a thioredoxin family member. In addition to these flagellar genes, it is thought that many signal transduction, membrane protein and metabolic enzyme encoding genes are involved sperm ciliopathies that result in low (<10%) sperm motility or complete asthenospermia. The best described among them are *CATSPER1* and *GALNTL5* which are crucial for proper function of sperm calcium-dependent voltage channels that govern sperm motility and hyperactivity.

Besides defined syndromic causes of asthenospermia, there are also two general classes of sperm structural defects defined by electron microscopy and that present clinically with severely compromised sperm motility (<10%). This first of these are the nonspecific flagellar anomalies that present as random, heterogeneous, microtubular alterations to the sperm axoneme. These anomalies arise from correctable disorders such as varicocele, reactive oxygen species, and gonadotoxin exposure, and there is typically no evidence of familial occurrence. The second is termed dysplasia of the fibrous sheath, which is usually associated with near-complete or total immotility. It has a more homogenous

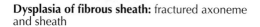

Normal flagellar axoneme

Primary ciliary dyskinesia:
Absent outer dynein arms (*arrows*)

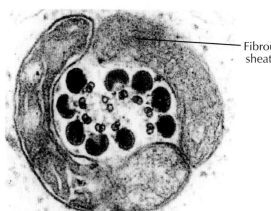

Dysplasia of fibrous sheath: fractured axoneme and sheath

Dysplasia of fibrous sheath: abnormal fibrous sheath

From Chemes HE. Phenotypes of sperm pathology: genetic and acquired forms in infertile men. J Androl. 2000;21(6):799-808.

and distinctive phenotype characterized by sperm fibrous sheath, axonemal, and periaxonemal distortions. There is a strong familial incidence, suggesting that such conditions are genetic in origin; indeed, those with Kartagener syndrome are grouped in this category.

More commonly, asthenospermia is due to acquired rather than genetic causes. Many of the medical conditions, medications, and lifestyle choices that result in oligospermia (see Plate 5.4) also cause asthenospermia. And unlike genetic asthenospermia, the effect of toxicants on

sperm motility is dose dependent, in which the effect is greater with higher exposure levels. This is no more aptly demonstrated than by examining the relationship between the intrinsic (fevers) and extrinsic (hot baths or tubs) heat exposure and sperm motility: the higher the dose (temperature) and duration or frequency of exposure, the more profound the decrease in sperm motility. Second, the effects of acquired causes of asthenospermia are typically reversible with discontinuation of toxicants, unlike that due to genetic causes.

Plate 5.6

Sperm and Ejaculation

Normal spectral cytogenetic or karyotype analysis

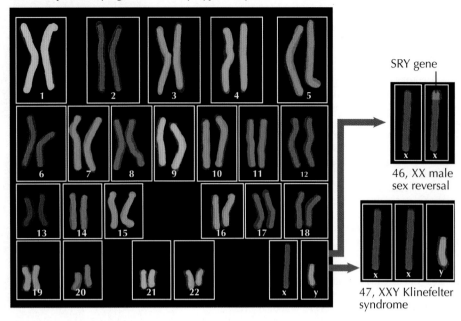

SRY gene

46, XX male
sex reversal

47, XXY Klinefelter
syndrome

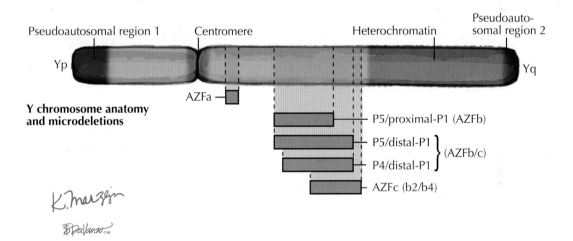

Pseudoautosomal region 1 Centromere Heterochromatin Pseudoauto-somal region 2

Yp Yq

AZFa

Y chromosome anatomy and microdeletions

P5/proximal-P1 (AZFb)

P5/distal-P1 } (AZFb/c)
P4/distal-P1 }

AZFc (b2/b4)

AZOOSPERMIA: SPERM PRODUCTION PROBLEMS— GENETIC AND ACQUIRED CAUSES

Azoospermia is defined as the absence of sperm in the ejaculate. When diagnosed as part of a male infertility evaluation, this condition is due to testicular failure in 75% and obstruction in 25% of cases. Similar to oligospermia, testicular failure causing azoospermia is commonly either genetic or acquired in nature. Ten percent to 15% of men who are infertile with azoospermia harbor a chromosomal abnormality on either the sex chromosomes or autosomes. Klinefelter syndrome (47,XXY) is the most frequently detected sex chromosomal abnormality among men with azoospermia (see Plate 3.22). In addition, syndromes such as myotonic dystrophy, Noonan syndrome, 46,XX male syndrome and mixed gonadal dysgenesis, sickle cell anemia, congenital adrenal hyperplasia, Kallmann syndrome (see Plate 3.18), Prader-Willi syndrome, and Kennedy disease are rare but well-described genetic causes of azoospermia.

Isolated, nonsyndromic point mutations are also a common cause of azoospermia and testicular failure. The most common among these are small, underlying deletions in one or more gene regions on the long arm

of the Y chromosome (Yq) that occur in 15% of men with azoospermia. Deletion of the DAZ (Deleted in Azoospermia) gene in the AZFc region is the most commonly observed microdeletion in azoospermia. Less common but well-recognized Y chromosome mutations are found in USP9Y, UTY, and DBY in the AZFa region of Yq; RBMY1, HSFY, PRY (1 and 2), EIFA1Y, and KDM5D in the AZFb region; and BPY2 and CDY1 in the AZFc locus. Interestingly, the male X chromosome is also thought to harbor mutations and deletions that are thought to cause spermatogenic failure. These include *AKAP3, AKAP4, NXF2, TAF7L, USP26,* and *TEX11.* Finally, there are known autosomal mutations linked to spermatogenic failure, including *SOHLH1, SYCP3* and *DPY19L2,* and *SPATA16,* the latter of which also results in acrosomeless sperm.

Acquired causes of primary testicular failure are as prevalent as their genetically defined counterparts as causes of azoospermia. Cryptorchidism (see Plate 3.16), especially when occurring bilaterally, is a very common cause of acquired nonobstructive azoospermia. Mumps orchitis presenting during puberty or bacterial epididymo-orchitis classically induces inflammation, testicular

parenchymal necrosis, and azoospermia. By the same mechanisms, testicular torsion or trauma can result in primary testis failure, even with timely surgical correction. Testicular failure is also common after chemotherapy (alkylating agents in particular) or radiotherapy treatment for malignancy or benign disease. Interestingly, durable azoospermia is not strongly associated with either COVID-19 or Zika viral infections, although temporary azoospermia can occur in the setting of high fevers.

Despite the lack of effective treatments to treat most cases of genetic and acquired testicular failure and azoospermia, many men who are affected can have usable "pockets" of mature sperm in their testicles. Great advances in testicular sperm retrieval techniques (see Plate 5.11) now allow for the detection and use of this sperm for biologic fatherhood with IVF and intracytoplasmic sperm injection (ICSI). Although more commonly observed with genetic rather than acquired azoospermia, a progressive deterioration in testicular sperm production with advancing chronologic age can be a barrier to fatherhood with nonobstructive azoospermia.

Plate 5.7

Reproductive System: VOLUME 1

AZOOSPERMIA: EXCURRENT DUCT OBSTRUCTION

The lack of ejaculated sperm in semen can result from anatomic blockage of the ductal system leading sperm away from the testicle in the setting of normal spermatogenesis and is termed obstructive azoospermia. The posttesticular ducts include the epididymis, vas deferens, seminal vesicles, and associated ejaculatory apparatus (see Plate 3.3). Ductal obstruction can be due to congenital or acquired causes. In cases of idiopathic or unexplained obstruction, 65% of blockages will be found in the epididymis, 30% in the vas deferens, and 5% at the level of the ejaculatory duct. Rarely, intratesticular obstruction of testis efferent ductules (see Plate 3.3) may occur.

The most common congenital cause of obstruction is cystic fibrosis (CF) or its variant, congenital absence of the vas deferens (CAVD, see Plate 4.22). CF is the most common autosomal recessive genetic disorder in the United States. The diagnosis is made on physical examination and confirmed by transrectal ultrasound (TRUS; see Plate 4.12) showing seminal vesicle, ampullary vas deferens, or ejaculatory duct agenesis or hypotrophy. Most cases are not microsurgically reconstructable, and sperm retrieval (see Plate 5.11) is required with assisted reproduction to conceive.

Idiopathic epididymal obstruction is a relatively uncommon condition found in otherwise healthy men. It may be linked to prior occult infection, but has also been shown to be related to CF in that one-third of men who are affected harbor CF gene mutations. The role of prior tuberculosis epididymitis infection with resulting scar tissue causing blockage is likely an underestimated cause of idiopathic obstruction. This is especially true given that 20% of tuberculosis cases are of genitourinary origin and present with few to no systemic manifestations. It is often amenable to microsurgical reconstruction. Young syndrome presents with a triad of chronic sinusitis, bronchiectasis, and obstructive azoospermia. The pathophysiology of the condition is unclear but may involve abnormal ciliary function or abnormal mucus quality, resulting in fluid concretion and blockage in the fine epididymal ducts. Spermatogenesis is usually normal, and microsurgical procedures can be performed to reestablish reproductive tract continuity.

Adult polycystic kidney disease is an autosomal dominant disorder associated with numerous cysts of the kidney, liver, spleen, pancreas, epididymis, seminal vesicle, and testis. Disease onset usually occurs in the 20s or 30s with symptoms of abdominal pain, hypertension, and renal failure. Infertility is usually secondary to obstructing cysts in the epididymis or seminal vesicle, which may be amenable to microsurgery.

Ejaculatory duct obstruction involves blockage of the ejaculatory ducts—the delicate, paired, collagenous tubes that connect the vas deferens and seminal vesicles to the urethra. It is the cause of infertility in 5% of men with azoospermia. It can be congenital, resulting from müllerian duct (utricular) cysts, wolffian duct (diverticular) cysts, or congenital atresia or acquired from seminal vesicle calculi or postsurgical or inflammatory scar tissue. It presents as hematospermia, painful ejaculation, or infertility. The diagnosis is confirmed by finding a low-volume ejaculate, and TRUS reveals dilated seminal vesicles or dilated ejaculatory ducts. Treatment with endoscopic unroofing of the ejaculatory ducts can restore fertility and reduce symptoms (see Plate 4.9). A substantial proportion of idiopathic cases are associated with CF mutations.

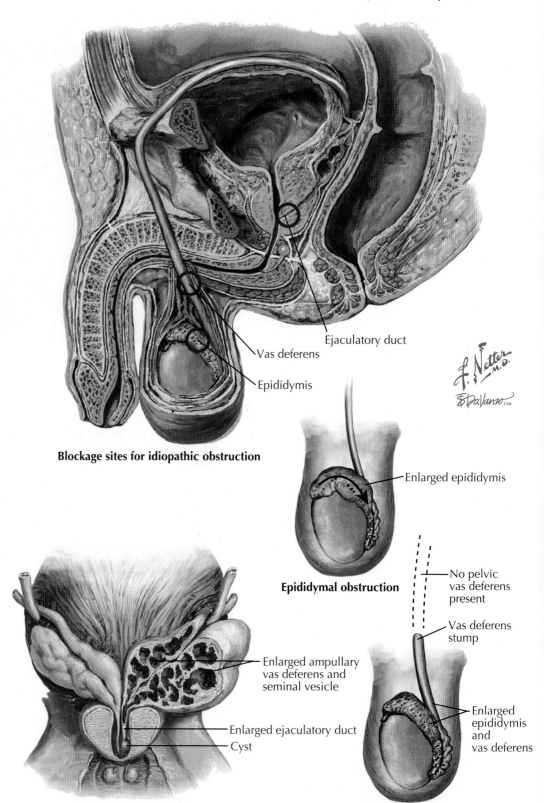

Blockage sites for idiopathic obstruction

Ejaculatory duct

Vas deferens

Epididymis

Enlarged epididymis

Epididymal obstruction

No pelvic vas deferens present

Vas deferens stump

Enlarged ampullary vas deferens and seminal vesicle

Enlarged ejaculatory duct

Cyst

Enlarged epididymis and vas deferens

Unilateral ejaculatory duct obstruction

Congenital absence of vas deferens (CAVD)

The most common cause of acquired ductal obstruction is due to vasectomy. Vasectomies are performed on 1 to 3 million US men annually for contraception, and approximately 5% of men desire to have the vasectomy reversed, most commonly because of remarriage. Groin and hernia surgery can result in inguinal vas deferens obstruction, especially in cases in which the polypropylene mesh is used in repair. This is thought to be due to perivasal inflammation causing vasal obstruction. Bacterial infections such as

Escherichia coli (in men age >35) or *Chlamydia trachomatis* may involve the epididymis or vas deferens, with scarring and obstruction that may or may not be amenable to microsurgical repair. Commonly, a testis biopsy (see Plate 5.8) is needed to distinguish between a failure of sperm production and obstruction in men with azoospermia. If normal, obstruction is confirmed, and formal surgical investigation of the reproductive tract begins with a vasogram followed by microsurgical reconstruction.

Plate 5.8

Sperm and Ejaculation

AZOOSPERMIA: DIAGNOSTIC PROCEDURES

The evaluation of the infertile, azoospermic man involves a direct assessment of spermatogenesis. This provides definitive evidence of either obstructive or nonobstructive azoospermia. The testis biopsy is most commonly used to assess sperm production. The technique involves a small, open incision in the scrotal wall and testis tunica albuginea under local anesthesia. A small wedge of testis tissue is removed, examined histologically, and seminiferous tubule architecture and cellular composition are assessed (for patterns, see Plate 3.22). Alternatively, percutaneous sampling of testis tissue with a biopsy gun can be used, similar to that employed for prostate biopsy. Although several excellent descriptions of testis seminiferous epithelium histology have been reported, no individual classification has been uniformly adopted as a standard approach.

A testis biopsy is not usually indicated for cases of oligospermia (low sperm count), as partial reproductive tract obstruction is very rare. In addition, although a single, unilateral testis will define excurrent ductal obstruction, the finding of two asymmetric testes may warrant bilateral testis biopsies to best define the pathology.

With normal sperm production, formal investigation of the reproductive tract for obstruction is warranted, beginning with a vasogram (see Plate 5.9). Abnormal sperm production defines the problem as nonobstructive azoospermia. The testis biopsy may also indicate the premalignant condition, intratubular germ cell neoplasia, that tends to occur globally within the affected testis. This condition exists in 5% of men with a contralateral germ cell testis tumor and is more prevalent in men who are infertile than those who are fertile.

Since the advent of in vitro fertilization and intracytoplasmic sperm injection (IVF-ICSI), a relatively recent indication for testis biopsy is to determine whether men with nonobstructive azoospermia have mature sperm present in the testis that may be used for assisted reproduction. A single testis biopsy will detect the presence of sperm in 30% of men with nonobstructive azoospermia. Other surgical and nonsurgical approaches have sought to improve the "yield" of sperm in cases of testis failure.

It is now clear that men with nonobstructive azoospermia can have "patchy" or "focal" areas of sperm production in a testis otherwise devoid of mature sperm. This has led to the development of more sophisticated approaches to testis biopsy, including multibiopsy techniques and percutaneous fine-needle aspiration (FNA) testis "mapping." As a single testis biopsy is subject to sampling error, the principle underlying these advanced approaches is to reduce this error by more intensive sampling. In return, sperm detection rates of 60% or more are obtained. With the multibiopsy method, four to six individual testis biopsies are taken from different areas of the testis to increase the odds of finding sperm in any particular tissue sample.

Similar to other "open" or percutaneous testis biopsy methods, FNA mapping is performed under local anesthesia. Unlike these techniques, however, smaller tissue samples are obtained that are then examined cytologically instead of histologically. It is also a diagnostic procedure that creates a geographic "map" of the testis to justify future and potentially more invasive attempts at sperm retrieval. FNA mapping involves wrapping the testis and scrotal skin with a gauze wrap posteriorly. The "testicular wrap" is a convenient handle to manipulate

the testis and also fixes the scrotal skin over the testis for the procedure. Percutaneous aspiration sites are marked on the scrotal skin, 5 mm apart, according to a template. The number of aspiration sites varies with testis size and ranges from 4 (to confirm obstruction) to 18 per testis (for nonobstructive azoospermia). FNA is performed with a sharp-beveled, small-gauge needle using the established suction cutting technique. Precise, gentle in-and-out movements are used to aspirate tissue

fragments. After aspiration, the tissue fragments are expelled onto a slide, gently smeared, and fixed in 95% ethyl alcohol. Pressure is applied to each site for hemostasis and a routine Papanicolaou stain is performed and the slides read by a cytologist for the presence or absence of mature sperm with tails. If sperm are detected, then sperm retrieval can proceed at the time of IVF-ICSI with a very high possibility of finding sufficient sperm for all oocytes retrieved.

Testicular biopsy

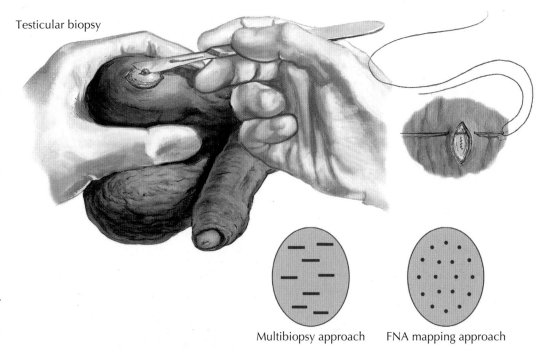

Multibiopsy approach   FNA mapping approach

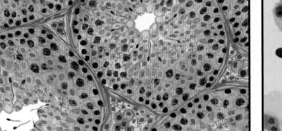

Testis biopsy histology   FNA mapping cytology

FNA technique

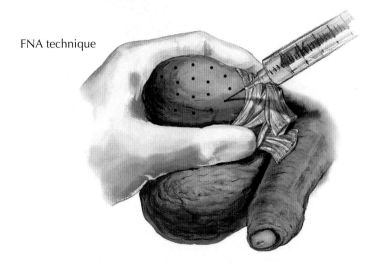

Plate 5.9

Reproductive System: VOLUME 1

AZOOSPERMIA: REPRODUCTIVE MICROSURGERY

The role of microsurgery in the treatment of male infertility is well established and cost-effective compared with assisted reproduction, including IVF-ICSI. Surgery also attempts to reverse specific pathology and, as such, allows for conception at home rather than in the laboratory. The rise of microsurgery as a surgical discipline followed three advances: (1) refinements in optical magnification, (2) the development of more precise microsuture and microneedles, and (3) the ability to manufacture smaller and more refined surgical instruments. In urology, microsurgery was first applied to renal transplantation and vasectomy reversal. Techniques evolved quickly from humble beginnings using borrowed forceps from the local jewelry store (the "jeweler's forceps") and using human hair for fine suture material, to its current highly refined state.

The most commonly performed microsurgical procedure in urology is vasectomy reversal. The most common reason for vasectomy reversal is remarriage and the desire for more children. Occasionally, an individual will have chronic pain after vasectomy or have lost a child and desire another. Infection, congenital deformities, trauma, and previous surgery are less frequent indications for vasovasostomy or epididymovasostomy. Reproductive tract obstruction is suspected in men with normal FSH and testosterone levels, normal testis size, and azoospermia.

Vasal obstruction is generally corrected by vasovasostomy. Although there are several methods for performing vasovasostomy, including a modified single-layer anastomosis and a strict two-layer anastomosis, neither is proven superior to the other. Importantly, optical magnification with an operating microscope improves outcomes as smaller sutures can be used, reducing cicatrix formation and failure rates. However, surgeon experience is the most critical factor for success. In the best hands, 95% to 99% of patients have a return of sperm after vasovasostomy.

At the time of vasectomy reversal, the vas deferens is transected below the vasectomy site. If the fluid egressing from the vas deferens contains no sperm, a second acquired obstruction may exist in the delicate tubules of the epididymis. As more time passes after vasectomy, the greater will be the "back-pressure" behind the blocked vas deferens, causing a "blowout" at some point in the 18-foot-long microscopic epididymal tubule. A blowout results in blockage of the tubule as it heals. In this case the abdominal vas deferens must be connected to the epididymis proximal to the blowout to bypass both sites of obstruction and to reestablish reproductive tract continuity in a procedure termed *epididymovasostomy.*

For epididymovasostomy, the epididymis is exposed by opening the tunica vaginalis that surrounds the testis. The epididymis is inspected and an individual tubule selected that appears dilated and is proximal to the obstruction. Two different approaches to epididymovasostomy are now popular: the mucosa-to-mucosa end-to-side method and the invagination approach. With the traditional mucosal approach, the opened epididymal tubule is connected to the cut end of the vas deferens, with four to six small microsutures placed radially around the circumference of each. This "inner" layer is buttressed with another, "outer" layer of radially

placed microsutures to strengthen the delicate connection. With the invagination method, one, two, or three "vest" microsutures are placed near but not into the opening of the epididymal tubule to allow the epididymal tubule to be drawn into, or "invaginated" into, the lumen of the vas deferens, theoretically creating an improved watertight seal. After epididymovasostomy, approximately 60% to 80% of men will have sperm in the ejaculate.

In cases of idiopathic epididymal obstruction, a similar approach as that taken for vasectomy reversal is employed, except for an important difference. Because there is no iatrogenic blockage of the vas deferens with idiopathic obstruction, the fluid within the vas deferens

is sampled from, and the vas deferens inspected by, vasography instead. After puncturing or hemitransecting the straight segment of the scrotal vas deferens, diluted dye or contrast medium is injected into the vas deferens toward the bladder from the scrotum. In plain-film radiographs, contrast delineates the proximal vas deferens, seminal vesicle, and ejaculatory ducts and the site of obstruction can be determined. In addition, the finding of no sperm in the vasal fluid from the testis side of the vas deferens implies that there is an obstruction present in the epididymis. With this information, the site of obstruction can be accurately determined and the system microsurgically reconstructed with either vasovasostomy or epididymovasostomy.

Two-layer

Modified one-layer

Microsurgical vasovasostomy approaches

Microsurgical two-layer vasovasostomy

Inner layer closure

Outer layer closure

Mucosa to mucosa epididymovasostomy

"Vest" suture placement

Vasal fluid sampling

Invagination epididymovasostomy

Vasostomy closure after vasogram

Plate 5.10   Sperm and Ejaculation

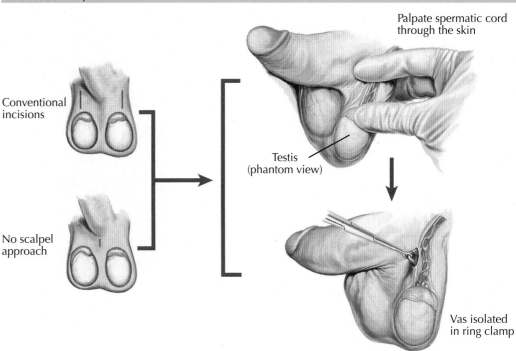

Vas delivery methods

Conventional incisions

No scalpel approach

Testis (phantom view)

Palpate spermatic cord through the skin

Vas isolated in ring clamp

VASECTOMY

Male contraceptives seek to prevent live sperm from entering the female reproductive tract. There have been unique innovations in male contraceptive technology for almost 5000 years:

- 3000 BCE: Evidence of condom use made from animal bladder or intestine or linen cloth in Crete and Egypt.
- 1800 BCE: Spermicides made by combining crocodile feces and fermented dough in Egypt.
- 1830: First vasectomy performed in a human by R. Harrison in London. Its popularity rose dramatically after World War II. The first national program for vasectomy was launched in India in 1954.
- 1855: The first rubber condom is made by Charles Goodyear, who later invented the rubber tire.

The most effective male contraceptive developed yet is the vasectomy, first performed almost 200 years ago. The goal of vasectomy is to interrupt sperm flow from the epididymis to the prostate and thereby prevent sperm from entering the semen during ejaculation. This is accomplished by physically occluding the vas deferens on each side where it is most easily accessible, within the scrotum. The keys to its success are the facts that it is a permanent sterilization method and that host compliance is not required to enable contraception with each sexual event.

There are two key portions to the vasectomy technique: delivery of the vas deferens and occlusion of the vas deferens. The vas deferens can be delivered either through traditional incisions or by using a "no scalpel" puncture technique employing sharp forceps instead of a scalpel. Techniques used to occlude or seal the vas deferens include division of the vas deferens, segmental vasal resection, ligation with surgical clips or suture, fascial interposition, or cauterization. An "open-ended" vasectomy is also used but will typically occlude by cicatrix formation over time. Applying combinations of these occlusive techniques is also popular to reduce the failure rate to fewer than 1 in 500 cases.

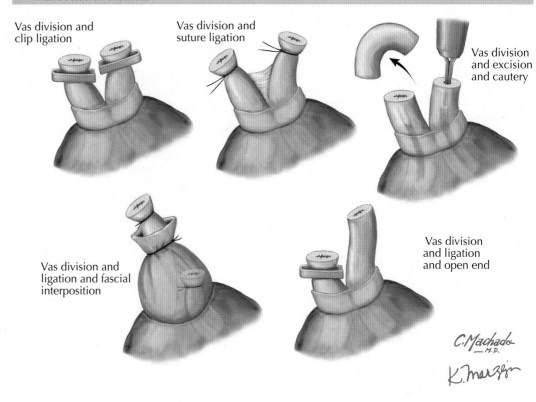

Vas occlusion methods

Vas division and clip ligation

Vas division and suture ligation

Vas division and excision and cautery

Vas division and ligation and fascial interposition

Vas division and ligation and open end

C. Machado —M.D.

K. Marzejon

Complications of vasectomy include hematoma formation, infection, sperm granulomas, short-term pain, and chronic pain syndrome. In experienced hands, the overall complication rate is typically <1% to 5%. Although rare, pregnancies after vasectomy usually occur in the first several months after the procedure, as the residual downstream vasal tubing contains millions of motile sperm that require expulsion with repeated ejaculation before sterility is attained. Roughly 30 ejaculations or 3 months of time is needed after vasectomy to acquire sterility. The long-term safety of vasectomy is well established, despite unsubstantiated claims that rates of cardiovascular disease, low testosterone, sexual dysfunction, prostate cancer, and dementia due to progressive aphasia are increased after the procedure. Notably, ejaculate volume typically decreases by 10% or less and its gross appearance is unchanged. And, although considered a permanent form of contraception, the vast majority of vasectomies can be successfully reversed with advanced microsurgical techniques (see Plate 5.9).

Plate 5.11

Reproductive System: VOLUME 1

THERAPEUTIC SPERM RETRIEVAL

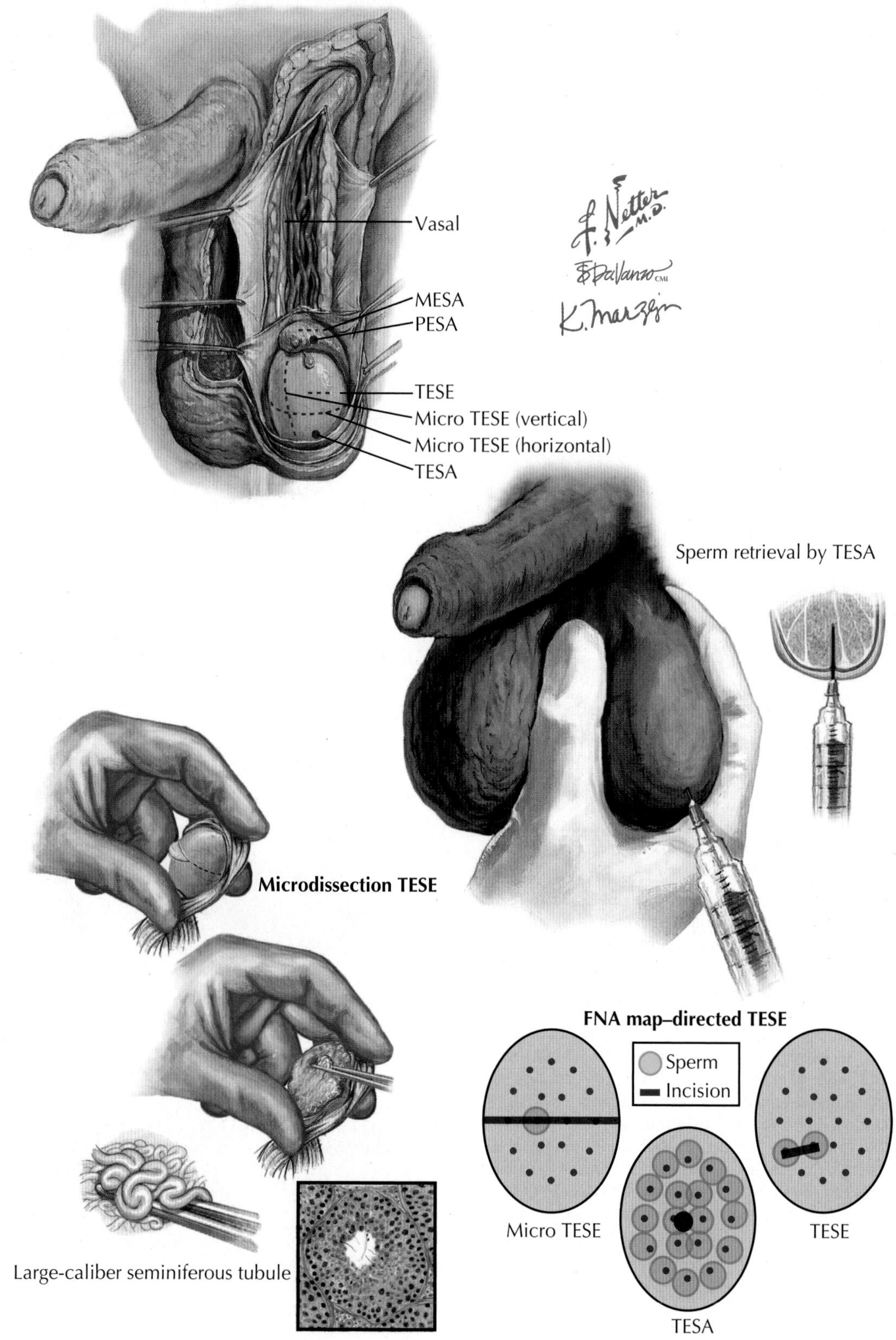

Sperm retrieval techniques collect sperm from organs within the male genital tract. Developed in 1985, 10 years before the description of ICSI, sperm retrieval combined with IVF and ICSI allows men with severe infertility the opportunity for fatherhood. Candidate organs for sperm retrieval include the vas deferens, epididymis, and testicle in men with obstruction and the testis in men with nonobstructive azoospermia. Although it is not difficult to retrieve sperm from men with normal sperm production, it can be very difficult to find sperm in men with testicular failure and nonobstructive azoospermia.

Patients with congenital or acquired obstruction of the excurrent ductal system at the level of the prostate or the pelvic portions of the vas deferens are candidates for vasal sperm aspiration. Also included are men with ejaculatory failure due to diabetes or spinal cord injury. Vasal aspiration is performed either coincident with, or a day in advance of, IVF egg retrieval and is undertaken in a manner similar to a vasectomy. Through a scrotal puncture, the vas deferens is identified. Using optical magnification, a small incision or puncture is made in the delicate wall of the vas deferens until the lumen is entered. Sperm and fluid are aspirated and, after sufficient sperm are obtained, the vas deferens wall is closed microsurgically; no closure is needed for a puncture vasotomy. Vasal sperm is the most "mature" or fertilizable of all retrieved sperm, having passed through epididymal maturation. This is reflected in the fact that pregnancies have been achieved with vasal sperm and intrauterine insemination (IUI) and IVF without ICSI.

Epididymal sperm aspiration is performed when the vas is either absent, such as with CAVD, or is scarred from prior surgery, trauma, or infection. Two different approaches to epididymal sperm aspiration are microscopic epididymal sperm aspiration (MESA), in which the epididymis is explored microsurgically and sperm aspirated from individual epididymal tubules, and percutaneous epididymal sperm aspiration (PESA), in which sperm are aspirated blindly from the epididymis after percutaneous puncture. The most important difference between these techniques is that individual epididymal tubules are sampled for sperm with MESA, but multiple epididymal tubules are sampled with PESA; thus the overall yield and bankability of sperm is less with PESA than MESA. As epididymal sperm are not as "mature" as vasal sperm, they require IVF-ICSI for pregnancy success.

The newest of the three sperm aspiration techniques, testicular sperm retrieval, was first reported in 1993, 1 year after ICSI. It demonstrated that sperm do not have to "mature" and pass through the epididymis to be able to fertilize an egg (with ICSI). Testicular sperm extraction is indicated for patients who are "obstructed" and is also useful for many men with nonobstructive azoospermia. In men with obstruction, testis sperm can be retrieved by needle aspiration (TESA) or percutaneous or open surgical biopsy (TESE). TESA involves holding the testis with the epididymis located posteriorly followed by insertion of a hollow needle (16- to 23-gauge) into the testis through the stretched skin of the scrotum.

In men with nonobstructive azoospermia, TESE is usually needed to retrieve sufficient sperm for IVF-ICSI. To improve the likelihood of finding sperm, a multibiopsy TESE has been described in which many biopsies are taken until enough sperm are obtained. A variant of multibiopsy TESE is microdissection TESE, which involves taking multiple testis biopsies through a

large incision that exposes the entire testis parenchyma. With an operating microscope, the entire bed of testis tissue is examined for sperm-containing seminiferous tubules that are larger in diameter and more opaque, or whiter, than tubules without active spermatogenesis.

FNA map–directed TESE employs a diagnostic mapping procedure (see Plate 5.8) to guide subsequent sperm retrieval for IVF-ICSI. Information obtained from the map "directs" the TESE, taking advantage of the a priori knowledge that sperm are present in men

with nonobstructive azoospermia before IVF-ICSI. Depending on the location, density, and quantity of sperm found on the map, sperm retrieval may involve TESA, TESE, or microdissection TESE.

The ability to freeze and thaw retrieved sperm is a significant advance in the care of men with azoospermia. It simplifies the timing and orchestration of fertility procedures, adds convenience to reproductive urologists' schedules, and allows multiple opportunities to conceive with IVF-ICSI without repeating surgical sperm retrieval.

Vasal
MESA
PESA
TESE
Micro TESE (vertical)
Micro TESE (horizontal)
TESA

Sperm retrieval by TESA

Microdissection TESE

Large-caliber seminiferous tubule

FNA map–directed TESE

○ Sperm
▬ Incision

Micro TESE

TESA

TESE

Plate 5.12

Sperm and Ejaculation

Ejaculatory Disorders

Although commonly viewed as a single event, ejaculation is actually two separate processes: emission and ejaculation. During emission, the semen is "loaded" into the prostatic urethral chamber. After this, ejaculation is the forcible expulsion of semen from the penis in a series of spurts caused by rhythmic contractions, about 1 second apart, of the pelvic muscles. Ejaculation is different from orgasm or climax, the latter being an event that is centered in the brain that is closely associated with ejaculation.

Disordered ejaculation in which there is no semen produced at the time of climax is called *aspermia*. This is different from azoospermia (see Plate 5.6), in which semen is present but contains no sperm. In the absence of ejaculate, there can be failure of ejaculation (anejaculation) or ejaculation into the bladder (retrograde ejaculation). Failure of ejaculation can be a lifelong, primary event (congenital anorgasmia) or an acquired problem (secondary anorgasmia). The treatment of these conditions is different and important to distinguish.

Similar to a sneeze, ejaculation is a spinal reflex. With both, there is a "point of no return" that occurs after the reflex is stimulated. Ejaculation is under control of two nervous systems: the sympathetic (autonomic) nervous system governs emission and the somatic nervous system controls ejaculation. Sympathetic nerves arise from thoracolumbar spine at levels T10–L2. They form the superior hypogastric plexus and run in front of the aorta in the back and pelvis. Expulsion of the ejaculate is governed by the somatic nervous system through the pudendal nerve (S2–S4). Interruption of either nervous system input can result in ejaculatory disorders.

PREMATURE EJACULATION.

The average time from vaginal penetration to ejaculation in men is 9 minutes. Premature ejaculation is present when orgasm occurs within 1 minute after vaginal penetration, or when ejaculation occurs too early for female partner satisfaction. This problem occurs in 30% of adult men, and it is the most common form of male sexual dysfunction. It can be due to erectile dysfunction, anxiety, and nerve hypersensitivity and is treatable. Importantly, although medications can "control" the problem and delay ejaculation, "curing" the problem usually requires sex education to learn control and satisfaction. Secondary premature ejaculation can be improved by normalizing erection function in many cases.

RETROGRADE EJACULATION.

This is a straightforward diagnosis that requires a history of aspermia, with a postejaculate urine sample showing sperm. Causes include medical conditions such as diabetes mellitus, multiple sclerosis, spinal cord injury, tethered spinal cord, spina bifida, medications such as alpha-blockers, tricyclic antidepressants and finasteride, and surgical procedures such as transurethral prostatic resection (see Plate 4.17), V-Y plasty of the bladder neck, rectal, anterior spinal, and retroperitoneal procedures. The treatment of retrograde ejaculation depends on its cause. If drug induced, then the offending medication should be discontinued. Oral therapy with α-agonist agents can help close the bladder neck and avoid entry of the semen into the bladder during ejaculation. Sperm can also be "harvested" from the bladder and used for fertility procedures if needed.

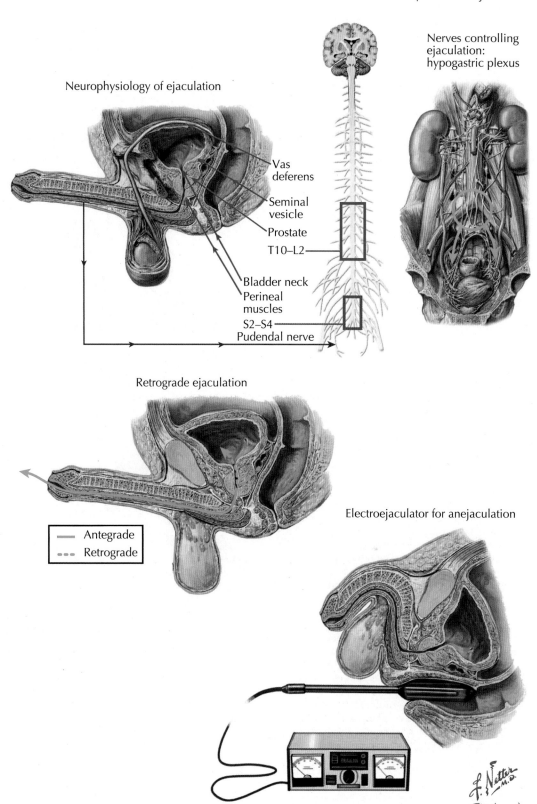

Neurophysiology of ejaculation

Nerves controlling ejaculation: hypogastric plexus

Vas deferens
Seminal vesicle
Prostate
T10–L2
Bladder neck
Perineal muscles
S2–S4
Pudendal nerve

Retrograde ejaculation

—— Antegrade
∙∙∙ Retrograde

Electroejaculator for anejaculation

ANEJACULATION.

This condition can be congenital or acquired. Congenital anorgasmia occurs in about 1 in 1000 men. Despite the lack of orgasm, nocturnal emissions during sleep may occur. Treatment of primary anejaculation is difficult, as individuals who are affected often lack sensual awareness. Generally, treatment is sought when the couple desires a pregnancy, as erections and sexual performance are otherwise unaffected. Again, sex education has the highest chance of curing this problem.

Fertility issues can be bypassed with prostatic massage for sperm, collection and insemination of nocturnal semen emissions, penile vibratory stimulation or rectal probe electroejaculation, or sperm retrieval (see Plate 5.11). Secondary or acquired anejaculation can be due to the same medications that cause retrograde ejaculation. Anejaculation can also be caused by diabetes, multiple sclerosis, and spinal cord injury. In these cases, penile vibratory stimulation, rectal probe ejaculation, or surgical sperm retrieval techniques can be used to achieve fertility.

Plate 5.13

Reproductive System: VOLUME 1

**Epigenetic
(Methyl group)(Acetylation)**

Possible epigenetic disorders in
offspring associated with advanced
paternal age:
• Schizophrenia
• Autism spectrum disorder
• Dyslexia
• Bipolar disorder
• Alzheimer disease

Chromatin

DNA base pair

Single-Gene Point Mutation

Single-gene dominant disorders in
offspring and genes associated with
advanced paternal age:

Achondroplasia	FGFR3
Apert syndrome	FGFR2
Crouzon syndrome	FGFR2
Pfeiffer syndrome	FGFR2
Aniridia	PAX6
Wilms tumor	WT1
Bilateral retinoblastoma	RB1
Hemophilia A	F8
Fibrodysplasia ossificans	ACVR1
Lesch-Nyhan syndrome	HPRT1
Marfan syndrome	FBN1
Multiple endocrine neoplasia	RET
Neurofibromatosis 1	NF1
Oculodentodigital syndrome	GJA1
Osteogenesis imperfecta	COL1A1/2
Polycystic kidney disease	PKD1/2
Gardner syndrome	APC
Progeria syndrome	LMNA
Thanatophoric dysplasia	FGFR3
Treacher-Collins syndrome	TCOF1
Tuberous sclerosis	TSC1,2
Wardenburg syndrome 1&3	PAX3

Histones
Protamines
(sperm)

DNA helix

**Numerical or Structural
Chromosomal Disorder**

Numerical or structural chromosomal
disorders in offspring associated with
advanced paternal age:

Sex chromosome aneuploidy (XXY, XYY)
• Trisomy 21
• Robertsonian translocations

PATERNAL AGE EFFECTS ON OFFSPRING

Unlike any other cell in the body, the sperm DNA payload is responsible for transgenerational inheritance. It is also true that the quality of the DNA packaged in sperm changes with chronologic age of the host male. Therefore any qualitative changes occurring in sperm with advanced paternal age are likely to be made manifest in offspring and are termed *paternal age effects*. Given that life expectancy in the U.S. averaged 45 years in 1900 and 70 years in 1950, the concept of the older father and paternal age effects on offspring are entirely new to us as a species over the last two generations.

The way male and female gametes are produced differs dramatically in mammals. All female gametes are made by birth and are ovulated throughout life. On the contrary, male gametes begin production at puberty and constantly regenerate throughout adulthood. This difference in gamete manufacture has major implications for heritable genetic alterations in offspring. There is some debate regarding whether the continuous cell division during spermatogenesis places male gametes at risk for chromosomal injury with advanced paternal age. We now know that numerically, there is a slightly higher incidence of sperm sex chromosomal aneuploidy with advanced age, but not necessarily autosomal aneuploidy. In addition, increases in chromosome structural anomalies have not been reliable demonstrated with paternal age. Thus there is not a strong relationship between advanced paternal and increased numerical or structural chromosomal issues in offspring.

Another source of heritable genetic defects are single-gene mutations. In sperm, these could result from errors in DNA replication that are associated with the continuous process of spermatogonial cell division. By puberty in humans, 30 such cell divisions have occurred. After puberty, 23 divisions occur annually. The simple fact that the spermatogonia of older men have undergone numerous cell divisions could increase the chance of errors in DNA transcription, which are the source of single-gene mutations. Indeed, the effect of advanced paternal age on conditions in offspring associated with single-gene mutations is well established.

These disorders consist of autosomal dominant diseases that have known associations with advanced paternal age and are termed *sentinel phenotypes* because they occur with significant frequency and low fitness, and stem from highly penetrant mutations. Formal risk estimates suggest that the risk of inherited autosomal dominant mutations doubles in fathers from age 25 to 44 years old and then increases logarithmically from the fifth to subsequent decades of paternal age.

Recent evidence also suggests that DNA methylation marks in sperm that control gene expression, termed *epigenetics*, are altered with paternal age. Sperm appear to accumulate hundreds of DNA methylation defects with age that localize to specific genomic sites, many of which control genes associated with neurodevelopment (i.e., schizophrenia, bipolar disorder, autism, and mood

disorders). In a study of sperm donated twice by men, once when young and again when older, the rate of epigenetic change in sperm doubled that estimated for other body tissues. Even more intriguing, the epigenetic changes that occur in sperm as men age tend to cluster in genes associated with schizophrenia and bipolar disorder, diseases known to occur more in offspring with advanced paternal age. Thus there also appear to be paternal age–related disorders in offspring that are a consequence of epigenetic alterations transmitted in sperm.

There are other risks to offspring that appear to correlate to advanced paternal age, but their underlying mechanisms are not well understood. These include higher rates of miscarriage, fetal loss, congenital anomalies, and certain birth defects.

VULVA

Plate 6.1

Reproductive System: VOLUME 1

EXTERNAL GENITALIA

The vulva includes those portions of the female genital tract that are externally visible in the perineal region. The mons veneris, overlying the symphysis pubis, is a fatty prominence covered by curly sexual (pubic) hair that functions as a dry lubricant during intercourse. From the mons, two longitudinal folds of skin, the labia majora, extend in elliptical fashion to enclose the vulval cleft. They contain an abundance of adipose tissue, sebaceous glands, and sweat glands, and are covered by hair on their upper outer surfaces. The anterior commissure marks their point of union at the mons. Posteriorly, a slightly raised connecting ridge, the posterior commissure or fourchette, joins them. Between the fourchette and the vaginal orifice, a shallow, boat-shaped depression, the fossa navicularis, is evident. The labia minora are thin, firm, pigmented, redundant folds of skin, which anteriorly split to enclose the clitoris; laterally, they bound the vestibule and diminish gradually as they extend posteriorly. The skin of the small labia is devoid of hair follicles, poor in sweat glands, and rich in sebaceous glands. The skin of the labia majus, and to a lesser extent the labia minus, is subject to most of the same dermatologic pathologies as other areas of skin.

The clitoris, a small, cylindrical, erectile organ, situated at the lower border of the symphysis, is composed of two crura, a body and a glans. The crura lie deeply, in close apposition with the periosteum of the ischiopubic rami. They join to form the body of the clitoris, which extends downward beneath a loose prepuce to be capped by the acorn-shaped glans. Only the glans of the clitoris is generally visible externally between the two folds formed by the bifurcation of the labia minora. When the clitoris is abnormally enlarged due to exposure to excess androgens, the clitoral index (the product of the sagittal and transverse diameters of the glans, in millimeters, normal <35 mm^2) is used to grade the degree of enlargement.

The vestibule becomes apparent on separation of the labia. Within it are found the hymen, the vaginal orifice, the urethral meatus, and the opening of Skene and Bartholin ducts. The external urethral meatus is situated upon a slight papilla-like elevation, 2 cm below the clitoris. In the posterolateral aspect of the urinary orifice, lie the openings of Skene ducts. They run below and parallel to the urethra for a distance of 1 to 1.5 cm. Bartholin ducts are visible on each side of the vestibule, in the groove between the hymen and the labia minora, at about the junction of the middle and posterior thirds of the lateral boundary of the vaginal orifice. Each duct, approximately 1.5 cm in length, passes inward and laterally to the deeply situated vulvovaginal glands. The Bartholin glands are situated posterior to the 3 and 9 o'clock locations, which is important clinically when a Bartholin gland abscess is considered in patients with labial swelling.

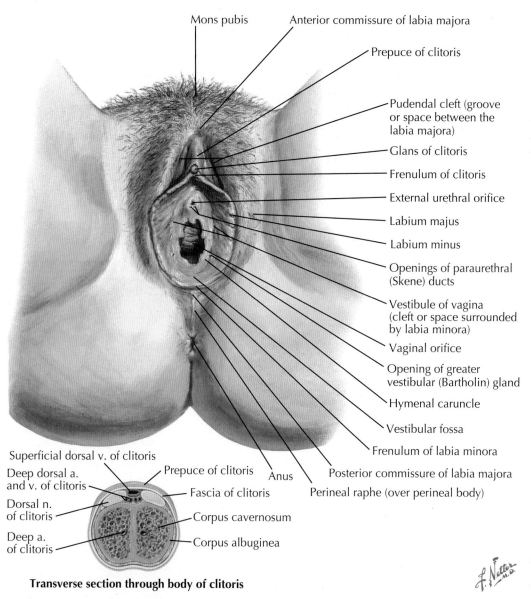

Mons pubis
Anterior commissure of labia majora
Prepuce of clitoris
Pudendal cleft (groove or space between the labia majora)
Glans of clitoris
Frenulum of clitoris
External urethral orifice
Labium majus
Labium minus
Openings of paraurethral (Skene) ducts
Vestibule of vagina (cleft or space surrounded by labia minora)
Vaginal orifice
Opening of greater vestibular (Bartholin) gland
Hymenal caruncle
Vestibular fossa
Frenulum of labia minora
Posterior commissure of labia majora
Anus
Perineal raphe (over perineal body)

Superficial dorsal v. of clitoris
Deep dorsal a. and v. of clitoris
Dorsal n. of clitoris
Deep a. of clitoris
Prepuce of clitoris
Fascia of clitoris
Corpus cavernosum
Corpus albuginea

Transverse section through body of clitoris

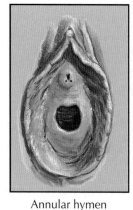

Annular hymen

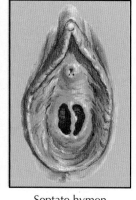

Septate hymen

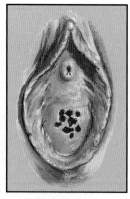

Cribriform hymen

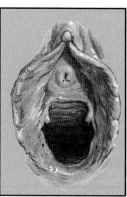

Parous introitus

The vestibula fossa, the frenulum of labia minora, and the posterior commissure of labia majora occupy the posterior boundaries of the vulvar structures. These are most at risk for sexual or obstetric trauma. This is also the location where pain is most often mapped in cases of vulvar vestibulitis.

The hymen is a thin, vascularized membrane that separates the vagina from the vestibule. It is covered on both sides by stratified squamous epithelium. As a rule, it shows great variations in thickness and in the size and shape of the hymenal openings (e.g., annular, septate, cribriform, crescentic, fimbriate). After tampon usage, coitus, and childbirth, the shrunken remnants of the hymen are known as *carunculae hymenales* or *hymeneal caruncles*. The presence or absence of the hymen is insufficient to determine the presence or absence of past sexual activity.

Plate 6.2

Vulva

PUDENDAL, PUBIC, AND INGUINAL REGIONS

The superficial fascia of the anterior abdominal wall has been cut away, exposing the aponeurosis of the external oblique muscle, with the linea alba in the midline and the linea semilunaris laterally outlining the rectus compartment beneath. Below are the inguinal ligaments, continuous with the fascia lata of the thighs, and the structures of the perineum superficial to the inferior fascia of the urogenital diaphragm. The fascial layers of the canal of Nuck emerge from the superficial inguinal ring and descend toward the lateral margin of the labium majus. These layers are composed of fibers both from the aponeurosis of the external oblique and from the transversalis fascia. The innermost layer is closely applied to the round ligament, which becomes more attenuated as it descends and eventually terminates by fine, fingerlike attachments in the labium majus. Within this sac is a vestigial remnant of peritoneum, the homologue of the tunica vaginalis in the male. The canal of Nuck may persist in the child or the adult in a patent form and may then give rise to inguinal hernias or the so-called hydrocele feminae. Adjacent to the terminal portion of this process on the right side is Colles fascia, attached laterally to the ischiopubic ramus and inferiorly to the fascia covering the superficial transverse perineal muscle, which forms the upper margin of the ischiorectal fossa.

Lateral to the subcutaneous inguinal ring and below the inguinal ligament lies the fossa ovalis surrounding the femoral artery and vein. Close to the fossa are the origins of the inferior epigastric, iliac circumflex, and superficial external pudendal vessels.

To expose the superficial muscles and inferior fascia of the urogenital diaphragm or triangular ligament, Colles fascia has been cut away on the left side. Closely applied to the left lateral wall of the vagina and lying below the labium majus is the bulbocavernosus muscle, which passes from the central tendinous point of the perineum to be attached in the corpus cavernosum and suspensory ligament of the clitoris. This muscle also is a constrictor of the introitus. At right angles to the bulbocavernosus muscle and similarly attached to the central tendinous point is the superficial transverse perineal muscle, which runs laterally to the tuberosity of the ischium and helps support the midportion of the pelvic floor. The ischiocavernosus muscle is the hypotenuse of the triangle formed by the bulbocavernosus and the superficial transverse perineal muscles and runs from the tuberosity of the ischium upward to be inserted in the crus of the clitoris, which it covers for most of its length. Within the triangle is the inferior fascia of the urogenital diaphragm, which blends with the deep fibers of Colles fascia. The triangular shape of the whole urogenital diaphragm stands out clearly in this view, with the apex at the symphysis pubis, the ischiopubic rami forming the sides and the transverse perineal muscles connected by the central tendinous point of the perineum, the base. The external anal sphincter sends interdigitating fibers to join those of the transverse perineal, bulbocavernosus, and pubococcygeus muscles in the central perineum. Knowledge of these relationships, along with that of the underlying levator ani muscular plate, is important when dealing with obstetric lacerations or other trauma.

The lateral view illustrates the manner in which the muscles and fasciae of the urogenital diaphragm are applied to and support the pelvic viscera. The urogenital fascia is composed of a superior and an inferior layer joining to form a single ligament anterior to the urethra and posterior to the vagina. Elements from these cover the outer surfaces of the pelvic viscera, where they are known as the *endopelvic fascia*. Composed of smooth muscle and fibrous tissue, they are thin superiorly where they lie just beneath the reflections of the pelvic peritoneum, but they become thicker as they approach their attachments to the upper fascia of the urogenital diaphragm and levator ani muscles.

Superficial fatty (Camper) layer
Deeper membranous (Scarpa) layer
} Subcutaneous tissue
Rectus sheath (anterior layer)
Aponeurosis of external oblique muscle
Superficial inguinal ring
Anterior superior iliac spine
Round ligament of uterus and coverings (cut)
Inguinal ligament (Poupart)
Pubic tubercle
Saphenous opening
Pubic symphysis
Fascia lata of thigh
Suspensory ligament of clitoris
Ischiopubic ramus
Superficial perineal (Colles) fascia (cut away) to open superficial perineal space
Ischiocavernosus muscle
Perineal membrane
Deep perineal (investing or Gallaudet) fascia (partially cut away)
Ischial tuberosity
Fat body of ischioanal fossa
Superficial perineal (Colles) fascia (cut edge turned down)
Superficial transverse perineal muscle
Bulbocavernosus muscle (covers bulb of vestibule)
Round ligament of uterus and coverings
Superficial perineal (Colles) fascia

Peritoneum
Urachus
Vesical fascia
Transversalis fascia
Uterovaginal fascia
Subcutaneous tissue { Fatty / Membranous
Rectus abdominis muscle
Rectal fascia
Rectus sheath (anterior layer)
Uterus
Pubic symphysis
Bladder
Inferior (arcuate) pubic ligament
Transverse perineal ligament
Levator ani muscle
Suspensory ligament of clitoris
Vagina
Rectum
Sphincter urethrae and sphincter urethrovaginalis muscles
Perineal membrane
Anococcygeal body
Superficial perineal space
Superficial perineal (Colles) fascia
Inferior fascia of pelvic diaphragm
Perineal body
Superior fascia of pelvic diaphragm
External anal sphincter muscle

Plate 6.3

Reproductive System: VOLUME 1

PERINEUM

The mons veneris in front, the buttocks behind, and the thighs laterally bound the perineum. More deeply, it is limited by the margins of the pelvic outlet, namely the pubic symphysis and arcuate ligament, ischiopubic rami, ischial tuberosities, sacrotuberous ligaments, sacrum, and coccyx. A transverse line joining the ischial tuberosities divides the perineum into an anterior urogenital and a posterior anal triangle.

The perineal floor is composed of skin and two layers of superficial fascia—a superficial fatty stratum and a deeper membranous one. The former is continuous anteriorly with the superficial fatty layer of the abdomen (Camper fascia) and posteriorly with the ischiorectal fat. The deeper, membranous layer of the superficial perineal fascia (Colles fascia) is limited to the anterior half of the perineum. Laterally, it is attached to the ischiopubic rami; posteriorly, it blends with the base of the urogenital diaphragm; and anteriorly, it is continuous with the deep layer of the superficial abdominal fascia (Scarpa fascia).

The urogenital diaphragm is a strong, musculomembranous partition stretched across the anterior half of the pelvic outlet between the ischiopubic rami. It is composed of superior and inferior fascial layers between which are located the deep perineal muscles, the sphincter of the membranous urethra, and the pudendal vessels and nerves. It is pierced by the urethra and vagina.

The anal triangle is delineated by the superficial perineal muscles anteriorly, the sacrotuberous ligaments and margins of the gluteus maximus laterally, and the coccyx posteriorly. It contains the anal canal and its sphincters, the anococcygeal body, and the ischiorectal fossae.

The ischiorectal fossae are prismatic in shape. The lateral wall of each is formed by the obturator internus fascia, and its medial wall by the fascia overlying the levator ani, the coccygeus, and the external anal sphincter muscles. The tendinous arch marks its apex. Anteriorly, the fossa extends between the urogenital and pelvic diaphragms. Posteriorly, the sacrotuberous ligament and gluteus maximus muscle limits it. The contents of the ischiorectal fossa include an abundance of fat, the inferior hemorrhoidal vessels and nerves, and the internal pudendal vessels and nerves within the Alcock canal.

The muscles of the perineum include the bulbocavernosus, the ischiocavernosus, the superficial and deep transverse perineal muscles, the sphincter of the membranous urethra, and the external anal sphincter. These muscles, in general, correspond to their homologues in the male. The ischiocavernosus muscles are smaller than in the male. They overlie and insert into the crura of the clitoris instead of into the crura of the penis, as in the male. The bulbocavernosus muscles surround the orifice of the vagina and cover the vestibular bulbs. They are attached posteriorly to the central tendinous point of the perineum and to the inferior fascia of the urogenital diaphragm and insert anteriorly into the corpora cavernosa clitoridis. They are sometimes termed the *sphincter vaginae*. Spasms in this muscle

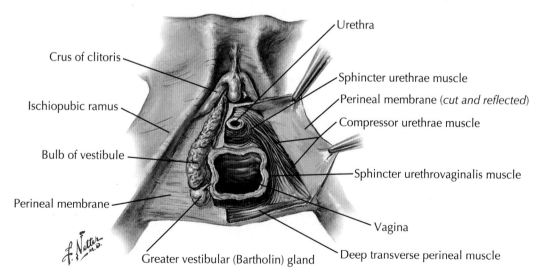

group are often found in patients with genital pelvic pain/penetration disorder (formerly known as *vaginismus*). The pair of deep transverse perineal muscles (within the urogenital diaphragm) are interrupted near the midline by the vagina, into which they insert.

The central point of the perineum lies at the base of the urogenital diaphragm between the vaginal and anal orifices. It is a common fibrous point of attachment for

the bulbocavernosus, the superficial and deep transverse perineal, the levator ani, and the external anal sphincter muscles. This area is often referred to as the *perineal body*.

The anococcygeal body is of fibromuscular consistency and extends from the anus to the coccyx. It receives fibers from the external anal sphincter and the levator ani muscles and serves as a support for the anal canal.

Plate 6.4

Vulva

LYMPHATIC DRAINAGE: EXTERNAL GENITALIA

A network of lymphatic anastomoses drains the external genitalia, the lower third of the vagina, and the perineum. Bilateral or crossed extension and drainage is common. The superficial femoral nodes are reached through the superficial external pudendal lymphatic vessels, although the superficial external epigastrics may also play a role. From the region of the clitoris, deeper lymphatic vessels may pass directly to the deep femoral nodes, particularly to the Cloquet node in the femoral canal, or through the inguinal canal to the external iliac nodes. Sometimes, intercalated nodes may be encountered in the prepubic area or at the external inguinal ring. The lowermost portion of the vagina, like the vulva, may drain to the femoral nodes. This complex network of lymph nodes is clinically important, for these are the nodes to which cutaneous and vulvovaginal gland malignancies may drain. Regional lymph node dissections are routinely performed in the surgical treatment of vulvar cancer as the status of regional lymph nodes is essential for therapeutic planning and overall prognosis. Superficial nodes in the groin may also become enlarged when significant inflammation is present in the vulvar structures (e.g., Bartholin gland infections).

The inguinal lymph nodes, both superficial and deep, lie within the subcutaneous tissue roughly overlying the femoral triangle ("femoral" lymph nodes). Lymphatic vessels tend to follow the course of veins draining a particular region. The lymph nodes are arranged in groups or chains in close relation to the vessels. The nodes found in this region are generally further referred to as the *superficial and deep inguinal lymph nodes*.

The superficial femoral nodes are a group of nodes found in the loose, fatty connective tissue of the femoral triangle between the superficial and deep fascial layers. These nodes receive lymphatic drainage from the external genitalia of the vulvar region, the gluteal region, and the entire leg, including the foot: the saphenous vein nodes drain the lower extremities, whereas the superficial circumflex vein nodes drain the posterolateral aspect of the thighs and buttocks.

Afferent vessels from the lower abdominal wall and the upper superficial aspects of the genitalia extend to the superficial epigastric vein nodes in the abdominal wall above the symphysis. The superficial external pudendal vein nodes drain the external genitalia, the lower third of the vagina, the perineum, and the perianal region. Efferent lymphatic vessels from all the superficial femoral nodes drain to the more proximal superficial inguinal (femoral) nodes, the deep inguinal (femoral) nodes, and the external iliac nodes. Efferent lymphatics from this group of nodes penetrate the fascia lata to enter the deep femoral nodes and represent the greatest concentration of lymph nodes in the female.

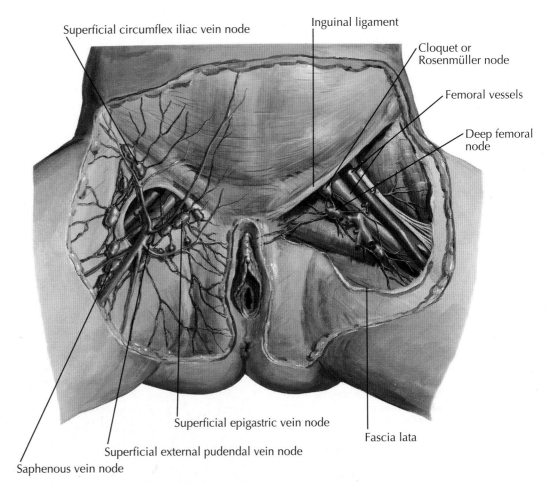

Superficial circumflex iliac vein node

Inguinal ligament

Cloquet or Rosenmüller node

Femoral vessels

Deep femoral node

Superficial epigastric vein node

Fascia lata

Superficial external pudendal vein node

Saphenous vein node

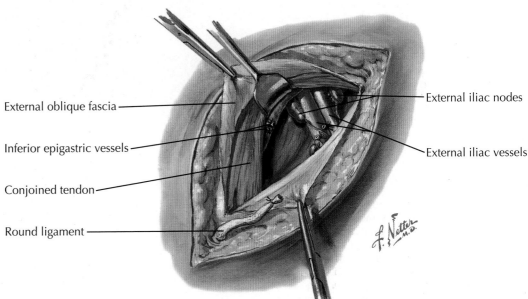

External oblique fascia

Inferior epigastric vessels

Conjoined tendon

Round ligament

External iliac nodes

External iliac vessels

Exposure of external iliac nodes through inguinal canal

A few constant nodes are usually associated with the deeper lymphatic trunks along the femoral vessels. These may be situated on the mesial aspect of the femoral vein, above and below its junction with the saphenous vein. The highest of the deep femoral nodes lies within the opening of the femoral canal (Cloquet or Rosenmüller node). The deep femoral nodes receive afferent lymphatics directly or indirectly from the parts drained by the superficial femoral lymphatics and send efferent vessels to nodes higher in the chain and to the external iliac nodes.

Knowledge of the lymphatic drainage of the perineum can be especially helpful in the assessment of and treatment of patients with vulvar cancers. Lymphatic mapping and sentinel lymph node biopsy may be applied in these patients. The sentinel node(s) are those nodes that directly drain the primary tumor and are thought to predict the metastatic status of the upper nodes in the groin.

Plate 6.5

Reproductive System: VOLUME 1

BLOOD SUPPLY OF PERINEUM

The perineum and vulva are richly supplied with blood vessels, which become clinically important during childbirth and surgical procedures. Blunt trauma to the area, such as straddle injuries in children, can result in significant bleeding or hematoma formation when vessels are ruptured and bleeding into the loose compartments of the perineum occurs.

The internal pudendal artery in the female is a far smaller vessel than it is in the male, although its course is generally the same in both sexes. When leaving the lesser pelvis through the lower part of the greater sciatic foramen, it enters the ischiorectal fossa through the lesser sciatic foramen. Here, accompanied by its venae comites and the pudendal nerve, it lies in a fibrous canal (Alcock canal) formed by the fascia covering the obturator internus muscle. The branches of the internal pudendal artery include small ones to the gluteal region, the inferior hemorrhoidal artery, the perineal artery, and the artery of the clitoris. The pudendal artery (and vein) is closely associated with the pudendal nerve as it passes the ischial spine near the insertion of the sacrospinous ligament (on the dorsal aspect of the coccygeal muscle), placing it at risk when sacrospinous colpopexy is performed. (A rare complication of this operation is massive hemorrhage from the inferior gluteal or pudendal arteries.)

The inferior hemorrhoidal artery pierces the wall of the Alcock canal and passes medially through the ischiorectal fat to supply the anal canal, anus, and perineal area. The perineal artery pierces the base of the urogenital diaphragm to enter the superficial perineal compartment, where it supplies the ischiocavernosus, bulbocavernosus, and transverse perineal muscles. A constant transverse perineal branch runs along the superficial transverse perineal muscle to the central point of the perineum. The terminal branches of the perineal artery, the posterior labial arteries, pierce the deep layer of the superficial perineal fascia (Colles fascia) to the labia.

The artery of the clitoris enters the deep compartment of the urogenital diaphragm and runs along the inferior ramus of the pubis in the substance of the deep transverse perineal muscle and the sphincter of the membranous urethra, ending in four branches, which supply chiefly the erectile tissue of the superficial perineal compartment. The artery of the bulb passes through the inferior fascia of the urogenital diaphragm to supply the cavernous tissue of the vestibular bulb and

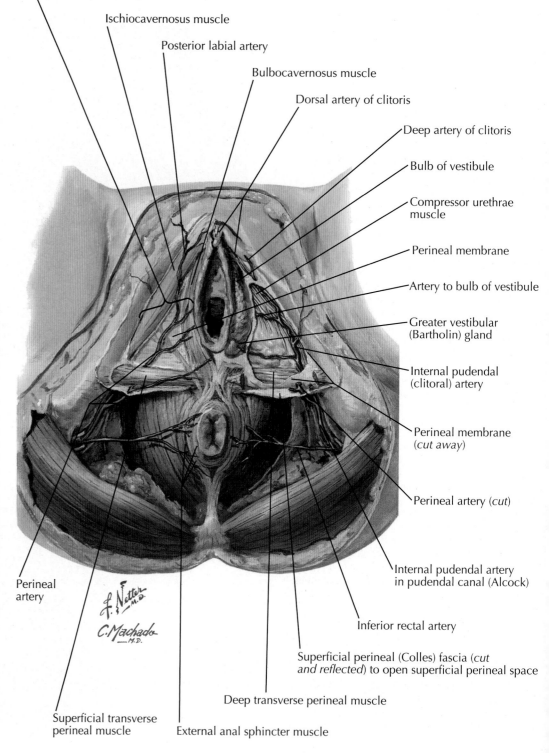

the Bartholin gland. The urethral artery runs medialward toward the urethra and anastomoses with branches from the artery of the bulb. The deep artery of the clitoris pierces the fascial floor of the deep compartment just medial to the corpus cavernosum of the clitoris, which it enters. The dorsal artery of the clitoris leaves the deep perineal compartment just behind the transverse pelvic muscle and runs over the dorsum of the clitoris to the glans.

Note: Deep perineal (investing or Gallaudet) fascia removed from muscles of superficial perineal space.

The blood supply of the vulva and perineum is richly connected to the vascular supply of the entire vaginal barrel, the cervix, and the uterus through a number of ascending and descending anastomoses. This vascular net surrounds the vaginal canal with major trunks running in the lateral vaginal wall at the 3 and 9 o'clock locations. Trauma to these areas, as with a vaginal delivery, can result in significant blood loss that may be difficult to control.

Plate 6.6

Vulva

Innervation of External Genitalia and Perineum

The musculature and integument of the perineum are innervated mainly by the pudendal nerve. Derived from the anterior rami of the second, third, and fourth sacral nerves, it leaves the pelvis through the greater sciatic foramen, between the piriformis and coccygeus muscles, and crosses beneath the ischial spine on the mesial side of the internal pudendal artery. It then continues within the Alcock canal in the obturator fascia on the lateral wall of the ischiorectal fossa, toward the ischial tuberosity. The pudendal nerve divides into three branches: (1) The inferior hemorrhoidal nerve pierces the medial wall of the Alcock canal, traverses the ischiorectal fossa, and supplies the external anal sphincter and perianal skin. (2) The perineal nerve runs for a short distance in the Alcock canal and divides into a deep and a superficial branch. The deep branch sends filaments to the external anal sphincter and levator ani muscles and then pierces the base of the urogenital diaphragm to supply the superficial and deep perineal muscles, the ischiocavernosus and bulbocavernosus muscles, and the membranous urethral sphincter. The superficial branch divides into medial and lateral posterior labial nerves, which innervate the labium majus. (3) The dorsal nerve of the clitoris passes through the urogenital diaphragm to the glans of the clitoris.

A number of nerves innervate the perineal skin. The anterior labial branches of the ilioinguinal nerve (L1) emerge from the external inguinal ring to be distributed to the mons veneris and the upper portion of the labium majus. (Extreme flexion of the leg during childbirth or vaginal operative procedures can result in temporary or permanent loss of function of this nerve.) The external spermatic branch of the genitofemoral nerve (L1, 2) accompanies the round ligament through the inguinal canal and sends twigs to the labium. The perineal branches of the posterior femoral cutaneous nerve (S1, 2, 3) run forward and medialward in front of the ischial tuberosity to the lateral margin of the perineum and labium majus. Branches of the perineal nerve (S2, 3, 4) include the dorsal nerve of the clitoris and the medial and lateral posterior labial branches to the labium majus. The inferior hemorrhoidal branch of the pudendal nerve (S2, 3, 4) contributes to the supply of the perianal skin and accounts for the sensory portion of the "anal wink" reflex. The perforating cutaneous branches of the second and third sacral nerves perforate the sacrotuberous ligament and turn around the inferior border of the gluteus maximus to supply the buttocks and contiguous perineum. The anococcygeal nerves (S4, 5, and coccygeal nerve) unite along the coccyx and then pierce the sacrotuberous ligaments to supply the anococcygeal area.

The course and distribution of the pudendal nerve make it an ideal candidate for safe and effective regional nerve blockade. A pudendal nerve block can be accomplished through either a transcutaneous or transvaginal approach, although the former has generally fallen out of

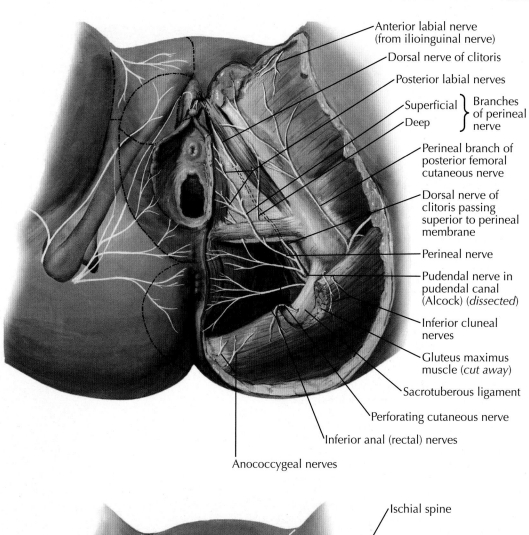

- Anterior labial nerve (from ilioinguinal nerve)
- Dorsal nerve of clitoris
- Posterior labial nerves
- Superficial ⎱ Branches of perineal nerve
- Deep ⎰
- Perineal branch of posterior femoral cutaneous nerve
- Dorsal nerve of clitoris passing superior to perineal membrane
- Perineal nerve
- Pudendal nerve in pudendal canal (Alcock) (*dissected*)
- Inferior cluneal nerves
- Gluteus maximus muscle (*cut away*)
- Sacrotuberous ligament
- Perforating cutaneous nerve
- Inferior anal (rectal) nerves
- Anococcygeal nerves

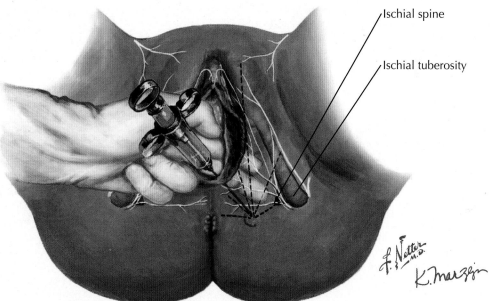

- Ischial spine
- Ischial tuberosity

Produces anesthesia of pudendal and other nerves of perineal area

favor. In the transcutaneous approach, intradermal wheals are made bilaterally, midway between the rectum and the ischial tuberosities. With the middle and index fingers of the clinician's left hand (for a block on the patient's left side) in the vagina, a 10-cm needle is guided to a point just under and beyond the ischial spine, where 10 to 15 mL of a 0.5% to 1.0% local anesthetic solution is deposited. This blocks the internal pudendal nerve, as

it passes dorsal to the spine just before entering the Alcock canal. The clinician's right hand is used to guide placement of a block on the patient's right side.

In the transvaginal approach to a pudendal nerve block, the needle is placed within a needle guide and directed to the ischial spine by traversing the lateral vaginal wall. This approach is often faster and better tolerated than a transcutaneous route.

Plate 6.7

Reproductive System: VOLUME 1

DERMATOSES

The skin of the vulva is subject to the same dermatoses that occur over the rest of the body surface. Those described here, and subsequently, are only a few of the more common lesions.

Folliculitis refers to a papular or pustular inflammation about the apertures of hair follicles, caused by *Staphylococcus aureus* or mixed organisms. Furuncles are larger and more deeply situated and exhibit the typical signs of inflammation about a central core of purulent exudate. Contributory factors for a *staphylococcus pyoderma* infection include the irritation of tight underclothes or vulvar pads, lack of cleanliness, diabetes, and lowered immune competence (natural or iatrogenic). Abundant inflammation helps to separate folliculitis from seborrheic dermatitis. Topical therapy with sitz baths, topical antibiosis, and interim drying and ventilation is usually sufficient. Systemic antibiotic therapy may be appropriate in selected cases.

Sebaceous cysts may form in any of the hair-bearing portions of the vulva. They can be differentiated from folliculitis by their limited number, distribution, and reduced or absent signs of inflammation. Sebaceous cysts will often spontaneously drain or may be opened and drained if large or symptomatic.

Herpes genitalis is a herpes simplex infection of the vulva similar to that which occurs about the lips, nose, cornea, or, in the male, on the penis. It is a superficial, localized, and frequently recurring lesion, caused by the herpes virus. Either or both herpes simplex virus 1 (HSV-1) and 2 (HSV-2) can cause genital herpes, although most cases of recurrent genital herpes are caused by HSV-2. Herpetic vulvitis appears as groups of vesicles on an edematous, erythematous base. The blisters tend to break, with the formation of small ulcers, or they dry and become covered with crusts. Initial infections are often extremely painful, even to the extent of causing urinary retention in females. Symptoms of recurrent infections are usually limited to local pruritus or burning. Herpes zoster is differentiated by the distribution of vesicles along a nerve trunk and the occurrence of a prodromal period of fever, malaise, and localized pain. The clinical diagnosis of genital herpes should be confirmed by laboratory testing.

Tinea cruris is a fungus infection or ringworm of the groin, usually caused by *Epidermophyton floccosum*. The lesions consist of discrete patches, which may cover the vulva, pubis, lower abdomen, groins, and inner thighs. They are pink or red in color, scaly, and sharply demarcated from normal skin. Secondary inflammatory changes may be superimposed as the result of scratching, moisture, and irritation. The condition may be spread by direct contact or through use of contaminated clothing. The diagnosis may be corroborated by culture on Sabouraud medium or by examination of superficial scales placed in a hanging drop of 10% sodium or potassium hydroxide to establish the presence of the characteristic branching mycelia.

Psoriasis of the vulva is not uncommon, affecting up to 2% of the general population. The most common presentation is persistent vulvar itching. The presence of

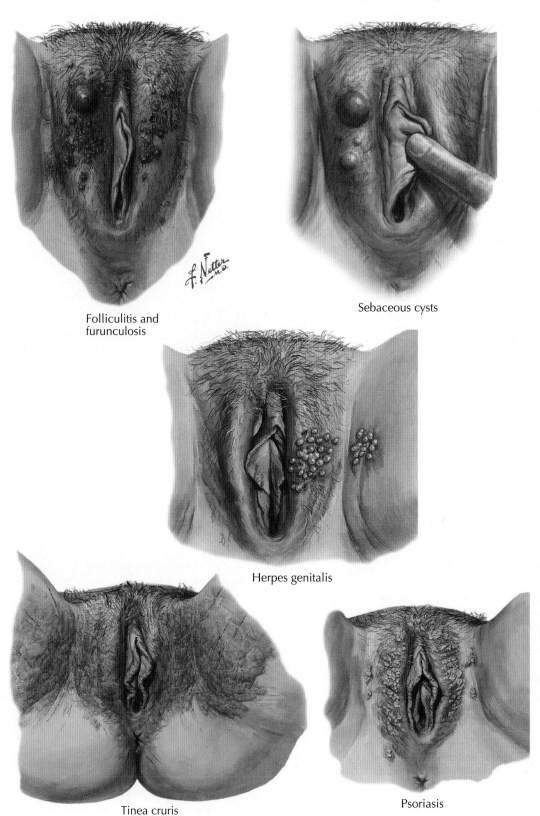

Folliculitis and furunculosis

Sebaceous cysts

Herpes genitalis

Tinea cruris

Psoriasis

similar lesions on the scalp and extensor surfaces of the extremities is helpful in establishing the diagnosis. The general characteristics of psoriasis include (1) reddened, slightly elevated, dry, and sharply demarcated patches covered with silvery-white scales, (2) a characteristic distribution, (3) the presence of nail changes, (4) history of chronicity or recurrence, and (5) a familial tendency. The diagnosis is usually established by its characteristic appearance and distribution, although the silver scales, typical of psoriasis, are generally only found on the

mons and not elsewhere on the vulva. A biopsy may be required to confirm the diagnosis. Initial treatment begins with avoidance of irritants, the use of emollients and moisturizers, and limited use of topical steroids. Topical antibiotics or antifungal therapy is prudent when significant skin cracking has occurred. Many of the treatments used to treat psoriasis elsewhere are too harsh to use on genital skin. Unfortunately, there is no true cure for psoriasis, but it can be controlled with phototherapy, systemic therapies, and immune

Plate 6.8

Vulva

DERMATOSES (Continued)

modulation treatments. (Drugs targeting the interleukin [IL]-17 pathway have demonstrated efficacy for psoriasis.)

Acne inversa (formerly hidradenitis suppurativa) is a chronic, unrelenting, refractory infection of the skin and subcutaneous tissue that is fourfold more common in females than in males. It is initiated by the obstruction and subsequent inflammation of follicles and apocrine glands, with resultant sinus and abscess formation. This process may involve the axilla, vulva, and perineum. The most effective therapy is based on early, aggressive, wide excision of the affected area. Topical therapy with antibiotics, topical steroids, oral contraceptives, antiandrogens, and isotretinoin may be used in early or mild cases.

Contact vulvitis is characterized by vulvar irritation caused by contact with an irritant or allergen. Irritants may be primary or immunologic in character. The list of potential irritants can be extensive, including excessive hygiene ("feminine hygiene" sprays, deodorants and deodorant soaps, tampons, or pads—especially those with deodorants or perfumes), tight-fitting undergarments or those made of synthetic fabric, colored or scented toilet paper, and laundry soap or fabric softener residues. Even topical contraceptives, latex condoms, lubricants, "sexual aids," or semen may be the source of irritation. Soiling of the vulva by urine or feces can also create significant symptoms. Severe dermatitis of the vulva resulting from contact with poison ivy or poison oak is occasionally observed. Diffuse reddening of the vulvar skin is accompanied by itching or burning. Symmetric, red, edematous change in the tissues is seen with occasional ulceration with weeping sores and secondary infection possible. Skin changes are limited to those areas exposed to the allergen. Identification and removal of the irritant, along with perineal care, is generally sufficient to resolve the symptoms. If symptoms are particularly severe or persistent, administer wet compresses or soaks using Burow solution (aluminum acetate 2.5%–5% solution), three to four times daily for 30–60 minutes), followed by air drying or drying with a hair dryer on cool setting. Loose-fitting clothing and the sparing use of a nonmedicated baby powder may facilitate the drying process. Further evaluation is warranted (including biopsy) if initial therapy does not produce significant improvement.

Genital intertrigo is a superficial inflammation of the external genitalia and upper thighs. It appears as a red or brownish discoloration, particularly of the interlabial sulci, the furrows between the vulva and thighs, and the inner aspect of the thighs. It commonly includes moist erythema, malodor, weeping, pruritus, and tenderness. It is caused by chafing, especially in females with obesity, and during hot weather. Anything that contributes to local moisture, such as a persistent vaginal discharge or urinary incontinence, will prolong the irritation. A dermatophytosis frequently is superimposed.

Acute aphthous ulcers (acute genital ulceration, Lipschütz ulcers, non–sexually acquired genital ulceration [NSAGU], and vulvar aphthae) are similar to the more common oral ulcers known as *canker sores*. These ulcers are the result of a localized vasculitis caused, in

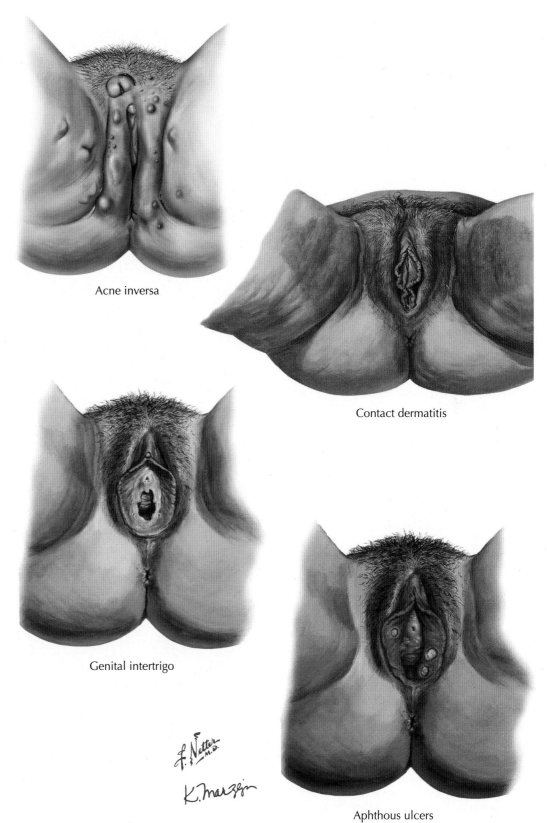

Acne inversa

Contact dermatitis

Genital intertrigo

Aphthous ulcers

about one-third of cases, by various infections. The most common precursors are Epstein-Barr virus, *Mycoplasma pneumoniae*, and viral respiratory infections (parvovirus, influenza, paramyxovirus). These painful ulcers appear quickly, evolving from a purpuric area that rapidly becomes necrotic and then ulcerates over 1 to 2 days. The majority of patients have flulike symptoms that precede or accompany the ulcers. Lesions are sharply marginated (punched out) and may have a white coagulum or adherent, black crust at the base of

the ulcer. Multiple ulcers are common. Although the pain is similar to that of acute herpetic infections, the absence of vesicles and the larger size (up to 3 cm) of aphthous ulcers make the diagnosis apparent. Biopsy is seldom needed. Treatment is primarily supportive and includes reassurance, local hygiene, sitz baths, wound care, and pain control. Oral analgesics or topical anesthetics (lidocaine 2% viscous solution) may be required for pain control. Ulcers can take up to 6 weeks to fully heal, but they generally heal without scarring.

Plate 6.9

Reproductive System: VOLUME 1

ATROPHIC CONDITIONS

Atrophy may follow natural or surgical menopause, or loss of ovarian function by chemotherapy (alkylating agents) or x-ray therapy. Because the condition causes both vaginal and urinary symptoms, the term *genitourinary syndrome of menopause* (GSM) is the preferred term to describe vaginal atrophy and its accompanying symptoms. It is the result of the loss of estrogen stimulation to the genital tract. The skin changes are variable in degree and slowly progressive. With the loss of subcutaneous fat beneath the mons veneris and labia majora, the vulva assumes an increasingly shrunken appearance. The pubic hair becomes thin, sparse, and brittle. The labia minora, clitoris, and prepuce are reduced in size. The skin becomes thin, inelastic, shiny, and occasionally depigmented. Microscopically, the stratified squamous epithelium is reduced in thickness and there is a loss of elastic fibers. The underlying connective tissue shows evidence of decreased vascularity and increased fibrosis.

In the past, the terms *kraurosis vulvae* and *leukoplakia* were applied to similar atrophic changes. Leukoplakia was primarily an inflammatory process, whereas kraurosis vulvae was essentially an extreme degree of atrophy. These terms have been discarded in part because abnormal lesions of the vulva require biopsy to establish a correct diagnosis and to rule out the possibility of an occult malignancy (present in 4%–6% of cases of lichen sclerosus).

Atrophic vulvitis (the former kraurosis vulvae) is a progressive sclerosing atrophy of marked degree, resulting in stenosis of the vaginal opening and effacement of the labia minora and clitoris. Dyspareunia is a common complaint because of dryness and the shrinkage of the vaginal introitus and canal. The vulvar skin is thin, dry, shiny, depigmented, and yellow-white. The tension of parts often causes cracks, excoriations, and annoying pruritus.

These atrophic changes must be differentiated from the changes of lichen sclerosus. Lichen sclerosus is a benign, chronic, progressive condition characterized by marked inflammation, epithelial thinning, and distinctive dermal changes. It is often accompanied by symptoms of pruritus and pain. Microscopically, the epithelium becomes markedly thinned with a loss or blunting of the rete ridges. In some cases, there is also a thickening or hyperkeratosis of the surface layers. Inflammation is usually present, and an autoimmune etiology has been postulated. When lichen sclerosus is present, there is usually a diffuse whitish change to the vulvar skin. Lichen sclerosus often presents as white, atrophic papules that may coalesce into plaques. The vulvar skin often appears thin, and there may be scarring and contracture beyond what is seen with simple estrogen deprivation. In addition, fissuring of the skin is often present, accompanied by excoriation secondary to itching. As the disease progresses, the labia are flattened and the clitoris becomes buried under the fused prepuce. It is nonneoplastic and involves glabrous skin as well as the vulva. Areas of squamous hyperplasia (formerly called *hyperplastic dystrophy without atypia*) also appear as whitish lesions in general, but the tissues of the vulva usually appear thickened and the process tends to be more focal or multifocal than diffuse. (The term *lichen sclerosus et atrophicus* was dropped because the epithelium is metabolically active, not atrophic.) The diagnosis should be confirmed by biopsy.

Vulvar atypia (formerly leukoplakia) may present as a slowly progressing, chronic, inflammatory, hypertrophic process involving the epidermis and subepithelial tissues. It may occur as single or multiple discrete plaques or as a

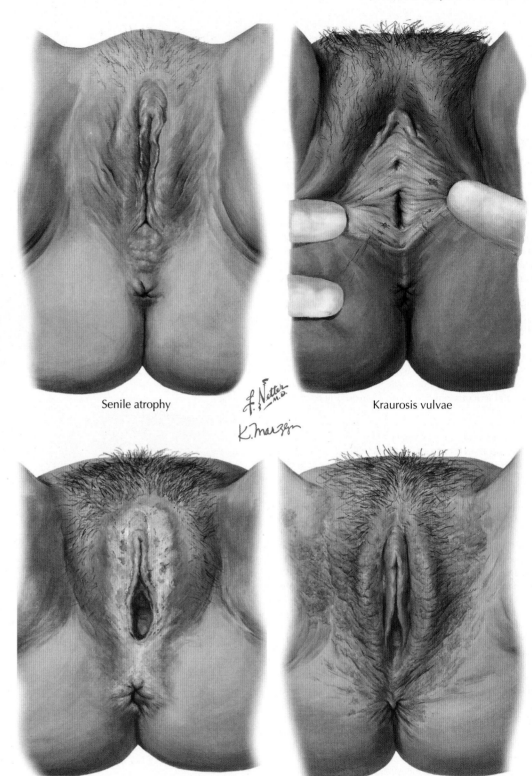

Senile atrophy

Kraurosis vulvae

Leukoplakia

Lichenification

generalized lesion involving the clitoris, prepuce, labia minora, posterior commissure, perineum, and perianal areas. The lesion is grayish-white in color, thickened, and almost asbestos-like in appearance. Fissures and ulcerations are common. The histologic picture includes hyperkeratosis, increase in the stratum granulosum, acanthosis, lymphatic infiltration of the cutis, and destruction of the elastic fibers of the corium. Differentiation of this from other lesions of the vulva is important because squamous cell carcinoma of the vulva is preceded by these changes in almost 50% of cases.

Prolonged scratching may provoke lichenification (hypertrophic vulvar dystrophy, lichen simplex chronicus), a secondary change in the skin. The skin has a thickened, leathery appearance in which the normal markings appear accentuated. When moisture is present, the lesion assumes a grayish-white, soggy appearance. Hyperkeratosis, parakeratosis, acanthosis, and prolongation of the retial pegs can be seen histologically, but the subepithelial elastic fibers are not destroyed. The condition is common, representing 40% to 45% of nonneoplastic epithelial disorders.

Plate 6.10

Vulva

CIRCULATORY AND OTHER DISTURBANCES

Varices of the vulva occur most often during pregnancy, as an aftermath of repeated pregnancies, or the result of any processes that increase intraabdominal pressure such as a chronic cough. They are usually associated with varicose veins of the lower extremities. A primary factor in their development is the presence of retarded venous flow caused by increased intrapelvic or intraabdominal pressure. The veins of the labia and prepuce are most commonly involved, either unilaterally or bilaterally. They may form subcutaneous convolutions, which sometimes reach the size of a fist. Subjectively, there may be an annoying full, "dragging," or heavy sensation. The varices become prominent when the patient is standing or straining and tend to disappear when in the supine position. Those that occur during pregnancy are apt to subside, to a great extent, after delivery. A varix may rupture as a result of direct trauma, injury during labor or delivery, excessive coughing, or other straining. Rarely, a venous thrombosis may ensue. When symptomatic, resection, fulguration, sclerosis, or embolization therapies may be required.

Angioneurotic edema is an allergic reaction that may involve the vulva as it does other areas. The condition is a self-limited, localized subcutaneous swelling that results from extravasation of fluid into interstitial tissues. It may occur in isolation, accompanied by urticaria, or as a component of wider allergic response including anaphylaxis. The diagnosis is suggested by the sudden appearance, without apparent cause, of a large, noninflammatory, painless vulvar swelling that is transient and generally asymmetric. Differentiation should be made from nephrotic or cardiac edema, or that which results from increased intrapelvic pressure secondary to neoplasm or large pelvic exudates. The possibility of a patent canal of Nuck giving rise to an inguinal hernia should also be considered. Because of the loose texture of the subcutaneous tissue of the labia, marked edematous swelling may accompany small local infections or contact with allergens. The list of potential irritants can be extensive, including "feminine hygiene" sprays, deodorants and deodorant soaps, tampons or pads (especially those with deodorants or perfumes), tight-fitting or synthetic undergarments, colored or scented toilet paper, and laundry soap or fabric softener residues. Even topical contraceptives, latex condoms, lubricants, "sexual aids," or semen may be the source of irritation. Soiling of the vulva by urine or feces can also create significant symptoms. Severe dermatitis of the vulva resulting from contact with poison ivy or poison oak is occasionally found. Frequently, no specific causation is apparent. Spontaneous resolution over the course of a few hours to a few days is typical and is hastened by the removal of the inciting allergen or cause.

The term *elephantiasis* is applied to chronic, hypertrophic tissue changes secondary to excessive lymph stasis. In the tropics, it is known as *lymphatic filariasis* with the

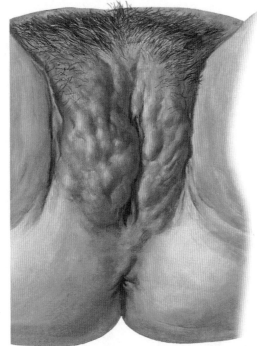

Varicose veins

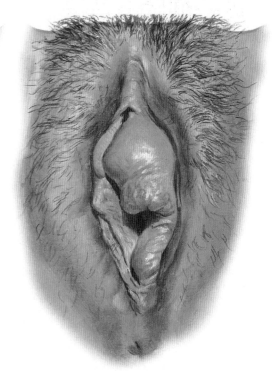

Angioneurotic edema

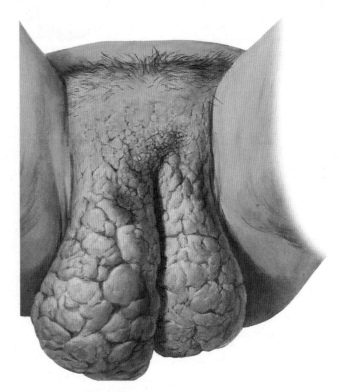

Elephantiasis

most common cause a parasitic worm, *Wuchereria bancrofti* (90%). *Brugia malayi* and *Brugia timori* may also cause this condition. These infections are spread by mosquitoes, and humans are the definitive hosts. Other diseases, particularly lymphogranuloma venereum, may cause obstruction of the lymph channels of the vulva. Histologically, the lymph vessels appear greatly dilated, and the subcutaneous tissue is thickened, edematous, and inflamed. The skin surface may be pale, smooth, nodular, or warty. The labia may be converted into large, pachydermatous, sessile, or pedunculated tumors. Prevention relies on mass drug administration to the populace. In many areas around the world, this has resulted in dramatic reductions or elimination of these infections. Once vulvar skin changes have occurred, no specific treatment is available to reverse the findings. Rarely, partial excision is required for large or particularly symptomatic cases.

Plate 6.11

Reproductive System: VOLUME 1

VULVAR TRAUMA AND LACERATIONS

A hematoma of the vulva may be secondary to a fall or blow, surgical or obstetric trauma, or rupture of a varix. The blood from minor extravasations is slowly absorbed and requires only supportive care. A hematoma of the vulva that occurs during or after labor, however, may be of vital significance, because it may extend paravaginally and pararectally to the subperitoneal space and be associated with significant loss of circulating blood volume. A large collection of blood may distend the labia and infiltrate into the ischiorectal fossa and buttock. The most common source of vulvar hematomas in young patients is blunt trauma from straddle injuries. Sexual abuse, rape, and water skiing accidents that result in impact to the perineum can also result in vulvar trauma and hematoma formation. Based on the presumed cause, the possibility of an accompanying laceration must always be considered. The presence of hematuria suggests a more extensive injury and requires additional evaluation. Analgesics, pressure, and ice are appropriate initial therapies. Warm sitz baths may provide comfort after the first 24 hours. Surgical drainage for rapidly expanding hematomas or those >10 cm in diameter may be required, although surgical intervention should generally be avoided as the likelihood of finding and controlling the source of bleeding in the loose, highly vascular tissues of the vulva is low. Most hematomas gradually resolve with conservative management only and leave no lasting sequelae.

Laceration of the external genitalia can occur as a result of blunt or sharp trauma, childbirth, or in the course of surgical access and repair. Because vulvar lacerations can also result from sexual activity, including rape or abuse, great care must be taken in evaluating the circumstances reported surrounding the clinical presentation. Straddle injuries, such as falling on the crossbar of a brother's bicycle, will generally cause symmetric trauma and usually involves the anterior and posterior portions of the vulva and surrounding perineum, the mons, clitoral hood, and the labia minora. They are generally located anterior or lateral to the hymen. The possibility of tears to the clitoral hood should be explored. Trauma restricted to the 3 to 9 o'clock positions of the vulva or hymen (posterior fourchette) is suggestive of abuse but is not diagnostic. In young girls, such injuries may indicate vaginal penetration and possible vaginal injury, warranting assessment for deeper damage including rectum or vaginal perforation. If sexual abuse or rape is suspected, great care must be taken to preserve evidence, provide contraceptive and sexually transmissible infection prophylaxis, and provide appropriate emotional support and follow-up.

The blunt trauma that can cause hematomas can result in burst injuries to the skin of the labia or perineum. These lacerations tend to be superficial, and stellate or jagged in character. If there is minimal bleeding, and the extent of the laceration can be fully ascertained, they may be allowed to heal by primary or secondary intention. Small, absorbable synthetic sutures may also be used to approximate the edges and give a better cosmetic result. Examination under general anesthesia

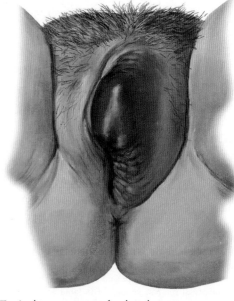

"Straddle" injury is common cause of vulvar hematoma.

Typical appearance of vulvar hematoma, a hematoma involving one or both labia

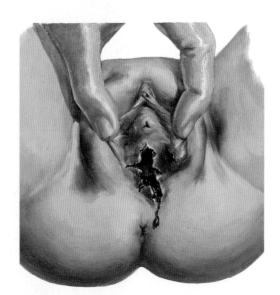

Presence of vulvar hematoma in children most often due to "straddle" injury, but should raise concern of sexual abuse, especially if lacerations are present

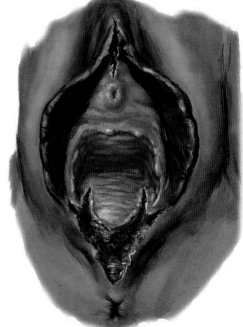

Obstetric lacerations can be midline, lateral, or bilateral and can extend well into the vaginal barrel.

may be indicated any time the patient is unable to urinate or there is hematuria, lower abdominal tenderness, or signs of occult blood loss such as hypovolemia. This is warranted to exclude injuries of the upper vagina and intrapelvic viscera. Any penetrating injury that results in vulvar lacerations must be thoroughly evaluated to ascertain the extent of any possible injury to internal structures, including entry into the peritoneal cavity.

Perineal lacerations (lateral or posterior to the vulva) may only involve the perineal skin or may extend into deeper tissues including the perineal body, levator plate, rectal sphincter, and rectal mucosa. Even moderate-sized hemostatic superficial lacerations may be left open, but actively bleeding lacerations should be closed with fine absorbable synthetic suture. When the lacerations are deep and potentially involve the supporting musculature or perineal body, the placement of deeper sutures for hemostasis or approximation of support structures is appropriate. This should be performed with regional or general anesthesia and adequate visualization.

Plate 6.12

Vulva

DIABETES, TRICHOMONIASIS, MONILIASIS

Vulvovaginal infections are a common occurrence and frequent cause for clinical evaluation. Although most frequently these are not associated with any underlying risk factor, females who are immunocompromised or have diabetes mellitus are at increased risk for opportunistic infections such as yeast infections.

Even without infection, vulvar itching is a common occurrence in females with diabetes. It may persist with or without a varying degree of dermatitis secondary to scratching. Frequently, a mycotic vulvitis or vulvovaginitis is superimposed and gives the characteristic picture of diabetic vulvitis. This is manifested by an inflamed, dark-red, or beefy appearance, which first involves the vestibule and labia minora and then spreads to adjacent parts. The elevated levels of sugar in the secretions bathing the vulva are thought to favor the growth of various fungi. As a result of irritation, excoriations and furuncles are common.

Moniliasis is a vulvovaginal infection caused by ubiquitous fungi found in the air or as common inhabitants of the vagina, rectum, and mouth. (*Candida* species are part of the normal flora of approximately 25% of females.) Vulvovaginitis caused by yeast belonging to the *Candida albicans* group has been variously designated as mycotic vaginitis, vulvovaginitis, yeast vulvovaginitis, vaginal thrush, or moniliasis. On speculum examination, white, cheesy, irregular plaques are found, partially adherent to the congested epithelium of the vagina and cervix. These are easily wiped off, sometimes leaving a red margin or shallow ulceration. The associated vaginal discharge may resemble curds and whey and may have a characteristic yeasty odor. The presence of most yeast species elicits a strong allergic response, resulting in the vestibule and lower portions of the labia becoming edematous, inflamed, and covered by minute vesicles, pustules, or ulcerations. Moniliasis may occur during childhood, sexual maturity, and after the menopause, but it is most common during the reproductive years. It has a definite predilection for pregnant females and females with diabetes, in whom it may be particularly resistant to treatment. Although often suspected by the typical clinical appearance, the diagnosis must be established with the addition of the microscopic demonstration of mycelia and yeast buds in the wet smear under high dry power. The thread-like mycelia and conidia may be more apparent after the use of 10% potassium hydroxide solution or in stained smears. If further confirmation is desired, a culture may be made on special culture media, although this is seldom necessary. Perineal hygiene (keeping the perineal area clean and dry, avoiding tight or synthetic undergarments), education regarding prevention, and encouraging completion of the prescribed course of antifungal therapy are all appropriate interventions.

A vaginal infection by the sexually transmitted single-celled anaerobic flagellate protozoan *Trichomonas vaginalis* accounts for approximately one quarter of all

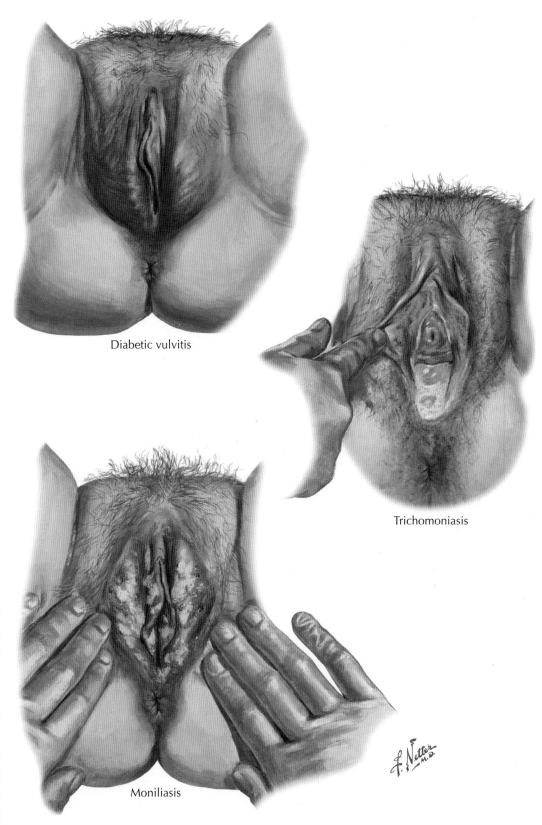

Diabetic vulvitis

Trichomoniasis

Moniliasis

vaginal infections. It is the most common nonviral sexually transmitted disease worldwide. In the acute stage of trichomoniasis, a vulvitis is usually also present, as evidenced by congestion of the vestibule and the inner aspects of the labia minora. On separating the inflamed labia, a thick, odoriferous, bubbly discharge may be seen in the vestibule. Presenting symptoms suggestive of trichomoniasis include a sudden increase in vaginal discharge, itching about the vulva, a burning sensation as urine passes over the inflamed area, and

dyspareunia. A wet mount examination of secretions from the vulva or vagina suspended in saline will demonstrate a fusiform protozoon slightly larger than a white blood cell with three to five flagella extending from the narrow end. These provide active movement. Culture, positive nucleic acid amplification test (NAAT), or positive rapid antigen or nucleic acid probe test can confirm the diagnosis but is seldom necessary. Evaluation for concomitant sexually transmissible infections should be strongly considered.

Plate 6.13

Reproductive System: VOLUME 1

Vulvodynia is a syndrome of intense sensitivity of skin of posterior vaginal introitus and vulvar vestibule resulting in dyspareunia and pain on attempted use of tampons.

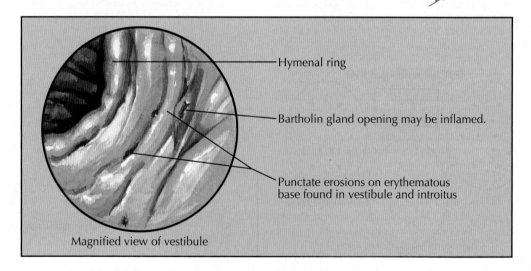

Area most commonly involved is posterior to Bartholin glands.

Opening of minor vestibular glands

Orifice of Bartholin gland

Bartholin gland

Level of discomfort is usually out of proportion to degree of physical findings, which include 1 to 10 small (3–10 mm) areas of punctate inflammation, some with ulceration in perineal and vaginal epithelium.

Involved area may be demarcated by light touch with cotton-tipped applicator.

JOHN A. CRAIG—AD
D. Mascaro

Hymenal ring

Bartholin gland opening may be inflamed.

Punctate erosions on erythematous base found in vestibule and introitus

Magnified view of vestibule

VULVODYNIA

Vulvodynia (previously referred to as *vulvar vestibulitis, provoked vulvodynia, vestibulodynia, vulvar vestibulitis, chronic vulvar pain of unknown etiology,* and *focal vulvitis*) is an uncommon syndrome of intense sensitivity of the skin of the posterior vaginal introitus and vulvar vestibule, characterized by progressive worsening, which leads to dyspareunia, vulvar pain, and loss of sexual function. Some estimates place its prevalence at 15% of all females, but significant, disabling symptoms are much less common. Although the median age of occurrence is 36 years, it can occur at any time after the late teenage years. New onset of symptoms is uncommon after menopause.

By definition, vulvodynia has an unknown cause, but there does appear to be a high degree of association with human papillomavirus (HPV), although no causal link has been established. It has been postulated that the use of oral contraceptives may increase the risk or severity of vulvodynia and that patients with vulvodynia should switch to other methods of contraception. Strong evidence for either causation or significant improvement is lacking. Despite the implication of the term *vulvitis,* widespread true inflammation is not a characteristic of this process.

The most common symptom is intense pain and tenderness at the posterior introitus and vestibule, most often present for 2 to 5 years. (Some authors suggest that symptoms must be present for 3–6 months before the diagnosis is made.) Most patients are unable to use tampons (33%) or to have intercourse (entry dyspareunia, 100%). The appearance of focal inflammation, punctation, and ulceration of the perineal and vaginal epithelium is common, although erythema is no longer included in the diagnostic criteria.

On physical examination, punctate areas (1–10) of inflammation 3 to 10 mm in size may be seen between the Bartholin glands, hymenal ring, and middle perineum. Colposcopy of the vulva (using 3% acetic acid) may reveal the characteristic small, inflammatory punctate lesions varying in size from 3 to 10 mm, often with superficial ulceration and acetowhite areas. The Bartholin gland openings may be inflamed as well. The area involved may be demarcated by light touching with a cotton-tipped applicator, although the level of discomfort is often out of proportion to the physical findings. If a biopsy is performed (not necessary for diagnosis), inflammation of minor vestibular glands may be seen.

Vulvodynia must be differentiated from cases of genital pelvic pain/penetration disorder (formerly known as *vaginismus*), chronic or atrophic vulvitis, hypertrophic vulvar dystrophy, and other vulvar dermatoses, including contact (allergic) dermatitis.

Initial management includes general perineal hygiene, cool sitz baths, moist soaks, or the application of soothing solutions such as Burow solution (aluminum acetate 2.5%–5%). Patients should be advised to wear loose-fitting clothing and keep the area dry and well ventilated. Pelvic floor physical therapy has been reported to be successful in many studies. Cognitive behavioral therapy and antidepressants have also been used to assist with symptom control. Spontaneous remission may occur in one third of patients over the course of 6 months.

More specific suggestions include topical anesthetics (lidocaine 2% jelly [or 5% cream] as needed or overnight) and antidepressants (amitriptyline hydrochloride), which may reduce pain and itch. Interferon injections may provide relief in up to 60% of patients but cannot be used in females who are pregnant. (Patients should be warned that interferon injections are associated with flulike symptoms and a clinical response may not be seen for up to 3 months. Patients should abstain from intercourse during the series of injections.) Refractory disease may require surgical resection or laser ablation. Surgical therapy is associated with 50% to 60% success rates.

Plate 6.14

Vulva

GONORRHEA

It is estimated that the rate of infection with gonorrhea from one act of intercourse with an infected partner is 20% for males but 60% to 80% for females. This rate increases to 60% to 80% for both sexes with four or more exposures. The symptoms of acute gonorrhea of the vulva may appear from 1 day to several days after contact, are often mild or transitory, and may be overlooked. The patient may experience burning on urination, urinary frequency, leukorrhea, and itching in the vestibule. Occasionally, however, the first suggestive manifestation of disease is not apparent until the following menses or shortly thereafter, when the ascending infection has resulted in an acute salpingitis. Examination of the external genitalia may reveal a congested vestibule bathed in pus and an inflammation of the urethra and Skene and Bartholin ducts. The acute infection ascends via the mucosa and epithelium of the urogenital tract and may give rise to an endometritis, peritonitis (pelvic inflammatory disease), and tuboovarian abscess. By lymphatic absorption and hematogenous spread, it may result in septicemia, endocarditis, arthritis, and tenosynovitis. Although if untreated, gonorrheal infection may, at times, be uncomplicated and self-limited, the tendency for establishment of deep-seated chronic foci is strong. These occur particularly within compound tubular glands and structures lined by columnar epithelium, such as the periurethral and Bartholin glands and the endocervix.

In acute urethritis, the mucosa of the external urethral meatus is reddened and edematous. On gentle stripping of the urethra, a few drops of thick yellow pus escape. The inflammatory reaction results in urinary frequency, urgency, and dysuria.

Acute skenitis is evident in the swollen, slightly raised, injected ostia of Skene ducts, which expel pus when milked. The ducts may harbor gonorrheal organisms over long periods of time. Thickened ducts and conspicuous orifices from which beads of pus can be expressed suggest a chronic infection.

In acute bartholinitis, the openings of the Bartholin ducts, normally inconspicuous, become more apparent because of the surrounding inflammation. On palpation, the Bartholin gland may be enlarged and tender. The infection can progress rapidly, resulting in an extremely painful swelling of the lower half of the labia. Eventually, a tender, red fluctuant abscess may develop, with taut, congested overlying skin, edema of the labia, and regional lymphadenopathy. This abscess may persist or may lead to a chronic infection, evidenced by enlargement of the gland, recurrent abscesses, and cyst formation.

Chronic urethritis may be manifested by a palpable induration of the posterior urethral wall mainly due to a persistence of infection within the shallow posterior urethral glands, seen endoscopically as small, granular areas on the urethral floor. The only symptom may be a burning sensation on urination.

In vulvovaginitis of childhood gonorrhea, the vagina and the vestibule of the vulva are inflamed and edematous and are covered by a creamy, yellow-green

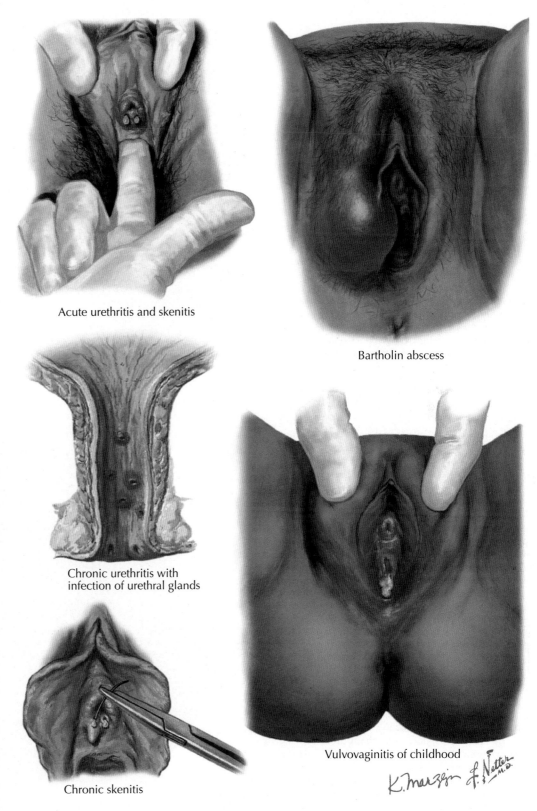

Acute urethritis and skenitis

Bartholin abscess

Chronic urethritis with infection of urethral glands

Chronic skenitis

Vulvovaginitis of childhood

discharge. The profuse leukorrhea results in secondary irritation of the labia and perineum. The adult vaginal epithelium, by virtue of its thickness and acidic environment, is more resistant to the gonococcus, but in childhood and after menopause, the vagina is far more susceptible to infection because of its thin epithelial layer and its alkaline environment.

Traditional culturing on Thayer-Martin agar plates maintained in a CO_2-rich environment has been replaced by NAAT as the preferred method. Cervical tests provide 80% to 95% diagnostic sensitivity. Specimens should also be obtained from the urethra and anus, although these additional samples do not significantly increase the sensitivity of testing. A Gram stain of any cervical discharge for the presence of gram-negative intracellular diplococcus supports the presumptive diagnosis but does not establish it (sensitivity, 50%–70%; specificity, 97%). Even when the diagnosis is established by other methods, all cases of gonorrhea should have cultures obtained to assess antibiotic susceptibility, although therapy should not be delayed pending the results.

Plate 6.15

Reproductive System: VOLUME 1

SYPHILIS

Since antiquity, syphilis has been the prototypic venereal disease. Syphilis presents with an easily overlooked first stage and, if left untreated, can slowly progress to a disabling disease noted for central nervous system, cardiac, and musculoskeletal involvement. The primary lesion of syphilis, although readily noted by the male, is not infrequently overlooked by the female. It appears most commonly on the labia majora, mons veneris, clitoris, fourchette, and vaginal epithelium but can also be seen on the anus, rectum, pharynx, tongue, lips, fingers, or the skin of almost any part of the body. The initial lesions first appear 10 to 60 days (average, 21 days) after infection as a fissure, abrasion, or nodule with slight erosion and may then develop the characteristics of a Hunterian chancre: an orange-red, granular ulcer, round or oval in shape, 1 or 2 cm in diameter, with sharp margins and an indurated base. Multiple chancres are sometimes seen, particularly within the labial folds.

Inguinal lymphadenopathy begins slowly, and by the sixth week after infection is usually well delineated. It appears as firm, painless, nonsuppurating nodes, from the size of a cherry to that of a walnut. Histologically, the chancre shows edema, congestion, and infiltration with lymphocytes, plasma cells, epithelioid, and giant cells. The initial lesions heal and may be associated with progression to a low-grade fever, headache, malaise, sore throat, anorexia, generalized lymphadenopathy, and a diffuse, symmetric, asymptomatic maculopapular rash over the palm and soles ("money palms"), mucous patches, and condyloma lata.

The Venereal Disease Research Laboratory (VDRL) and rapid plasma reagin tests are nonspecific tests that are good screening tests because they are rapid and inexpensive. The fluorescent treponemal antibody absorption or microhemagglutination *Treponema pallidum* tests are specific treponemal antibody tests that are confirmatory or diagnostic. They are useful to rule out a false-positive screening test, and reductions in the cost of these tests has changed their role to one of screening as well as confirmation. False-positive screening results may occur in patients with lupus, hepatitis, sarcoidosis, recent immunization, drug abuse, or during pregnancy. These test results may be falsely negative in the second stage of the disease as a result of high levels of anticardiolipin antibody that interferes with the test (prozone phenomenon). Up to 30% of patients with a primary lesion have negative test results. (Approximately 15%–25% of patients treated during the primary stage revert to being serologically nonreactive after 2–3 years.) If neurosyphilis is suspected, a lumbar puncture with a VDRL performed on the spinal fluid is required. (Unless clinical signs or symptoms of neurologic or ophthalmic involvement are present, cerebrospinal fluid analysis is

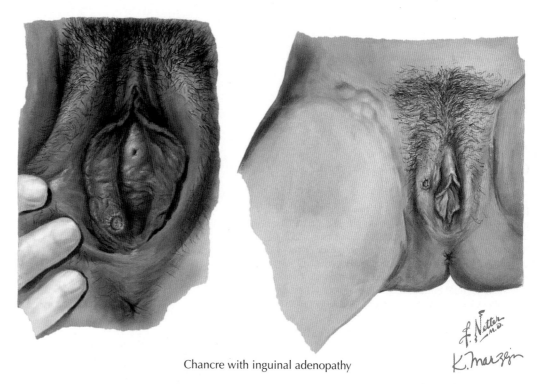

Chancre with inguinal adenopathy

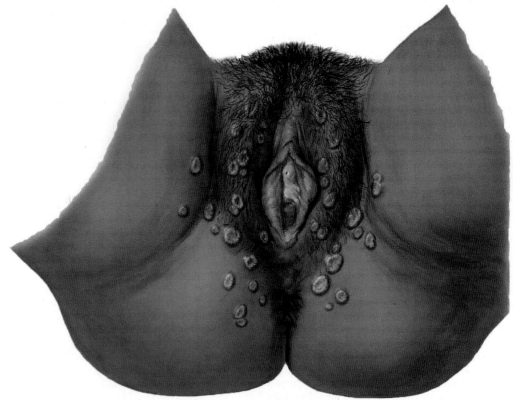

Condylomata lata

not recommended for routine evaluation of patients who have primary or secondary syphilis.) Screening for HIV infection should also be strongly considered.

The moisture, warmth, and irritation of the opposing surfaces of the vulva tend to modify the papules of secondary syphilis, which appear in this region. Through coalescence, hypertrophy, maceration, and ulceration, the typical condylomata (moist papules, syphilitic warts) are produced. These appear as multiple slightly elevated, disc-shaped, round or oval lesions, of sizes varying up to that of a dime. They are often confluent or

in clusters, with a moist, slightly depressed, necrotic surface. Condylomata lata may cover the vulva, perineum, perianal region, inner thighs, and buttocks and grow during pregnancy. The lesions are highly infectious.

Ulcerated and hypertrophic gummas of the vulva, as manifestations of tertiary syphilis, are rare. They are firm, massive growths, which may extend deeply into underlying tissues or may appear as multinodular ulcerated tumors involving part or most of the vulva. Secondary infections are common.

Plate 6.16

Vulva

CHANCROID AND OTHER INFECTIONS

Infection by *Haemophilus ducreyi* (a small, fastidious, gram-negative rod) results in chancroid, one of a group of infrequently encountered sexually transmitted infections. Chancroid is more common than syphilis in some areas of Africa and Southeast Asia but uncommon in the United States (roughly 20 cases per year). After incubation of 4 to 10 days, a papule or pustule, surrounded by a vivid areola of inflammation, may be noted within the vestibule, at the fourchette, or on the labia minora. This develops into one or more typical "soft chancres." The chancroid appears as a pinkish-red, granular ulcer with punched-out, uneven, undermined edges and a necrotic, purulent floor. The ulceration is painful and destructive and lacks the characteristic induration seen in the primary chancre of syphilis. Suppurative inguinal nodes or "buboes" are common. The combination of a painful ulcer and tender inguinal adenopathy suggests chancroid; when accompanied by suppurative inguinal adenopathy, they are almost pathognomonic. A definitive diagnosis of chancroid requires identification of *H. ducreyi* on special culture media that is not widely available; even using these media, sensitivity is ≤80%. Gram stain of material from open ulcers can also be confirmatory.

Lymphogranuloma venereum is caused by one of a number of serotypes (L-1, L-2, L-3) of *Chlamydia trachomatis*. Although uncommon in the United States, this infection causes significant morbidity. The initial lesion appears a few days after exposure as a papule, pustule, or erosion on the vulva or within the vagina. It is of short duration, inconspicuous, and therefore almost always overlooked. Within 1 to 3 weeks the tendency toward lymphatic spread becomes evident in the slow development of inguinal adenitis progressing until a painful, matted mass of glands is present, with periadenitis and occasional suppuration and draining sinuses. The extent and severity of inguinal lymphadenitis in the female is less than in the male. When the pelvic and perirectal lymphatics become involved, rectal stricture may result from progressive inflammation and ulceration about the entire circumference of the rectum, with subsequent fibrosis and cicatrization. At times, hypertrophic changes with extensive infiltration and ulceration may involve the vulva, vagina, urethra, and perineum. The destructive process may give rise to fistulae and blockage of lymph channels may cause elephantiasis. The lymph node pathology is that of a granuloma with multiple abscesses and masses of epithelioid and giant cells. Diagnosis is by complement fixation testing—80% of patients have a titer of 1:16 or greater. Genital and lymph node specimens (i.e., lesion swab or bubo aspirate) may be tested for *C. trachomatis* by culture, direct immunofluorescence, or NAAT, which has improved sensitivity and specificity for diagnosis compared with other types of testing.

Granuloma inguinale (also called *Donovanosis*) is relatively common in the tropics, New Guinea, and Caribbean areas, but it accounts for fewer than

Chancroid

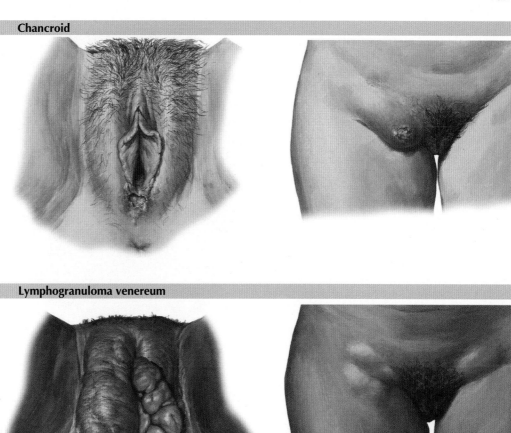

Lymphogranuloma venereum

Granuloma inguinale

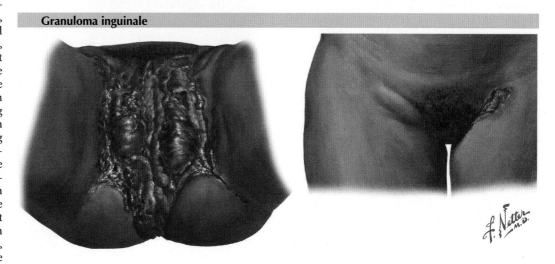

100 cases per year in the United States. This infection is caused by the intracellular gram-negative bacterium *Klebsiella granulomatis* (formerly known as *Calymmatobacterium granulomatis*). The incubation period varies. The primary lesion may be seen as a vivid, circumscribed, granulomatous nodule on the vulva, vaginal epithelium, cervix, or in such extragenital sites as the face or neck. The initial lesion spreads by peripheral extension rather than through the lymphatics. The skin and mucous membranes are primarily involved. The disease does not penetrate deeply but may gradually extend to the groin, inner thigh, perianal region, and buttock. The characteristic picture is that of a red, exuberant, granulomatous surface, with well-defined serpiginous margins. The "pseudobubo" sometimes seen is usually a subcutaneous granuloma. Healing occurs slowly, the lesion persisting many months or years. The diagnosis is established by the appearance of the typical lesions and by demonstration of Donovan bodies in surface smears or biopsies. Chancroid, syphilis, tuberculosis, and carcinoma must be excluded in the differential diagnosis.

Plate 6.17

Reproductive System: VOLUME 1

CYSTS

A Bartholin cyst results from the occlusion of the excretory duct or one of its subdivisions. Etiologic factors include specific or nonspecific infections and accidental or operative trauma. Most often an infection in one or both Bartholin glands results in swelling and/or abscess formation. Usually, the acute process is unilateral and marked by pain and swelling. Systemic symptoms are minimal except in advanced cases. Once the acute infection has passed, stenosis and scarring of the duct may result in the formation of a chronic cyst.

The cyst appears as fluctuant swelling in the posterior aspect of the labia. When palpated between the thumb and index fingers, it is quite movable beneath the overlying skin. The cysts may be clear, yellow, or bluish in color, and the size may vary from that of a marble to that of a large egg. Unless secondarily infected, it causes little or no discomfort. (More than 80% of cultures of material from Bartholin gland cysts are sterile.) The contents of the cyst are usually clear and mucoid. Microscopic examination usually reveals evidence of the transitional cell epithelium, derived from the duct wall, and Bartholin gland tissue. The cyst lining is usually transitional epithelium, but the pathologic diagnosis is made by the additional presence of compound mucinous glands in the wall.

Of all Bartholin gland cysts, 85% occur during the reproductive years (peak, 20–29 years). Asymptomatic cysts in females younger than 40 do not need treatment. (Above this age, biopsy is indicated.) Excision of the gland is often difficult and is associated with significant risk of morbidity, including intraoperative hemorrhage, hematoma formation, secondary infection, scar formation, and dyspareunia. Therefore excision is not generally recommended. When treatment must be instituted, marsupialization of the cysts is usually the best course: a 1- to 2-cm vertical or "stab" incision is made, usually within the hymeneal ring; sutures are generally not required. A Word catheter should then be placed through the incision and inflated with a few milliliters of saline. The catheter is left in place for 6 weeks. As an alternative, iodoform gauze packing may be placed within the cavity with a 2- to 3-cm "tail" left outside the incision to facilitate eventual, gradual removal. Unless cellulitis is present, antibiotic therapy is not required.

The labia majora and minora contain numerous sebaceous glands. When occlusion of a duct occurs, a cystic enlargement may result from retention of sebum and epithelial debris. Sebaceous cysts are usually small but may reach the size of a walnut. They may be single or multiple. They are moderately firm, quite movable, and may be asymptomatic when uninfected. When secondary infection occurs, the cyst becomes tense, red, swollen, tender, and painful, resembling a furuncle.

Inclusion cysts are sometimes noted in the perineum, at the fourchette, and within the vaginal wall. They are usually quite small, varying in size from a pea to a walnut. They may result as an aftermath of a reparative operation for perineal laceration or from a laceration that is allowed to heal spontaneously but without good apposition of the dermal edges. When a portion of epithelium is buried beneath the surface, it usually becomes encysted, with an accumulation of desquamated and degenerated epithelium.

A cyst of the canal of Nuck refers to a cystic dilatation of an unobliterated peritoneal pouch, the analog to the processus vaginalis in the male. This may extend for a varying distance along the round ligament, which this pouch accompanies during fetal life. The cyst may develop in the upper half of the labium majus with a pedicle leading into the inguinal canal. An excised specimen may present a wall composed of fibrous and muscular tissue. A lining epithelium of low cuboidal or cylindrical cells (persistent endothelium) may or may not be present.

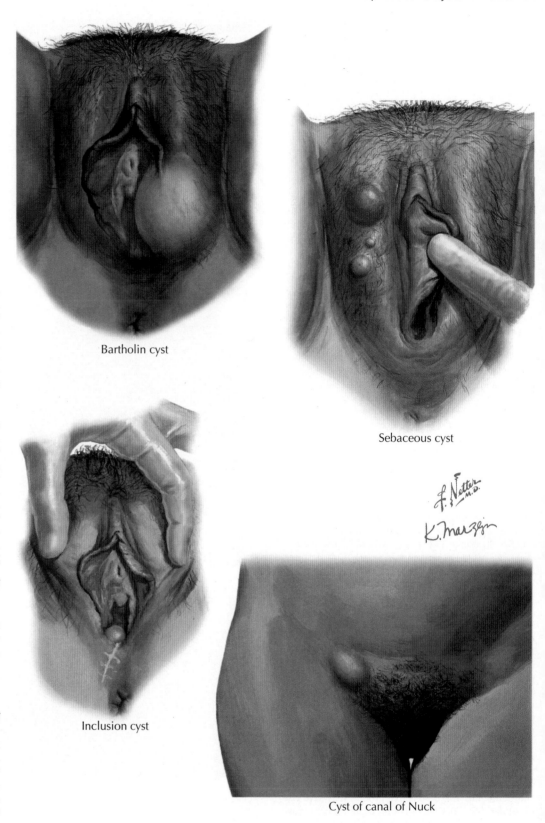

Bartholin cyst

Sebaceous cyst

Inclusion cyst

Cyst of canal of Nuck

Plate 6.18

Vulva

BENIGN TUMORS

Benign tumors of the vulva include the fibroma, fibromyoma, lipoma, papilloma, condyloma acuminatum, urethral caruncle, hidradenoma, angioma, myxoma, neuroma, and rarely endometroid growths.

Condylomata acuminata are a form of papilloma commonly known as *venereal warts*. These are caused by several serotypes (most frequently serotypes 6 and 11; 90%) of HPV. This double-stranded DNA virus is found in 2% to 4% of all females, and up to 60% of patients have evidence of the virus when polymerase chain reaction techniques are used. The virus is hardy and may resist even drying, making transmission and autoinoculation common. The virus is most commonly spread by skin-to-skin (generally sexual) contact and has an incubation period of 3 weeks to 8 months, with an average of 3 months. Roughly 65% of patients acquire the infection after intercourse with an infected partner. There is some evidence that fomite transmission could rarely occur. The papillomas usually appear as multiple, soft, pointed, warty excrescences about the labia and perineum. The lesions are often symmetric across the midline due to autoinoculation. When numerous, they may give rise to a confluent, cauliflower-like growth. Histologically, they present a central stroma of congested and infiltrated connective tissue covered by hypertrophied, stratified squamous epithelium with deep papillary projections, and a thick, superficial, cornified zone.

Fibromas arising from the connective tissue of the vulva are usually small to moderate in size. They tend to become pedunculated as they increase in size and weight. Their consistency depends in part on the degree of edema due to degeneration or deficiency of the circulation. They may originate from the region of the round ligament or the deeper pelvic structures and present themselves at the vulva. Occasionally, microscopic section reveals an apparent fibroma to be a fibromyoma. Sarcomatous changes may occur, although rarely.

Lipomas of the vulva are less common than fibromas. They are softer and have a more homogeneous consistency. They may occasionally reach large proportions.

The hidradenoma is a benign, relatively rare tumor of sweat gland origin. It appears usually as a small nodule on the labium majus or in the interlabial sulcus. The skin over the surface of the tumor may ulcerate and bleed, giving rise to a grayish or red fungating tumor, sometimes mistaken for carcinoma. Histologically, the hidradenoma or sweat gland adenoma presents an edematous, tubular structure lined by nonciliated columnar cells with clear cytoplasm and dark-staining nuclei. In the smaller acini, cuboidal or rounded cells may be evident. Cystic changes and intracystic papillary proliferations are not infrequent.

Urethral caruncles are pedunculated or sessile, small to pea-sized, bright-red growths projecting from the posterior edge of the urethral meatus. They may be

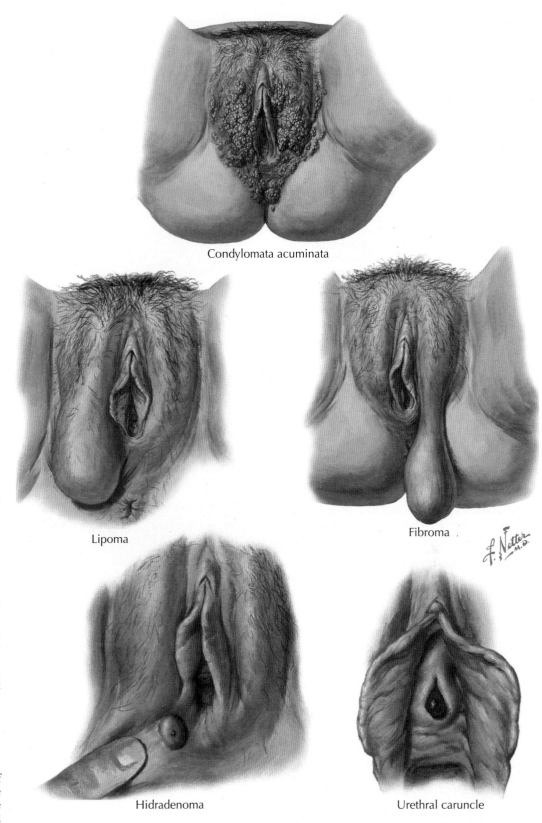

Condylomata acuminata

Lipoma

Fibroma

Hidradenoma

Urethral caruncle

granulomatous, angiomatous, or telangiectatic. They are extremely sensitive and often give rise to urinary frequency and dysuria. Because of the associated vascularity, edema, and inflammatory reaction, bleeding occurs readily. Repeated or chronic infections of the urethra or bladder may predispose toward the development of a caruncle. It is important to discriminate a caruncle from patulous or simple eversion of the external urethral meatus, prolapse of the urethral mucosa, and localized carcinoma of the urethra. Urethral

prolapse occurs most commonly in elderly females. The entire circumference of the urethral mucosa is seen to protrude through the external meatus, similar to that seen in prolapse of the rectal mucosa through the anus. Congestion and edema are marked. Localized thrombosis and necrosis may occur, accompanied by severe bleeding. A small carcinoma of the urethra may simulate or be superimposed upon a urethral caruncle. Errors in diagnosis may be avoided by biopsy or excision instead of destruction by cauterization.

Plate 6.19

Reproductive System: VOLUME 1

MALIGNANT TUMORS

About 5% of the malignant tumors of the female genital organs originate on the vulva. In the United States there are approximately 6100 new cases of and 1500 deaths from vulvar cancer each year. The incidence of vulvar cancer has risen in the last several decades, likely related to increased exposure to HPV. Primary carcinoma is almost always seen in elderly females with an average age for in situ tumors being 40 to 49 years, and 65 to 75 for invasive lesions. The median age at death is 78 years. The vast majority of these tumors are of the squamous cell variety. Histologic types include squamous cell (up to 90%), melanoma (5%), basaloid, warty, verrucous, giant cell, spindle cell, acantholytic squamous cell (adenoid squamous), lymphoepithelioma-like, basal cell, and Merkel cell. Sarcoma accounts for approximately 2% of vulvar cancers. Metastatic tumors from other sources are rare but do occur.

Squamous cell cancer of the vulva generally presents as an exophytic ulcer, hyperkeratotic plaque, or mass (fleshy, nodular, or warty). It may arise as a solitary lesion or develop hidden within hypertrophic or other vulvar skin changes, making diagnosis difficult and often delayed. Lesions are multifocal in 5% of cases. Known or suspected risk factors include infection with HPV (molecular analysis detected HPV DNA in >85% of vulvar cancers, primarily serotypes 16 and 33), smoking, immunosuppression, and lichen sclerosus.

Leukoplakia and venereal granulomatous lesions appear to be predisposing factors in the development of vulvar malignancy. It is estimated that about 50% of primary carcinomas are preceded by leukoplakia. The initial lesion may be a small, firm nodule or thickening, with slow but progressive enlargement, infiltration, and, finally, ulceration. The early symptoms may be insignificant, consisting merely of soreness and pruritus. In the neglected case the tumor may become large, nodular, hypertrophic, ulcerated, and foul-smelling. Additional prevailing complaints may then include a purulent, odoriferous leukorrhea and local irritation after urination. Lymphatic extension to the regional inguinal nodes occurs early and in a high percentage of cases. Distant metastases are rare. However, because pulmonary involvement is occasionally encountered, a routine x-ray examination of the chest is warranted. Because of neglect and lack of recognition, the average case is not brought to operation until about 1 year after the onset of symptoms.

Basal cell carcinoma of the vulva is relatively uncommon. A variable incidence of 1.2% to 13% of the epidermoid carcinomas has been reported. Basal cell carcinoma of the vulva is to be differentiated from the squamous cell variety. The age of appearance, the signs, and the symptoms are similar to those of early squamous cell carcinomas. A rodent ulcer or superficial erythematous type may be seen. Definite connections with other diseases or predisposing factors, such as leukoplakia or hypertrophic venereal lesions, have not been established. The neoplasms are slow growing and radiosensitive. Regional metastases are rare, but local extension and recurrence

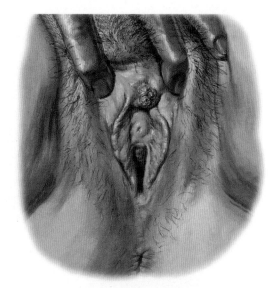

Carcinoma of the clitoris

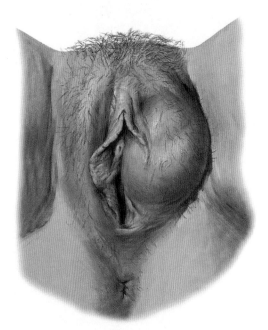

Sarcoma of the labium

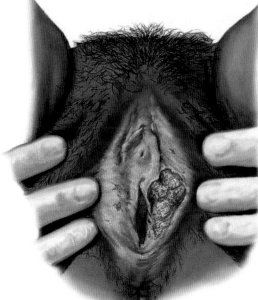

Carcinoma on leukoplakia

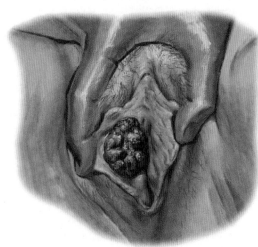

Metastatic hypernephroma

are characteristic. Wide local excision may suffice instead of the more radical vulvectomy and bilateral femoral and pelvic lymphadenectomy.

Occasionally, adenocarcinoma may develop from Bartholin glands, mucous glands, or sweat glands. Rarely, a medullary carcinoma may be seen. The sites of origin, in the order of their frequency, are the labia majora, prepuce of the clitoris, labia minora, Bartholin gland, posterior commissure, and urethral area.

Secondary carcinoma of the vulva (metastatic to) is uncommon but may occur. This is particularly true of

metastases from a hypernephroma of the kidney, chorioepithelioma of the uterus, and carcinoma of the uterine body or cervix. At times the vulvar lesion may be the first indication of the existence of a primary carcinoma elsewhere.

Sarcoma of the vulva is infrequent. Varieties include fibrosarcoma, spindle cell sarcoma, lymphosarcoma, myxosarcoma, liposarcoma, round cell, giant cell, and polymorphous cell sarcoma. These are usually very aggressive in character. Occasionally, their malignancy may be of low grade.

Plate 6.20

Vulva

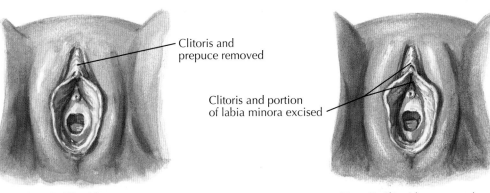

Clitoris and prepuce removed

Type I: Clitoridectomy

Clitoris and portion of labia minora excised

Type II: Clitoridectomy and partial excision of labia minora

FEMALE CIRCUMCISION

Female circumcision is an infrequently culturally determined practice of ritually cutting a female's external genitals that results in removal of part or all of the external genitalia including the labia majora, labia minora, and/or the clitoris. This activity is illegal in many locations. Female circumcision (female genital mutilation [FGM], infibulation) is generally performed as a ritual process, often without benefit of anesthesia and frequently under unsterile conditions, generally near the time of puberty or soon after. The resulting scarring may preclude intromission or normal vaginal delivery should pregnancy be achieved. In rare cases, scarring and deformity may be sufficient to result in amenorrhea or dysmenorrhea. The ritual is often performed to reinforce a female's place in her society, to establish eligibility for marriage and entry into womanhood. It is thought by some to be a religious custom, but no religion condones it. It is sometimes also performed to safeguard virginity or to paradoxically improve fertility. Although the ritual can have devastating effects on the woman's sexual pleasure, it is sometimes performed to enhance the husband's pleasure.

The amount and location of tissue removed determine the type of infibulation:

Type I—excision of the prepuce, with or without excision of part of or the entire clitoris.

Type II—excision of the clitoris with partial or total excision of the labia minora. (This is the most common form.)

Type III—excision of part or all of the external genitalia and stitching/narrowing of the vaginal opening (infibulation).

Type IV—pricking, piercing, or incising of the clitoris and/or labia; stretching of the clitoris and/or labia; cauterization by burning of the clitoris and surrounding tissue.

Other forms of FGM include the following:

Scraping of the tissue surrounding the vaginal orifice (angurya cuts) or cutting of the vagina (gishiri cuts).

The introduction of corrosive substances or herbs into the vagina to cause bleeding or for the purpose of tightening or narrowing the vagina.

Any other procedure that falls under the definition given previously.

It has been estimated that over 200 million females worldwide have undergone some form of female circumcision. Whereas FGM is uncommon in the United States (estimated at 168,000, with 48,000 younger than 18 years of age), over 95% of females in some countries (e.g., Somalia) have had one of these procedures. In 2013 the United Nations General Assembly passed a resolution to advise the elimination of female genital cutting.

These patients may experience bleeding and infection (including tetanus), urinary retention, and pain at the time of the original procedure. Long term, the patient may experience sexual dysfunction, difficulty with menstrual hygiene, recurrent vaginal or urinary tract

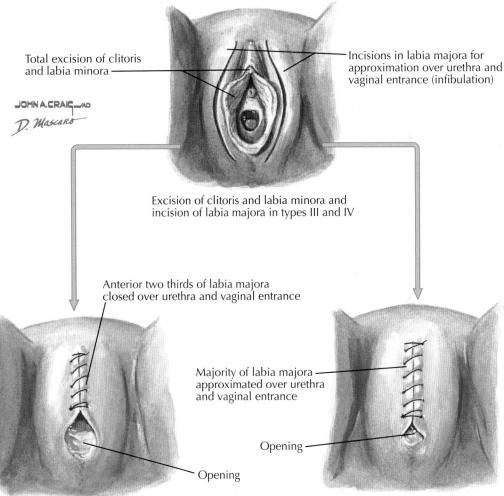

Total excision of clitoris and labia minora

Incisions in labia majora for approximation over urethra and vaginal entrance (infibulation)

JOHN A. CRAIG—MD
D. Mascaro

Excision of clitoris and labia minora and incision of labia majora in types III and IV

Anterior two thirds of labia majora closed over urethra and vaginal entrance

Majority of labia majora approximated over urethra and vaginal entrance

Opening

Opening

Type III: Modified (intermediate infibulation)—allows moderate posterior opening

Type IV: Total infibulation—allows only small posterior opening for urine and menstrual flow

infections, retrograde menstruation, hematocolpos, or chronic pelvic inflammatory disease. Excessive scarring, including keloid formation, adhesions, and pelvic and back pain are all common. Initiation of sexual activity may also present medical complications for the infibulated female. For example, if her narrow introitus tears "naturally" (by penile penetration), local infections and laceration of adjacent tissues may occur, leading to possible further complications. Increasingly, women are consulting physicians before initiating sexual activity and requesting deinfibulation.

Surgical opening of fused or scarred genital tissue may be necessary to allow for menstrual hygiene and sexual function. An anterior episiotomy, with or without subsequent repair, may be required at the time of childbirth. (Subsequent repair of the episiotomy is illegal in some locations, such as the United Kingdom and others, because this amounts to reinfibulation.) Sexual sequelae are often lifelong despite surgical revision (especially when clitoridectomy has been performed). Care for these patients must be provided in a nurturing, nonjudgmental way.

VAGINA

Plate 7.1

Reproductive System: VOLUME 1

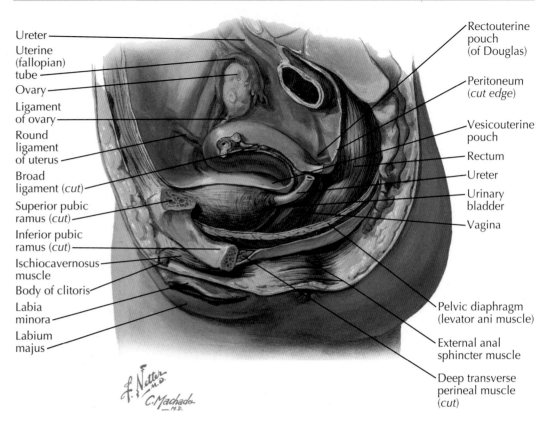

Paramedian (sagittal) dissection

Ureter
Uterine (fallopian) tube
Ovary
Ligament of ovary
Round ligament of uterus
Broad ligament (*cut*)
Superior pubic ramus (*cut*)
Inferior pubic ramus (*cut*)
Ischiocavernosus muscle
Body of clitoris
Labia minora
Labium majus

Rectouterine pouch (of Douglas)
Peritoneum (*cut edge*)
Vesicouterine pouch
Rectum
Ureter
Urinary bladder
Vagina
Pelvic diaphragm (levator ani muscle)
External anal sphincter muscle
Deep transverse perineal muscle (*cut*)

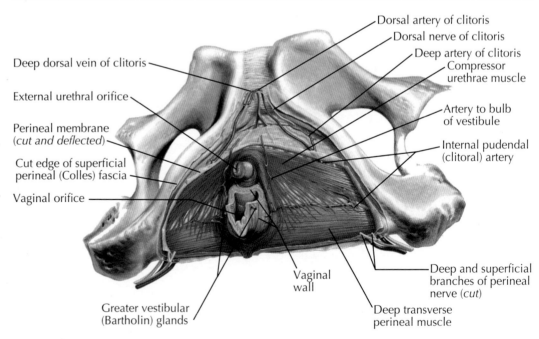

Deep perineal space

Deep dorsal vein of clitoris
External urethral orifice
Perineal membrane (*cut and deflected*)
Cut edge of superficial perineal (Colles) fascia
Vaginal orifice
Greater vestibular (Bartholin) glands

Dorsal artery of clitoris
Dorsal nerve of clitoris
Deep artery of clitoris
Compressor urethrae muscle
Artery to bulb of vestibule
Internal pudendal (clitoral) artery
Deep and superficial branches of perineal nerve (*cut*)
Deep transverse perineal muscle
Vaginal wall

VAGINA

The vagina (from Latin, literally "sheath" or "scabbard") serves as the portal to the internal female reproductive tract and a route of egress for the fetus during delivery. The viscera contained within the female pelvis minor include the pelvic colon, urinary bladder and urethra, uterus, uterine tubes, ovaries, and vagina. These structures surround the vagina and interact with it in the clinical setting. Therefore the vagina also provides a convenient portal to understanding the pelvic viscera of the female.

The vagina is a thin-walled, distensible, fibromuscular canal covered by specialized epithelium that extends from the vulva inward to the cervix and uterus. Under normal circumstances, the vagina is a potential space that is larger in the middle and upper thirds, giving it an inverted pear- or T-shape when viewed perpendicular to its long axis. The walls of the vagina are normally flattened in the anteroposterior diameter, giving the appearance of the letter H in cross section.

In its distal extreme, the vagina opens to the vulva at the hymeneal ring, opening at the caudal end of the vulva, behind the opening of the urethra. When upright, the vaginal tube points in an upward-backward direction with the axis of the upper portion of the vagina in close to the horizontal plane, curving toward the hollow of the sacrum. In most females an angle of at least 90 degrees is formed between the vagina and the uterus. The cervix is directed downward and backward to rest against the posterior vaginal wall. The spaces between the cervix and attachment of the vagina are called *fornices*, with the posterior fornix considerably larger than the anterior fornix.

Although there is wide variation, the length of the vagina is approximately 6 to 9 cm (2.5–3.5 in) along the anterior wall, and 8 to 12 cm (3–4.5 in) along the posterior wall. During sexual arousal, the upper portion of the vagina elongates and widens through a relative upward movement of the uterus and cervix. This is thought to facilitate capture and retention of sperm to enhance the chance of conception.

Throughout most of its length, the vagina lies directly on top of the descending rectum, separated by the rectovaginal septum. The upper one-fourth of the vagina is separated from the rectum by the rectouterine pouch (posterior cul-de-sac). The urethra and base of the urinary bladder lie above the anterior vaginal wall separated by the thin layers of endopelvic fascia. As they enter the bladder, the ureters pass forward and medialward close to the lateral fornices.

The vagina is held in position by the surrounding endopelvic fascia and ligaments: the lower third of the vagina is surrounded and supported by the urogenital and pelvic diaphragms. The levator ani muscles and the lower portion of the cardinal ligaments support the middle third of the vagina, whereas portions of the cardinal ligaments and the parametria support the upper third.

The vagina is supplied with an extensive anastomotic network of vessels that surround its length. The vaginal artery originates either directly from the uterine artery or as a branch of the internal iliac artery arising posterior to the origin of the uterine and inferior vesical arteries. There is an anastomosis with the descending cervical branch of the uterine artery to form the azygos arteries. Branches of the internal pudendal, inferior vesical, and middle hemorrhoidal arteries also contribute to the interconnecting network from below. These can be a significant source of bleeding with obstetric lacerations. They are also important in the development of vaginal transudate during sexual arousal, when the vagina produces lubrication to aid in penetration.

Plate 7.2

Vagina

PELVIC DIAPHRAGM FROM BELOW

Removing the superficial muscles and fasciae of the pelvic floor, the pelvic diaphragm, viewed from below, forms a hammock of muscle from the pelvic brim, investing the urethra, vagina, and rectum and attaching posteriorly to the sacrum and coccyx. The principal muscles of this group are the levatores ani, consisting of both medial and lateral components on each side and supplied by the pudendal nerve. The larger medial component, the pubococcygeus, arises from the posterior surface of the superior ramus of the pubis adjacent to the symphysis, whence the fibers pass downward and backward around the lateral walls of the vagina, with some fibers reaching the coccyx, some terminating in the fascia forming the central tendinous point of the perineum, and others blending with the longitudinal muscle coats of the rectum. The pubococcygei are separated medially by the interlevator cleft through which pass the dorsal vein of the clitoris, the urethra, vagina, and rectum. These organs are supported by musculofascial extensions from the pubococcygei, their inferior fascia being continuous with the superior fascia of the urogenital diaphragm.

The lateral component of the levatores ani, the iliococcygeus, arises from the ischial spine and from the tendinous arch, a condensation of the parietal pelvic fascia covering the inner surface of the obturator internus muscle, which extends from the posterior surface of the pubis to the spine of the ischium. The iliococcygeus inserts in the last two segments of the coccyx, but some elements cross the midline anterior to the coccyx to unite with those from the opposite side in a raphe, where they are joined at a more superficial level by fibers from the sphincter ani externus and the transverse perineal muscles.

Posteriorly, the main pelvic diaphragm is nearly completed by the triangular coccygeus muscle. The apex of the coccygeus is attached to the spine of the ischium and the sacrospinous ligament, which it directly overlies; the base is attached to the lower portion of the lateral sacrum and the coccyx. This is best seen in the lateral view. In addition to supporting the pelvic viscera, the muscles of the pelvic diaphragm aid in the constriction of the vagina during coitus, parturition, micturition, and defecation. The obturator internus and piriformis muscles round out the posterior pelvis before passing through the lesser and greater sciatic foramina, respectively, to insert on the femur. These muscles lie close to the lateral walls of the pelvis.

The obturator internus arises from the circumference of the obturator fossa by fibrous attachments directly to the bone and, to a lesser extent, from the obturator membrane, the tendinous arch, and the obturator fascia, which covers the inner surface of the muscle. The fibers pass downward and backward, forming tendinous bands as they near the lesser sciatic notch and then, passing through this notch, they insert outside the pelvis on the medial surface of the greater trochanter of the femur.

The piriformis, best seen in the lateral view, arises from the lower portion of the sacrum and the sacrotuberous ligament, with its fibers covering a large part of the greater sciatic notch, through which it passes out of the pelvis to attach in the superior portion of the greater trochanter of the femur. The piriformis is supplied by sacral nerves 1 and 2, and the obturator internus by sacral nerves 1, 2, and 3. They aid in external rotation and abduction of the hip and are not directly concerned with support of the pelvic floor. However, the fascia covering these muscles is continuous with the pelvic diaphragm and with the endopelvic fascia.

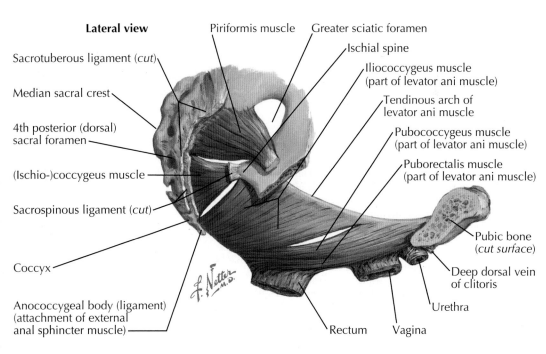

Inferior view

Pubic symphysis
Inferior (arcuate) pubic ligament
Inferior pubic ramus
Deep dorsal vein of clitoris
Urethra
Vagina
Rectum
Ischial spine
(Ischio-)coccygeus muscle
Piriformis muscle (cut)
Sacrospinous ligament (cut)
Sacrotuberous ligament (cut)
Sacrum
Tip of coccyx

Musculofascial extensions to urethra
Musculofascial extensions to vagina
Interdigitating fibers of perineum
Puborectalis muscle (part of levator ani muscle)
Pubococcygeus muscle (part of levator ani muscle)
Tendinous arch of levator ani muscle
Obturator internus muscle
Iliococcygeus muscle (part of levator ani muscle)
Ischial tuberosity
Obturator internus tendon
Ischial spine
Sacrospinous ligament
Piriformis muscle
Sacrotuberous ligament
Levator plate (median raphe) of levator ani muscle
Anococcygeal body (ligament) (attachment of external anal sphincter muscle)

Lateral view

Sacrotuberous ligament (cut)
Median sacral crest
4th posterior (dorsal) sacral foramen
(Ischio-)coccygeus muscle
Sacrospinous ligament (cut)
Coccyx
Anococcygeal body (ligament) (attachment of external anal sphincter muscle)

Piriformis muscle
Greater sciatic foramen
Ischial spine
Iliococcygeus muscle (part of levator ani muscle)
Tendinous arch of levator ani muscle
Pubococcygeus muscle (part of levator ani muscle)
Puborectalis muscle (part of levator ani muscle)
Pubic bone (cut surface)
Deep dorsal vein of clitoris
Urethra
Rectum
Vagina

Plate 7.3

Reproductive System: VOLUME 1

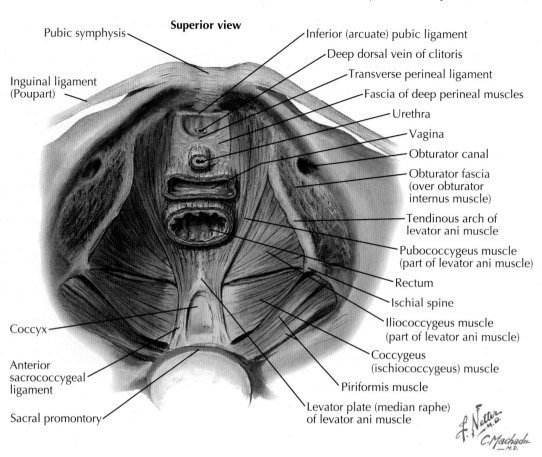

Superior view

Pubic symphysis

Inguinal ligament (Poupart)

Inferior (arcuate) pubic ligament

Deep dorsal vein of clitoris

Transverse perineal ligament

Fascia of deep perineal muscles

Urethra

Vagina

Obturator canal

Obturator fascia (over obturator internus muscle)

Tendinous arch of levator ani muscle

Pubococcygeus muscle (part of levator ani muscle)

Rectum

Ischial spine

Iliococcygeus muscle (part of levator ani muscle)

Coccygeus (ischiococcygeus) muscle

Piriformis muscle

Coccyx

Anterior sacrococcygeal ligament

Sacral promontory

Levator plate (median raphe) of levator ani muscle

PELVIC DIAPHRAGM FROM ABOVE

The pelvic diaphragm forms a musculotendinous, funnel-shaped partition between the pelvic cavity and the perineum and serves as one of the principal supports of the urethra, vagina, rectum, and pelvic viscera. It is composed of the levator ani and coccygeus muscles, sheathed in a superior and inferior layer of fascia. The muscles of the pelvic diaphragm extend from the lateral pelvic walls downward and medially to fuse with each other and are inserted into the terminal portions of the urethra, vagina, and anus. Anteriorly, they fail to meet in the midline just behind the pubic symphysis, exposing a gap in the pelvic floor, which is completed by the urogenital diaphragm. This gap is partially filled by the subpubic ligament that is pierced by the dorsal vein of the clitoris. In this area, the inferior fascia of the pelvic diaphragm fuses with the superior fascia of the urogenital diaphragm.

The levator ani muscles may be subdivided into an anterior pubococcygeus and a posterior iliococcygeus portion. They originate on each side at the posterior aspect of the pubis, the tendinous arch, and the ischial spine. They are inserted into the coccyx, the anococcygeal body, the lower end of the anal canal, the central point of the perineum, the lower vagina, and the posterolateral surface of the urethra. The levator ani muscles are primarily supporting structures, but they also contribute a sphincteric action on the anal canal and vagina. These muscles and their investing fascia are critical to maintaining support for the vagina and bladder. Rupture or stretch of this support system after pregnancy or childbirth is one of the major causes of pelvic support defects (hernias) and the attendant problems of urinary incontinence and fecal retention. It is to the tendinous arch (arcus tendineus) that some transabdominal approaches to the treatment of cysto-urethroceles provide anchorage or reattachment. The levator sling is also the plate on which pessaries must rest to provide mechanical support to prolapsing pelvic organs.

The pectineal ligament (also known as the *inguinal ligament of Cooper*) is an extension of the lacunar ligament that runs on the pectineal line of the pubic bone, seen as a ridge on the superior ramus of the pubic bone and forming part of the pelvic brim. Lying across it are fibers of the pectineal ligament and the proximal origin of the pectineus muscle. This fibrous line has been used clinically as an anchor point for incontinence procedures such as the Marshall-Marchetti-Krantz and Burch procedures.

The coccygeus muscles are triangular in shape, arise from the ischial spine, and are inserted into the lateral borders of the lower sacrum and upper coccyx. They lie on the pelvic aspect of the sacrospinous ligaments.

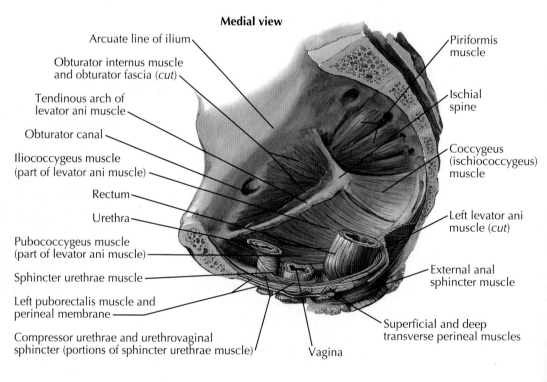

Medial view

Arcuate line of ilium

Obturator internus muscle and obturator fascia (cut)

Tendinous arch of levator ani muscle

Obturator canal

Iliococcygeus muscle (part of levator ani muscle)

Rectum

Urethra

Pubococcygeus muscle (part of levator ani muscle)

Sphincter urethrae muscle

Left puborectalis muscle and perineal membrane

Compressor urethrae and urethrovaginal sphincter (portions of sphincter urethrae muscle)

Piriformis muscle

Ischial spine

Coccygeus (ischiococcygeus) muscle

Left levator ani muscle (cut)

External anal sphincter muscle

Superficial and deep transverse perineal muscles

Vagina

The fasciae of the pelvic diaphragm are continuous with the fascial layers of the perineal compartments—the endopelvic fascia, the obturator fascia, the iliac fascia, and the transversalis fascia of the abdomen.

Aside from the muscles of the pelvic diaphragm, two muscles—the obturator internus and the piriformis—cover the walls of the true pelvis. The piriformis is triangular and lies flattened against the posterior wall of the pelvis minor. It originates from three or more processes lateral to the first, second, third, and fourth anterior sacral foramina and leaves the pelvis through the greater sciatic foramen above the ischial spine to be inserted by a rounded tendon into the upper border of the greater trochanter of the femur. The obturator internus muscles are fan-shaped and cover the side walls of the pelvis.

Plate 7.4

Vagina

SUPPORT OF PELVIC VISCERA

To clarify the relationships of muscles and fasciae in supporting the pelvis, with particular reference to the vagina and internal female genitalia, the uterus, in the accompanying picture, has been elevated upward and backward, resulting in alignment of the axes of the uterus and vagina. The plane chosen for the section (small upper diagram) runs from a point anterior to the body of the uterus down through the anterior vaginal fornix and along the longitudinal axis of the vagina to the perineum. At this level, the large iliac vessels run close to the superior pubic rami, which form the lateral pelvic walls. These pubic rami are connected to the ischiopubic rami across the obturator foramen by the obturator membrane, the obturator internus muscle, and the obturator fascia. The broad ligaments begin at the lateral pelvic walls as double reflections of the parietal peritoneum, forming large wings, which divide to include the uterus and separate the pelvic cavity into anterior and posterior compartments. They are continuous with the peritoneum of the bladder anteriorly and the rectosigmoid posteriorly. The broad ligaments contain fatty areolar tissue, blood vessels, and nerves, and at their apices invest the round ligaments, which are condensations of smooth muscle and fibrous tissue holding the uterus forward and inserting below and anterior to the fallopian tubes. The left ovary has been lifted up to demonstrate the uteroovarian and infundibulopelvic ligaments, the latter containing the ovarian blood supply. The bladder peritoneal reflection has been detached from the uterus, revealing the endopelvic or uterovaginal fascia, which runs laterally to the pelvic wall as the cardinal ligament, and with the associated blood vessels, nerves, and fat forms the parametrium. The uterine arteries and veins extend medially from their origins in the hypogastric vessels to the lateral vaginal fornices. The ureters (cross-sectioned) at this point pass beneath the uterine vessels and then continue in the uterovaginal fascia medially and anteriorly across the upper vagina into the bladder. The proximity of the ureters to the uterine blood supply and vagina explains why they may easily be injured during hysterectomy and in operations to repair lacerations of the upper vagina or endopelvic fascia.

The pelvic diaphragm is quite thin in cross section, contrasting sharply with its breadth. Although some of the fibers of the levators come directly from the pelvic brim, the main portion of the muscle originates from the tendinous arch formed by a condensation of the fascia of the obturator internus. The levators here are passing around the posterior vagina and enclosing the

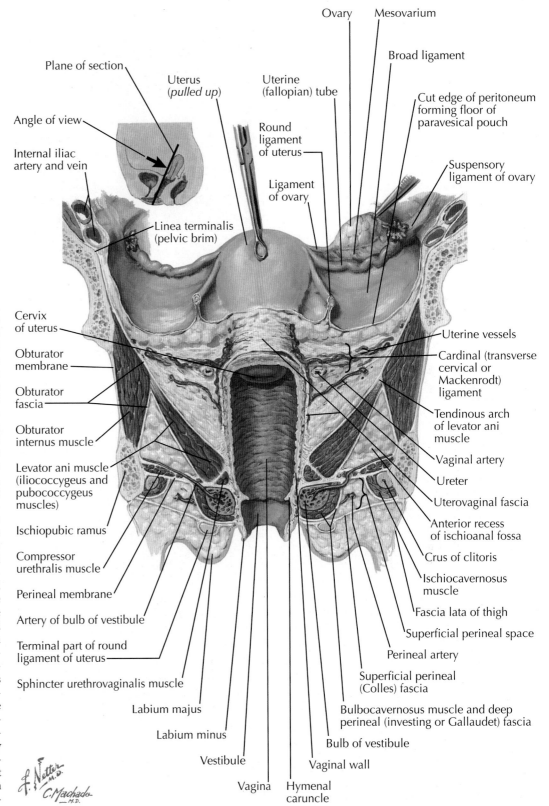

upper two-thirds of that organ. Below the levators and separated from them laterally by the upward extension of the ischiorectal fossa is the urogenital diaphragm or triangular ligament, containing at this level the deep transverse perineal muscle and the artery of the clitoris. The lower third of the vagina lies superficial to the pelvic diaphragm, and its opening into the vestibule is bounded by the hymen and farther laterally by the vestibular bulb and its covering bulbocavernosus muscle. Close to the ischiopubic rami at the margin of the bony outlet of the pelvis are the crura of the clitoris,

covered medially by the ischiocavernosus muscles and the fat pad in the superficial perineal compartment, which is limited below by Colles fascia. The labia (majora and minora) lie superficial to Colles fascia and between the thighs. The muscles and fasciae below the triangular ligament are concerned chiefly with coital function and play no part in the support of the pelvic viscera. This plate demonstrates the surgical implications of either the abdominal or vaginal approach to reconstruction of the elaborate supporting framework of the pelvic floor.

Plate 7.5

Reproductive System: VOLUME 1

Frontal section, anterior view

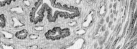

- Ureteric orifice
- Trigone of urinary bladder
- Neck of urinary bladder
- Detrusor muscle of bladder wall
- Cavernous venous plexus of urethra
- Levator ani muscle and Fibromuscular extension
- Urethra
- Sphincter urethrae muscle
- Perineal membrane
- Bulb of vestibule
- Bulbocavernosus muscle and deep perineal (investing or Gallaudet) fascia
- Round ligament of uterus (terminal part)
- Superficial perineal (Colles) fascia
- Labium majus
- Labium minus

Lacunae and openings of urethral glands

Openings of paraurethral (Skene) ducts

FEMALE URETHRA

The urethra, situated at the lowest portion of the bladder and passing downward and forward beneath the symphysis, varies from 3 to 5 cm in length and averages about 6 mm in diameter. The angle formed by the internal urethral orifice and the bladder at the bladder neck and surrounded by the intrinsic sphincter is critical to maintaining normal urinary continence; to withstand the hydrostatic pressure of the bladder, this area is further supported by the fascia and tensing muscles of the pelvic diaphragm. Its mucosal surface is thrown into longitudinal folds by the constricting action of the external supporting structures. The most prominent of these longitudinal folds, situated on the posterior aspect of the urethra, is sometimes referred to as the *urethral crest*. The endopelvic fascia that covers the bladder is continuous over the entire urethra just below the mucosal layer, and contiguous to it is a thin layer of erectile tissue formed by the cavernous venous plexus. The muscular coats that surround the bladder also cover the urethra but become thinner as it passes downward toward the external meatus. The upper two-thirds of the urethra lie behind the symphysis pubis and are referred to as the *intrapelvic urethra*. It is this portion that passes through the musculofascial attachments forming the interlevator cleft. The perineal portion extends from the superior fascia of the urogenital diaphragm to the meatus. As it passes through the urogenital diaphragm, the urethra is surrounded by the sphincter urethrae membranaceae, the homologue of the muscle of the same name in the male but a far weaker and less important structure. Near the external meatus, the urethra is adjacent to the upper ends of the vestibular bulbs and the surrounding bulbocavernosus muscles. At its meatus, the urethra lies in the anterior vaginal wall between the folds of the labia minora 2 to 3 cm below the clitoris. Along its entire length, but especially in its perineal portion, the urethra is perforated by the openings of numerous small periurethral glands, the homologues of the prostatic ducts in the male.

The schematic reconstruction of this duct system shows that although the ducts of the small glands may enter the urethra independently, the majority of them form an interdependent conducting system terminating in the large paraurethral (Skene) ducts, which open on either side of the midline, posterior to the urethral meatus. These are vestigial remnants that serve no specific purpose but are important in that their position predisposes them to infection, especially by the gonococcus,

and that their relatively poor drainage increases the risk of a chronic infection.

Cross sections through the lower urethra show the mucosal folds and the immediate supporting structures: the submucosal lamina propria is a loose network of fibrous and elastic tissue containing a prominent venous system, the cavernous plexus or corpus spongiosum, which accounts for the extreme vascularity in the area. The muscle coats consist of an inner longitudinal and an outer circular layer, both quite thin and mutually interdependent. A thin layer of striated muscle referred to as

the *external sphincter* and supplied by the pudendal nerve also surrounds the lower urethra, but these distal muscle groups have little to do with micturition. Under high-power microscopy, it can be seen that the epithelium of both the urethra and the periurethral ducts are of the stratified squamous type. The epithelium of the intrapelvic portion of the urethra, as it approaches the bladder neck, tends to be transitional. The glandular epithelium, on the other hand, is of the columnar type, not infrequently stratified. The submucosal connective tissue is relatively poor in cells.

Schematic reconstruction

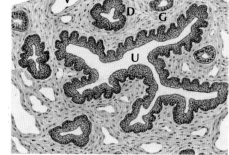

- Urethral glands
- Urethra
- External urethral orifice
- Paraurethral (Skene) duct
- Opening of paraurethral (Skene) duct
- Vaginal orifice
- Vagina

U	Urethral canal
D	Paraurethral duct
G	Periurethral gland
V	Thin-walled vein
LP	Lamina propria
LM	Longitudinal smooth muscle
CM	Circular smooth muscle
SM	Striated (extrinsic) muscle

Low power

High-power section through lower portion of urethra

Plate 7.6

Vagina

Vaginal wall

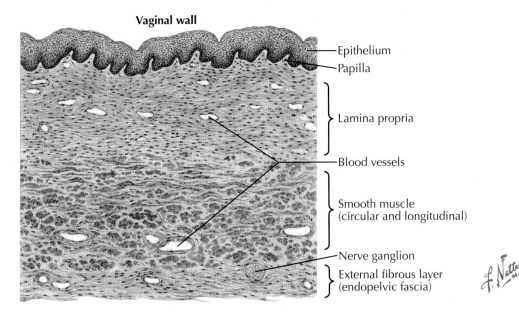

Epithelium
Papilla

Lamina propria

Blood vessels

Smooth muscle
(circular and longitudinal)

Nerve ganglion

External fibrous layer
(endopelvic fascia)

VULVA AND VAGINA HISTOLOGY

The vagina is lined by squamous epithelium (not a mucosa) and capable of dilation and constriction as a result of the action of its supporting muscles and erectile tissue. The three principal layers are easily recognized in the cross section through the vaginal wall. The epithelial surface is composed of stratified squamous epithelium divided into basal cell, transitional cell, and spinal or prickle cell layers, also referred to as *basalis*, *intraepithelial*, and *functionalis*, respectively. The superficial cells contain keratin but normally show no gross cornification in females of reproductive age. The epithelium is slightly thicker than the corresponding structure in the cervix and sends more and larger papillae into the underlying connective tissue, giving the basement membrane an undulating outline. These papillae are more numerous on the posterior wall and near the vaginal orifice. Beneath the epithelium, which has a thickness of 150 to 200 μm, a dense connective tissue layer known as the *lamina propria* is supported by elastic fibers crossing from the epithelium to the underlying muscle. These elastic fibers, here and throughout the pelvis, are critical to pelvic support and function. The lamina propria becomes less dense as it approaches the muscle, and in this area it contains a network of large, thin-walled veins, giving it the appearance of erectile tissue. The smooth muscle beneath this layer is divided into internal circular and external longitudinal groups, the latter being thicker and stronger and continuous with the superficial muscle bundles of the uterus. No dividing membrane or fascia separates these two interlacing muscle groups. The adventitial coat of the vagina is a thin, firm, fibrous layer arising from the visceral or endopelvic fascia. In this fascia and in the connective tissue between it and the muscle runs another large network of veins and, in addition, a rich nerve supply.

The Bartholin gland is situated just lateral to the vaginal vestibule and appears in cross section as a collection of small mucus-secreting glands lined by a single layer of columnar epithelial cells with basally placed nuclei. Occasionally, the columnar epithelium is stratified. The small glands tend to be oval and symmetric and are supported in a loose, vascular connective tissue. The main Bartholin duct is lined by columnar epithelium as it runs upward along the side of the vagina, but as it nears its opening in the midportion of the lateral wall of the vestibule, the epithelium takes on the stratified squamous characteristics of the vaginal epithelium. This transition accounts for the fact that malignant tumors of Bartholin gland may be of either the adenomatous or the squamous type.

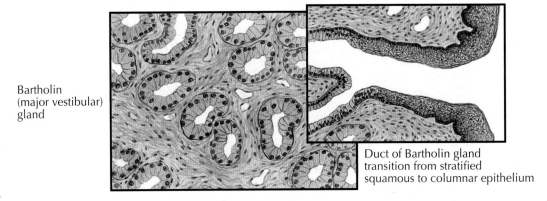

Bartholin
(major vestibular)
gland

Duct of Bartholin gland
transition from stratified
squamous to columnar epithelium

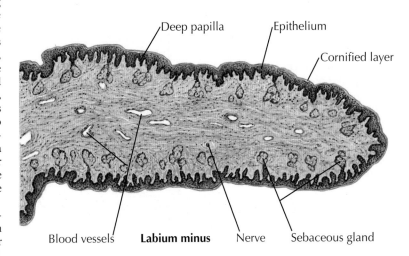

Deep papilla

Epithelium

Cornified layer

Blood vessels **Labium minus** Nerve Sebaceous gland

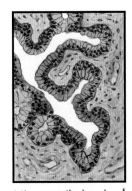

Minor vestibular gland

The minor vestibular glands, situated around the clitoris and urethra and aiding in the lubrication of the vaginal surface, are of a more racemose, branching type than Bartholin glands. The mucus-secreting epithelium of these glands is tall, columnar, and one or two cells deep.

The labium minus has an epithelium more deeply pigmented than that of the vagina. The superficial cells are more markedly keratinized and form a horny (cornified) layer, which is especially prominent in postmenopausal females. The papillae of the lamina propria push deeply into the overlying epithelium, but the surface layer is clearly demarcated from the underlying layers by its basement membrane and often by a thin area of edema. Close to the surface are located numerous small sebaceous glands but no hair follicles or fat cells, in contrast to the labia majora. The connective tissue supporting the labium is acellular but rich in nerves and small vessels. The veins are not so numerous or so large as those in the vagina and cannot be regarded as erectile tissue.

Plate 7.7

Reproductive System: VOLUME 1

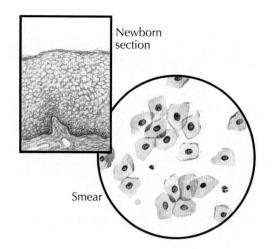

Newborn section

Smear

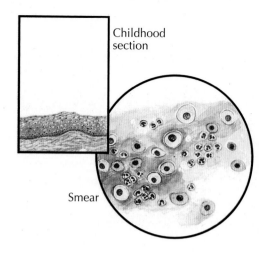

Childhood section

Smear

VAGINA: CYTOLOGY

The superficial cells of the vaginal epithelium are under the influence of ovarian hormones, changing in character over the course of a female's lifetime and the phases of the reproductive cycle. These variations are largely dependent on the amount of circulating estrogen.

In the newborn, the vaginal epithelium is lush as a result of the transfer of maternal estrogen across the placenta. The precornified and cornified cells shed from this epithelium are scattered but occasionally form loose clusters. A few polymorphonuclear leukocytes may be found but few, if any, lactobacilli (Döderlein bacilli) are present. After delivery, circulating estrogen levels fall rapidly and the vaginal epithelium quickly transitions to that of childhood.

In childhood, when the circulating estrogen is at a low level, the vaginal epithelium is thin, fragile, and at risk for infection. The cytologic smear is composed chiefly of basal cells, with a background of mucus and polymorphonuclear leukocytes. The basal cells are round or oval, with vesicular nuclei and a large nuclear/cytoplasmic ratio. The cytoplasm is, with only a few exceptions, basophilic. This smear is typical of an atrophic condition and similar to that seen after menopause.

During the reproductive years, the vaginal epithelium thickens and undergoes cyclic change in response to the varying hormone levels of the menstrual cycle. In the past, these changes from more immature, basaloid cells early in the cycle to a predominance of mature, precornified cells late in the cycle were used to help assess hormone levels and to provide indirect evidence of ovulation. Lactobacilli help maintain an acidic environment, stabilizing the vaginal flora and promoting cornification. A few white blood cells are normally present.

In pregnancy, as a result of the high levels of both estrogen and progesterone, the epithelium becomes a thick layer of superficial cells with marked keratinization. Desquamation of superficial precornified cells is associated with marked clumping and folding of the cells, which have elongated or oval vesicular nuclei. A few cornified cells with pyknotic nuclei, polymorphonuclear leukocytes, lactobacilli, and free nuclei are present in varying numbers. Near the 12th week of pregnancy, a change in the vaginal smear occurs: fewer cells are shed, clumping and folding have lessened, precornified cells predominate, and the overall appearance is similar to that seen in the normal early proliferative phase of the menstrual cycle. As pregnancy advances, the increased progesterone produces progressively smaller precornified cells, which are referred to as "navicular cells."

In the puerperium, after the sudden drop of steroid hormones before recurrence of normal menstrual cycles, the vaginal epithelium is thin. The puerperal vaginal

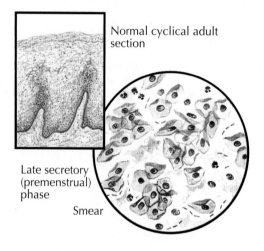

Normal cyclical adult section

Late secretory (premenstrual) phase

Smear

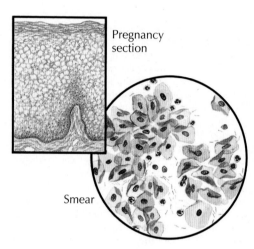

Pregnancy section

Smear

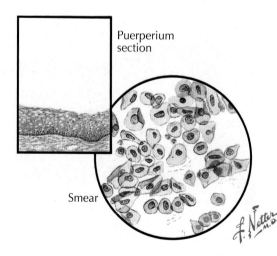

Puerperium section

Smear

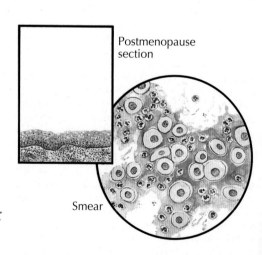

Postmenopause section

Smear

smear is characterized by the presence of a large number of basal cells, a few precornified and cornified cells, and some inflammatory debris in the background, but not to the same extent as in smears from atrophic epithelium. With the return of normal ovarian cycling, the epithelium will again rebound to its normal prepregnancy thickness and character.

In the postmenopausal years, the vaginal epithelium is very thin, smooth, and relatively pale as a result of the cessation of ovarian function and the significant decrease

in estrogen levels. The absence of this protection leads to bacterial invasion and a resulting inflammatory reaction in the supporting layers, with a thin layer of edema beneath the basement membrane. The atrophic smear is characterized by almost 100% basal cells dispersed in a thick background of mucus. Numerous polymorphonuclear leukocytes and some lymphocytes are present, but when these occur in excessive numbers, they usually indicate the presence of clinical infection. Most of the cells are basophilic, but a few pink acidophils are found.

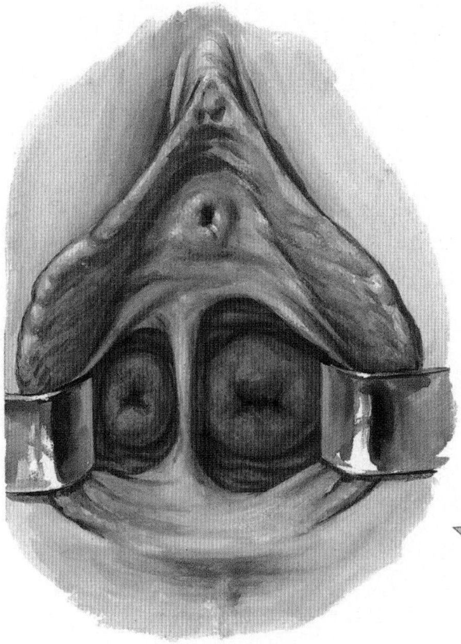

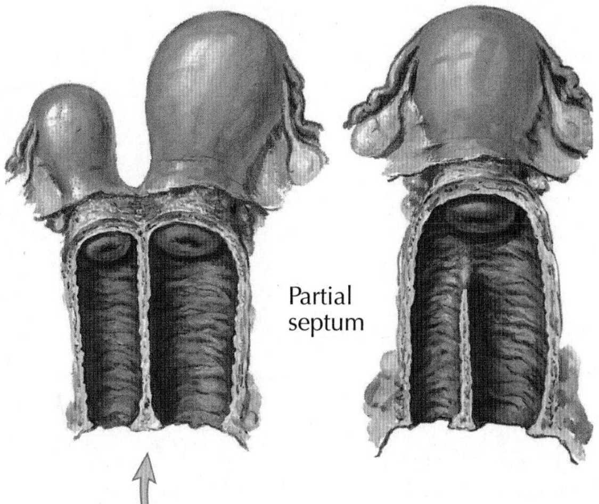

Plate 7.8

Vagina

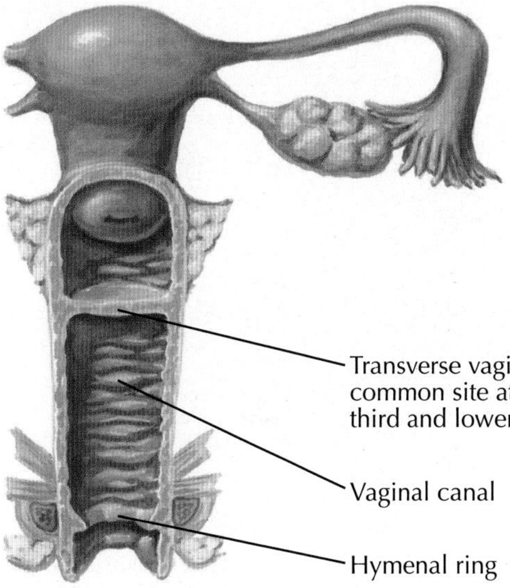

CONGENITAL ANOMALIES

The müllerian ducts first appear between the seventh and eighth weeks of embryonic life as invaginations of the coelomic epithelium overlying the genital folds. These ducts migrate caudally in the developing embryo, cross toward the midline, and fuse to form the anlage of the uterus, cervix, and upper three-quarters of the vagina. The unfused, cranial portions of the müllerian ducts develop into the fallopian tubes. The caudal fused column of cells moves further downward to join the urogenital sinus, which pushes in from the perineal surface. With the sloughing of the internal core of the cell column to form the vagina, the process is completed in 5 to 6 weeks, although full differentiation takes several weeks longer.

The majority of congenital anomalies of the uterus and vagina are caused by a failure of the müllerian ducts to fuse completely or to develop after fusion. The most extreme anomaly results from complete lack of union of the ducts as a result of inhibition in growth at a very early stage. (The HOX genes have been shown to play key roles in body patterning and organogenesis, and in particular during genital tract development.) The result of this failure of fusion in the adult is the complete absence of the uterus and vagina, but with a normal ovary (because it is derived from a different embryonic source). The fallopian tube may be well developed or rudimentary. The tube is connected near the midline to a small bulb of fibrous tissue attached anteriorly to the bladder peritoneum and posteriorly to the peritoneum of the rectosigmoid. This bulb, which has its counterpart on the opposite side, represents the abortive attempt to form a uterus and may occasionally contain an endometrial lining. Because the vagina is absent, drainage of menstrual flow is impossible, and blood is retained within the genital tract or must drain into the peritoneal cavity. The external genitalia and the vaginal vestibule are normally developed, distinguishing this condition from pseudohermaphroditism. Vaginal atresia is often unrecognized until the occurrence of amenorrhea after puberty or dyspareunia after the initiation of sexual activity. Above the vestibular dimple, between bladder and rectum, a potential space filled with loose areolar connective tissue may be found, which can be opened surgically. The eponymous term Mayer-Rokitansky-Küster-Hauser syndrome is sometimes applied to these cases of vaginal atresia, usually with absent cervix and uterus.

A less extreme degree of failure in müllerian fusion leads to a double vagina. In such instances the ducts have fused incompletely and have progressed independently to maturity. In the perineal view, the longitudinal septum dividing the vaginal compartments extends outward from the vestibule separating the two cervices. A longitudinal section through the vagina shows the appearance of the same anomaly from above, each

uterus having its own fallopian tube and ovary, and each theoretically fertile, although often associated with preterm delivery and other pregnancy complications. The partial septate vagina is a milder degree of congenital malformation, which is caused by a failure of the core of solid müllerian epithelium to slough completely at its lowermost portion.

The frequent occurrence of vaginal anomalies with other congenital malformations in the genitourinary tract results from their common embryonic heritage.

The possibility of associated lesions in the upper urinary tracts should always be investigated.

Incomplete canalization of the müllerian tubercle and sinovaginal bulb can result in a transverse vaginal septum. These patients will have a normal appearing introitus leading to a foreshortened blind vaginal pouch. After puberty, a large hematocolpos or hematometra may result from this outflow obstruction. Partial septa have been reported in females exposed in utero to diethylstilbestrol (DES).

Double vagina

Septum is usually less than one centimeter in thickness and may be complete or incomplete. Location is variable.

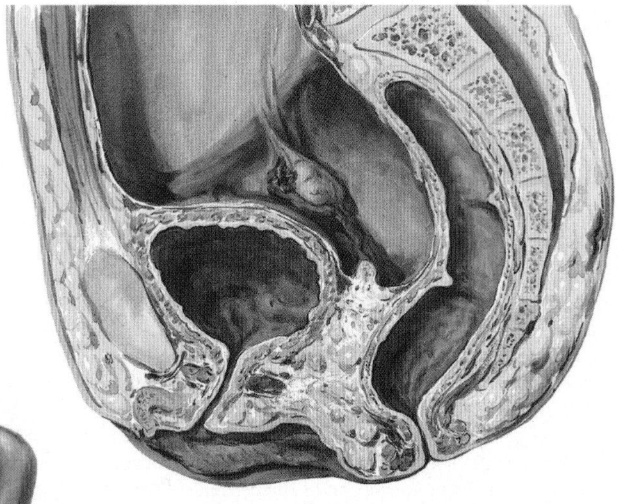

Partial septum

Complete septum with double uterus

Absence of vagina and uterus

Transverse vaginal septum—most common site at junction of upper third and lower two thirds of vaginal canal

Vaginal canal

Hymenal ring

Plate 7.9

Reproductive System: VOLUME 1

IMPERFORATE HYMEN, HEMATOCOLPOS, FIBROUS HYMEN

An imperforate hymen is the most commonly encountered anomaly resulting from abnormalities in the development or canalization of the müllerian ducts. It is caused by failure of the endoderm of the urogenital sinus and the epithelium of the vaginal vestibule to fuse and perforate during embryonic development. In addition to primary amenorrhea and coital dysfunction, an imperforate hymen may also be associated with hematocolpos, endometriosis, vaginal adenosis, infertility, chronic pelvic pain, and long-term sexual dysfunction.

The hymen, located at the junction of the vagina and the vestibule, is the product of the combined embryologic fusion of the urogenital sinus and the müllerian ducts. As the urogenital sinus advances upward like a diverticulum from the outside, it envelops the column of müllerian cells, which has already moved nearly four-fifths of the distance from the cervix down to the vestibule. The infoldings of the sinus at the point of union form the lateral walls of the hymen, but the posterior or dorsal portion is a composite of sinus cells externally and müllerian cells internally. The superficial epithelium of the hymen, as of the vagina and cervical portio vaginalis, is derived entirely from the epithelium of the urogenital sinus, which pushes up the vaginal tube and undergoes differentiation into the stratified squamous layer. The opening of the vagina may occur independently of the formation of the hymen.

It is obvious that the complexity of this embryologic development may lead to congenital hymenal malformations. The imperforate hymen is usually detected at birth or puberty. At birth, a hydromucocolpos may accumulate under the influence of maternal hormones. Hence at birth a bulging of the imperforate hymen may be noted between the labia, especially when there is an increase in intraabdominal pressure such as seen during crying. If there is a significant hydromucocolpos detected by rectal examination in the newborn, then the hymen should be excised (cruciate incision followed by excision of margins) to allow continued drainage. During childhood, the imperforate hymen may be asymptomatic before puberty and may go unrecognized unless detected by careful physical examination. However, with the beginning of menstruation and the entrapment of menstrual flow, the vagina gradually becomes distended with blood. From the pressure of retained blood within the vagina, the hymen bulges outward. As seen in the cross section, this situation may progress to the extreme, with the entire vagina engorged with old blood (hematocolpos), the uterus likewise enlarged by its own retained menstrual flow (hematometra), and blood passing through the tubal isthmus to form a large hematosalpinx, which occasionally drains into the peritoneal cavity. Because of the possible effects on the upper genital tract, ultrasonography to evaluate the upper genital tract is often indicated. These patients may seek medical assistance because of primary amenorrhea, pelvic pain (especially cyclic), a pelvic mass, or occasionally urinary retention with large masses. Incision with excision of the margins of the hymen and release of the retained blood quickly relieves the situation. Occasionally, the atresia involves not only the hymen but also the lowermost portion of the vagina and, in these patients, a somewhat deeper dissection and reconstruction must be done before the hematoma can be evacuated.

A different form of external vaginal atresia is a thick, fibrous, but not imperforate hymen, which can easily be incised to produce normal patency of the vaginal canal. This type of hymen is relatively uncommon. When it occurs, it may cause dyspareunia, impede tampon use, or completely prevent intromission. Although properly considered an anomaly, this malformation, unlike those of the upper vagina, is usually not associated with congenital anomalies elsewhere in the genitourinary tract.

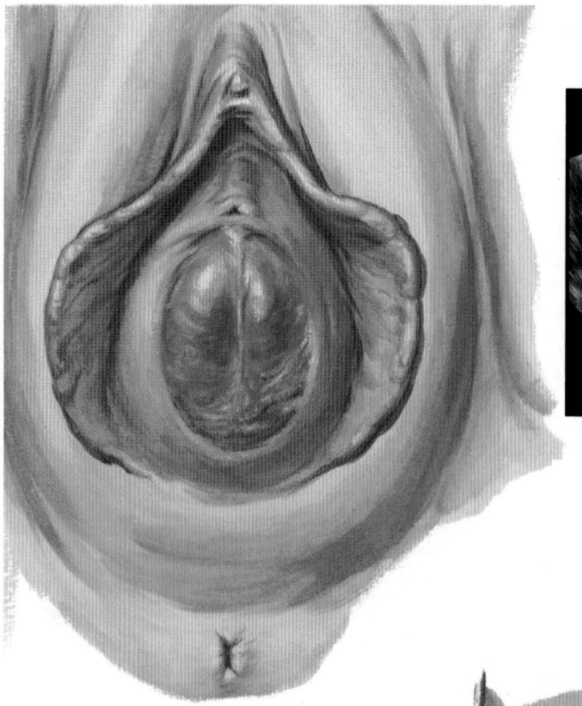

Imperforate hymen

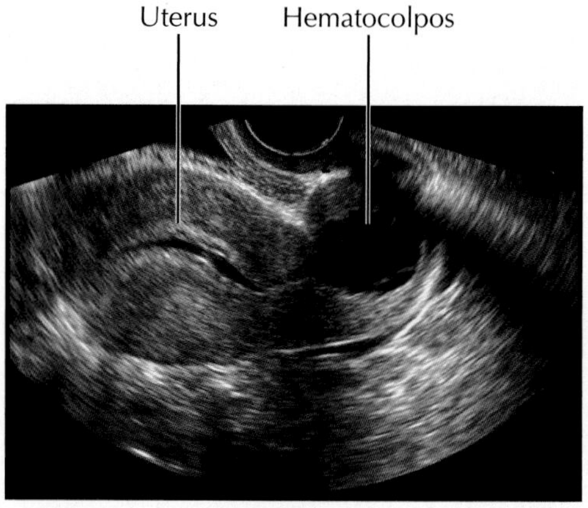

Uterus   Hematocolpos

Sagittal view

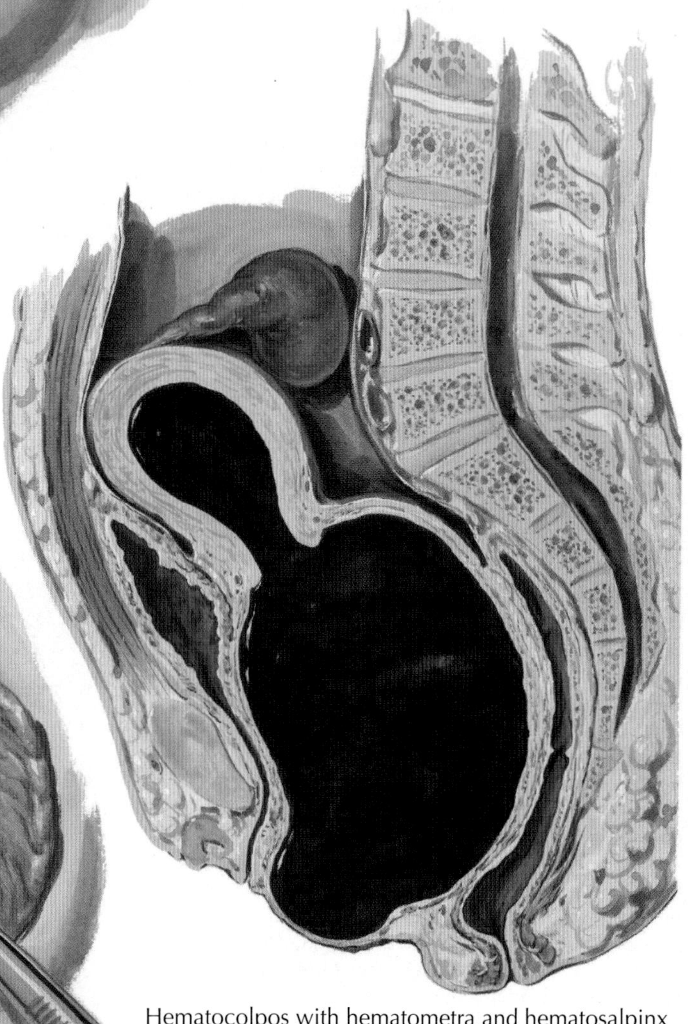

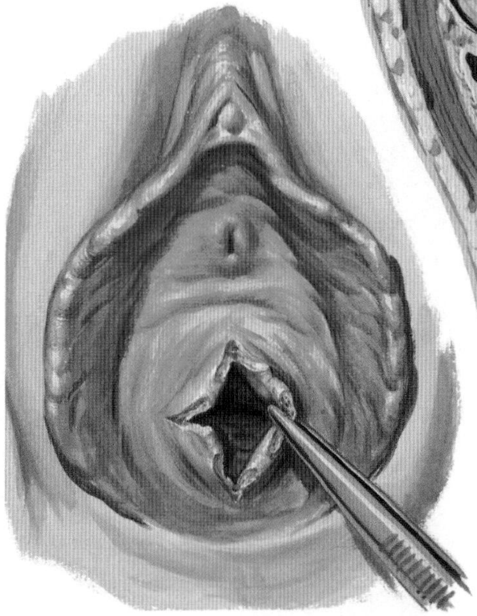

Thick, fibrous hymen (after cruciate incision)

Hematocolpos with hematometra and hematosalpinx

Plate 7.10

Vagina

VAGINITIS: *TRICHOMONAS*, *MONILIA*, BACTERIAL VAGINOSIS

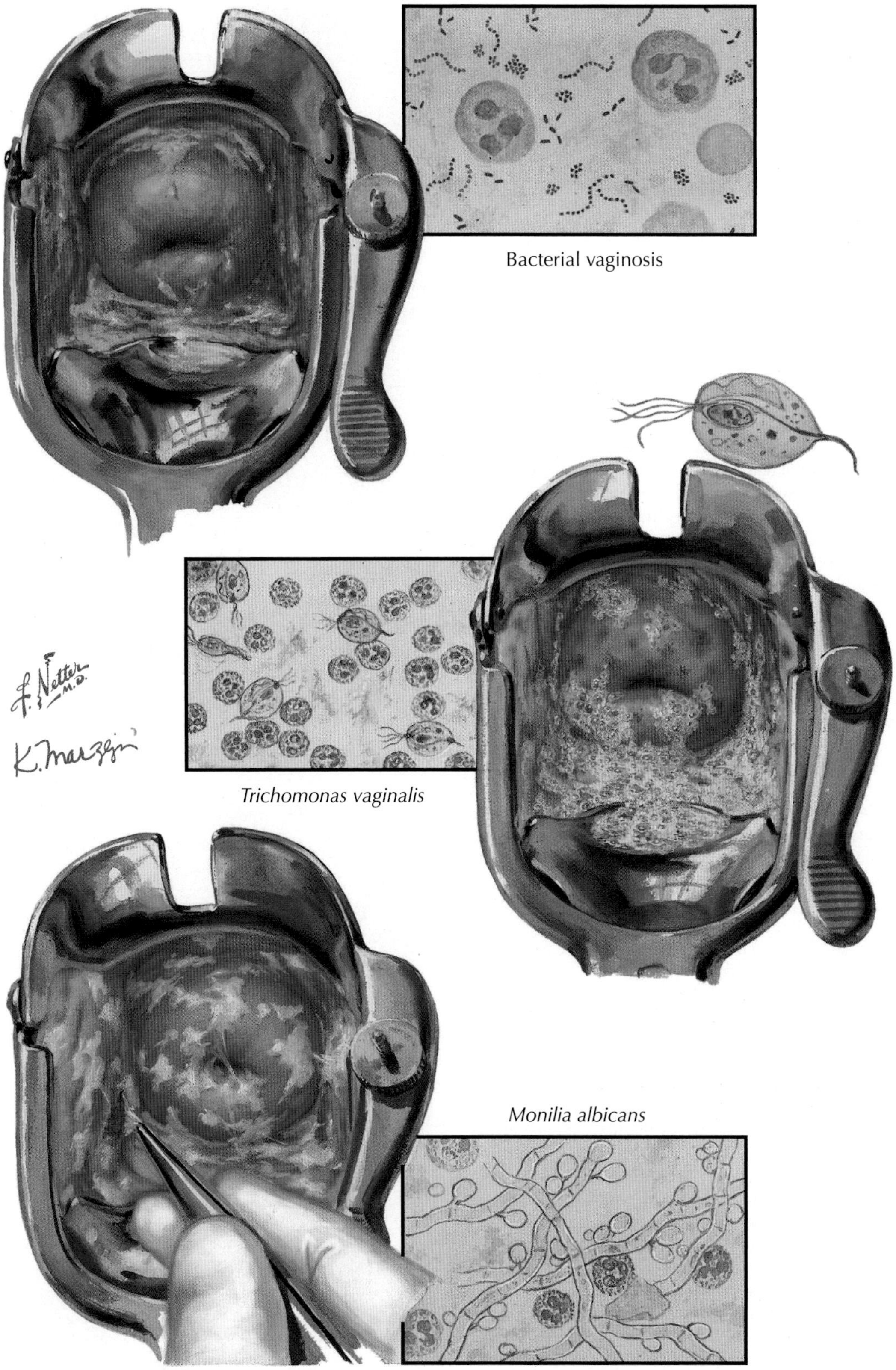

The vagina is a medium for many different types of bacteria, some of which, like lactobacilli, are necessary for normal vaginal metabolism and for maintenance of the vaginal pH at the normal level of 3.8 to 4.2. Also present in numbers, which may be altered by such conditions as age, debility, systemic disease, ovulation, menstruation, and pregnancy are a variety of potentially pathogenic organisms. Among these are streptococci, staphylococci, colon bacilli, and fungi.

Bacterial vaginosis is a condition caused by an overgrowth of normal or pathogenic bacteria that results in irritation, inflammation, and clinical symptoms. Bacterial vaginosis is a change in vaginal ecology caused by an overgrowth of anaerobic bacteria, often with an absence of clinical symptoms. It should be noted that bacterial vaginosis does not engender an inflammatory response and is therefore technically not a type of vaginitis. Bacterial vaginosis is a polymicrobial process that involves the loss of normal lactobacilli, an increase in anaerobic bacteria (especially *Gardnerella vaginalis*, *Bacteroides* sp., *Peptococcus* sp., and *Mobiluncus* sp.), and a change in the chemical composition of the vaginal secretions. There is a 1000-fold increase in the number of bacteria present, and a 1000:1 anaerobic:aerobic bacteria ratio (normal 5:1), high levels of mucinases; phospholipase A_2, lipases, proteases, arachidonic acid, and prostaglandins are all present. Amines (cadaverine and putrescine) are made through bacterial decarboxylation of arginine and lysine. These amines are more volatile at an alkaline pH, such as that created by the addition of 10% KOH or semen (roughly a pH of 7), giving rise to the odor found with the "whiff test" or reported by these patients after intercourse. The vaginal pH will be from 5 to 5.5.

The second most common type of specific vaginal infection (between one quarter to one third of cases) is due to fungal causes. These are ubiquitous fungi found in the air or as common inhabitants of the vagina, rectum, and mouth. The most common species responsible are *Candida albicans* (80%–95%), *Candida glabrata, Candida tropicalis,* or others (5%–20%). These infections are more common when there is an altered vaginal ecosystem (stress, antibiotic use, pregnancy, diabetes, depressed immunity, topical contraceptives, and warm and moist environment). The diagnosis is established by clinical examination and demonstration of the branching, club-shaped filaments in an unstained, wet preparation. The vaginal pH will be normal, from 4 to 4.5. Culture (Nickerson's or Sabouraud media) or monoclonal antibody staining may be obtained but are seldom necessary. Except when the identification of the species involved in recurrent or resistant infections is desirable, culture has generally been replaced by more rapid DNA probe tests, polymerase chain reaction (PCR) tests, or a combined molecular test for all three of the common vaginitis causes. Clinically, the infection causes an aphthous ulcerative infection with a patchy, white exudate, which leaves a raw, bleeding surface when it is removed. The discharge may be thick or watery and is irritating to the external surfaces.

Infections caused by *Trichomonas vaginalis*, a protozoan parasite, are found in approximately 25% of gynecologic patients. *Trichomonas* is a fusiform protozoon slightly larger than a white blood cell with three to five flagella, which provide active movement, extending from the narrow end. On examination, the vaginal walls are

Bacterial vaginosis

Trichomonas vaginalis

Monilia albicans

red and edematous with small petechial hemorrhages, producing the so-called "strawberry" appearance. The thin, greenish-yellow discharge contains many small bubbles, giving it a foamy appearance, which is almost pathognomonic. The discharge is irritating to the external genitalia and causes severe burning and itching. Diagnosis is established by physical examination, with microscopic examination of vaginal secretions in normal saline (sensitivity of 60%–70%). The vaginal pH will be from 6 to 6.5 or higher. Culture or monoclonal antibody

testing may be obtained but is seldom necessary. Nucleic acid amplification tests detect RNA by transcription-mediated amplification (PCR or reverse transcriptase), are highly sensitive and specific, and have become the accepted gold standard for the diagnosis. Rapid antigen and DNA hybridization probes may also be used but carry a higher false-positive risk when prevalence is low. Because this infection is almost exclusively transmitted sexually, evaluation for concomitant sexually transmissible infections should be strongly considered.

Plate 7.11

Reproductive System: VOLUME 1

Urethral opening

Chancre on wall of vagina

Mucous patches and ulcers

Ulcer on cervix and vaginal wall

Ulcerated lesion in the posterior vagina

Cervix

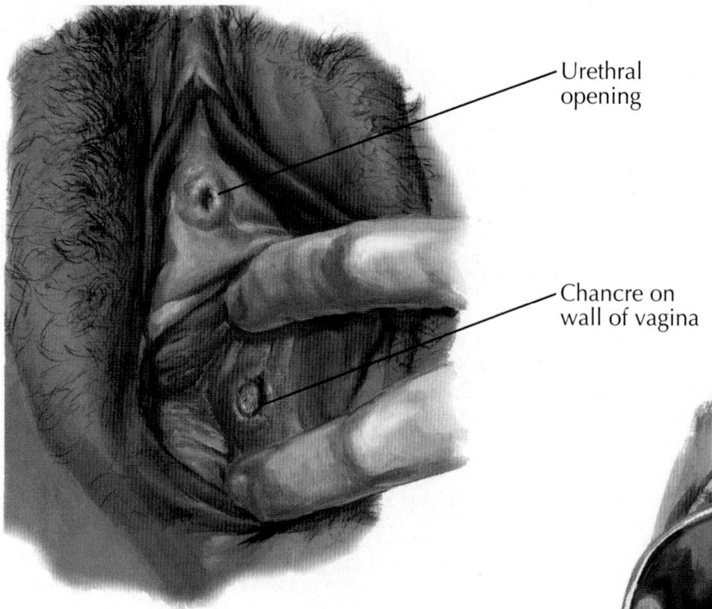

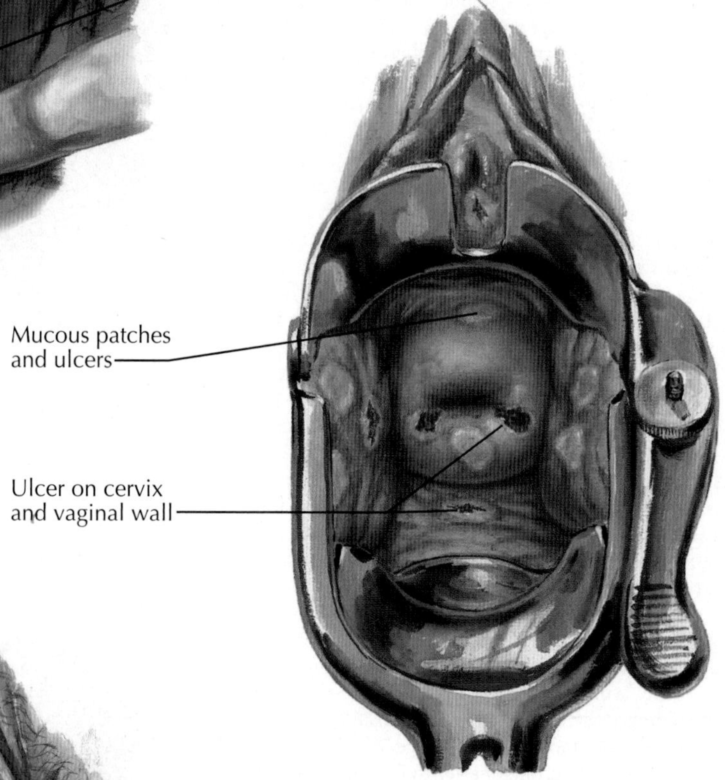

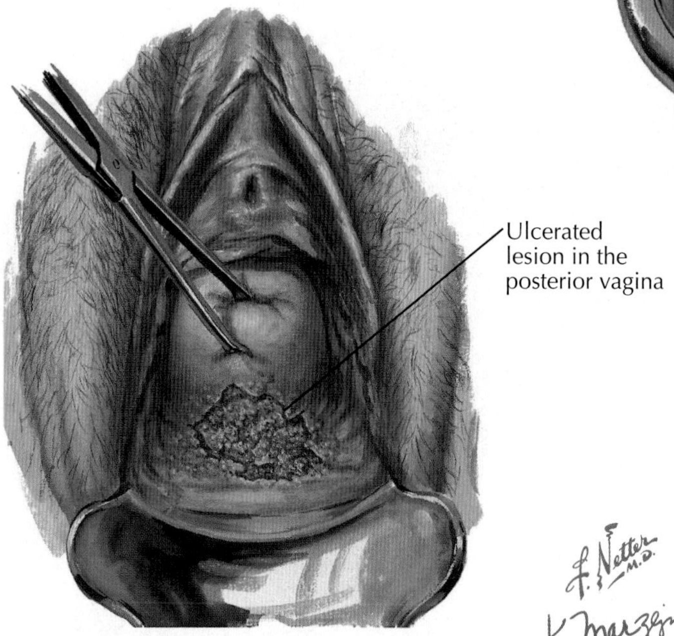

Tuberculosis

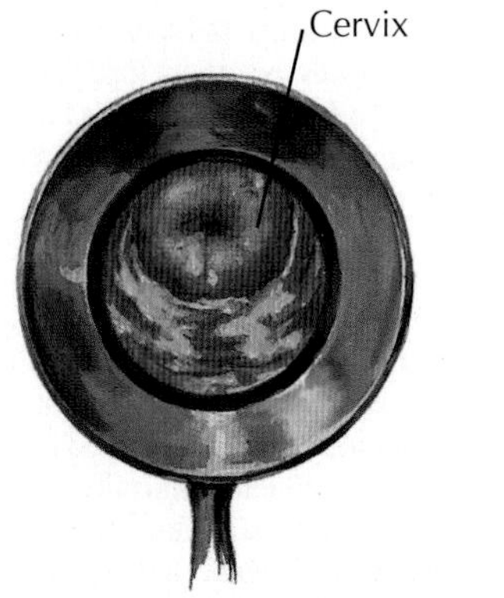

Gonorrhea in childhood

VAGINITIS: VENEREAL INFECTIONS

In clinical practice an occasional case is seen in which the differential diagnosis of a lesion in the lower genital tract involves the exclusion of syphilis. In the female, primary lesions occur more often on the external genitalia and less frequently in the vagina or on the cervix. If in the vagina, a chancre is most likely to be near the vestibule, with no predilection for anterior, posterior, or lateral walls. It has the characteristic raised, indurated border surrounding a shallow ulceration. Because the disease is most often in the lower third of the vagina, associated inguinal lymphadenopathy may be present. Although routine serologic tests are frequently negative at this stage, serologic testing (or dark-field examination if available), should lead to the proper diagnosis, and a biopsy can rule out other granulomas, carcinoma, or various infections. The mucous patches of late syphilis also occur in the vagina as well as on the external genitalia. They are white, vesicular lesions that may coalesce and break down to form shallow ulcers and are not to be confused with the firm, raised condylomata lata that are also late manifestations of syphilis. At this stage, a positive serologic test should indicate the probable diagnosis; a dark-field examination of scrapings is usually positive for *Treponema pallidum*. The Venereal Disease Research Laboratory and rapid plasma reagin tests are good screening tests, and the fluorescent treponemal antibody absorption or microhemagglutination *T. pallidum* tests are specific treponemal antibody tests that are confirmatory or diagnostic. Screening for HIV infection should also be strongly considered.

Because of the resistance of the thick vaginal epithelium during reproductive life to neisserial organisms, gonorrhea in the vagina is less common than in Bartholin and Skene glands or in the upper genital tract. However, at the extremes of age, in the postmenopausal period and especially in childhood, gonorrheal vaginitis is a definite clinical entity. Vaginitis in a child can be evaluated through the use of a cystoscope or hysteroscope, which is easily introduced through the small introitus and affords an excellent view. The yellow, purulent exudate, which is frequently the presenting symptom, covers the inflamed vaginal walls, and the cervix often shows extensive erosion around the external os. A malodorous, purulent discharge from the urethra, Skene duct, cervix, vagina, or anus (even without rectal inoculation) 3 to 5 days after exposure (40%–60%) may also be present. The diagnosis can be made by smears or cultures, although negative results are not conclusive.

Tuberculosis seldom affects the vagina, although the increase in individuals who are immunocompromised (natural or iatrogenic) as well as the rise in international travel have resulted in an increase in the incidence of this infection. At one time, it constituted approximately

2% of disease of the upper genital tract and appeared occasionally on the external genitalia as lupus vulgaris. When found in the vagina, it is secondary to tuberculosis of the fallopian tubes, uterus, and cervix and is usually located in the posterior vaginal fornix, which is most likely to receive the infected discharge from the uterine cavity. A rare case may result from coitus with an individual who harbors acid-fast organisms in his seminal tract. Vaginal lesions are of the miliary type, with

the white seedings eventually coalescing to form a large ulceration and producing a foul discharge. Diagnosis is made by smears and cultures, as in other forms of tuberculosis, but a biopsy is a quick and accurate way of securing the correct answer. A careful search should be made for tuberculosis elsewhere in the body, and treatment should include the use of the systemic drugs, plus resection of foci in the upper genital tract and of the vaginal lesion if it is not too extensive.

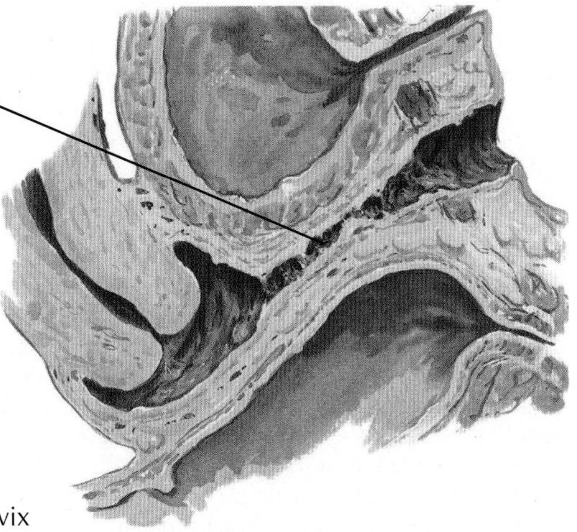

Plate 7.12

Vagina

Vaginitis: Chemical, Traumatic

Some vaginal inflammations, in addition to those due to direct bacterial invasion, are caused by the ill-advised introduction of foreign objects or substances. Vaginal douches and solutions have been used for a variety of gynecologic conditions, and an incalculable number of proprietary douche powders or fluids have been devised to alleviate or cure different types of real or perceived disturbances. Although it is doubtful that the brief contact of the vaginal epithelium with the materials contained in a commercial douche produces a salutary effect other than a cleansing one, the practice continues to be widespread. When homemade solutions or other agents are used, the risk is increased. The danger of such a procedure is the possibility of producing a chemical burn, with marked redness, swelling, and ulceration of the vaginal walls. Under these circumstances, a purulent exudate soon appears, and the patient has intense local pain. Such accidents were particularly perilous when, during early pregnancy, various solutions were used to induce abortion. Even with the availability of elective pregnancy terminations, cases of this nature are still encountered. If the immediate damage has not been too severe, the inflammation may subside spontaneously or with mild palliative therapy, but if a necrotizing agent has been applied, adhesions may form that scar or occlude the vagina. Even when scarring is relatively mild, chronic pain and sexual dysfunction may result.

Foreign bodies in the vagina can also lead to infection and ulceration of the vaginal epithelium, whereas the symptoms may be referred to the bladder or rectum. Pins, coins, marbles, and many other objects have been recovered from the vaginas of children or those temporarily or permanently impaired. The insertion of these articles may be the result of attempted masturbation or abuse. The purulent discharge that eventually results brings the child and her caregiver to the clinic. A history of the sudden onset of profuse leukorrhea in an infant or child should alert the physician to the possibility of a foreign body in the vagina, and a hysteroscope or cystoscope may be valuable for obtaining the exposure necessary to examine the vagina and remove the offending object. If it is embedded in the vaginal wall because of long neglect, removal may be difficult, but the inflammatory process quickly subsides once its cause has been eliminated.

On occasion, the retention of a foreign body is explained by neglect of a situation originally established for a specific therapeutic purpose. Tampons inserted to control menstrual flow and forgotten may be responsible for inflammation and leukorrhea. When tampons are used toward the end of menstrual flow or the patient is in the habit of infrequent tampon changes, there is a greater risk that the tampon will be forgotten, leading to irritation and secondary bacterial infection.

Pessaries are designed to correct displacements of uterus, bladder, or rectum, but if they become neglected, infection or other damage may result. This is particularly true if the patient has a poor memory or for those who may be remiss in their personal hygiene. Hard rubber or metal ring pessaries used for uterine prolapse are especially likely to give trouble, because if not regularly taken out and cleaned, with simultaneous inspection of the vagina, they give rise to severe local infection, cystitis, and pyometra, or they may even become embedded deep in the vaginal wall. Gross hemorrhage also may occasionally occur. Removal of foreign bodies is usually a simple office procedure, but in an exceptional case general anesthesia and an operating room environment may be required. To avoid these complications, follow-up of pessary users should occur at regular intervals.

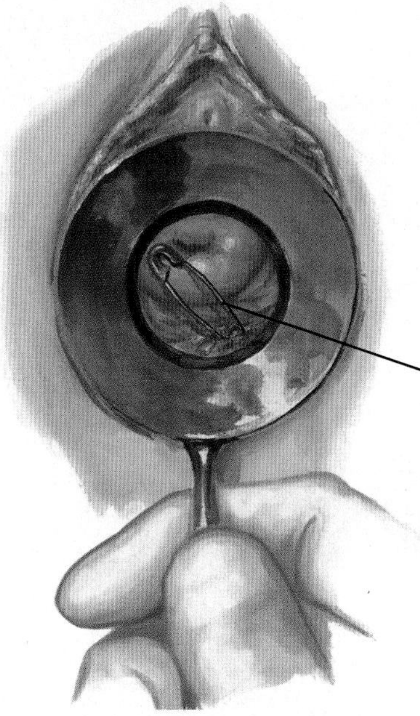

Adhesions in vagina

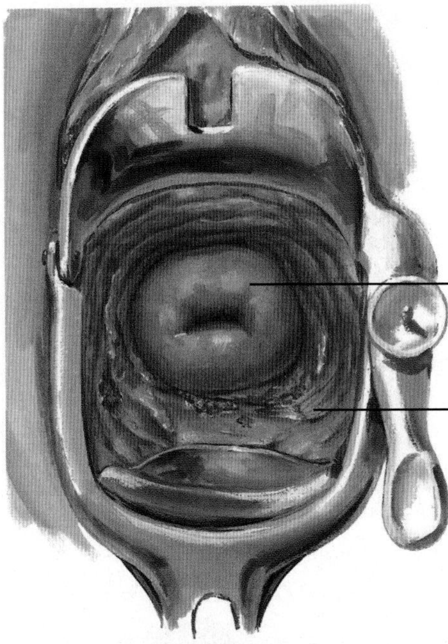

Cervix

Vaginal wall

Chemical vaginitis

Adhesions after severe chemical erosion

Safety pin in vagina of child

Foreign body

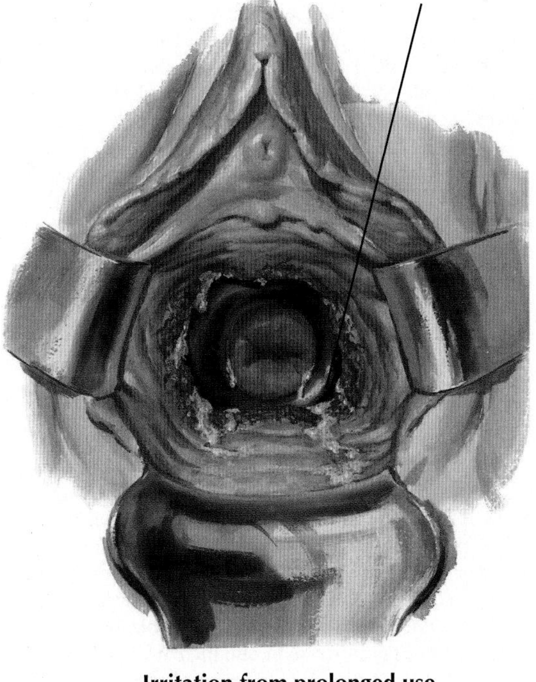

Pessary

Irritation from prolonged use of pessary and poor hygiene

Plate 7.13

Reproductive System: VOLUME 1

TOXIC SHOCK SYNDROME

Toxic shock syndrome (TSS) is an uncommon, potentially life-threatening condition caused by toxins produced by an infection with *Staphylococcus aureus*. First described in a series of pediatric cases in 1978, TSS is rare, being seen in only 1 to 2 of 100,000 females 15 to 44 years old. The incidence rose sharply in 1980 when roughly 800 cases where reported, all associated with menstruation. There was a sharp decline with recognition and withdrawal of some highly absorbent tampon products. Up to 60% of cases seen now are not related to menstruation.

TSS requires infection by *S. aureus* (generally methicillin susceptible) and at its peak was associated with the use of super absorbency tampons, prolonged use of regular tampons, or barrier contraceptive devices. Although most commonly associated with prolonged tampon use, about 60% of TSS cases are associated with other conditions, including postoperative staphylococcal wound and skin infections, and nonsurgical focal infections. Postpartum cases (including transmission to the neonate) have been reported. Even the use of laminaria to dilate the cervix has been reported to be associated with rare cases. Overall, the prevalence of TSS has declined with newer menstrual hygiene products and awareness of more appropriate use patterns.

Patients with TSS experience rapid onset of fever higher than 38.9° C (102° F), hypotension, and a diffuse rash that is commonly absent in places where clothing presses tightly against the skin. The hypotension seen may progress to severe and intractable hypotension and ventilatory and multisystem dysfunction or failure. Patients may also exhibit agitation, arthralgias, confusion, and diarrhea. Nonspecific symptoms also include headache, myalgias, nausea, and vomiting. Desquamation, particularly on the palms and soles, can occur 1 to 2 weeks after onset of the illness. Many of these symptoms can mimic other exanthems or gastrointestinal illnesses, making a high degree of suspicion a prerequisite to establishing the correct diagnosis. The characteristics that define TSS are shown below.

The pathophysiology of TSS involves exotoxins produced by *S. aureus;* TSS toxin-1 (TSST-1); and enterotoxins A, B, C, D, E, and H. For toxic shock to develop, three conditions must be met: there must be colonization by the bacteria, it must produce toxin, and there must be a portal of entry for the toxin. The presence of foreign bodies, such as a tampon, is thought to reduce local magnesium levels, which promotes the formation of toxin by the bacteria. Most individuals develop antibodies to TSST-1 by early adulthood, but patients with TSS do not seem to develop a sufficient antibody response to TSST-1.

The management of patients with TSS consists of rapid evaluation and supportive intervention. Aggressive support and treatment of the attendant shock are paramount. (Frank shock is common by the time the patient is first seen for care.) The site of infection must be identified and drained, by surgery or by removing the contaminated tampon. Antibiotic therapy with a β-lactamase–resistant antistaphylococcal agent should be started early, but it does not alter the initial course of the illness. Other support (e.g., mechanical ventilation or pressor agents) may be needed. Acute respiratory distress syndrome is a common sequela of TSS, and patients must be monitored for the development of this complication. Acute renal failure, alopecia, and nail loss may also occur in these patients.

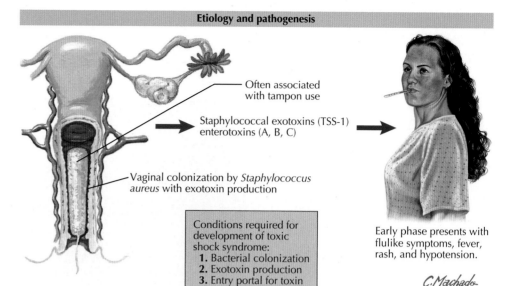

Etiology and pathogenesis

Often associated with tampon use

Staphylococcal exotoxins (TSS-1) enterotoxins (A, B, C)

Vaginal colonization by *Staphylococcus aureus* with exotoxin production

Conditions required for development of toxic shock syndrome:
1. Bacterial colonization
2. Exotoxin production
3. Entry portal for toxin

Early phase presents with flulike symptoms, fever, rash, and hypotension.

C. Machado M.D.
JOHN A. CRAIG AD

Clinical features of toxic shock syndrome

Spectrum of disease ranges from mild, flulike symptoms to rapid loss of function in various organ systems.

Fever greater than 102°F

Diffuse, macular erythematous rash—appearance similar to "sunburn"

General measures of organ support and shock therapy should be instituted.

Headache, irritability, and confusion

Adult respiratory distress syndrome may complicate condition.

Hypotension (may be severe)

Nausea and vomiting

Diarrhea

Complete blood count, liver and renal function studies

Desquamation of palms and soles (occurs late)

Culture for *Staphylococcus aureus*

Tampon removal

CHARACTERISTICS THAT DEFINE TOXIC SHOCK SYNDROME

- Fever >38.9°C (102°F)
- Diffuse, macular, erythematous rash
- Desquamation of palms and soles 1 to 2 weeks after onset
- Hypotension (<90 mm Hg systolic or orthostatic change)
- Negative blood, pharyngeal, and cerebrospinal fluid cultures
- Negative serologic tests for measles, leptospirosis, Rocky Mountain spotted fever
- Findings in three or more of the following organ systems:
  - Gastrointestinal: Vomiting or diarrhea at onset of illness
  - Muscular: Severe myalgia or creatine phosphokinase elevation >2 times the upper limit of normal
  - Mucous membranes: Vaginal, oropharyngeal, or conjunctival hyperemia
  - Renal: Blood urea nitrogen or serum creatinine >2 times the upper limit of normal or pyuria (>5 leukocytes/high-power field) in the absence of urinary tract infection
  - Hepatic: Bilirubin or transaminases >2 times the upper limit of normal
  - Hematologic: Platelets <100,000/μL
  - Central nervous system: Disorientation or alterations in consciousness without focal neurologic signs when fever and hypotension are absent

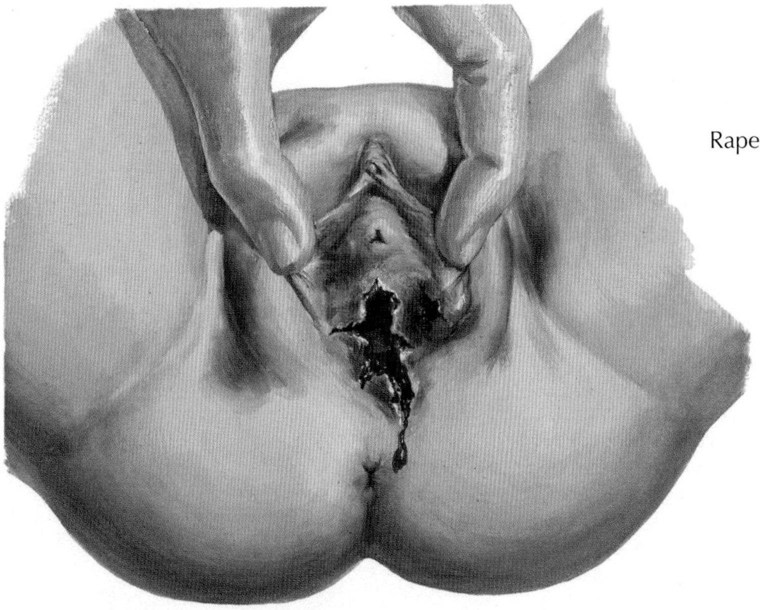

Plate 7.14

Vagina

Rape injury in a child

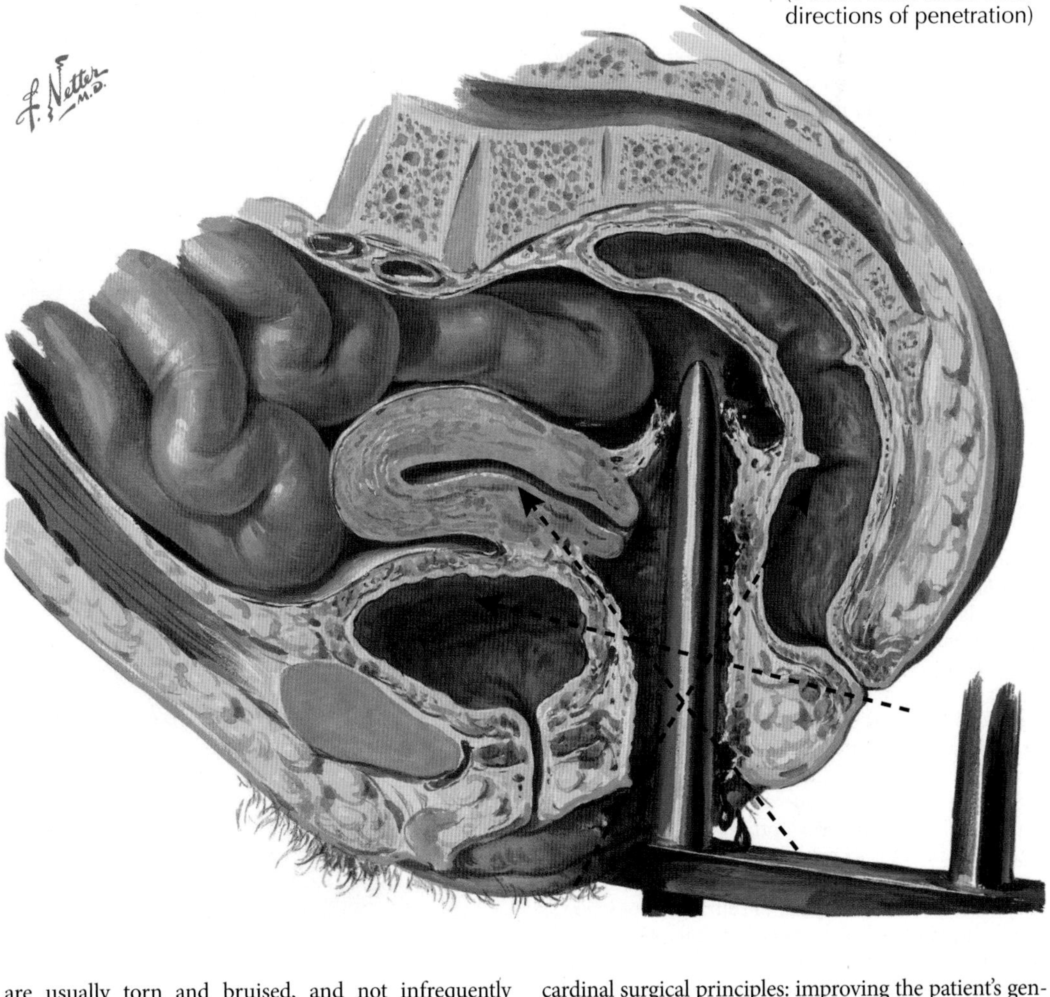

TRAUMA

Nonobstetric lacerations of the vaginal wall or introitus are most often the result of sexual trauma (consensual or otherwise). This may occur from intercourse (80%), saddle or water skiing injury, sexual assault, or penetration by foreign objects. A rape injury, in particular, may be a potentially serious one, because it is often associated with psychological trauma (rape trauma syndrome), damage to adjacent vital organs, and even surgical shock. This is especially true when the injury occurs in a child. Inspection of the vestibule and vagina in such a case often reveals a jagged laceration, which has ruptured the hymen, torn the labia minora, and extended down the perineum toward the anus. The external genitalia may also be badly damaged, with contusions and abrasions as far as the medial surfaces of the thighs. In more severely traumatized victims, the tears may compromise the integrity of the urethra, bladder, and rectum or breach the peritoneum. Such individuals may be brought into the hospital in a state of profound shock requiring immediate blood and fluid replacement before definitive surgical treatment can be instituted. In adults, common sites of lacerations are the vaginal wall, the lateral fornices, and the cul-de-sac. Rape injuries are dangerous in elderly, postmenopausal females who, because of vulvar and vaginal atrophy and the attendant increased fragility of the vaginal wall, are predisposed to more extensive damage. In younger females, the trauma to the vagina from rape is usually not so grave, although during pregnancy and in the immediate postpartum period, the tissues are vascular, delicate, and liable to injury.

Vigorous self-instrumentation during masturbation occasionally causes vaginal lacerations in children or older females, especially when a sharp or breakable object is used. Similarly, some practices in association with a sexual partner may result in accidental injury. Patients may be reluctant to report the presence or circumstances of the injury and may present with abdominal or low back pain as their chief complaint.

Because of its relatively protected position between the thighs and inside the external genitalia, the vagina is seldom subject to trauma by other than sexual means. When it does occur, it is most frequently the so-called picket fence injury caused by falling astride a sharp object that penetrates the vagina. This type of impalement, like a rape injury, may produce a dangerous surgical condition, depending on the extent of the damage to the adjacent pelvic viscera. In the lower picture, the arrows indicate the various possible lines of perforation, and it must be remembered that the lesions may be multiple. The spike of the metal fence has passed upward through the vagina, lacerating the posterior wall and piercing the peritoneum of the posterior cul-de-sac. Such a wound may cause peritonitis, intestinal injury, or prolapse of the small intestine into the vagina. The external genitalia

Impalement with perforation of fornix (*broken lines*: some other directions of penetration)

are usually torn and bruised, and not infrequently hematomas propagate upward in the loose connective tissue between the pelvic viscera and especially within the leaves of the broad ligament, where suppuration may ensue.

There are three basic responsibilities in the care of someone who may have been raped or abused: the detection and treatment of serious injuries, the preservation of evidence, and protection against sequelae. Treatment of all types of vaginal trauma is governed by the following

cardinal surgical principles: improving the patient's general condition, controlling the local hemorrhage, and repairing the laceration. The latter may involve several different stages, depending on which organs are involved, but the steps can be taken in logical sequence once the patient has been made safe for surgery. Any time there is a suspicion that the abdominal cavity has been entered, exploratory laparoscopy or laparotomy should be carried out to assess the possibility and perform any needed repairs.

Plate 7.15

Reproductive System: VOLUME 1

CYSTOCELE, URETHROCELE

A cystocele or urethrocele (anterior compartment pro-lapse) results from a loss of support for the anterior vagina, through rupture or attenuation of the pubovesi-cocervical fascia, manifested by descent or prolapse of the urethra (urethrocele) or bladder (cystocele). With stretch or rupture of the principal muscular supports of the vagina and the breach of the pelvic fascia in the pubovesicocervical plane during parturition, the bladder may push forward and downward through the anterior vaginal wall to form the hernia known as *cystocele*. Although a minor defect of this type is the rule rather than the exception in parous females (10%–15% of reproductive age females, 30%–40% after meno-pause), the size of such hernias depends on a variety of factors, among them the number and difficulty of pre-vious deliveries, the general condition of the individual before delivery, and the quality of pre- and postpartum care. The cystocele may undergo further exacerbation between pregnancies, or in the postmenopausal period as a result of conditions that tend to increase the intraabdominal pressure such as obesity, chronic cough, heavy lifting, intrinsic tissue weakness, or atrophic changes caused by estrogen loss. Some authors include smoking as a risk factor. There is some experimental evidence that changes in gene activation after child-birth can affect elastin production and repair, increas-ing the risk of pelvic support defects.

Several classification systems are used for defining the extent of the support defect encountered. Small cystoceles, involving only a slight deviation from the normal, are referred to as first degree; those that advance nearly to the introitus are second degree; those that come to the introitus or beyond are third degree. Other classifications use a four-step designation with the differentiation between the third and fourth degrees being the level of the hymenal ring. The POP-Q assess-ment system is a much more detailed and reproducible method of quantification that is used extensively for research and in the urogynecologic field but has failed to gain universal clinical usage.

A cystocele does not necessarily cause symptoms. If the hernia is large enough to produce incomplete void-ing, the stasis leads to recurrent attacks of cystitis with dysuria, frequency, nocturia, and stress incontinence. The individual may complain of suprapubic pressure, a dragging sensation in the pelvis, or the presence of a vaginal mass. Pain and dyspareunia are rare symptoms.

Stress urinary incontinence is a common presenting complaint for those with anterior compartment pro-lapse. Anterior support failures are best demonstrated by having the patient strain or cough while observing the vaginal opening through the separated labia. When a urethrocele or cystocele is present, a downward move-ment and forward rotation of the vaginal wall toward the introitus is demonstrated. A double-ended specu-lum or the lower half of a Graves, Peterson, or other vaginal speculum may be used to retract the posterior

Large cystocele

Urethrocele with moderate cystocele

vaginal wall, facilitating the identification of the support defect. Occasionally, it is necessary to have the patient stand to determine the degree of herniation and incon-tinence present. An evaluation of urinary function is advisable, especially if surgical therapy is being consid-ered. In the past, the functional significance of a cysto-urethrocele was gauged by elevating the bladder neck (using fingers or an instrument) and asking the patient to strain (referred to as a *Bonney* or *Marshall-Marchetti*

test). This test has fallen out of favor as nonspecific and unreliable.

Treatment generally consists of weight reduction, treatment of chronic cough (if present), and any infec-tions. Topical or systemic estrogen therapy is often prescribed, but the evidence is controversial. Specific measures include pessary therapy, pelvic muscle exer-cises, and surgical repair. There is a limited role for medical therapy.

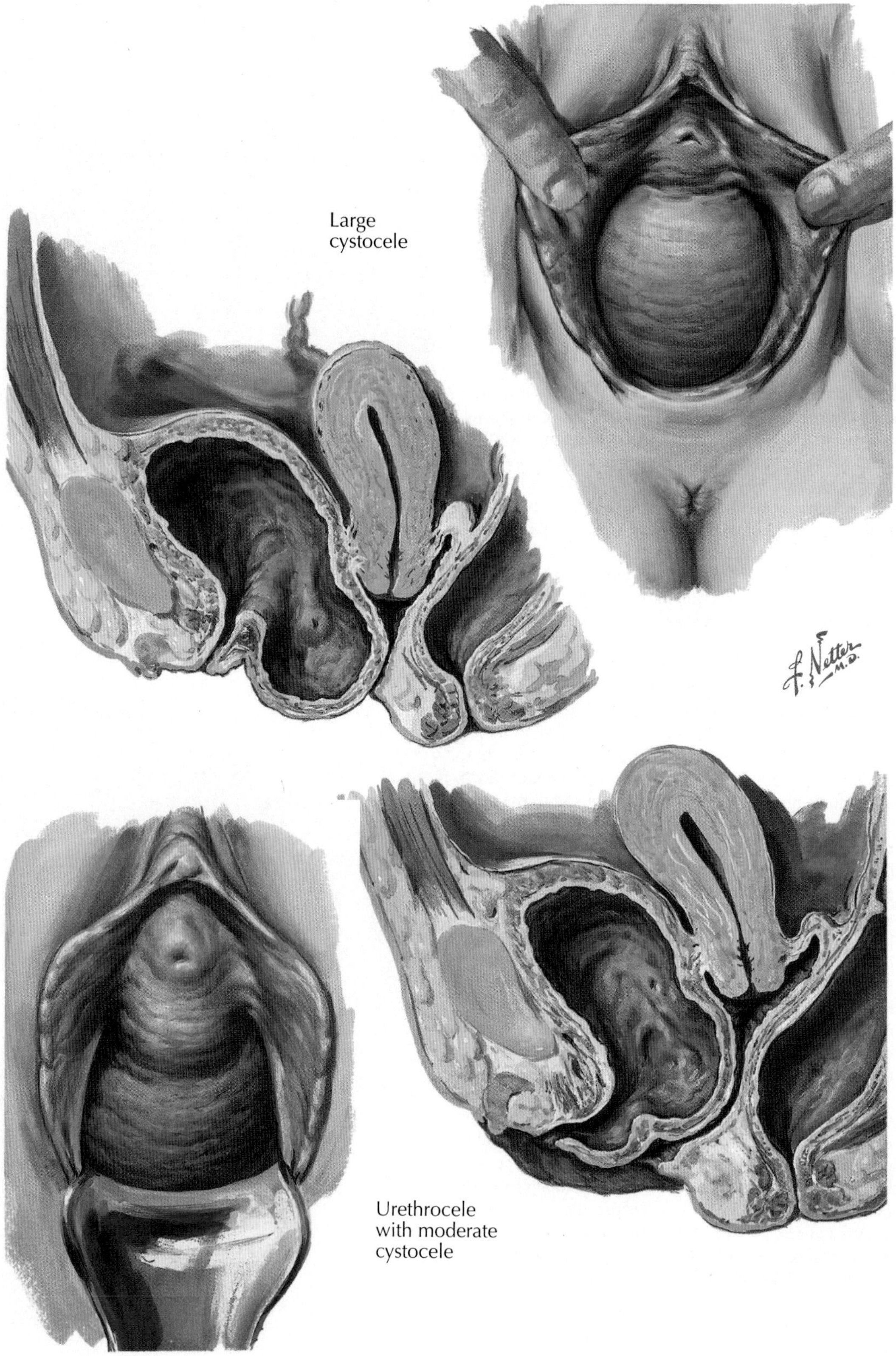

Plate 7.16

Vagina

RECTOCELE, ENTEROCELE

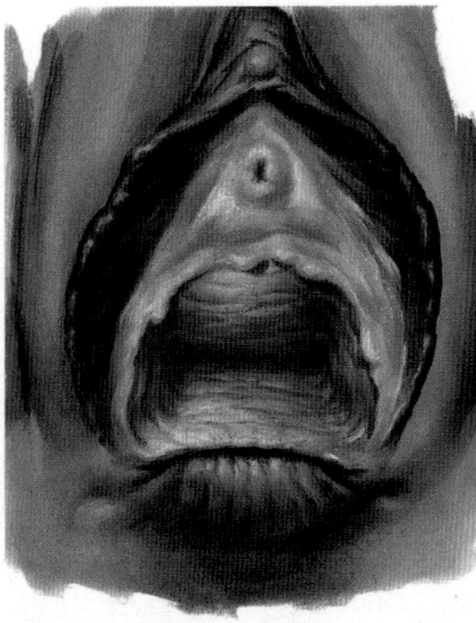

Failure of the normal support mechanisms between the rectum and the vagina results in herniation of the posterior vaginal wall and underlying rectum into the vaginal canal and eventually to, and through, the introitus. The clinical end result of posterior obstetric trauma may be a rectocele or enterocele (posterior compartment prolapse). They can ensue after multiple pregnancies in the absence of severe trauma or, as in cystocele, from any situation that tends to increase the intraabdominal pressure over a long period of time. Congenital weakness, poor health, and poor care predispose to the development of rectocele. Some authors include smoking as a risk factor. A rectocele may be found in 10% to 15% of reproductive age females, rising to 30% to 40% of females after menopause.

Rectocele seldom occurs alone. When it does, it is usually asymptomatic, although the patient may complain of a dragging sensation and difficulty evacuating the rectum when it is full because of the obstruction offered by the bulging ampulla. However, constipation is more often a contributing cause than an effect. Rectoceles can be graded by the POP-Q system or by their size, with third degree denoting a hernia to or beyond the introitus. Hemorrhoids, prolapse of the rectal mucosa, and local infections about the anus may occur in association with large rectoceles. A rectocele does not cause fecal incontinence if the anal sphincters are intact.

Surgical repair is indicated when the hernia causes severe symptoms or is of very large size. It is usually done for first- or second-degree rectocele in the course of a vaginal plastic operation devised for anterior compartment prolapse, because good levator approximation further buttresses the anterior wall. If done from below, the operation should include complete dissection and inversion of the hernial sac (enterocele), plication of the perirectal fascia, and realignment of the pubococcygeus muscles. In difficult cases, it is occasionally necessary to make an abdominal approach and suspend the rectum by suturing it to the posterior vaginal wall and uterosacral ligaments. The use of natural materials (such as fasciae) or synthetic mesh to augment surgical repairs has become common, although documentation of their superiority is not available.

Congenital elongation of the cul-de-sac of Douglas with prolapse of the intestine or omentum can produce inversion of the pelvic floor in the absence of obstetric trauma in the condition known as *primary enterocele*. Because both rectocele and enterocele present in the posterior vagina, the two conditions may be difficult to differentiate when they occur together. A horizontal retraction line in the vaginal epithelium between the hernias may lead to the correct diagnosis, or reduction of the rectocele may demonstrate another bulge higher in the vagina. Palpation of intraperitoneal structures and the presence of peristaltic activity in the sac are more conclusive evidence. Transvaginal ultrasonography may be used to assess the presence of an enterocele if not clinically apparent. To overlook and therefore fail to repair an enterocele is a common cause of recurrence of prolapse after surgery. Such recurrences are referred to as *secondary enteroceles*, but in those cases that have had previous inadequate surgical treatment of a primary enterocele, the term is a misnomer.

As in the other vaginal hernias, the presence of a mass, pelvic pressure, and sometimes pain cause a female with an enterocele to seek relief. Intestinal symptoms are rare, and obstruction seldom occurs because of the width of the neck of the sac. High ligation and excision of the peritoneal sac with closure of the uterosacral ligaments by the vaginal approach is the treatment of choice, but an abdominal operation with complete obliteration of the posterior cul-de-sac is sometimes indicated after an unsuccessful vaginal operation.

Lacerated perineum (healed)

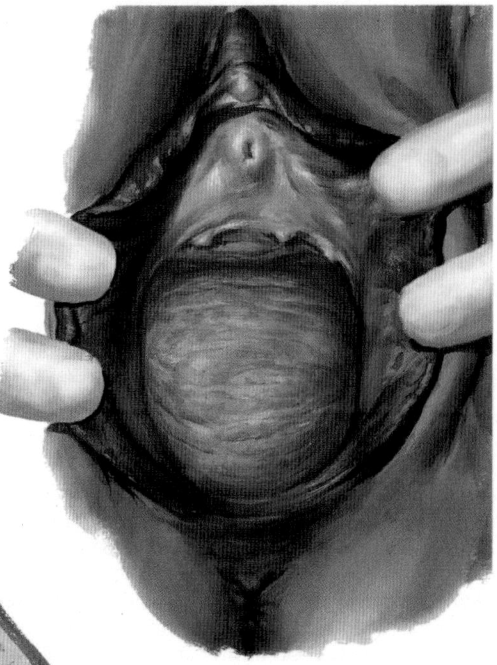

Large rectocele

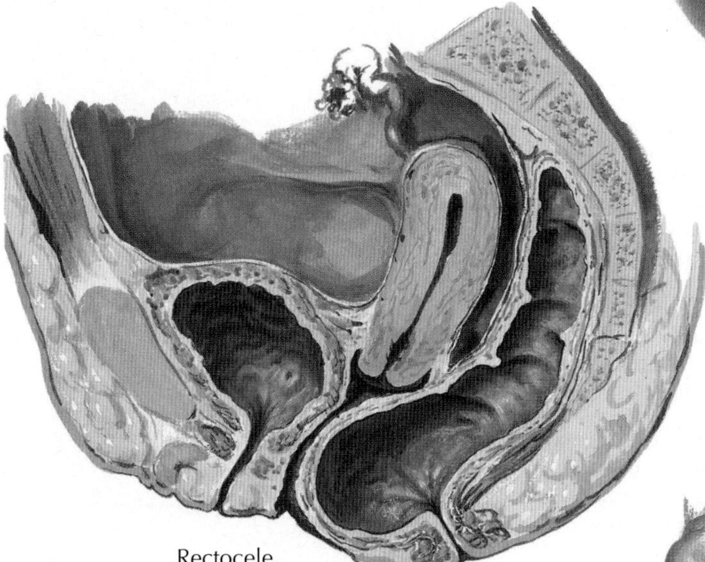

Rectocele

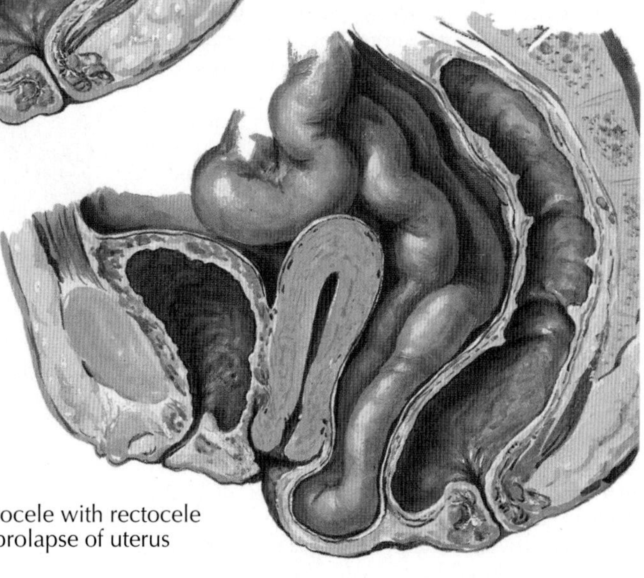

Enterocele with rectocele and prolapse of uterus

Plate 7.17

Reproductive System: VOLUME 1

Dilated ureter

Uterus

Bladder

Vagina

Rectum

Types of fistulae
1. Vesicovaginal
2. Urethrovaginal
3. Vesicocervicovaginal
4. Rectovaginal
5. Enterovaginal
6. Ureterovaginal (inset)

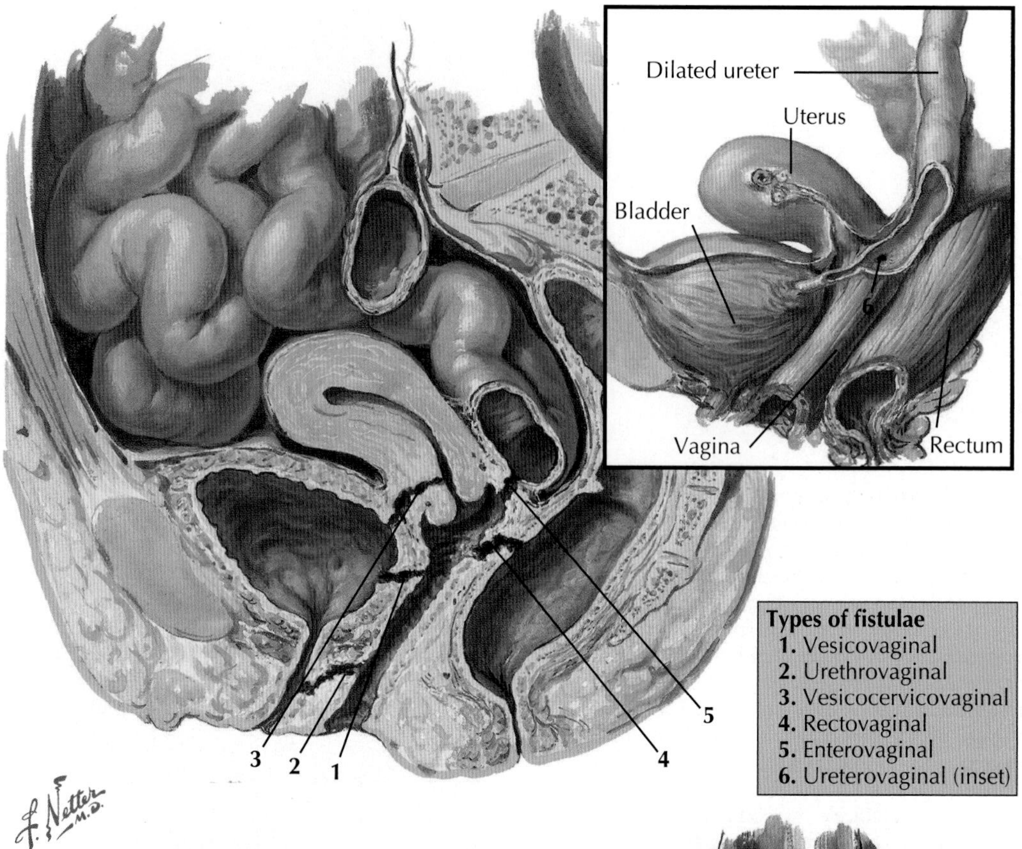

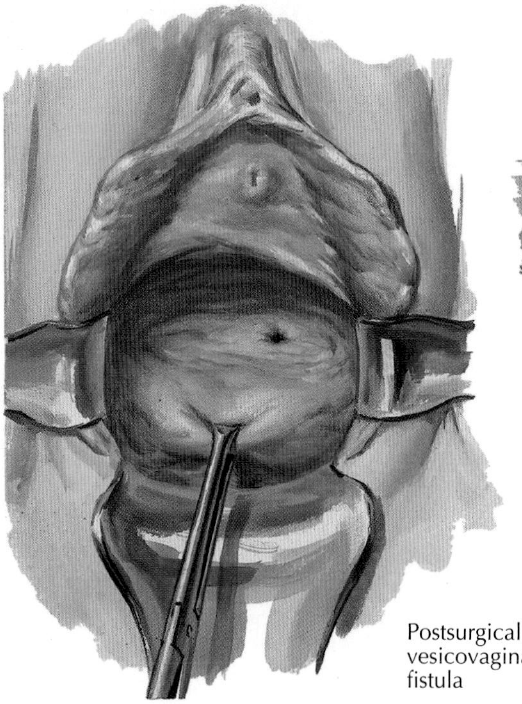

Postsurgical vesicovaginal fistula

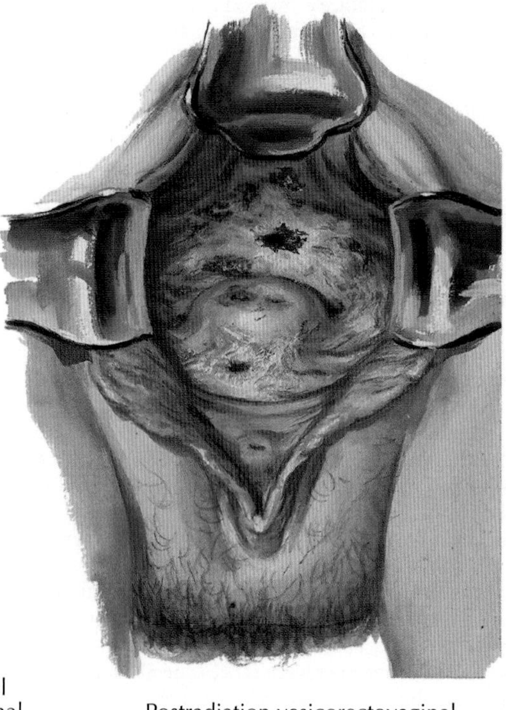

Postradiation vesicorectovaginal fistula (patient in knee-chest position)

FISTULAE

A fistula is an abnormal communication between two cavities or organs. In gynecology, this usually refers to a communication between the gastrointestinal or urinary tracts and genital tract. Because of its anatomic location in close apposition to the bladder and rectum, the vagina is occasionally the site of fistulae, which divert the urinary and fecal streams, causing incontinence. These fistulae may occur in any part of the vaginal canal and are sometimes multiple.

Urinary tract fistulae may result from surgical or obstetric trauma, irradiation, or malignancy, although the most common cause by far is unrecognized surgical trauma. Roughly 75% of urinary tract fistulae occur after abdominal hysterectomy. Urinary tract fistulae are most common after uncomplicated hysterectomy, although pelvic adhesive disease, endometriosis, or pelvic tumors increase the individual risk. Signs of a urinary fistula (watery discharge) usually occur from 5 to 30 days after surgery (average 8–12), although they may be present in the immediate postoperative period. If the defect is small, it may spontaneously heal with simple catheter drainage of the bladder (20%–30% of patients). More severe defects should not be repaired until the tissues have returned to normal condition. Final repair may be by the transvaginal, transvesical, or transperitoneal routes, depending on the size and position of the opening. Cystoscopy may be required to evaluate the location of a urinary tract fistula in relation to the ureteral opening and bladder trigone and to exclude the possibility of multiple fistulae.

The majority of urethrovaginal fistulae are due to obstetric injury. However, they may be congenital, the most common form being hypospadia. Unlike vesicovaginal fistulae, which almost invariably cause urinary incontinence, urethrovaginal fistulae may be associated with no symptoms, especially if the defect is located well forward of the vesical neck and near the introitus.

Vesicocervicovaginal fistulae are relatively uncommon and are usually caused by cancer of the cervix or surgical injury to the bladder in the course of a subtotal hysterectomy. A fistulous tract in this area is often difficult to identify and to repair.

Fistulae between the gastrointestinal tract and vagina may be precipitated by the same injuries that cause genitourinary fistulae; most common are obstetric injuries and complications of obstetric lacerations (lower third of vagina). Fistulae may also follow hysterectomy or enterocele repair (upper third of vagina). Inflammatory bowel disease or pelvic radiation therapy may hasten or precipitate fistula formation. Although Crohn disease, lymphogranuloma venereum, or tuberculosis are recognized risk factors, these are uncommon. For those that do not heal spontaneously (75% of fistulae), the only effective treatment is surgical. Repair of these fistulae may necessitate diversion of the fecal stream by colostomy before definitive closure. The scarring and puckering of surrounding tissues produced by radiation therapy greatly reduces the chances of successful closure. Such lesions must always be biopsied to rule out the possibility of residual malignancy. Surgical treatment of these defects is complicated, because the underlying pathologic process is usually still progressing and the results are poor.

Surgical mismanagement accounts for most ureterovaginal fistulae. In the course of hysterectomy, the ureter may be compressed by clamp or suture just before it enters the bladder wall, resulting in obstruction, necrosis, and formation of a new urinary outlet through the upper vagina. Urinary incontinence of this type can be differentiated from that due to vesicovaginal fistula by observing the vagina after the introduction of a dye into the bladder. Ureterovaginal fistulae are of serious significance because measures to restore the continuity of the urinary tract may be unsuccessful with loss of the involved kidney.

Occasionally, a combined vesicorectovaginal fistula converts the vagina into a cloaca.

Plate 7.18

Vagina

ATROPHIC CONDITIONS

With the cessation of ovarian follicular activity, blood estrogen levels become much lower than during normal reproductive life. This decrease has just as an important effect upon the vulvar and vaginal tissues as upon the uterine lining. This is a normal physiologic process and, in the early stages, may give rise to no subjective manifestations, although it can usually be observed clinically as a general shrinking in the caliber of the vaginal canal, with shortening of the fornices. The rugae become less prominent, and the epithelium is of a pale rather than a rosy hue and is increasingly friable. Cracking, vulvar itching, dyspareunia, and postcoital bleeding may be early signs of estrogen loss. Because the vagina normally harbors many different pathogenic bacteria in a quiescent state, as a result of estrogen deficiency the progressive decrease in the resistance of the vaginal epithelium often leads to inflammation and an increased risk of infection. There is a change in vaginal pH toward the alkaline as the normal vaginal flora are lost.

The histology of the vagina after the menopause is characterized by a thin superficial epithelium. In the subepithelium is found a diffuse infiltration of both polymorphonuclear leukocytes and lymphocytes. The stroma is edematous. Correspondingly, a cytologic smear from the postmenopausal vagina shows cells typical of complete atrophy, with a heavy influx of polymorphonuclear leukocytes.

The clinical picture of atrophic vaginitis (genitourinary syndrome of menopause) is quite characteristic. The vagina is narrowed, especially near the apex, making visualization of the cervix difficult. The thin epithelium is covered with numerous small petechial hemorrhages; in some areas, these have coalesced with breakdown of the superficial epithelium and the formation of small ulcerations. The epithelium around the hemorrhages and denuded areas exhibits marked pallor and almost complete absence of rugae. A thin, pale, malodorous, and irritating discharge is commonly present. Clinically, the condition may be confused with a *Trichomonas* infection, and infestation with *T. vaginalis* is not infrequently superimposed upon atrophic vaginitis. Almost any type of bacterial organism may be involved, and the infection is usually mixed.

As the condition advances, attempts at regeneration and repair lead to the formation of adhesions, which at first are filmy and friable but which eventually become firm and fibrous and may occlude a part of or the entire vagina. A speculum view of this type of case is seen in the middle of the plate, with trabecular adhesions running across the upper vagina, like stalactites, completely obliterating the canal and obscuring the cervix.

Significant atrophic vaginitis, both in the early and in the late stages, may lead to postmenopausal bleeding and is one of the commonest causes of this symptom.

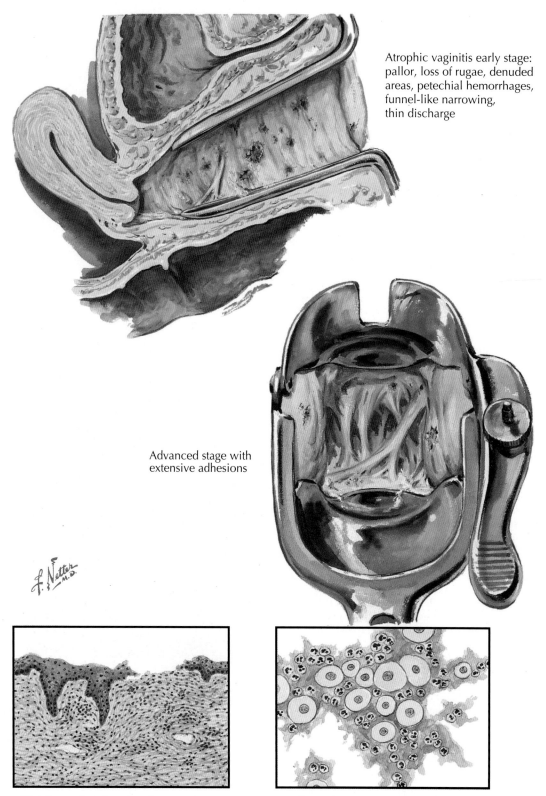

Atrophic vaginitis early stage: pallor, loss of rugae, denuded areas, petechial hemorrhages, funnel-like narrowing, thin discharge

Advanced stage with extensive adhesions

Histology of vagina after the menopause

Smear from postmenopausal vagina

In the milder forms, a pinkish discharge may result from chafing of denuded areas, whereas in the advanced stage, rupture of one of the adhesions as a result of trauma may result in profuse hemorrhage. The latter is to be particularly avoided during pelvic examinations on elderly females or in the course of a vaginal preparation for an operative procedure. A tear of one of these adhesions may extend upward into the broad ligament and cause direct injury to the uterine vessels.

Therapy consists of estrogen replacement, either topically or systemically. Care must be exercised with topical therapy in these patients, for up to 25% of estrogen placed in the vagina may be absorbed into the circulation. This amount may be even greater for patients with atrophic changes. Continuous estrogen exposure without periodic or concomitant progestins increases the risk of endometrial carcinoma six- to eightfold when the uterus is present.

Plate 7.19

Reproductive System: VOLUME 1

CYSTS AND BENIGN TUMORS

Vaginal tumors are relatively rare, but it is likely that the actual occurrence is more common than recognized, because many of these tumors are asymptomatic and therefore go unnoticed and untreated. Benign tumors are more prevalent than malignant and, of these, cysts are the most prevalent. Vaginal cysts are formed chiefly from embryonic epithelial remnants, which may be derived from either the müllerian or wolffian ducts, the latter giving rise to the Gartner duct cysts found on the anterolateral vaginal walls. Gartner duct cysts are blind pouches formed at the branching lower ends of the primitive mesonephric tubules. They may be single or multiple and seldom attain large size. Occasionally, a cyst of this type is large enough to occlude the vaginal canal and resemble a cystocele. In such cases, the patient may have pain, dyspareunia, bladder pressure, or even dystocia during parturition. Because the wolffian duct crosses the anlagen of the broad ligament and the uterus before entering the anterolateral vaginal wall, it is not unusual for cysts of mesonephric origin to extend well upward between the leaves of the broad ligament, increasing the hazard of surgical excision. These cysts, often an incidental finding on routine pelvic examination, need not always be excised, although some uncertainty as to the exact histologic nature of the lesion must exist when the physician decides on conservative management. The histologic architecture is extremely variable. The epithelial lining may consist of a single layer of cuboidal or high columnar epithelium, or either of these types may be stratified. Occasionally, they are lined by stratified squamous epithelium. A few inflammatory cells may be present in the stroma, and, in a very rare exception, the cyst may undergo acute infection and suppuration but never malignant degeneration.

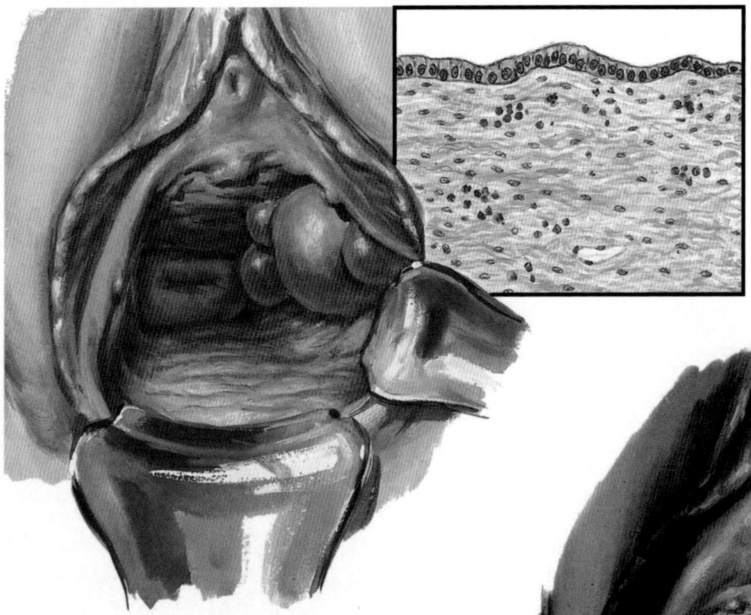

Congenital cysts of müllerian origin may occur in the fornices or lower in the vagina and are often referred to as *inclusion cysts.* They are remnants that have been pushed aside and buried by the advancing superficial epithelium of the urogenital sinus. Some inclusion cysts are formed when the adult vaginal epithelium is turned into the subepithelial tissues as a result of the trauma of delivery, vaginal surgery, or trauma repair. These are usually in the posterior wall near the introitus. Inclusion cysts average less than 1 cm in diameter and are seldom larger than 3 cm. They are often asymptomatic but may cause dyspareunia or make the patient conscious of the presence of a lump. The excised specimens are usually of bluish color and firm consistency and, when opened, contain thick, glairy mucus in contrast to the thin secretion of Gartner duct cysts. The lining cells may be columnar or squamous. Inclusion cysts can be easily removed but, when asymptomatic, need no treatment.

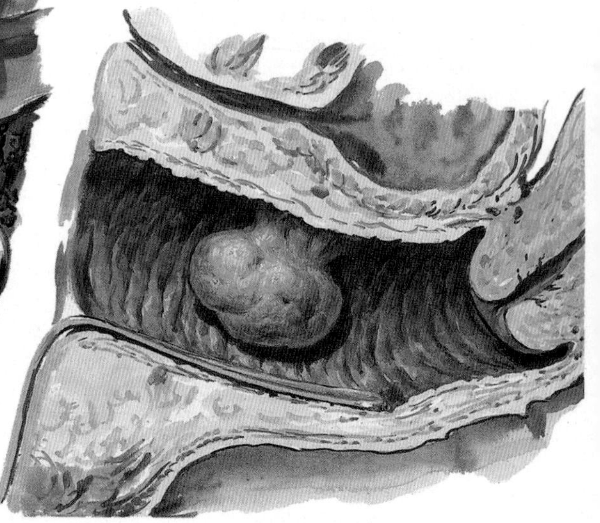

Papilloma and condylomata acuminata occur in the vagina as well as on the external genitalia. Their gross and microscopic characteristics are not modified by their vaginal location. Condylomata are grouped near the vestibule on the posterior and lateral walls or high

in the posterior fornix. They produce a foul discharge, especially when they become large and infected, and must be carefully differentiated from malignancy and the venereal granulomas before appropriate treatment is instituted. Local application of podophyllin, trichloroacetic acid, or other topical therapies eradicates the majority of small lesions, but care must be exercised to avoid damaging adjacent normal tissues.

Fibroma and myoma are quite common in the vagina but are seldom of a size sufficient to produce symptoms. The rare case may be large and pedunculated. These tumors are usually insensitive but may occasionally cause local discomfort. Surgical excision is indicated, because malignancy cannot be excluded grossly.

Other benign vaginal tumors, such as lymphangioma and mole, are extremely rare.

Gartner duct cyst, section of wall with columnar and cuboidal epithelium

Multiple Gartner duct cysts

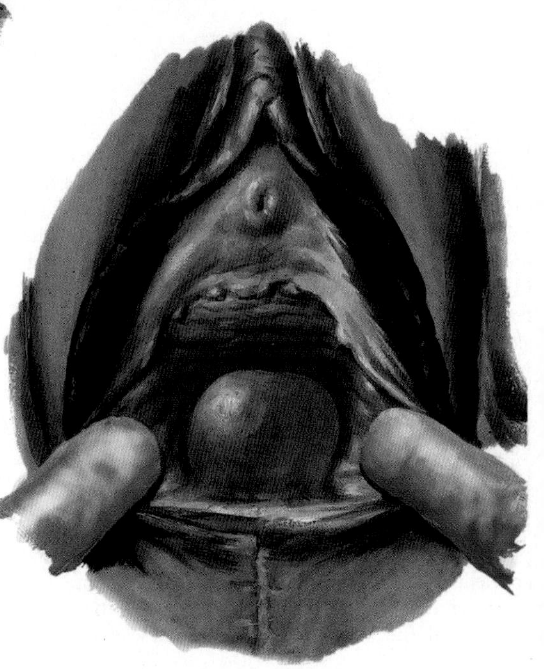

Inclusion cyst

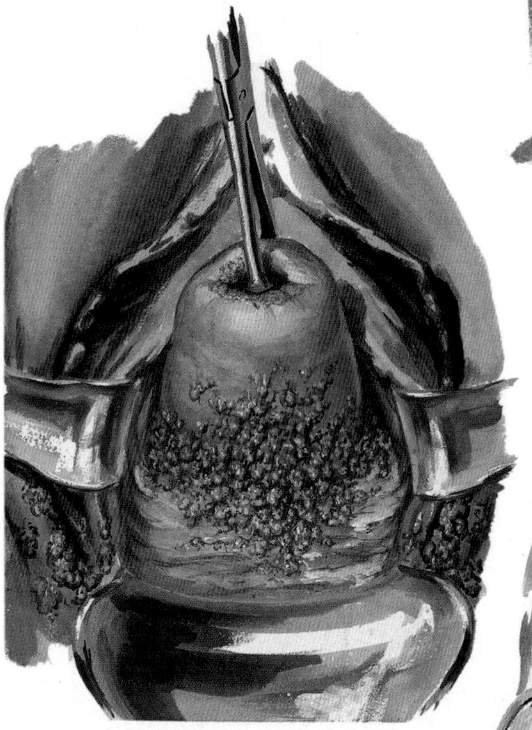

Condylomata acuminata

Fibroma

Plate 7.20

Vagina

ENDOMETRIOSIS: VULVA, VAGINA, CERVIX

Endometriosis is a benign but progressive condition characterized by endometrial glands and stroma found in locations other than the endometrium. It is estimated that between 5% and 15% of females, 20% of gynecologic laparotomies, 30% to 70% of patients with chronic pain, and 30% to 50% of patients with infertility have endometriosis. It is most common during the third and fourth decades of life, with 5% of cases diagnosed after menopause. The occurrence of the disease in the vagina ranks ninth in order of frequency behind the ovary, uterine ligaments, rectovaginal septum, pelvic peritoneum, umbilicus, laparotomy scars, hernial sacs, and appendix. In most females, lesions are found in multiple locations. Almost invariably, vaginal endometriosis is associated with similar lesions in the ovary and rectovaginal septum. The relative frequency of implants in these areas lends support to the theory of Sampson that the etiology of the disease is from retrograde menstruation through the fallopian tubes, because gravity would tend to spread the endometrial particles in this manner. However, it is also true that these structures are covered by tissue derived from primitive coelomic epithelium, which, in response to inflammatory or hormonal stimuli, might undergo metaplasia, as suggested by Robert Meyer. Although up to 90% of females have retrograde menstruation, most females do not develop endometriosis, which suggests that additional factors are involved. Instances of presumed iatrogenic spread (surgical) have been reported, whereas a role for an immunologic defect is debated but remains to be conclusively established.

The large sagittal section shows a small area of endometriosis on the surface of the ovary and other implants on the adjacent peritoneum of the posterior cul-de-sac and lateral pelvic wall. Typical blue-domed endometrial cysts extend down the rectovaginal septum, causing agglutination of the anterior rectal wall to the posterior surface of the uterus. The thickest concentration of endometrial cysts is usually about the attachments of the uterosacral ligaments to the cervix. The presence of endometrium in the septum and its response to the cyclic influence of the ovarian hormones produce a dense, fibrous reaction, which is technically difficult to manage during surgery. The aberrant endometrium rarely penetrates the anterior rectal wall to involve the mucous membrane but more often invades the posterior vaginal fornix. Its presence in the rectum may cause cyclic rectal bleeding or partial obstruction and, in the vagina, dyspareunia or postcoital bleeding. Similar lesions in the anterior vaginal wall may directly involve the bladder, causing cyclic hematuria. The vaginal epithelium around involved areas is puckered and densely adherent, making attempted surgical dissection, or even biopsy, hazardous because of the possibility of damage to the rectum or bladder. Conservative operations may grossly remove the disease from the ovaries and pelvic peritoneum, but complete surgical excision of posterior cul-de-sac, uterosacral, and vaginal lesions is technically impossible, even if a total hysterectomy is performed. If annoying bleeding, dyspareunia, dyschezia, or pelvic pain develop and cannot be controlled, treatment with gonadotropin-releasing hormone agonists, oral

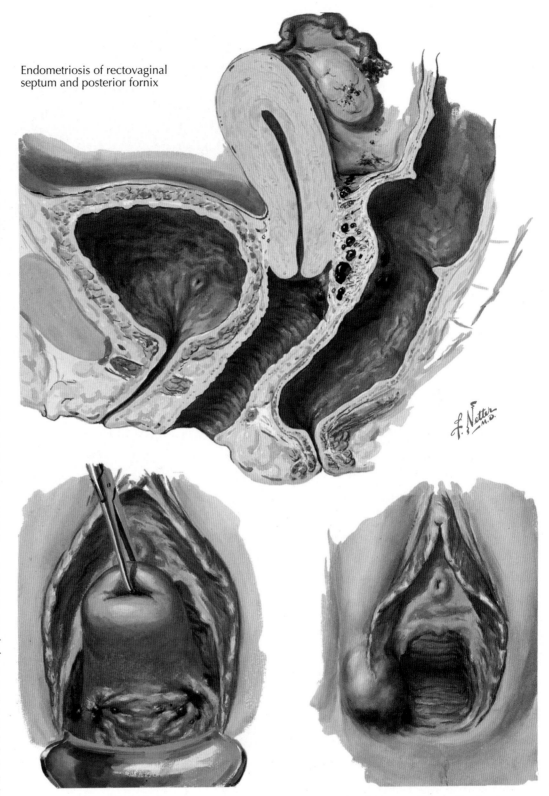

Endometriosis of rectovaginal septum and posterior fornix

Vaginal view

Involvement of Bartholin gland

contraceptives, or progestins suppresses the menstrual hormonal changes, which often control the disease symptom and progression.

Although the occurrence of endometriosis is understandable in areas where coelomic metaplasia or gravitational fall of regurgitated endometrial particles may be the exciting cause, its growth in areas far removed from the pelvis is harder to explain. Occasionally, the disease is found in the vulva or perineum. In the former case, it is assumed that migration is

downward through the canal of Nuck, because this tube is lined by coelomic epithelium; but in the perineum, such an explanation does not hold. Perhaps, in this instance, the spread of endometrium has been by way of the pelvic lymphatics, as suggested by Halban.

A rare case shows involvement of the Bartholin gland. In the absence of external endometriosis elsewhere, local excision of this lesion is indicated, if only for purposes of accurate microscopic diagnosis.

Plate 7.21

Reproductive System: VOLUME 1

Malignant Tumors: Primary

Primary carcinoma of the vagina represents approximately 1% of all malignancies in the female genital tract and ranks after carcinomas of the cervix, endometrium, ovary, and vulva in order of frequency. (In the United States, vaginal carcinoma is more common than vulvar carcinoma.) The lesion is most often located on the posterior vaginal wall and in the upper half of the vagina. Its early stage may be a small, irregular ulceration or a papillary, friable growth. The disease spreads by direct extension and gradually infiltrates the lateral and anterior walls of the vagina, extends into the rectovaginal or vesicovaginal septum, and eventually invades adjacent pelvic viscera. Later, the tumor disseminates by way of the pelvic lymphatics to the lymph glands in the iliac, obturator, and hypogastric areas. Distant metastases are rare.

The differential diagnosis must exclude the venereal granulomas and the possibility that the tumor is secondary. Laboratory diagnosis by vaginal biopsy is conclusive. Nearly always, vaginal cancer is of the squamous cell type and may be either a well-differentiated epithelioma or a wildly growing anaplastic tumor. Melanoma, sarcoma, adenocarcinoma, and other histologic types rarely occur. The strongest association is between squamous cell carcinoma and human papilloma virus types 16 and 18 infections, with 50% of cancers demonstrating evidence of this infection. The exceedingly rare adenocarcinoma of the vagina probably arises in aberrant cervical glands of müllerian origin or in remnants of the mesonephric duct.

Radiation is generally the best overall type of therapy except in very earliest stage disease. External beam radiation, supplemented with intracavitary or interstitial brachytherapy radiation, depending on the thickness of the primary tumor is typical. This should be followed by deep x-ray therapy to the pelvis. Treatment may be augmented by chemoradiation or chemotherapy. In the rare case where radical surgery is undertaken, it may be possible to remove the vaginal lesion with a wide margin, but a satisfactory excision frequently necessitates the sacrifice of the adjacent bladder or rectum as well as the pelvic and inguinal lymphatic drainage from the area. The 5-year salvage after either form of treatment is very low when the tumor is advanced.

Even more uncommon than carcinoma of the vagina are malignant tumors of connective tissue origin. Vaginal sarcomas are of two main histologic types. One occurs chiefly in adults and occupies a typical position in the muscle or submucosal layers of the posterior vaginal wall, elevating and ulcerating the epithelium above it. Because these tumors tend to outgrow their blood supply, a wide area may slough. Growth proceeds by direct extension to involve the entire vagina, but hematogenous spread may also occur, with metastases to the lungs and other distant organs. Microscopically, these sarcomas may be of spindle cell, round cell, or mixed cell types.

A rare form of sarcoma (embryonal rhabdomyosarcoma) is generally found in the vaginas of young girls. Rarely, these tumors may arise from the cervix. Although the cervical form of sarcoma is histologically similar to

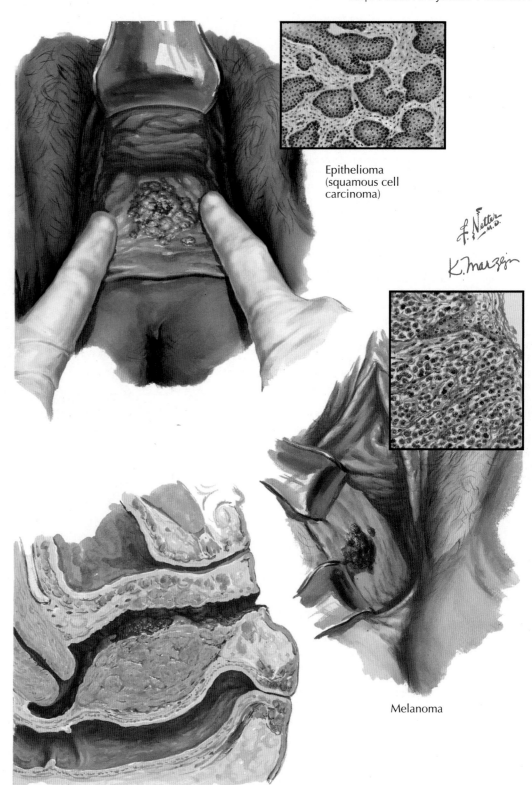

Epithelioma
(squamous cell
carcinoma)

Melanoma

Sarcoma

the vaginal form, the prognosis for the cervical form is better. Grossly, it forms large, grapelike clusters of tissue, which eventually protrude from the vaginal orifice and cause bleeding and foul discharge as a result of superficial necrosis. The tumor is often multicentric, with loose myxomatous stroma containing malignant pleomorphic cells and eosinophilic rhabdomyoblasts that have characteristic cross-striations (strap cells). Treatment is surgical excision combined with multiagent chemotherapy. Adjunctive radiation therapy has also been advocated but is generally reserved for those with residual disease.

Melanoma of the vagina is unusual, but an occasional case is reported. A primary focus elsewhere must be sought, because disease in this area is more often secondary. It does not differ in its gross or microscopic appearance from melanomas elsewhere. The large, anaplastic, pigmented cells are pathognomonic. Melanoma in the vagina is almost uniformly fatal.

Other rare primary malignancies of the vagina have been reported, including teratomas and clear cell carcinomas, the latter associated with maternal use of diethylstilbestrol during pregnancy.

Plate 7.22

Vagina

Cervical carcinoma

Nests composed predominantly
of atypical cytotrophoblasts

MALIGNANT TUMORS:
METASTASES AND EXTENSION

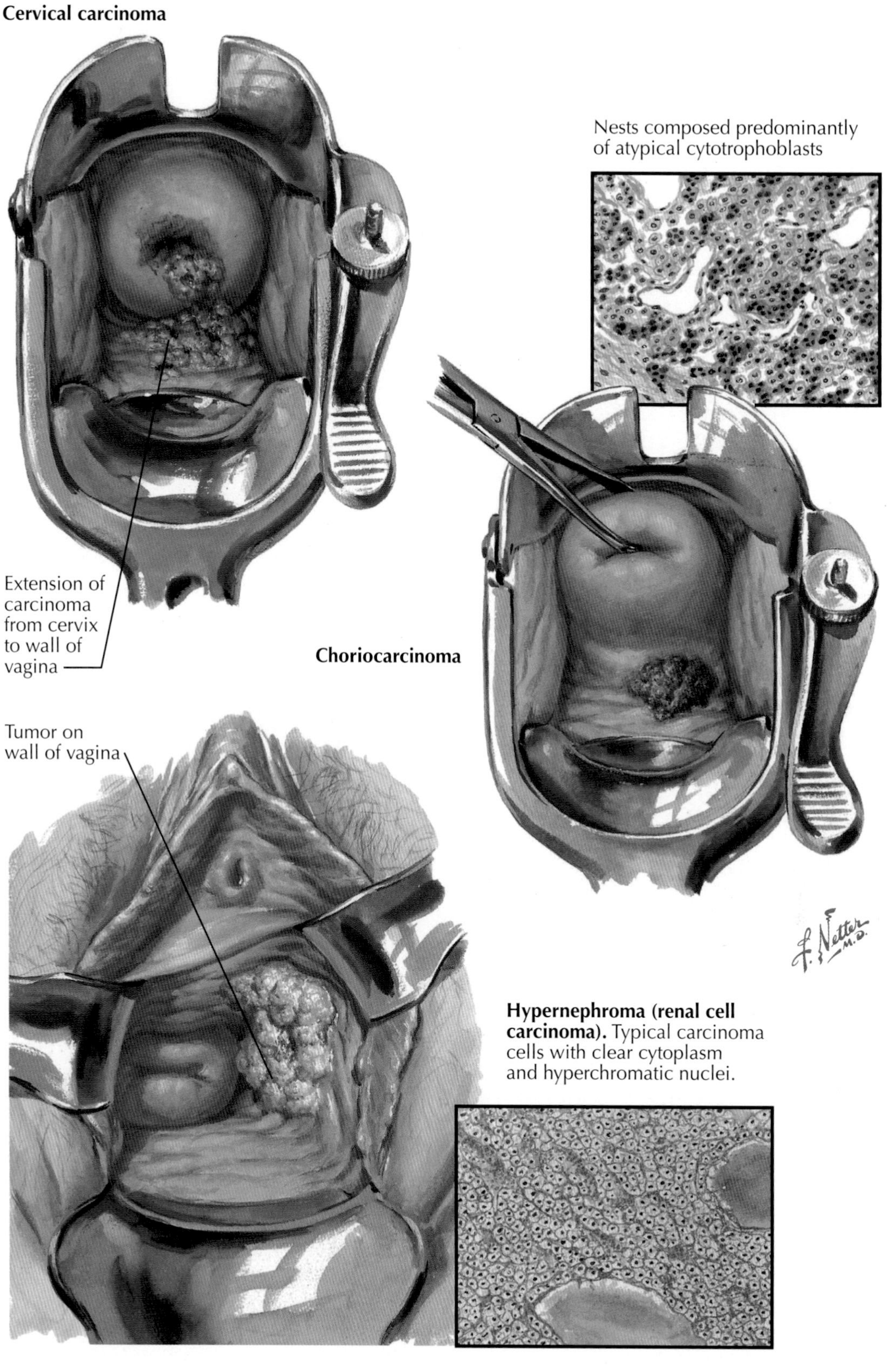

The majority of vaginal malignancies are secondary to tumors arising elsewhere in the body, often arising from the endometrium, cervix, vulva, ovary, breast, rectum, and kidney. The relatively high incidence of secondary lesions is due chiefly to the frequent extension of carcinomas of the cervix to the adjacent vaginal epithelium and supporting structures. This may occur with all grades and in all clinical stages, even including the so-called intraepithelial carcinomas. In the usual case, the earliest extension from a primary site on the cervix would be into one of the fornices and, in the absence of lymphatic or more distant spread, this would be classified as a Stage II carcinoma of the cervix, carrying a much graver prognostic significance than a Stage I. By convention, tumors involving the vagina and cervix are classified as cervical in origin; tumors involving the vulva and vagina are similarly classified as vulvar in origin.

Carcinoma of the endometrium is likely to implant upon the vaginal epithelium adjacent to the cervical canal; after hysterectomy for this disease, the vaginal vault is one of the most common sites of recurrence. Vulvar carcinomas may grow inward to involve a part or the entire vagina, and it is sometimes difficult to distinguish the point of origin.

The vagina is the most frequent site of metastases from uterine chorionepithelioma, and a speculum view of the dark-purple hemorrhagic growth is often the earliest manifestation of the presence of this disease. The tumor is papillary and friable, and bleeds easily on contact. Diagnosis is made by biopsy, which may be associated with considerable hemorrhage. A history of recent pregnancy or abortion is of aid to the pathologist, but the microscopic picture of the lesion is too characteristic to be missed, although some confusion may result from points of similarity with malignant hydatidiform mole. Columns of undifferentiated trophoblastic cells invade the smooth muscle of the vaginal wall. The large hyperchromatic nuclei of these trophoblastic cells are frequently in mitosis. Both Langhans and syncytial layers are present in about equal proportion. In spite of its extreme vascularity, the tumor tends to undergo infection and necrosis in some areas.

Another rare secondary vaginal neoplasm is the hypernephroma, or renal cell carcinoma, which forms a nodular, yellow, tumor mass, firmly fixed and puckering the overlying epithelium. A biopsy of this lesion shows the unmistakable alveolar arrangement of the large, pale-staining cells. A virtually unique vaginal metastatic malignancy is the case of a carcinoma of the thyroid that metastasized to the rectovaginal septum.

Pigmented vaginal lesions may occur, including nevi and melanoma, which account for 9% of vulvar and 5% of vaginal malignant lesions. Many of these may be

Extension of
carcinoma
from cervix
to wall of
vagina

Choriocarcinoma

Tumor on
wall of vagina

Hypernephroma (renal cell carcinoma). Typical carcinoma cells with clear cytoplasm and hyperchromatic nuclei.

metastatic from the vulva or other areas of the lower body. Prognosis and therapy of these lesions is predicated on the site and stage of the originating lesion.

Metastases or extensions from carcinomas of the ovary, bladder, or rectum are found in the vagina either before or after treatment of the primary disease. It would be unlikely that these extensions would provide the first indication of disease, but nearly all secondary vaginal neoplasms cause foul leukorrhea and bleeding

and, if unchecked, may eventually produce urinary or fecal fistulae. Treatment is aimed at the primary malignancy, but irradiation or local excision of the secondary sometimes offers temporary palliation when vaginal findings or symptoms prompt intervention. Overall, the prognosis is generally poor because, by definition, the primary tumor source is already advanced. Specific prognosis is determined by the tumor type, tissue of origin, and stage.

UTERUS AND CERVIX

Plate 8.1

Reproductive System: VOLUME 1

Paramedian (sagittal) dissection

Uterine (fallopian) tube — Ureter — Vesicouterine pouch

Ovary

Ligament of ovary

Round ligament of uterus

Broad ligament (*cut*)

Superior pubic ramus (*cut*)

Body of clitoris

Ischiocavernosus muscle

Labia minora

Rectouterine pouch (of Douglas)

Peritoneum (*cut edge*)

Rectum

Ureter

Pelvic diaphragm (levator ani muscle)

Vagina

External anal sphincter muscle

Labium majus — Urinary bladder

Inferior pubic ramus (*cut*) — Deep transverse perineal muscle (*cut*)

PELVIC VISCERA

The interrelationships between the uterus and the surrounding muscles, nerves, vessels, and organs determine both the pathophysiology of uterine function and dysfunction in addition to the therapeutic modalities available when pathologies exist. The viscera contained within the female pelvis minor include the pelvic colon, urinary bladder and urethra, uterus, uterine tubes, ovaries, and vagina. As with the pictures illustrating the structures of the male pelvis, the topography of the female pelvis is demonstrated in two sections.

The pelvic colon is surrounded by peritoneum and attached by its mesocolon to the medial border of the left psoas muscle and the sacrum, down to the third sacral vertebra. Its greater part lies in a horizontal plane, although it may occupy many positions, including the superior surface and posterior aspect of the uterus. The rectum extends from the third sacral vertebra to just beyond the tip of the coccyx. It is covered by peritoneum in front and at the sides in its upper third and in front only in its middle third; its lower third is devoid of peritoneum. During pregnancy, this close apposition between the uterus and rectosigmoid often contributes to or worsens the effects of constipation.

The ureter enters the true pelvis by crossing in front of the bifurcation of the common iliac artery and descends to the pelvic floor on the lateral pelvic wall. At the level of the ischial spine, it runs forward and medially, beneath the broad ligament, between the uterine and vaginal arteries to the lateral vaginal fornix. At this point it is approximately 2 cm lateral to the cervix, a point of potential injury during hysterectomy. The ureter then ascends in front of the vagina for a short distance to reach the base of the bladder, where it opens into the lateral angle of the trigone by piercing the bladder wall obliquely.

The urinary bladder lies behind the symphysis, in front of the uterus and the vagina. Its base is in direct contact with the anterior vaginal wall. The neck of the bladder lies on the superior surface of the urogenital diaphragm and is continuous with the urethra. The superior surface is covered by peritoneum and is in contact with the body and fundus of the anteflexed uterus. It is this reflection that must be mobilized during the course of cesarean delivery. The space of Retzius lies between the pubis and the bladder and is filled with extraperitoneal adipose tissue.

The topographic relationships of the uterus are observed in the cross sections as depicted on this page. The superior surface of the uterus is convex and generally directed forward. The anterior surface is flat and looks downward and forward, resting on the bladder.

Median (sagittal) section

Suspensory ligament of ovary — Sacral promontory — Vesicouterine pouch

Uterine (fallopian) tube — Ureter — Uterosacral ligament

Ovary

External iliac vessels

Ligament of ovary

Body of uterus

Round ligament of uterus (ligamentum teres)

Fundus of uterus

Urinary bladder

Pubic symphysis

Urethra

Sphincter urethrae

Crus of clitoris

Deep dorsal vein of clitoris

Labium majus

External urethral orifice

Labium minus

Vaginal orifice

Superficial transverse perineal muscle

Rectouterine pouch (of Douglas)

Cervix of uterus

Posterior part of vaginal fornix

Anterior part of vaginal fornix

Rectum

Vagina

Levator ani muscle

Anal canal

External anal sphincter muscle

Anus

Perineal membrane

Deep transverse perineal muscle

f. Netter M.D.
C. Machado M.D.

Its peritoneal covering is reflected at the level of the isthmus to the upper aspect of the bladder, creating the vesicouterine pouch. The posterior surface of the uterus is convex and lies in relation to the pelvic colon and rectum. The peritoneum of the posterior wall covers the body and upper cervix and then extends over the posterior fornix of the vagina to the rectum, to form the rectouterine pouch or cul-de-sac of Douglas. Laterally,

the visceral peritoneum becomes the anterior and posterior leaves of the broad ligament.

The cervix is directed downward and backward to rest against the posterior vaginal wall, entering at roughly a right angle. Only the upper half of its posterior surface is covered by peritoneum. The external os of the cervix lies at about the level of the upper border of the symphysis pubis in the plane of the ischial spine.

Plate 8.2

Uterus and Cervix

PELVIC VISCERA AND SUPPORT FROM ABOVE

Although the muscular hammock of the levator plate provides the caudal (inferior) floor for the pelvic viscera, the organs of the pelvis have their own mechanisms of support. When either or both of these two support systems fail, this failure can result in clinical symptoms. Understanding these supports can not only explain pathologies when present but also the therapeutic strategies that may be applied in their correction.

The term *endopelvic fascia* (actually a *pseudofascia*) refers to the reflections of the superior fascia of the pelvic diaphragm upon the pelvic viscera. At the points where these hollow organs pierce the pelvic floor, tubular fibrous investments are carried upward from the superior fascia as tightly fitting collars, which blend with and may even become inseparable from their outer muscle coat. Thus three tubes of fascia are present, encasing, respectively, the urethra and bladder, the vagina, and the lower uterus and the rectum. These fascial envelopes, with interwoven muscle fibers, are used in the repair of cystoceles anteriorly and rectoceles posteriorly. It is also within this fibrous tube investing the lower uterine segment that the so-called *intrafascial hysterectomy* is performed in an effort to protect the support of the remaining vaginal cuff. The vesical, uterine, and rectal layers of endopelvic fascia are continuous with the superior fascia of the pelvic diaphragm, the obturator fascia, the iliac fascia, and the transversalis fascia.

Uterine support is maintained directly and indirectly by a number of peritoneal, ligamentous, fibrous, and fibromuscular structures. Of these, the most important are the cardinal ligaments and the pelvic diaphragm with its endopelvic fascial extensions. The vesicouterine peritoneal reflection is sometimes referred to as the *anterior ligament of the uterus*, and the rectouterine peritoneal reflection as the *posterior ligament*. These are not true ligaments and they provide only limited additional support. The round ligaments are flattened bands of fibromuscular tissue invested with visceral peritoneum that extend from the angles of the uterus downward, laterally, and forward, through the inguinal canal to terminate in the labia majora.

The sacrouterine (uterosacral) ligaments are true ligaments of musculofascial consistency that run from the upper part of the cervix to the sides of the sacrum. At the uterine end, they merge with the adjacent posterior aspect of the cardinal ligaments and the endopelvic fascial tube. The broad ligaments consist of winglike double folds of peritoneum reflected from the lateral walls of the uterus to the lateral pelvic walls. Their superior margins encase the uterine tube and round ligaments.

They then continue as the infundibulopelvic ligaments as they progress laterally and superiorly. Inferiorly, the ensheathed uterine vessels and cardinal ligaments may be felt. Within the two peritoneal layers are to be found loose areolar tissue and fat, the fallopian tube, the round ligament, the ovarian ligament, the parametrium, the epoöphoron, paroöphoron and Gartner duct, the uterine and ovarian vessels, lymphatics, and nerves.

The cardinal or transverse cervical ligaments (of Mackenrodt) are composed of condensed fibrous tissue and some smooth muscle fibers. They extend from the lateral aspect of the uterine isthmus in tentlike fashion toward the pelvic wall to become inserted, fan-shaped, into the obturator and superior fasciae of the pelvic diaphragm. This triangular septum of heavy fibrous tissue includes the thick connective tissue sheath, which invests the uterine vessels. Medially and inferiorly, the cardinal ligaments merge with the uterovaginal and vesical endopelvic fascial envelopes. Posteriorly, they are integrated with the uterosacral ligaments.

The vesical and rectal endopelvic fasciae maintain bladder and rectum support, respectively.

Superior view with peritoneum intact

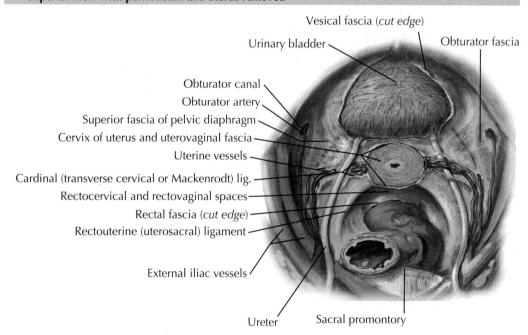

- Vesicouterine pouch
- Median umbilical fold (urachus)
- Urinary bladder
- Paravesical fossa
- Fundus of uterus
- Deep inguinal ring
- Round ligament of uterus
- Body of uterus
- Broad ligament
- Ligament of ovary
- Mesosalpinx
- Ovary
- External iliac vessels
- Sigmoid colon
- Uterine (fallopian) tube
- Suspensory (infundibulopelvic) ligament of ovary contains ovarian vessels.
- Sacral promontory
- Uterosacral ligament
- Ureteric fold
- Median sacral vessels
- Pararectal fossa
- Cervix of uterus
- Abdominal aorta
- Rectouterine pouch (of Douglas)

Superior view with peritoneum and uterus removed

- Vesical fascia (*cut edge*)
- Urinary bladder
- Obturator fascia
- Obturator canal
- Obturator artery
- Superior fascia of pelvic diaphragm
- Cervix of uterus and uterovaginal fascia
- Uterine vessels
- Cardinal (transverse cervical or Mackenrodt) lig.
- Rectocervical and rectovaginal spaces
- Rectal fascia (*cut edge*)
- Rectouterine (uterosacral) ligament
- External iliac vessels
- Ureter
- Sacral promontory

Plate 8.3

Reproductive System: VOLUME 1

Anterior view

Renal artery and vein

Renal artery and vein

Kidney

Ovarian artery and vein

Abdominal aorta

Ureter

Inferior mesenteric artery

Psoas major muscle

Ovarian artery and vein

Common iliac artery

Ureter

Median sacral vessels

Inferior vena cava

Superior rectal artery (cut)

Psoas major muscle

Round ligament of uterus (cut)

Peritoneum (cut edge)

Ovarian artery

Internal iliac artery

Suspensory (infundibulopelvic) ligament of ovary contains ovarian vessels

Anterior division

External iliac artery

Obturator artery and nerve

Umbilical artery (patent part)

Rectum

Middle rectal artery

Ovary

Uterine artery

Vaginal artery

Uterine (fallopian) tube

Round ligament of uterus (cut)

Inferior vesical artery

Round ligament of uterus

Inferior epigastric artery and vein

Uterus

Superior vesical arteries

Medial umbilical fold

Umbilical artery (occluded part)

Medial umbilical ligament

Urinary bladder

Vagina

Median umbilical ligament (urachus)

Blood Supply of Uterus and Pelvic Organs

With the exception of the ovarian, superior hemorrhoidal, and middle sacral arteries, the hypogastric divisions of the common iliac arteries supply the pelvic viscera.

The ovarian arteries arise from the aorta just below the origin of the renal vessels, at the same level at which the internal spermatic artery departs from the aorta in the male. The ovarian arteries course obliquely downward and laterally over the psoas major muscle and the ureter. They enter the true pelvis by crossing the common iliac artery just before its bifurcation. The ovarian artery enters the broad ligament at the junction of its superior and lateral borders. Continuing beneath the fallopian tube, it enters the mesovarium to supply the ovary. In addition to broad anastomoses with the ovarian rami of the uterine arteries, branches extend to the ampullar and isthmic portions of the tube, the ureter, and the round ligament.

The middle (median) sacral artery is embryologically the continuation of the aorta, which, owing to the strong development of the two common iliac arteries, has become a very thin vessel. It passes in the midline downward over the anterior surface of the fourth and fifth lumbar vertebrae, the sacrum and the coccyx, and terminates in the glomus coccygeum, after giving off lumbar, lateral, sacral, and rectal branches, which anastomose with branches of the iliolumbar artery and supply muscular and bony structures of the posterior pelvic wall.

The common iliac arteries are divisions of the abdominal aorta, which bifurcates at the left side of the body of the fourth lumbar vertebra. An important clinical landmark is that the right common iliac artery crosses anterior to the left common iliac vein, which can unilaterally compress the iliac venous system, resulting in relative venous stasis. This venous stasis increases the risk of venous thrombosis in the left iliac venous system, known as *May-Thurner syndrome*. The common iliac arteries diverge and divide into the external iliac and hypogastric (internal iliac) arteries. The ovarian vessels, the ureter, and the sympathetic nerve fibers descending to the superior hypogastric plexus cross the right common iliac artery. The left common iliac artery, in addition, is covered by the sigmoid colon and mesocolon and by the termination of the inferior mesenteric artery.

The external iliac artery is the larger of the two subdivisions of the common iliac. It extends downward along the superior border of the true pelvis to the lower margin of the inguinal ligament. It lies upon the medial border of the psoas major muscle. Midway between the symphysis pubis and the anterior superior iliac spine, it enters the thigh as the femoral artery.

The uterine artery arises from the anterior division of the hypogastric artery close to, or in common with, the middle hemorrhoidal or vaginal artery. It courses slightly forward and medialward on the superior fascia of the levator ani muscle to the lower margin of the broad ligament. The uterine artery, after entering the broad ligament, is surrounded in the parametrium by the uterine veins and a condensed sheath of connective tissue. It arches over the ureter about 2 cm lateral to the cervix. This topographic relationship is of extreme surgical importance. At the level of the isthmus, it gives off a descending cervical branch, which surrounds the cervix and anastomoses with branches of the vaginal artery. The main uterine vessels follow a tortuous course upward along the lateral margin of the uterus, giving off spiral branches to the anterior and posterior surfaces of the uterus. The uterine artery terminates in a tubal branch within the mesosalpinx, and an ovarian ramus, which anastomoses with the ovarian artery in the mesovarium.

Plate 8.4

Uterus and Cervix

LYMPHATIC DRAINAGE: PELVIS

The lymph nodes of the pelvis receive lymphatic drainage from the pelvic organs and the groin. They tend to follow the course of the larger vessels and are named accordingly. The pelvic lymph nodes are shown in the upper picture as they may be visualized in the most frequent surgical approaches, namely, the intraperitoneal and extraperitoneal radical dissection for neoplastic lymph node involvement. More and more, this view is not what is seen surgically because of a growing use of laparoscopic or robotically assisted laparoscopic lymph node dissection. These allow magnification and a dexterity of dissection that makes up for the more restricted overall field of view.

Located in the pelvis, the external iliac nodes are situated about the external iliac vessels superiorly and inferiorly. There are two distinct groups: one situated lateral to the vessels and the other posterior to the psoas muscle. The distal portion of the posterior group is enclosed in the femoral sheath. These nodes receive afferent vessels from the femoral nodes, the external genitalia, the deeper aspects of the abdominal wall, the uterus, and the hypogastric nodes. Some efferent lymphatics extend to the hypogastric nodes, but for the most part they pass upward to the common iliac and periaortic nodes. The majority of lymphatic channels to this group of nodes originate from the vulva, but there are also channels from the cervix and lower portion of the uterus. The external iliac nodes receive secondary drainage from the femoral and internal iliac nodes.

The hypogastric nodes (internal iliac group) lie in close relation to the hypogastric veins. The internal iliac nodes are found in an anatomic triangle whose sides are composed of the external iliac artery, the hypogastric artery, and the pelvic side wall. Included in this clinically important area are nodes with special designation, including the nodes of the femoral ring, the obturator nodes, and the nodes adjacent to the external iliac vessels. This rich collection of nodes receives channels from every internal pelvic organ and the vulva, including the clitoris and urethra.

The number of nodes and their locale are variable; rather constant nodes can be found at the junction of the hypogastric and the external iliac veins, in the obturator foramen close to the obturator vessels and nerve (the obturator node), and at the base of the broad ligament near the cervix, where the ureter runs beneath the uterine artery (ureteral node). The middle sacral nodes (node of the promontory) lie alongside the middle sacral vessels. Lateral sacral nodes may be found in the hollow of the sacrum in relation to the lateral sacral vessels. The hypogastric nodes receive afferents from the external iliac nodes, the uterus, vagina, bladder,

lower rectum, and some vessels from the tubes and ovaries. Efferent lymphatics pass to the common iliac and periaortic nodes.

The common iliac nodes lie upon the mesial and lateral aspects of the common iliac vessels and just below the bifurcation of the aorta. Most of these nodes are found lateral to the vessels. Besides those afferents just mentioned, they also receive primary afferents from the viscera, including the cervix and the upper portion of the vagina. Secondary lymphatic drainage

from the internal iliac, external iliac, superior gluteal, and inferior gluteal nodes flows to the common iliac nodes. Efferent lymphatics extend upward to the periaortic nodes.

The periaortic chain of nodes lies in front of and lateral to the aorta. These drain into the lumbar trunks, which terminate in the cisterna chyli. They receive afferents from the iliac nodes, the abdomen and pelvic organs, the tubes and ovaries, and the deeper layers of the pelvic wall.

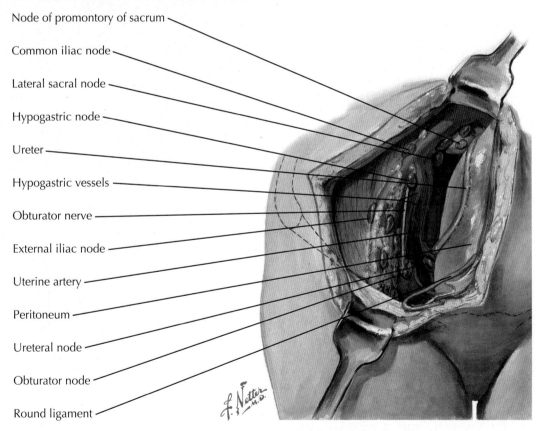

Intraperitoneal pelvic lymph nodes

- Bladder
- Vagina
- Ureteral node
- Uterine artery
- Obturator node
- Ureter
- Uterosacral ligament
- Obturator nerve
- External iliac node
- Hypogastric node
- Infundibulopelvic ligament

Extraperitoneal iliac lymph nodes

- Node of promontory of sacrum
- Common iliac node
- Lateral sacral node
- Hypogastric node
- Ureter
- Hypogastric vessels
- Obturator nerve
- External iliac node
- Uterine artery
- Peritoneum
- Ureteral node
- Obturator node
- Round ligament

Plate 8.5

Reproductive System: VOLUME 1

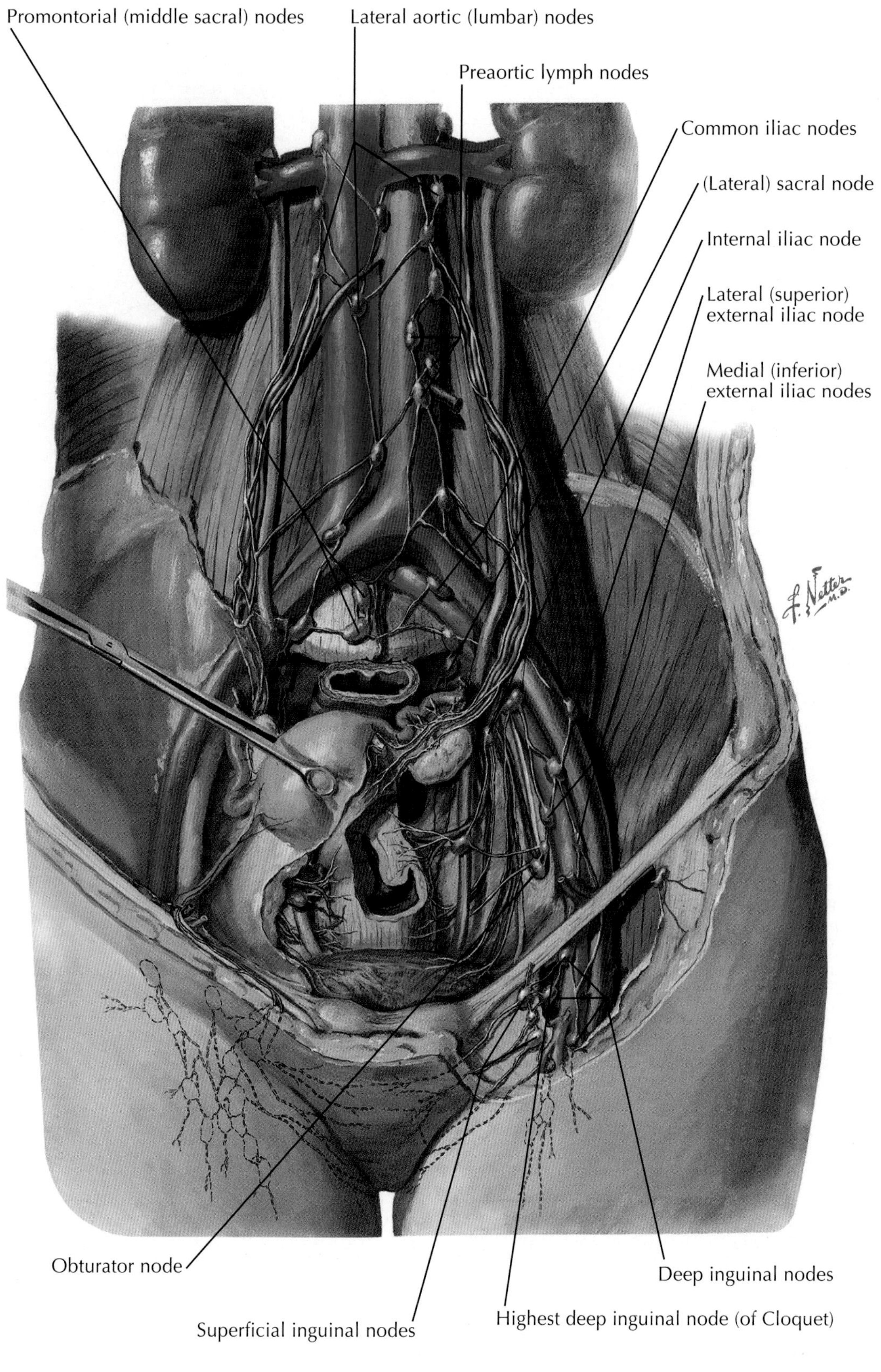

Promontorial (middle sacral) nodes

Lateral aortic (lumbar) nodes

Preaortic lymph nodes

Common iliac nodes

(Lateral) sacral node

Internal iliac node

Lateral (superior) external iliac node

Medial (inferior) external iliac nodes

Obturator node

Superficial inguinal nodes

Deep inguinal nodes

Highest deep inguinal node (of Cloquet)

LYMPHATIC DRAINAGE: INTERNAL GENITALIA

The lymphatics of the uterus are contained within three main networks or plexuses—one at the base of the endometrium, another in the myometrium, and a third subperitoneally. No lymphatics, surprisingly, have been detected in the superficial parts of the endometrium. The principal collecting trunks pass outward at the isthmus along the course of the uterine vessels. Drainage from the uterine body and from the cervix is similar, except that, in the region of the fundus, lymphatics are more likely to pass directly along with the ovarian lymphatics to the periaortic nodes. Occasionally, also, lymphatics may extend along the inguinal ligament to the femoral nodes. The number of lymph nodes in the group of parauterine nodes is small; most frequently there is a single node immediately lateral to each side of the cervix and adjacent to the pelvic course of the ureter. Although anatomists frequently do not comment about the parauterine nodes, the group receives special attention in radical surgical operations to treat uterine or cervical malignancy. Primary drainage to this node originates in the vagina, cervix, and uterus. Secondary drainage from this node is to the internal iliac nodes on the same side of the pelvis.

In lesions of the cervix, lymphatic drainage to the ureteral nodes, the lateral sacral nodes, and the nodes of the promontory may occur early. This drainage path allows for the evaluation of so-called *sentinel nodes* in patients with cervical cancer. The premise of this is that if the sentinel node is free of disease, the chance that the remaining regional lymph nodes are also disease free is more than 95%. This technique identifies the most likely first site of nodal metastases in a regional lymph node basin. Sentinel lymph node biopsy can be performed laparoscopically or as part of an open procedure. Although pelvic lymphadenectomy remains the standard for patients with cervical cancer, the use of sentinel lymph node biopsy for these patients is increasing.

From the uterus as a whole, afferent lymphatics may extend to the ureteral, obturator, hypogastric, external and common iliac, periaortic, lateral and middle sacral, and femoral nodes. Occasionally, intercalated nodes may also be involved between uterus and bladder or rectum. Although the afferent collecting lymphatics in the broad ligament are equipped with valves, the lymphatics of the uterus proper have none.

The ovarian lymphatics pass through the infundibulo-pelvic ligament along with the ovarian vessels to the lateral periaortic lymph nodes. On the left side, primary nodes may be situated between the left ovarian and left renal veins. On the right side, they may be found between

the right renal vein and the inferior vena cava. Shorter lymphatic pathways may also lead to the hypogastric nodes.

The tubal lymphatic drainage is similar to that of the ovaries. In addition, afferents drain to the common iliac nodes and those of the sacral promontory. The sacral nodes are found over the middle of the sacrum in a space bounded laterally by the sacral foramina. These nodes receive lymphatic drainage from both the cervix

and the vagina. Secondary drainage from these nodes runs in a cephalad direction to the subaortic nodes.

The lymphatics of the vagina share the lymphatic pathways of the cervix to the ureteral, hypogastric, obturator, external iliac, lateral sacral, and promontory nodes. Intercalated nodes between the vagina and bladder or vagina and rectum may also be present. The lowermost portion of the vagina, like the vulva, may drain to the femoral nodes.

Plate 8.6

Uterus and Cervix

INNERVATION OF INTERNAL GENITALIA

The pelvic organs are predominantly supplied by the autonomic nervous system. The sympathetic portion of the autonomic nervous system originates in the thoracic and lumbar portions of the spinal cord, and sympathetic ganglia are located adjacent to the central nervous system. In contrast, the parasympathetic portion originates in cranial nerves and the middle three sacral segments of the cord, and the ganglia are located near the visceral organs. Although the fibers of both subdivisions of the autonomic nervous system frequently are intermingled in the same peripheral nerves, their physiologic actions are usually directly antagonistic: sympathetic fibers in the female pelvis produce smooth muscle contraction, including the smooth muscle of the vascular system (vasoconstriction), whereas parasympathetic fibers cause the opposite effect on muscles and vasodilation.

Although autonomic nerve fibers enter the pelvis by several routes, the majority are contained in the superior hypogastric plexus, a caudal extension of the aortic and inferior mesenteric plexuses. From the inferior aspect of the celiac plexus at the level of the superior mesenteric artery, two or three intermesenteric nerves, connected by communicating branches, descend over the antero-lateral surface of the aorta, receiving fibers from the inferior mesenteric and lumbar sympathetic ganglia. At the bifurcation of the aorta, they join to form the superior hypogastric plexus or presacral nerve. The superior hypogastric plexus is found in the retroperitoneal connective tissue. It extends from the fourth lumbar vertebra to the hollow over the sacrum. In its lower portion, the plexus divides to form the two hypogastric nerves that run laterally and inferiorly. These pass downward and laterally near the sacral end of each uterosacral ligament and then forward over the lateral aspect of the rectal ampulla and upper vagina. In this vicinity they are known as the *pelvic plexuses*. These nerves spread out to form the inferior hypogastric plexus in the area just below the bifurcation of the common iliac arteries. A middle hypogastric plexus, overlying and just below the sacral promontory, may sometimes be present.

Each pelvic plexus is composed of interlacing nerve fibers and numerous minute ganglia spread over an area of 2 or 3 cm². They receive branches from the sacral ganglia of the sympathetic trunk and parasympathetic fibers from the second, third, and fourth sacral spinal nerves (nervi erigentes or pelvic nerves). The pelvic plexus of nerves is subdivided into secondary plexuses, which follow the course of the visceral branches of the hypogastric vessels. These include the rectal plexus (to rectum), the uterovaginal plexus (to inner aspect of fallopian tubes, uterus, vagina, and erectile tissue of vestibular bulb), and the vesical plexus (to bladder).

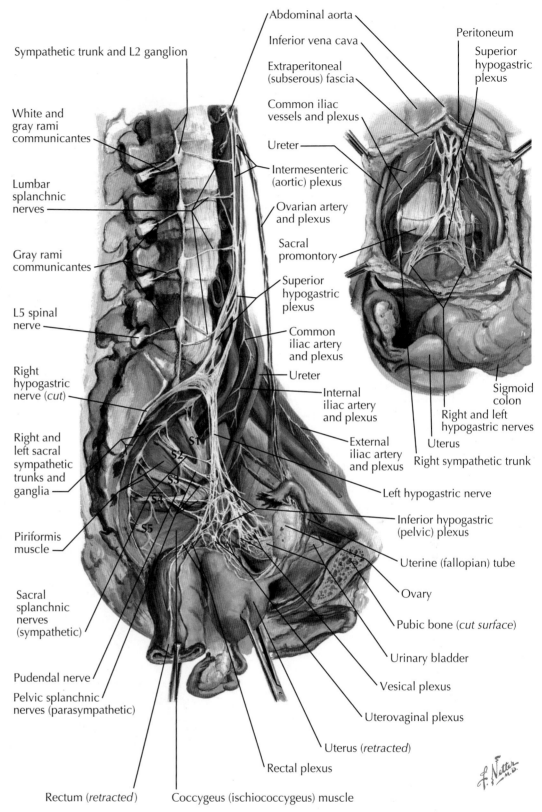

The ovarian plexuses are composed of a meshwork of nerve fibers, which arise from the aortic and renal plexuses and accompany the ovarian vessels to supply the ovaries, the outer aspect of the fallopian tubes, and the broad ligaments.

The anatomic relations of the presacral nerve, or superior hypogastric plexus, are of importance because its resection is sometimes performed for the relief of intractable pelvic pain. Beneath the peritoneum at the level of the bifurcation of the aorta, the superior hypogastric plexus will be found embedded in loose areolar tissue, overlying the middle sacral vessels and the bodies of the fourth and fifth lumbar vertebrae. Usually, a broad, flattened plexus, consisting of two or three incompletely fused trunks, is found. In 20% to 25% of cases, a single nerve is present. Fine nerve strands pass from the lumbar sympathetic ganglia beneath the common iliac vessels to the presacral nerve. The right ureter is visualized as it courses over the iliac vessels at the brim of the pelvis.

Plate 8.7

Reproductive System: VOLUME 1

Posterior view

Suspensory (infundibulopelvic) ligament of ovary

Mesosalpinx

Epoöphoron

Ligament of ovary

Fundus of uterus

Uterine (fallopian) tube

Isthmus   Ampulla   Infundibulum

Vesicular appendix (hydatid of Morgagni)

Fimbriae

Abdominal ostium

Corpus luteum

Ovary

Body of uterus

Mesometrium (broad ligament)

Ureter

Uterosacral ligament

Suspensory ligament of ovary

Ovary

Mesovarium

Ligament of ovary (uteroovarian)

Rectouterine pouch (of Douglas)

Frontal section

UTERUS AND ADNEXA

The uterus is a pear-shaped, thick-walled, hollow, muscular organ situated between the bladder and rectum. The fundus is the dome-shaped portion above the level of entrance of the fallopian tubes. The body, or corpus, lies below this and is separated from the cervix by a slight constriction, termed the isthmus. The cavity of the uterine body is a flattened potential space, triangular in shape. The uterine tubes open into its basal angles. Its apex is continuous with the cervical canal at the internal os. The uterine wall is composed of an outer serosal layer (peritoneum); a firm, thick, intermediate coat of smooth muscle (myometrium); and an inner mucosal lining (endometrium).

The cervix is cylindric, slightly expanded in its middle, and about 2.5 cm in length. Its canal is spindle-shaped and opens into the vagina through the external os. On the anterior and posterior walls, the endocervical mucosa is raised in a series of palmate folds. The cervical wall is more fibrous than that of the corpus. The oblique line of attachment of the vagina to the cervix divides the latter into supra- and infravaginal segments. About one-third of the anterior surface and one-half of the posterior surface of the cervix constitute the vaginal portion.

The peritoneum covers the fundus and corpus uteri on both its anterior and posterior aspects, reflecting at the cervicouterine junction to cover the vesicouterine excavation in front and the rectouterine excavation (cul-de-sac, pouch of Douglas) in back, from where it spreads over the bladder and rectum, respectively. At its lowest part, the peritoneum covers the cardinal ligament, which stretches laterally across the pelvic floor to the lateral pelvic walls.

The peritoneal layers that sheathe the fundus and uterine body unite on both sides of the uterus to form the broad ligament, which separates the vesicouterine and rectouterine pouches. The upper borders of the broad ligaments are folds of the peritoneum coming into existence when the anterior sheath turns to become the posterior sheath. These folds enclose the fallopian tubes. The broad ligaments expand downward from the lower edges of the tubes, assuming the function of a mesentery to the tubes, the mesosalpinx, in which the vessels to and from the tube take their course. In the mesosalpinx are also found the vestigial remnants of the mesonephric ducts.

The extreme lateral parts of the tube—the fimbriated infundibulum and ampulla—are not enclosed by the broad ligament and open into the peritoneal cavity. However, the latter forms in this region a band, the infundibulopelvic ligament, which attaches the posterior surface of this end of the tube to the lateral wall of the

Uterine (fallopian) tube

Fundus of uterus

Tubal ostium

Ampulla

Uterine part   Isthmus

Body of uterus

Infundibulum

Folds of uterine tube

Fimbriae

Isthmus of uterus

Ligament of ovary

Suspensory ligament of ovary (contains ovarian vessels)

Endometrium

Internal os

Myometrium

Vesicular appendix (hydatid of Morgagni)

Epoöphoron

Mesometrium (broad ligament)

Follicle (graafian)

Corpus albicans   } of ovary

Cervix of uterus

Uterine vessels

Corpus luteum

Cardinal (transverse cervical or Mackenrodt) ligament

External os

Vaginal fornix

Vagina

Cervical canal with palmate folds

pelvis. Another peritoneal fold, the suspensory ligament of the ovary, crosses the iliac vessels and runs medially to the free ends of the tubes. It contains the ovarian vessels and provides an attachment of the lateral pole of the ovary. This fold is not to be confused with the ligament of the ovary, a cord within the broad ligament running from the lateral angle of the uterus just below the uterine end of the tube downward to the lower or uterine margin of the ovary. The ovary is not

wrapped by the broad ligament. Only its lateral surface lies upon the parietal pelvic peritoneum, where the external iliac vessels, the obliterated umbilical artery, and the ureter form a shallow depression called the *ovarian fossa*. The anterior border of the ovary is attached to the posterior layer of the broad ligament by a short fold through which the blood vessels pass to reach the hilum of the ovary. For this reason, the fold has been named the mesovarium.

Plate 8.8

Uterus and Cervix

UTERINE DEVELOPMENT AND MUSCULATURE

In response to the ebb and flow of estrogenic secretions, the uterus exhibits two patterns of growth and development—one a lifelong curve from infancy to senility, and the other a transient recurrent increment and recession due to the swings of ovarian activity in each menstrual cycle.

Up to the seventh month of fetal life, the uterus grows in proportion to the rest of somatic development. Thereafter, a disproportionate acceleration in size takes place; this is considered to be a specific response to the high level of estrogens present in the mother as she approaches term.

Within a few days after birth, the infant's uterus shrinks somewhat because of the abrupt withdrawal of maternal hormones, which may even, at times, be sufficient to result in some vaginal spotting or frank bleeding. Thereafter, the size of the uterus remains static until, as a prelude to the menarche, the ovaries start to produce hormones.

Uterine growth is one of the earliest signs of puberty and generally precedes the menarche by 1 or 2 years. In 60% of girls, the uterus reaches adult size by the 15th year. By this time, a difference in proportion of length of the cervix to that of the fundus becomes evident. In the newborn and prepuberal uterus, the ratio of cervical length to that of the corpus is approximately 1:1. However, in the adult this ratio becomes 1:2 or greater. Measuring the distance from the external to the internal cervical os using a uterine probe and then measuring the total length of the uterine canal may confirm the diagnosis of an infantile organ in the adult. Ultrasonography has become a much less invasive way to accomplish the same measurements.

When mature, the uterus is about 8 to 10 cm long. The uterine width at the top measures 7 by 5 cm. It narrows to a diameter of 2 to 3 cm at the cervix.

Repeated pregnancies leave the uterus larger than in the nulliparous female. After the menopause, and its associated loss of hormonal stimulation, shrinking and atrophy progress. The senile uterus, with its thinned-out myometrium, often retrogresses to the size of the preadolescent stage. The ratio of cervical length to overall size often regresses to that found before puberty.

Because the uterus is formed by fusion of the müllerian ducts, its muscular structure is rather complex. The external longitudinal and internal circular fibers in the tubes are confluent with those in the uterus. Indeed, although the deep, spiraling, circular fibers sweep around the uterus in both clockwise and counterclockwise directions, each set is motivated independently by contractions that originate in each of the tubes. It appears that peristaltic waves initiated in the tubal walls act as lateral pacemakers for uterine contractions, which sweep down the fundus to the cervix. During labor, an element of rhythmicity results from a wandering pacemaker system of independent foci of initiator signals and strong interconnections between the cells through cellular gap junctions.

Smooth muscle bundles contained in the supportive ligaments interdigitate with the circular muscle system of the uterus. The importance of this complicated and interlaced system, embracing tubes, uterus, and ligaments, is realized during the menstrual cycle, where smooth muscle contractions are found to be a function of ovarian activity. They occur with greater force and frequency during the preovulatory peak of estrogen production. This coordination of muscular contractions in the three different structures may also serve to orient properly the ovary with the infundibulum of the tube at the time of ovulation. Any pathologic condition interfering with the coordination or strength of contractions from the tubes may be an important cause for uterine dysrhythmia, labor inertia, or dysmenorrhea.

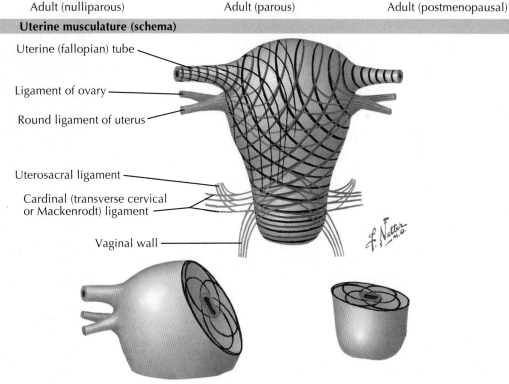

Uterine development

Newborn

4 years

Puberty

Adult (nulliparous)

Adult (parous)

Adult (postmenopausal)

Uterine musculature (schema)

Uterine (fallopian) tube

Ligament of ovary

Round ligament of uterus

Uterosacral ligament

Cardinal (transverse cervical or Mackenrodt) ligament

Vaginal wall

Spiral fibers pass deeply into wall and interlace (schema).

Plate 8.9

Reproductive System: VOLUME 1

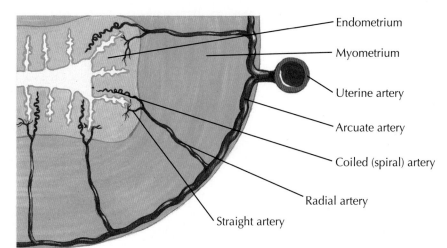

ENDOMETRIAL BLOOD SUPPLY

The arcuate arteries, which arise from the ascending and descending branches of the uterine arteries, circle the uterus just beneath the serosal surface. At intervals, they give off radial branches, which penetrate directly inward through the myometrium. Before entering the endometrium, the terminal branches of the radials divide into two distinct types of arteriole: straight and spiral.

The short, straight arterioles supply only the deepest third of the endometrium, ending in a more or less horizontal arborization of terminal twigs. These arterioles are not affected by cyclic hormonal changes; therefore they maintain a continuous circulation, and the area that they supply (the deepest third of the endometrium) does not take part in the menstrual necrosis and desquamation. The basal layer, thus continuously nourished and left intact during menstruation, provides the glands with remnants from which regrowth of the entire epithelial thickness takes place during the intermenstrual period.

The spiral arterioles, on the other hand, reach to the surface of the endometrium and exhibit marked changes in response to hormonal changes through the normal cycle. Branches are given off to invest glands and to supply the stroma. Arteriovenous and venovenous anastomoses have been demonstrated that develop particularly during the secretory phase of the cycle. In the superficial layer, a diffuse arteriovenous capillary network terminates in venous lakes or sinusoids.

This complicated vascular pattern, unique to the endometrium, was once believed to be the mainspring of the processes that enact the rhythmic necrosis and hemorrhage called *menstruation*. The spiral arterioles undergo extraordinary lengthening during the first or proliferative phase of the cycle. The stromal elements proliferate also, but at a much slower rate. As a result of this difference in growing speed, the spiral arteries are thrown into complex kinks and coils. This coiling would be even more marked were it not for the simultaneous accumulation of interstitial edema fluid that starts with the first preovulatory peak of estrogen production. A second period of fluid retention is found at the height of steroid production by the corpus luteum later during the cycle. This "waterlogging" of the uterine mucosa may reflect the sodium- and chloride-retaining action of progesterone via renal mechanisms, which is an attribute held in common by all steroid hormones. As a result, the spiral arteries are somewhat stretched during the time of greatest luteal activity. In the absence of a fertilized, implanted ovum, the corpus luteum begins to degenerate a few days before the end of the cycle. This then is accompanied by the fall in blood levels of estrogen and progesterone and, consequently, by a resorption of the interstitial fluid. The endometrium shrinks, becomes denser, and forces the spiral arteries to kink and "buckle." A slowed-down circulation, or even stasis, ensues.

From 4 to 24 hours preceding the onset of menstrual bleeding, an intense vasoconstriction and vascular

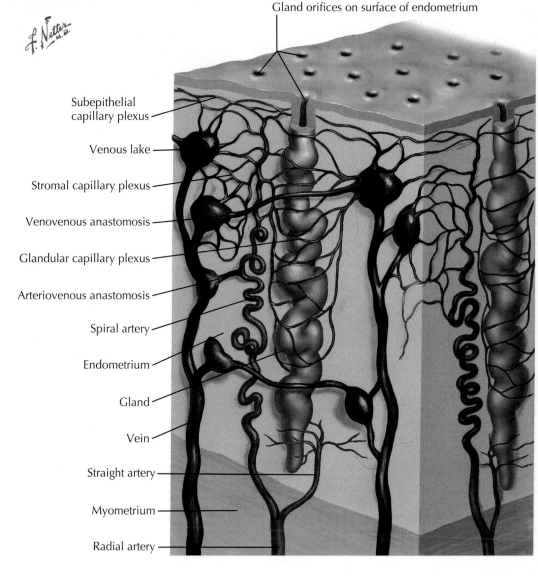

clotting are seen. The vasoconstriction, together with the antecedent buckling, was thought to lead to severe ischemia and therewith necrosis of the superficial parts of the endometrium, progressing to the actual desquamation of menstruation. Based on human perfusion studies, we know that this is not the underlying mechanism of menstruation. Rather, the initiation of menstrual sloughing occurs as a result of direct enzymatic digestion of the superficial tissues, which is hormonally dependent in that progesterone withdrawal induces the expression of matrix metalloproteinases. At the end of this digestive process, coagulation takes over: a platelet plug first occurs with the more organized coagulation cascade following; then vasoconstriction of vessels occurs and reepithelialization of endometrial tissues takes place, generated from the undisturbed basal layers.

Plate 8.10

Uterus and Cervix

ENDOMETRIAL CYCLE

In the early proliferative phase of the menstrual cycle the endometrium is thin and relatively homogeneous. The glands are simple and straight, leading directly from the base to the surface. Under high-power magnification, an occasional mitosis may be seen in the low columnar epithelial cells. A similar picture is found in prepubertal or postmenopausal endometrium, except that the endometrium is even thinner, consisting only of the basalis layer resting on the myometrium, and the glands are wholly inactive, the shrunken nuclei are pyknotic, and no mitoses appear to be present.

The late proliferative stage demonstrates marked growth in glands and stroma, with tortuosity of the glands and corkscrew convolutions. The stroma cells of the superficial layer may be separated by edema, and mitoses are frequently seen. The epithelium is higher and more columnar, and the nuclei are disorderly placed, both centrally and peripherally, at different levels in the cells.

Within 2 or 3 days after ovulation, the early signs of the secretory phase induced by progesterone are clearly visible. The endometrium shrinks slightly in thickness as the edema of the superficialis is lost. In the epithelial glands, the nuclei are now rounded and are arranged more or less in line in the middle of the cell. The cytoplasm of these cells is condensed toward the lumen by the accumulation of glycogen-rich secretions basally, but with hematoxylin and eosin staining this appears as a subnuclear empty space or vacuole. Mitoses are less common and disappear entirely by about day 20 of the cycle.

From day 21 through day 25, the endometrium is in active secretion; edema is now grossly apparent in the midlayer, so that the total thickness of the endometrium reaches a maximum. The glands take on a distinctive jagged or saw-toothed appearance. The round nuclei sink to a basal location, while secretions form vesicles at the luminal margin, which are disgorged into the gland lumen and leave the impression of a frayed and shaggy cellular edge. Arterioles exhibit a major increase in growth and tortuosity. Capillaries are prominent in the superficial layers, and contiguous stromal cells are first noted to become swollen and pale-staining.

Through the last 2 or 3 days (late secretory phase) of the cycle, regressive changes are found to coincide with a decrease and, finally, cessation of function of the corpus luteum. Endometrial intracellular edema is resorbed, causing shrinkage in total thickness of the endometrium. Superficially, the stroma cells accumulate cytoplasm in a dense layer called *predecidua*. The sectioned glands are widely dilated and filled with secretion and cellular debris. The glandular epithelium appears inactive, the cells are low columnar or cuboidal, and the nuclei are often pyknotic. With impending menstruation, an extensive diapedesis of red and white blood cells is seen in the stroma.

The process of menstruation first begins by a pooling of blood cells in intercellular spaces beneath the surface epithelium. Breaks in the surface occur, and pieces of stroma and broken glands are lifted off. Desquamation of the top layers down to the basalis takes place in 2 or 3 days. There are increased numbers of lymphocytes and polymorphonuclear leukocytes; the epithelial cells are characterized by pyknosis and fragmentation.

If conception has occurred, the secretory activity of the endometrium is maintained and increased by the corpus luteum of pregnancy. In a full-thickness specimen the thick, well-developed, true decidua extends well down into the midlayers, which are crowded with "saw-toothed" glands. The functioning cells are large, with basal, round, vesicular nuclei, filled with coarse granules except at the translucent luminal margin, where a distinct cell membrane balloons out into the gland lumen.

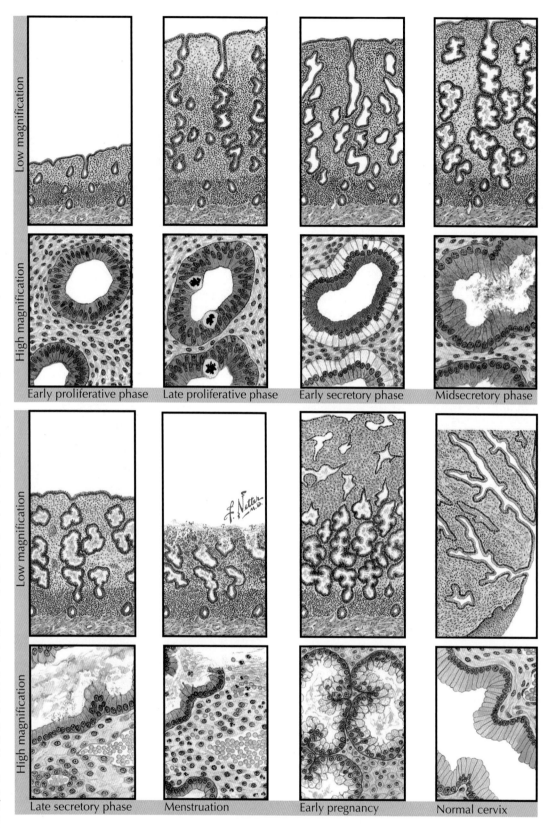

Low magnification | High magnification

Early proliferative phase | Late proliferative phase | Early secretory phase | Midsecretory phase

Low magnification | High magnification

Late secretory phase | Menstruation | Early pregnancy | Normal cervix

Plate 8.11

Reproductive System: VOLUME 1

ABNORMAL UTERINE BLEEDING

The endometrium is the only tissue in the body in which the regular, periodic occurrence of necrosis and desquamation with bleeding is usually a sign of health rather than of disease. A menstrual flow characterized by repeated regularity in timing, amount, and duration of bleeding bears witness to a normal and ordered chain of endocrine events for that individual. Irregularity in any of these characteristics suggests a functional disturbance or organic pathology. The major categories of pathologic states that can cause or be accompanied by either menorrhagia (heavy or prolonged flow, discussed separately) or metrorrhagia (spotting or bleeding between menstrual flows, discussed below) have been allocated to those that are uterine (intracavitary and intramural) and nonuterine (extramural).

In 2011, the International Federation of Gynecology and Obstetrics introduced an overarching classification system for all menstrual disturbances, known by the acronym PALM-COEIN. This classification system provided a unification of older, poorly defined terms and classifies uterine bleeding abnormalities by bleeding pattern: cyclic but heavy, AUB/HMB versus bleeding unrelated to, or independent of, the menstrual cycle, AUB/IMB. The system further classifies bleeding by etiology: structural versus nonstructural. This latter allocation of causes has many homologies to the older primary and secondary classifications, which were based upon clinically identifiable causation.

Despite the utility of this classification system, some limitations should be noted. All of the structural causes of abnormal uterine bleeding under this system affect the uterus and endometrium directly. The system presumes that vaginal, vulva, and rectal causes of perineal blood have been eliminated. Local uterine disorders include malignancy of the corpus or cervix, benign submucous fibroids and polyps, and adenomyosis. Infections such as endometritis or tuberculosis, although uncommon causes of abnormal uterine bleeding, are omitted or lumped into undifferentiated labels. Childbirth lacerations or erosions, only rarely the sole cause for undue bleeding, are similarly left unaddressed.

Local ovarian or adnexal structural disorders may involve primary malignancies, including those cystic or solid ovarian tumors that secrete steroid compounds. Pelvic inflammatory disease and endometriosis may also cause irregular bleeding. Ovarian structural entities such as these are generally allocated to the ovulatory dysfunction (AUB-O) category.

The more obvious members of the AUB-O classification are those processes that result in irregular or absent ovulation. Persistent estrogen without progesterone production, resulting from a continued failure to ovulate, tends to build up a hyperplastic endometrium in which nests of anaplastic glands may develop. Sporadic changes in circulating estrogen, spontaneously or through medication, undermines the support of the endometrium and initiates the changes inevitably followed by necrosis and bleeding. With the loss of ovarian function, the hypoplastic, estrogen-deficient endometrium sometimes breaks down and bleeds from a vulnerability to mild trauma or local infection.

A variety of systemic conditions may be responsible for abnormal bleeding and are lumped under the nonstructural classes. Conditions such as blood dyscrasias, leukemia, and purpura usually show signs of bleeding elsewhere but can cause abnormal uterine bleeding.

Chronic and debilitating disease states, including iron-deficiency anemia and either hypo- or hyperthyroidism, can produce abnormal flow as well as undermine placental function. Defects in steroid metabolism or excretion by the liver or kidneys may produce a buildup in circulating estrogen, with consequent endometrial effects. The PALM-COEIN system does not address these uncommon causes, relegating them to the AUB-N group.

Although not a cause of recurrent abnormal uterine bleeding, complications of pregnancy may present with abrupt heavy bleeding. Pregnancy disorders, due not only to placental dislocations or to deficiencies as illustrated under systemic conditions but also to miscarriage, ectopic gestation, or degenerative conditions such as hydatidiform mole or chorioepithelioma, constitute the most frequent causes of pregnancy-related uterine hemorrhage.

Functional and pathological causes of uterine bleeding

Cancer (or sarcoma) of uterine body
Tuberculosis
Fibroid (submucous)
Endometrial polyps
Adenomyosis
Cancer of cervix or endocervix
Endocervical polyps
Erosion
Trauma
Chancre

Local uterine disorders

Tubal or pelvic inflammation
Cysts
Endometriosis
Tumors – granulosa cell theca cell cancer

Local ovarian or adnexal disorders

Chorioepithelioma
Ectopic pregnancy
Abortion or premature separation of placenta
Placenta previa
Hydatidiform mole

Pregnancy disorders

Psychogenic states
Hypothyroidism, hyperthyroidism
Debilitating states
Defective enzymatic steroid metabolism
Blood dyscrasias

Systemic conditions

PALM-COEIN classification system for menstrual disturbances

Structural	Nonstructural
Polyp (AUB-P)	**C**oagulopathy (AUB-C)
Adenomyosis (AUB-A)	**O**vulatory dysfunction (AUB-O)
Leiomyoma (AUB-L)	**E**ndometrial (AUB-E)
• Submucous myoma (AUB-Lsm)	**I**atrogenic (AUB-I)
• Other myoma (AUB-Lo)	**N**ot yet classified (AUB-N)
Malignancy & hyperplasia (AUB-M)	

Plate 8.12

Uterus and Cervix

MENORRHAGIA

During the reproductive years, menstruation results in the loss of between 30 and 50 mL of blood each cycle. When this volume exceeds 80 mL, it is deemed abnormal. By the way the research description of menorrhagia was defined (population-based), only about 10% to 15% of menstruating females experience blood loss in excess of 80 mL per cycle. This level of blood loss was established as the threshold through the observations that anemia, without other apparent cause, was rarely seen with measured blood losses below 60 to 80 mL per cycle. In the clinical setting, quantifying the amount of menstrual bleeding experienced is very difficult and generally inaccurate. For this reason, most clinicians feel that the patient's complaint of heavy bleeding is all that is required to prompt an evaluation.

Menorrhagia (heavy menstrual flow) has traditionally been divided into primary and secondary: secondary is caused by (secondary to) some clinically identifiable cause; primary is caused by a disturbance of prostaglandin production. Menorrhagia is generally distinguished from acute vaginal bleeding (most often associated with pregnancy and pregnancy complications). Menorrhagia may result from an overproduction or an imbalance in the relative ratios of uterine prostaglandins (prostaglandin E_2, prostaglandin I_2, and thromboxane A_2). Some evidence suggests that patients with primary menorrhagia also have increased fibrinolysis, further enhancing a tendency to bleed.

The PALM-COEIN classification system of abnormal uterine bleeding generally resolves the traditional allocation of cases without clinically obvious causation (primary menorrhagia) into "dysfunctional uterine bleeding" ascribed to "ovulatory dysfunction" (AUB/HMB-O) or "endometrial" (AUB/HMB-E). However, the more physiologic attribution of primary menorrhagia to an endometrial prostaglandin-mediated process that occurs most often in a setting of normal ovulatory function and normal endometrial histology makes this system problematic for discussions of heavy menstrual bleeding.

Some authors classify the causes of secondary menorrhagia as those that are intrauterine (intracavitary), those that are intramural, and those that are systemic (extramural or extrauterine). Intrauterine causes for heavy menses closely match those listed in the PALM-COEIN system and include malignancy, polyps, and pedunculated myomata. Beyond these, endometrial hyperplasia, endomyometritis, and arteriovenous malformations would be lumped into the HMB-M group without further differentiation. Intrauterine contraceptive devices (IUCDs), especially copper-bearing ones, can also cause increased menstrual blood loss and would be classed as HMB-I. Intramural causes would include adenomyosis (HMB-A) and growths, benign or malignant, that distort the uterine cavity. Blood dyscrasias and platelet dysfunctions are examples of the extrauterine causes to be considered.

The evaluation of patients with heavy menstrual bleeding can be quickly accomplished with few, if any, laboratory or imaging studies. The first obligation in any episode of acute, large-volume bleeding is to stabilize the patient and evaluate for the possibility of an underlying pregnancy. When rhythmic heavy bleeding is the concern, the evaluation can be predicated on the age of the patient, the patient's contraceptive needs, and other factors. A careful history will generally suggest the presence of secondary causes. Absent these, a trial of empiric treatment is reasonable. Nonsteroidal antiinflammatory drugs (NSAIDs) have been shown to reduce menstrual loss by 30% to 50% when taken for the duration of menstrual flow. If the patient desires contraception, the use of combined oral contraceptives or a hormone-bearing IUCD may suffice on their own or may be supplemented by NSAIDs. (Levonorgestrel-releasing intrauterine systems have been shown to provide a comparable reduction in menstrual blood loss to that obtained by NSAIDs.) If an adequate clinical response is not evident within 1 to 3 cycles, the diagnosis should be reevaluated. Patients who are at a risk for endometrial hyperplasia or neoplasia or who do not show any response to initial therapy may require endometrial biopsy, hysteroscopy, or diagnostic curettage.

Primary menorrhagia

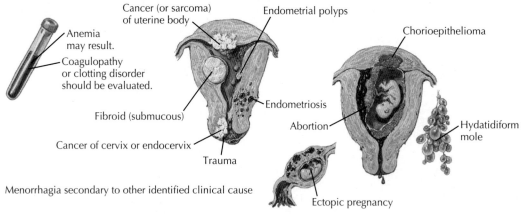

PGE_2 PGI_2
Thromboxane A_2

1° menorrhagia thought to result from imbalance or overproduction of uterine prostaglandins causing bleeding.

Menstrual loss of greater than 80 mL constitutes menorrhagia.

Secondary menorrhagia

Anemia may result.

Coagulopathy or clotting disorder should be evaluated.

Cancer (or sarcoma) of uterine body

Endometrial polyps

Chorioepithelioma

Fibroid (submucous)

Endometriosis

Cancer of cervix or endocervix

Abortion

Hydatidiform mole

Trauma

Ectopic pregnancy

Menorrhagia secondary to other identified clinical cause

Management flowchart for menorrhagia

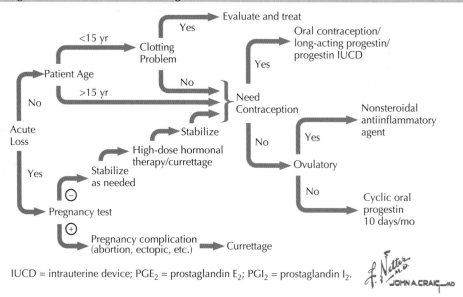

IUCD = intrauterine device; PGE_2 = prostaglandin E_2; PGI_2 = prostaglandin I_2.

Plate 8.13

Reproductive System: VOLUME 1

Dysmenorrhea

Painful menstruation (dysmenorrhea) affects an estimated 90% of females at some point during their reproductive years, with 10% to 15% of all females unable to function because of pain. Dysmenorrhea is generally divided into two broad classifications: primary dysmenorrhea is painful menstruation without a clinically identifiable cause, whereas secondary dysmenorrhea is recurrent menstrual pain resulting from a clinically identifiable cause or abnormality. Because the common causes of secondary dysmenorrhea (such as fibroids, pelvic adhesions, adenomyosis) are more frequent in older patients, the incidence of primary dysmenorrhea is greater in adolescents, whereas secondary dysmenorrhea presents later in reproductive life. (Dysmenorrhea that begins after the age of 25 is most often secondary.) Although dysmenorrhea is uncommon during the first 6 months of menstruation because of anovulation, 40% of females experience it in their first year. The abrupt onset of painful vaginal bleeding should suggest the possibility of a complication of pregnancy (abortion or ectopic pregnancy) rather than dysmenorrhea.

The underlying cause of primary dysmenorrhea is the overproduction of prostaglandin F_{2a} by the endometrium. Prostaglandin F_{2a} is a facilitator, if not originator, of nociceptive pain signals. In addition, it is a strong stimulator of uterine contractions, resulting in resting intrauterine pressures of 60 to 80 mm Hg and peak contractile pressures that sometimes exceed 400 mm Hg. The absence of an abnormality on pelvic examination, combined with historical characteristics, is diagnostic of primary dysmenorrhea.

The possible etiologies of secondary dysmenorrhea, like secondary menorrhagia, may be broadly classified as being intrauterine and extrauterine. Diffuse lower abdominal cramping, back or thigh pain, nausea, diarrhea, and headache may occur with either intrauterine or extrauterine sources of secondary dysmenorrhea, therefore these are not diagnostic. Extrauterine sources are more likely to provide hints of their presence through additional nonmenstrual symptoms. Intrauterine processes are more likely to be associated with other disturbances of menstruation, such as intermenstrual spotting or menorrhagia.

In secondary dysmenorrhea, the definitive treatment of the underlying cause may have to be modified by considerations such as the preservation of fertility. Although analgesics, antispasmodics, and oral contraceptives may have some temporary benefit, only specific therapy aimed at correcting the cause will ultimately be successful. When these are not practical, modification of the period itself (oral contraceptives, long-acting progestins, or gonadotropin-releasing hormone [GnRH] agonists) and analgesics (including continuous low-level topical heat, oral pain medications, and transcutaneous electrical nerve stimulation) should be considered and may be successful.

In primary dysmenorrhea, therapies directed toward the reduction of prostaglandins, or their effects, have proven the most effective. Oral contraceptives act to reduce the substrate available for formation of prostaglandins, whereas NSAIDs act to block the synthesis pathway at two later enzymatic steps (including cyclooxygenases [COX-1 and COX-2]). These drugs are generally well tolerated and need only be taken at the time of menstruation. NSAID therapy is generally so successful at improving, if not removing, symptoms that if no significant benefit is seen, the original diagnosis of primary dysmenorrhea should be reevaluated. Suppression of menstruation (depot medroxyprogesterone acetate, GnRH agonists) may be indicated for patients with severe pain.

Experience with continuous low-level (topical) heat therapy suggests that this modality provides pain relief that is comparable to NSAID therapy without the associated systemic side effects. The development of small, wearable, air-activated devices capable of supplying a low level of topical heat at a constant temperature over a prolonged period of time makes this a viable treatment option for many patients.

Symptoms of dysmenorrhea

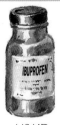

Pallor, perspiration

Collapse

Abdominal pain or cramps

Nausea, vomiting

Diarrhea

Causes of dysmenorrhea

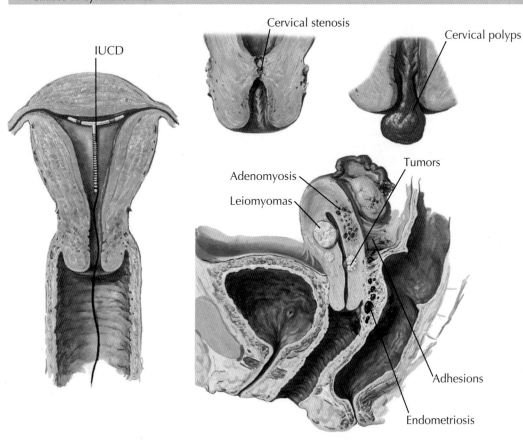

IUCD

Cervical stenosis

Cervical polyps

Adenomyosis

Tumors

Leiomyomas

Adhesions

Endometriosis

Treatment options for primary dysmenorrhea

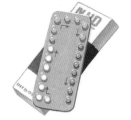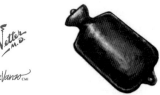

NSAIDs

Oral contraceptives

Heat therapy

Plate 8.14

Uterus and Cervix

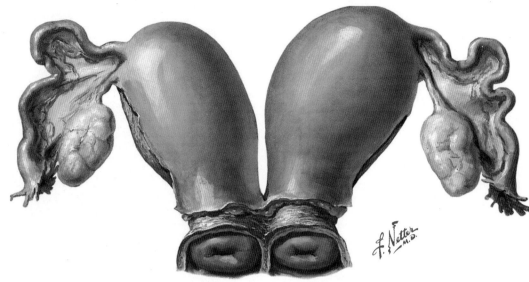

Uterus didelphys (uterus duplex separatus)

CONGENITAL ANOMALIES

The female genital tract develops from paired embryologic structures, the müllerian ducts, which give rise to the tubes and uterus as well as the upper two-thirds of the vagina. The upper or cephalic portion of the müllerian ducts, shortly after having made their appearance during the second month of fetal life, develop and course longitudinally, parallel and lateral to the wolffian (mesonephric) ducts. In the caudal region of the mesonephros, the müllerian ducts approach the midline, taking an oblique route for a short distance while crossing the wolffian ducts, then turn again, assuming a longitudinal direction now medial to the wolffian ducts. In this proximal part, the right and the left müllerian ducts approach each other and finally fuse to form the uterovaginal canal. The cephalic, originally longitudinal, part of the ducts are transformed and differentiate into the fallopian tubes. The short part, in the region where the wolffian duct is crossed in the early stages, gives rise to the uterine fundus and the uterine–tubal junction, whereas the uterine cervix and the vagina take their origin from the lower longitudinal portion of the müllerian ducts. The uterine corpus develops from a very small part of the müllerian ducts, a fact that explains the ratio of cervical length to the length of the entire uterus during fetal life and long after, until the ovarian hormones display their effect on the responsive tissue of the uterine body.

Incomplete fusion of the müllerian ducts will result in a variety of congenital anomalies of the reproductive organs. Anomalies of uterine development are relatively common, with the frequency ranging from about 1:200 to 1:600 females; however, septate or arcuate uterine anomalies may be present in up to 3% of females.

In its most extensive form with complete nonfusion of the müllerian ducts, duplication of the cervix and vaginal canal also may occur. When this occurs, one of the fallopian tubes is attached to the lateral angle of each hemiuterus. This form is called *uterus didelphys* or *uterus duplex separatus*. Each of these two organs may function separately and sustain a normal pregnancy, although there is a higher incidence of miscarriage, preterm labor and delivery, intrauterine growth restriction, and abnormal lie of the fetus. The two resulting halves may be of unequal size or volume.

This complete failure of the müllerian duct to fuse is rare. A more frequent abnormality occurs when there is only partial fusion of the ducts, as is the case in the uterus duplex bicornis or bicornuate uterus. Two uteri result that have in common a medial wall fully equipped with endometrial and myometrial structures. These two uterine bodies may be present with only a single cervix (uterus bicornis unicollis) or two cervices (uterus

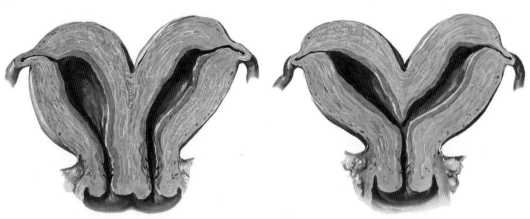

Uterus duplex bicornis (septus)   Uterus bicornis unicollis

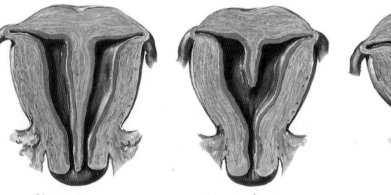

Uterus septus   Uterus subseptus   Uterus unicornis

bicornis bicollis), depending on the level of disrupted fusion.

In some cases, the uterine cavities are separated by a thin septum. When the septum entirely divides the uterine bodies, the organ is called *uterus septus* or *septate uterus*. Uterus subseptus is the term used to describe partial separation.

Occasionally, one müllerian duct may be very rudimentary, or it may even fail to develop at all. The half uterus (uterus unicornis, unicornuate uterus), arising from only one müllerian duct and its single attached tube, may be well formed and may function quite normally.

Uterine aplasia has been described repeatedly. Although in these cases the uterus is absent anatomically, rudimentary segments of the müllerian duct are usually found in varying degree, from a fibromuscular ribbon to minute particles of the former duct. The tubes in such cases may be present and end blindly.

Plate 8.15

Reproductive System: VOLUME 1

DISPLACEMENTS

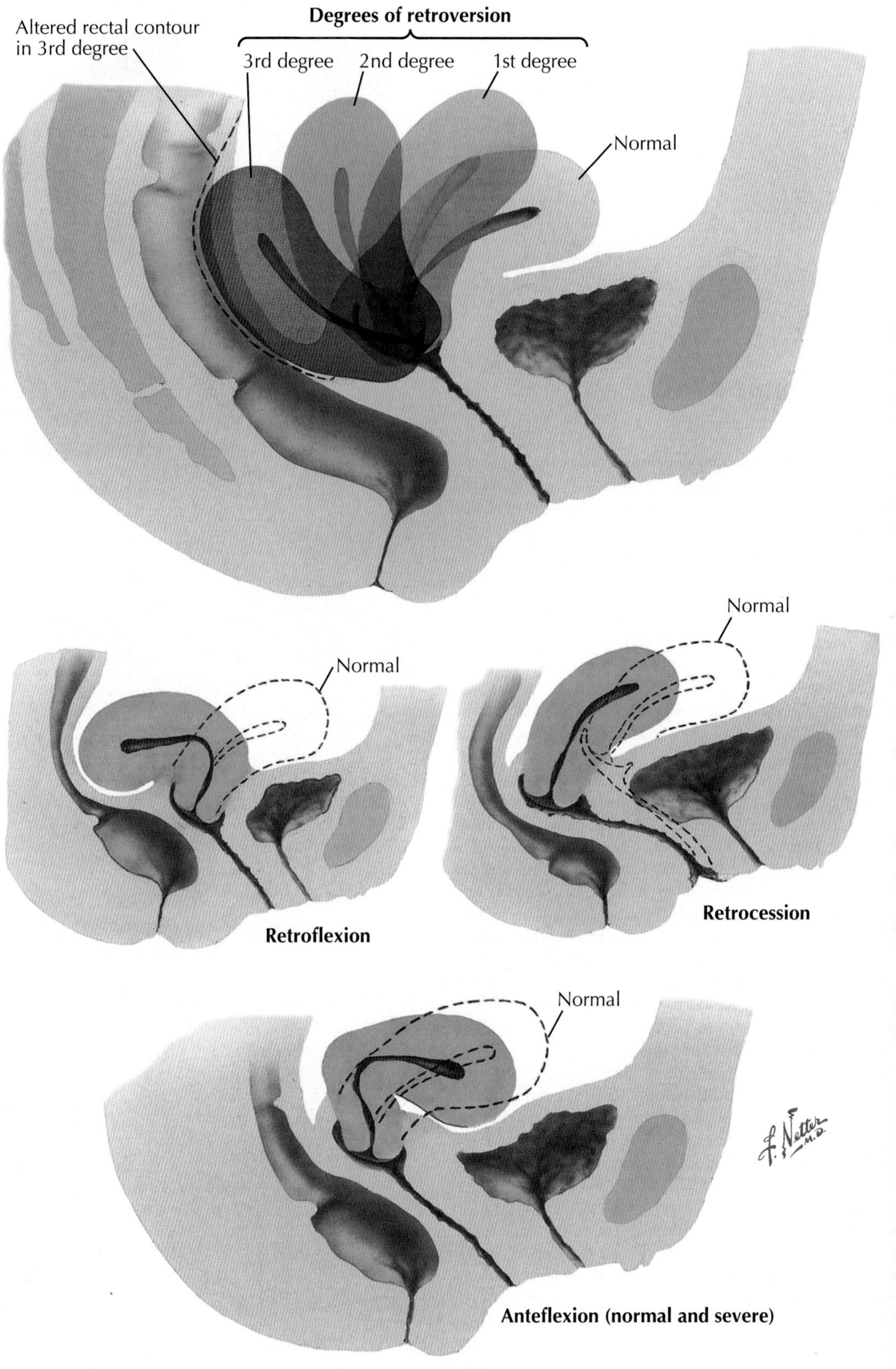

Minor variations in position of the uterus occur constantly with changes in posture, with straining, or with changes in the volume of bladder or rectal content. Only when the uterus becomes fixed or rests habitually in a position beyond the limits of normal variation should a diagnosis of displacement be made. Once thought to represent a pathology in itself, it should be considered pathologic only in those rare instances when such a position results in symptoms.

In the erect position, the cervix bends approximately at right angles to the axis of the vagina. The corpus curves slightly forward, and the uterus thus rests in an almost horizontal position on top of the bladder. It is maintained in this position by intraabdominal pressure exerted by the intestines against the posterior surface of the corpus while standing or sitting; the intrinsic tone of the uterine musculature and the specific fibromuscular bands or ligaments in the pelvis, namely, the round ligaments, the cardinal ligaments, and the uterosacral ligaments; and the fasciae and muscles of the perineum.

Three ligaments suspend the uterus: (1) the round ligaments, (2) the cardinal ligaments, and (3) the uterosacral ligaments, with the cardinal ligaments being the most significant. The round ligaments tend to pull the fundus to its anterior position, provided the cervix is held backward by the uterosacral ligaments. These and the round ligaments contribute to the correct position of the uterus in relation to the vagina, whereas the cardinal ligaments provide the cervix with lateral and axial stability.

Retrodisplacement most frequently occurs after parturition when the stretched ligamentous supports are no longer able to counteract the intraabdominal pressures and when the uterus, during involution, may be lacking in normal myometrial tone. The fundus is thus forced backward toward the sacrum.

Less frequently, retroposition of the uterus results from adhesions caused by endometriosis, tumors, or infections, such as pelvic inflammatory disease, that hold the uterine corpus in a fixed posterior position. Occasionally, in older females, backward displacement results from postmenopausal atrophy and loss of muscular tone of the uterine body and the suspensory structures.

Retroversion signifies a turning backward of the whole uterus without a change in the relationship of the corpus to the cervix. This is in contrast to retroflexion, where the relationship between cervix and uterus is altered. Retroflexion signifies a bending backward of the corpus on the cervix at the level of the internal os. In most cases, the cervix will have lost its normal right-angle relationship with the vaginal apex, and therefore some retroversion will be present as well.

First-degree retroversion includes all deviations from the anterior position in which the cervix-corpus axis points anterior to the axis of the vagina. This is common and of no clinical significance. When the cervix and corpus point directly along the axis of the vagina, the retroversion is designated as second degree or midplane. Any deviations beyond this point

Degrees of retroversion — Altered rectal contour in 3rd degree — 3rd degree — 2nd degree — 1st degree — Normal

Retroflexion — Normal

Retrocession — Normal

Anteflexion (normal and severe) — Normal

are termed third-degree, or true, retroversion. Clinically, the first-degree changes are of little consequence, are often transient, and no doubt occur physiologically. Second-degree displacements are very common, without referable symptoms.

In patients with obesity, this diagnosis often must be made by demonstrating that the endocervix extends straight back, whereas the fundus can be felt neither anteriorly over the symphysis nor posteriorly in the

cul-de-sac of Douglas. In third-degree retroversion, the examining finger comes upon the corpus lying directly back on the anterior surface of the rectum.

The term *retrocession* describes a slumping backward of the cervix and vaginal apex toward the coccyx, with the uterine relationships otherwise normal. It is generally associated with anteflexion, a forward bend of the corpus at the isthmus, which brings the fundus under the symphysis.

Plate 8.16

Uterus and Cervix

PROLAPSE

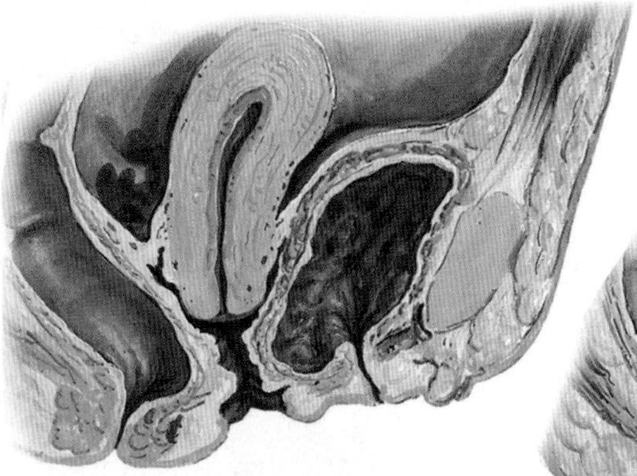

Prolapse is defined as any descent of the uterus down the vaginal canal, so that it lies below the normal position in the pelvis. In the extreme, this may result in the uterus descending beyond the vulva to a position outside the body (procidentia). Some degree of uterine descent is common in parous females.

The etiology and mechanism of a descensus of the uterus are fundamentally the same as those associated with retrodisplacement or the formation of a cystocele, enterocele, or rectocele: loss of normal structural support as a result of trauma (childbirth), surgery, chronic intraabdominal pressure elevation (such as obesity, chronic cough, or heavy lifting), or intrinsic weakness. The most common sites of injury are the cardinal and uterosacral ligaments, and the levator ani muscles that form the pelvic floor, which may relax or rupture. Rarely, increased intraabdominal pressure from a pelvic mass or ascites may weaken pelvic support and result in prolapse. Injury to or neuropathy of the S1 to S4 nerve roots may also result in decreased muscle tone and pelvic relaxation.

Retroversion of at least second degree is almost always concurrently present, as explained by plainly mechanical reasons: intraabdominal pressure forces the uterus directly downward, stretching all three sets of pelvic supporting structures, when the uterus, with the patient upright, is in a vertical or backward position.

Uterine prolapse can be graded by the POP-Q system or by degree of descent, with third degree denoting when the cervix is to, or slightly beyond, the introitus. Descent that does not involve protrusion of the cervix at the introitus is known as *first-degree* or *second-degree prolapse* based upon the distance toward the introitus. When only the cervix reaches the introitus or slightly protrudes, third-degree prolapse is present. If the entire uterus is pushed outside the introitus, a complete procidentia (fourth-degree prolapse in some numbering schemes) exists.

Because of the intimate association of the bladder with the cervix, prolapse of the uterus generally draws down the bladder and produces an accompanying cystocele. The laxity of structures constituting the pelvic floor, not being restricted to the uterovesical relations, leads to complete asthenia of the pelvic outlet, so that rectocele also is a frequent complication of prolapse. Enterocele is always present in procidentia, where the cul-de-sac of Douglas is brought down with the uterus and frequently contains loops of intestine or omental tabs. Because of chafing and irritation of the exteriorized cervix, ulcerations and erosions frequently occur. Surprisingly, cervix carcinoma is an uncommon finding in such irritated areas.

Prolapse may be associated with multiple complaints, ranging from functional bleeding and backache to the more common "heavy" or "bearing-down" feeling in the pelvis, urinary difficulties, and constipation. There may also be new-onset or paradoxical resolution of urinary incontinence. Each of these symptoms must be evaluated in the light of experience and judgment before attempting surgical correction. The patient's age, desire for fertility, and personal preferences should all enter into the equation in deciding upon correct management. It should be kept in mind that retroversion by itself is almost never a decisive factor in clinical complaints, that most backaches are due to reasons other than retrodisplacement, and that incontinence and urinary frequency may disappear following treatment of underlying urinary tract diseases. Surgical or pessary therapy may even make some symptoms (such as urinary incontinence) worse.

With these factors well in mind, the surgeon has a wide variety of procedures at their disposal to suspend the uterus, bladder, and vesicle neck and repair the pelvic diaphragm. Minimal prolapse does not require therapy. For those with more severe prolapse or symptoms, pessary therapy, surgical repair, or hysterectomy (with colporrhaphy) should be considered. Postmenopausal females should receive estrogen and progesterone replacement therapy for at least 30 days before pessary fitting or surgical repair.

Slight descent

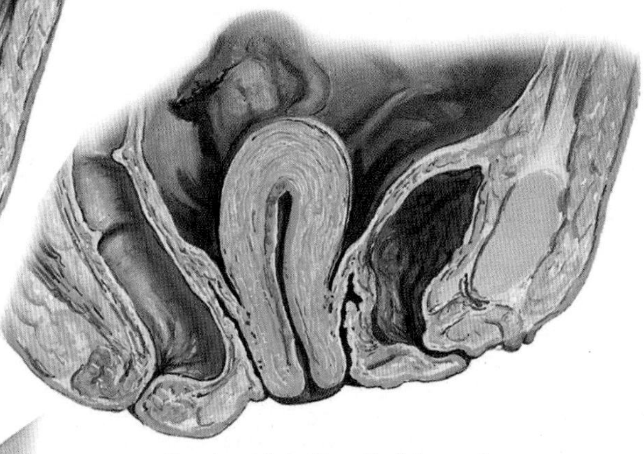

Cervix at introitus (3rd degree)

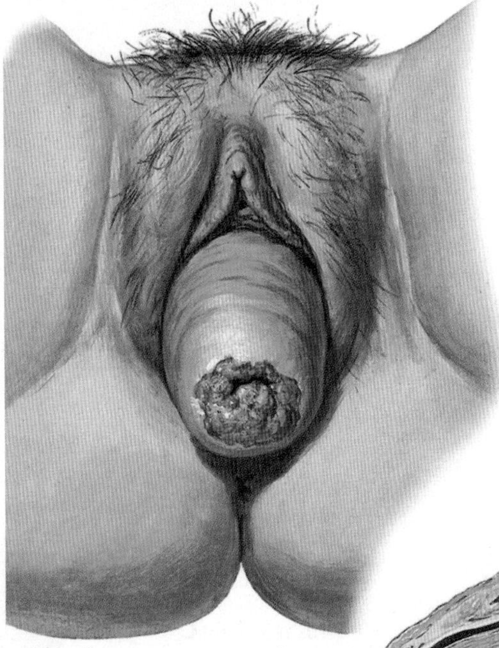

Clinical appearance procidentia

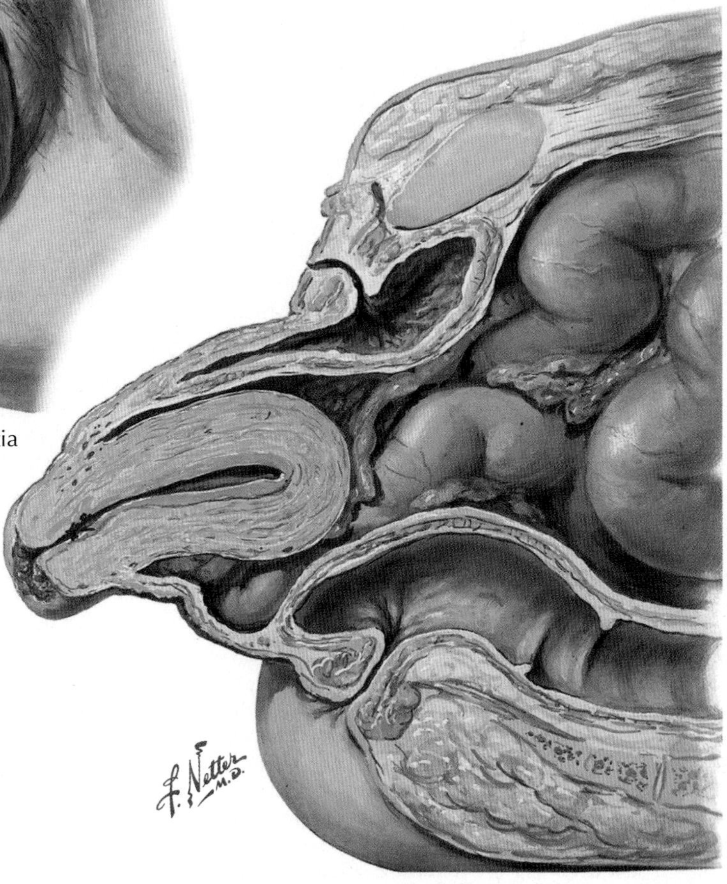

Complete prolapse cross section

Plate 8.17

Reproductive System: VOLUME 1

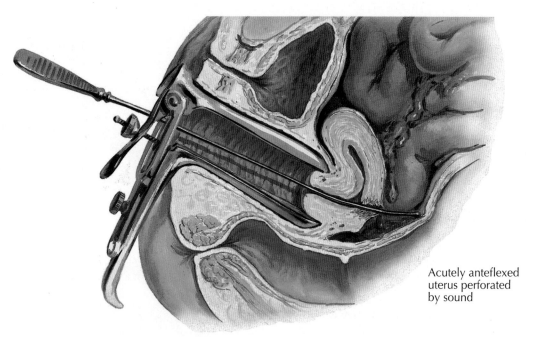

Acutely anteflexed
uterus perforated
by sound

RUPTURE AND PERFORATION

Spontaneous rupture of the uterus almost never occurs except during parturition. Such instances, however, seem to be extremely rare (estimated to be 1 in 15,000 deliveries) and are generally associated with significant uterine distension (polyhydramnios, multiple gestation). Rupture is found in 0.3% of patients with a previous cesarean delivery and up to 5% of patients for whom vaginal birth after cesarean delivery fails. The frequency of a rupture of the uterine scar before labor is, of course, far lower than in labor. These occurrences should be distinguished from uterine scar dehiscence in which there is separation of an old scar that does not penetrate the uterine serosa or result in complications. Rupture may also occur following surgery on the body of the uterus, such as after myomectomy. Surgical scars have also been found to represent a site of diminished resistance in accidents, such as a fall, which occasionally may cause a rupture of the normally well-protected organ. It is notable that traumatic rupture of the bladder is a far more frequent event than that of the uterus.

Surgical rupture of the corpus of the uterus results not infrequently from improper instrumentation of the uterus: passing a uterine sound, performing a dilation and curettage, or during a hysteroscopy. This complication occurs in 0.5% to 2% of procedures. This can easily happen when a dilation and curettage is performed for incomplete abortion when the uterine fundus is softened so it offers little resistance to the probing instrument. Perforation can also happen in the postmenopausal atrophic uterus when a thinned-out myometrium increases the risk almost eightfold. The loss of intrinsic muscle tone after the climacteric allows the corpus to bend sharply forward at the isthmus in acute anteflexion as a result of intraabdominal pressure. Bimanual examination may fail to detect the small fundus lying under the symphysis, and, in the mistaken impression that a second-degree retroversion is responsible for failure to feel the fundus, a straight uterine probe may be introduced. The end of the probe impinges promptly on the back wall of the canal. If this obstruction is wrongly interpreted as being due to stenosis at the internal os, added pressure may produce perforation through the posterior myometrium into the peritoneal cavity. When the uterus is in retroflexion, the anterior cervical wall offers a certain resistance to the dilating instrument, which, when forced, may enter the uterovesical pouch.

Perforation of the uterus at the time of IUCD placement may occur when there is significant anti- or retroflexion of the uterus. The incidence of perforation is reported to be 1 in 1000 insertions.

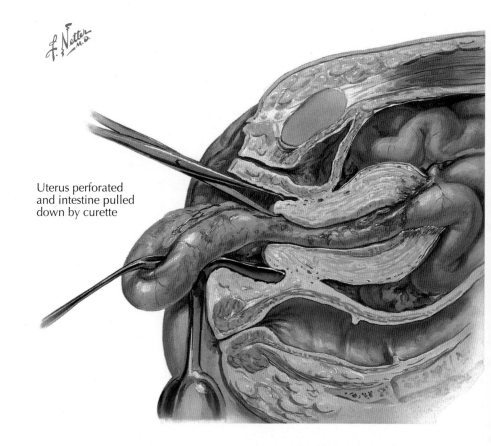

Uterus perforated
and intestine pulled
down by curette

Perforation of the uterine fundus can result from aggressive handling of a curette or excessive force during curettage. Inexperienced operators have occasionally pulled out a loop of intestine through such a rent. If a sound slips up to its hilt with no force applied and no resistance being felt, one must assume that a rupture of the uterus has been produced. When a perforation is suspected it must be confirmed, and any damage may need to be assessed by laparoscopic inspection of the pelvic organs.

The softness of the cervical and uterine tissues must be kept in mind whenever abortion is induced, when the uterine contents must be removed instrumentally as with an incomplete abortion, or when curettage is performed on the recently pregnant uterus (retained products after delivery). To decrease this risk, an experienced surgeon should use the largest curette accommodated by the dilated cervix for the procedure. When in doubt, ultrasonographic guidance can provide additional safety.

Plate 8.18

Uterus and Cervix

LACERATIONS, STRICTURES, AND POLYPS

Parturition rarely fails to leave its mark on the external cervical os. Linear or horizontal lacerations are common, and if no infection occurs, they may heal satisfactorily without specific surgical or postpartum care. More complex lacerations penetrating deeply into the gland-bearing portion of endocervical stroma or extending into the lateral fornix permit eversion of the lining of the endocervical canal. Infection frequently, if not always, results from such severe lacerations unless it is treated promptly and effectively. Lacerations of the cervix may even extend into the lower uterine segment or the parametria. Such lacerations are uncommon in spontaneous deliveries.

Stricture of the internal cervical os is seen after posttraumatic or postinfectious cicatrization as well as in the rare cases of partial or complete congenital atresia. If obstruction at the internal or external os is complete or if a narrowing (stenosis) of the cervical canal is present, the menstrual flow and endometrial debris are dammed up within the uterine cavity, producing hematometra. This type of stenosis is found after the radiation therapy of the cervix or uterine cavity. The presence of a large uterus distended with blood after the menopause should strongly suggest a diagnosis of carcinoma of the uterine body or cervix. During the childbearing ages, of course, the possibility of a pregnant uterus must always be considered before exploring with an instrument an assumed stricture of the cervical canal.

The uterine mucosa may give rise to the formation of polyps. These are fleshy tumors that arise as local overgrowths of endometrial glands and stroma and project beyond the surface of the endometrium. These are most common in the fundus of the uterus but may occur anywhere in the endometrial cavity. They are generally small (a few millimeters) but may enlarge to fill the entire cavity. Endometrial and endocervical polyps have, etiologically and clinically, a quite different significance. The etiology of cervical polyps remains unknown, although inflammation has been implicated. They arise from the mucous membrane of the cervix and histologically contain all the elements (columnar epithelium, fibrous stroma, and glands) of the endocervix. In the early stages, they cause no symptoms and remain undiagnosed, provided they are not detected by chance on the occasion of an examination prompted by other indications. As a rule, they are observed only when they extrude from the external os as soft, red, granular tabs, either single or multiple. Bleeding that is never profuse and often is only a slight staining or spotting induces the patient to seek care. The polyps tend to bleed readily on manipulation, particularly when the extruding parts of the polyp are ulcerated, which is frequently the case. The bleeding, when not caused by manipulation, is frequently in character and extent the same as that which may occur in cancer of the cervix, and it therefore is important not only that the polyps be removed completely at their bases to prevent

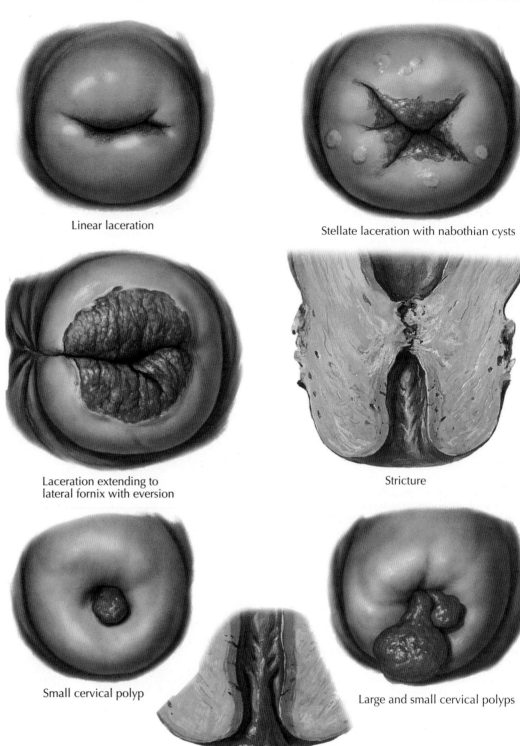

Linear laceration

Stellate laceration with nabothian cysts

Laceration extending to lateral fornix with eversion

Stricture

Small cervical polyp

Large and small cervical polyps

Section showing endocervical origin of a polyp

recurrence but also that a careful histologic examination of the obtained specimen(s) be made by an experienced pathologist.

Cervical polyps may spring also from the vaginal surface of the cervix (not illustrated). These far less frequently encountered polyps are gray rather than red, much firmer, and in some instances reach the size of several centimeters in diameter and pedicle length.

These are often difficult to distinguish from prolapsing fibromas or uterine fibroids (leiomyomata), and superficial condylomata.

Although the polyps are, as a rule, benign tumors, it should be kept in mind that carcinoma originating in a polyp has been infrequently reported. In all cases, one may expect recurrences if the polyps are not wholly removed at the base of their pedicles.

Plate 8.19

Reproductive System: VOLUME 1

CERVICITIS: EROSIONS, EXTERNAL INFECTIONS

Any exposure of the mucous glands in the endocervical canal predisposes the cervix to chronic low-grade infection. The most common causes of such exposure are eversions due to congenital defects or childbirth injuries. Congenital eversions are occasionally found in nullipara and present a concentric area of red, granular-appearing tissue about the external os. Exposure to increased levels of estrogen is thought to be a predisposing risk factor for such eversions.

The coarse, red appearance of this ectopic tissue is not primarily caused by infection but is due to the presence of a fine capillary network, which lies directly under and shines through the single layer of columnar cells. Indeed, one may find clinically very little infection, with neither ulceration nor true erosion at all, although evidence of irritation in the underlying stroma is generally histologically recognizable. In young girls, this anomaly often causes a noticeable thin, watery mucous discharge that may have been noted first even before the menarche. Thereafter, cyclic variations in the estrogen level cause increased activity of the endocervical glands and create a typical fluctuating pattern to the complaint of a nonodorous, colorless discharge. Such a characteristic story may alone be enough to suggest the diagnosis of the congenitally ectopic cervix in young females. Ulcerations or true erosions in such areas may result secondarily because of their vulnerability to saprophytic organisms.

The even, concentric appearance of the congenital lesions just described contrasts sharply with the jagged papillary eversions. These usually result from lacerations during childbirth. The gland-bearing surface of the endocervical canal pouts outward, and infection then may produce true erosions or loss of the overlying epithelial covering.

Spontaneous healing may fail to occur because inward growth of squamous epithelium does not adequately cover such exposed and infected areas. In areas where healing does occur, the epithelium blocks the exit of previously exposed glands, producing retention cysts of various sizes, the so-called *nabothian cysts*. Most healing occurs through squamous metaplasia and presents a smooth, characteristic appearance when the cervix is viewed through the colposcope. This metaplasia is stimulated by exposure to the more acidic environment of the vagina.

Monilial infections of the vulva and vagina almost invariably involve the cervix as well. Patches of white, cheesy discharge are found over the vaginal epithelium and cervix. The endocervical mucosa is fiery red and markedly inflamed. Generally, the infection causes an acute vulvovaginitis with intense itching. Diagnosis is usually possible from the characteristic appearance of the discharge, which is tenacious and difficult to wipe off.

The cervix is also involved in the *Trichomonas* infection of vulva and vagina. Similar to the epithelial changes in the vagina, the external orifice—as a matter of fact, the entire portio vaginalis of the cervix—assumes a

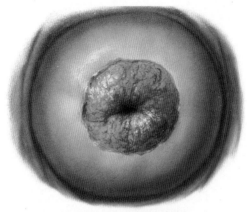

Congenital eversion in nulliparous cervix

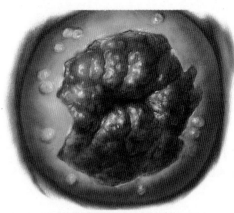

Extensive erosion with proliferation (papillary erosion); also nabothian cysts

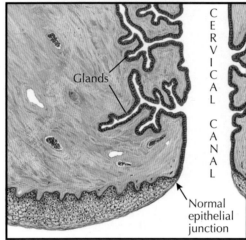

Section through normal portio vaginalis (schematic)

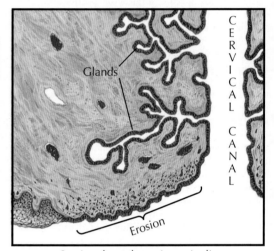

Section through portio vaginalis showing erosion (schematic)

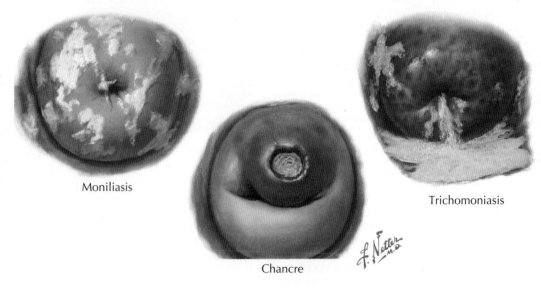

Moniliasis

Chancre

Trichomoniasis

spotted, "strawberry-like" or punctate appearance because of a typical arrangement of red spots on a pale background. This is present in about 15% of cases and, when seen, is considered pathognomonic. The slightly yellowish, creamy, profuse, and foul, sometimes frothy discharge from the orifice, indicating that the process has spread to the endocervical mucosa.

Chancre, the primary syphilitic lesion on the cervix, is relatively rare. It is said to account for not more than 1.5% of all primary lesions of the female genitalia. Chancre of the cervix consists of a sharply delimited ulceration on an indurated base, surrounded by an inflammatory reaction with marked edema. A grayish slough in the center of the ulcer may make difficult a diagnosis by dark-field examination. The lesion can always be correctly diagnosed by a biopsy from the indurated edge of the crater. Any exophytic lesion on the cervix should be biopsied to determine the diagnosis.

Plate 8.20

Uterus and Cervix

Cervicitis: Gonorrhea, Chlamydial Infections

Gonorrhea and chlamydial infections of the cervix are common and can ascend into the upper genital tract with potentially serious sequelae, including chronic pelvic pain, infertility, ectopic pregnancy, and an increased risk of hysterectomy. Infection by the obligate intracellular organism *Chlamydia trachomatis* is the second most common sexually transmitted disease (STD) and most common bacterial STD. More common than *Neisseria gonorrhoeae* by threefold, infections by *C. trachomatis* can be the source of significant complications and infertility. Twenty percent of pregnant patients and 30% of adolescent females who are sexually active experience chlamydial infections. Up to 40% of all females who are sexually active have antibodies, suggesting prior infection. The most common age for chlamydial infections is 15 to 30 years (85%), with a peak age of 15 to 19 years. The Centers for Disease Control and Prevention recommends screening all females who are sexually active and younger than 26 years. *Chlamydia* has a long incubation period (5–14 days, average 10 days) and may persist in the cervix as a carrier state for many years.

Gonorrheal infection is a common cause of clinically acute cervicitis. It is important to realize that this specific infection invades the lower reproductive tract first before ascending to the upper tract and pelvis. Infection by this gram-negative intracellular diplococcus remains common, with a rate of infection that is roughly 3 per 1000 females who are sexually active and as many as 7% of pregnant patients.

Acute infection of the deeply branching cervical and endocervical glands causes an outpouring of thick, tenacious, yellowish, mucopurulent discharge from a fiery red external os (leukorrhea). Skene glands near the urethral meatus are also commonly involved at this time, producing burning, frequency, and nocturia, whereas acute bartholinitis may be responsible for inflammation and edema of the vulva. These symptoms may appear singly or in any combination. Not infrequently, however, they are so mild as to pass unrecognized as danger signals—at the very time that treatment offers the most favorable prognosis.

Ascending, the organisms reach the tubes, which become swollen, inflamed, and tortuous. The endosalpinx is particularly vulnerable to specific infection, and pus drips from the edematous fimbriae into the posterior cul-de-sac, causing pelvic peritonitis. Lymphatic involvement in the mesosalpinx may be the forerunner of bacteremia or septicemia.

Although endometritis commonly coexists with salpingitis, endometritis is a distinct clinical syndrome. Chronic endometritis (not illustrated) is quite common. It accompanies all chronic adnexal infections, although its clinical significance is minor, particularly in view of the more significant symptoms and implications of tubal disease. Lower genital tract infections with *C. trachomatis*, *N. gonorrhoeae*, bacterial vaginosis, and *Trichomonas vaginalis* all increase the risk of histologically diagnosed endometritis. The ultimate diagnosis of endometritis is based on endometrial biopsy. The presence of plasma cells in the endometrial stroma combined with neutrophils in the superficial endometrial epithelium forms the histopathologic criteria for endometritis. In severe cases, diffuse lymphocytes and plasma cells in the endometrial stroma or stromal necrosis may be present.

The classic example of acute endometritis is the puerperal infection after delivery or infection after abortion.

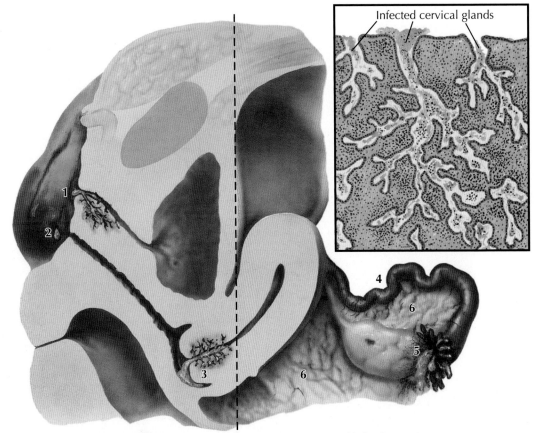

Infected cervical glands

Primary sites of infection
1. Urethra and Skene glands
2. Bartholin glands
3. Cervix and cervical glands

Subsequent sites of infection
4. Fallopian tubes (salpingitis)
5. Emergence from tubal ostium (tuboovarian abscess and peritonitis)
6. Lymphatic spread to broad ligaments and surrounding tissues (frozen pelvis)

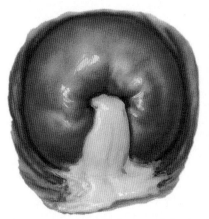

Appearance of cervix in acute infection

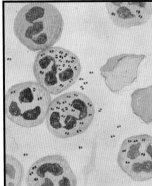

Gonorrheal infection (Gram stain)

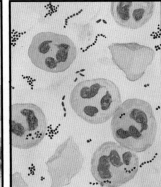

Nonspecific infection (Gram stain)

Mechanical irritation from pessaries and chemical irritation from caustic solutions and lesions after curettage may be followed by cervical or uterine infections. When pathogenic bacteria invade the myometrium, the uterus in acute endometritis or metritis is enlarged and very tender. The patients feel ill and complain of nausea and abdominal pains, and a thin, sanguineous, sometimes purulent, secretion appears at the external cervical os. Because many of the symptoms and signs associated with endometritis are subtle and nonspecific, a high degree of suspicion and a low threshold for performing an endometrial biopsy are required to establish the diagnosis. Treatment for endometritis is the same as that for outpatient salpingitis.

Because of the common coexistence of upper tract disease, the sequelae of endometritis distinct from salpingitis are difficult to determine.

Plate 8.21

Reproductive System: VOLUME 1

CERVICAL CELL PATHOLOGY IN SQUAMOUS TISSUE
•
Grades and cell types

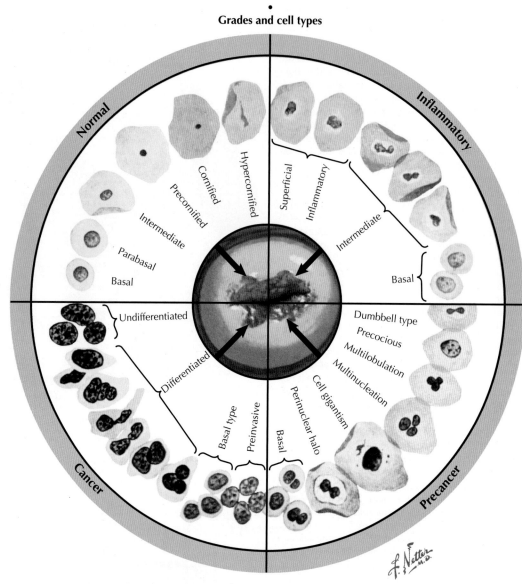

CANCER OF CERVIX: CYTOLOGY

In its early stages, cancer of the cervix is a curable disease. Essentially a slow-growing neoplasm, it is confined to the surface epithelium as a noninvasive growth for a period of several years. These in situ lesions are impossible to diagnose by gross examination. The Papanicolaou (Pap) smear dramatically changed both the diagnosis and treatment of cervical cancer. Enhanced understanding of the role of human papillomavirus (HPV) in cervical cancer is adding tools to the assessment of a female's risk of cervical cancer, but cervical cytology remains the mainstay of screening.

By a scraping technique, one obtains tissue from the external os, where the stratified squamous epithelium passes over into the columnar epithelium of the cervix. Because the squamocolumnar junction is, in the majority of cases, the original site of cervical cancer, an early diagnosis and a differentiation from inflammatory processes are possible. Only the most essential characteristics of normal and pathologic cells can be mentioned here.

For diagnostic purposes, the cells of the squamous epithelium have been classified according to the zones from which they derive—deep, middle, and superficial. The basal and the slightly larger parabasal cells of the deep layer are rather uniform in size, with fairly sharp nuclei. The intermediate and precornified cells of the

middle layer are larger than the deeper cells, with smaller nuclei, which stain less. The cornified cells of the superficial layer possess the characteristic staining qualities of cornification. The nuclei are small, often scarcely recognizable. These epithelial cells show some variable changes during inflammatory processes and are admittedly, in many instances, difficult to recognize as characteristic of inflammation. They cannot always be correlated with the clinical picture, and they return spontaneously to the cytologic characteristics of normal cells. Essentially, as seen in the diagrammatic drawing, the nuclei of the inflammatory cell type are larger and more irregular; the cytoplasm is more acidophilic, creating the impression of precornification and cornification, although evidence is available that this is not a true cornification ("pseudocornification"). The number of exfoliating cells is increased, as is also indicated by the schematic presentation. This results in the presence of more basal or immature cells.

The very earliest abnormalities associated with precancerous changes are nonspecific. The Bethesda ASC diagnosis has been developed to describe squamous cell changes that are more severe than reactive changes, but not as marked as those found in squamous intraepithelial lesions (squamous intraepithelial lesions [SIL], high and

low grade). The ASC designation has been subdivided into "atypical squamous cells—undetermined significance" (ASC-US) and "atypical squamous cells—cannot exclude HSIL" (ASC-H). The latter include those cytologic changes suggestive of high-grade squamous intraepithelial lesions (HSILs) but are insufficient for a definitive diagnosis. The category of "atypical glandular cells," by contrast, includes a range of findings from benign reactive changes in endocervical or endometrial cells to adenocarcinoma. The chief characteristics of the cells of all layers are the multilobulated, hyperchromatic nuclei and the greater number of cornified cells with distinct nucleus or nuclei as well as the appearance of giant cells.

The cellular changes in cancer of the cervix, whether it is clinically an early or a progressed growth, are in general the same as in carcinoma of all other organs. The lack of differentiation, the departure from the normal cell type to a more primitive (embryologic) type (anaplasia), the failure to cornify, the hyperchromatism, and the irregularity of the nucleus and its enlargement with relation to the size of the cell are demonstrated in the schematic drawing. The lack of cornified cells is also characteristic, but this does not mean that from the scrapings of normal tissue parts one might not obtain cornified elements.

Plate 8.22

Uterus and Cervix

CANCER OF CERVIX: VARIOUS STAGES AND TYPES

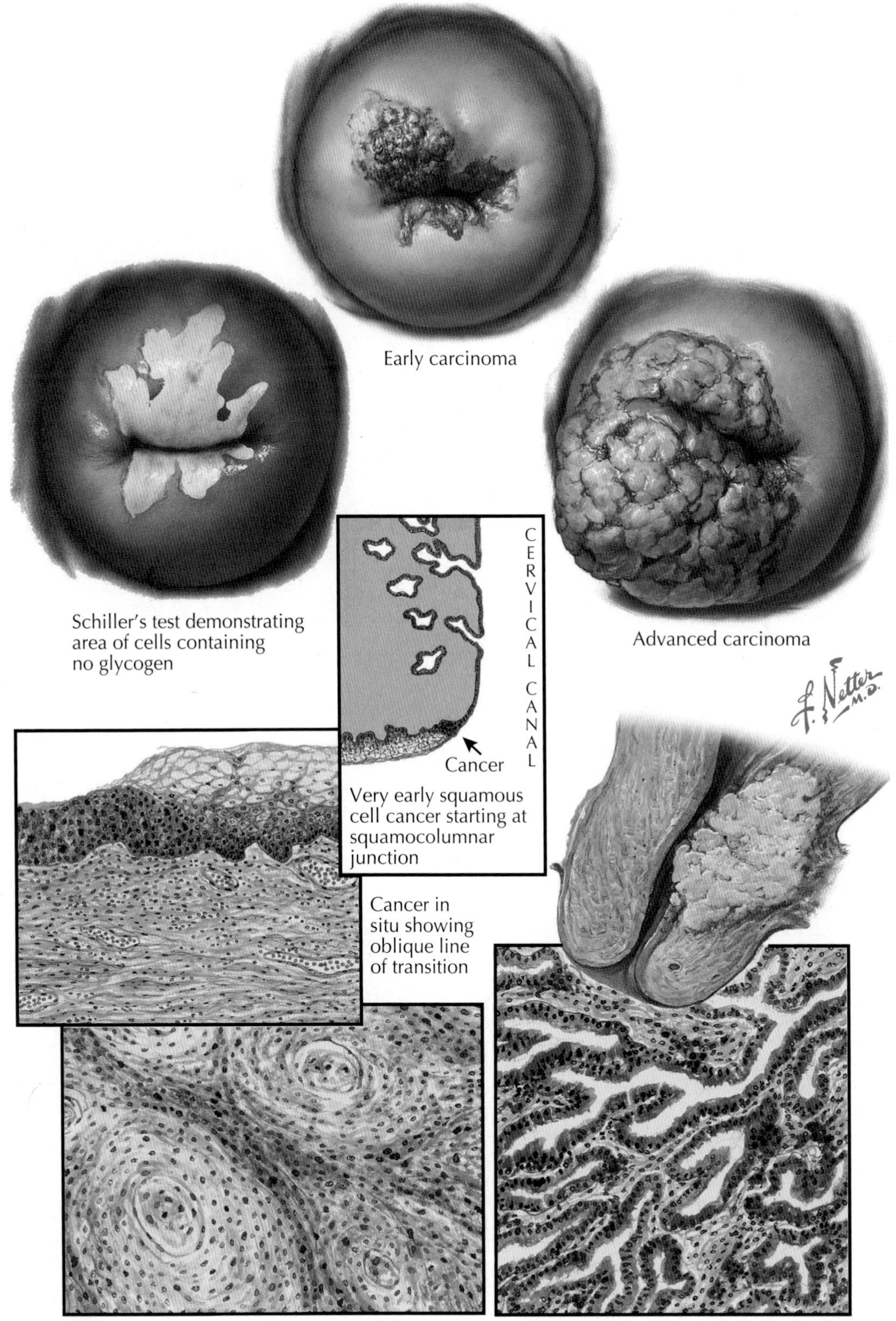

Almost all cancers of the cervix are carcinomas—85% to 90% are squamous carcinoma, and 10% to 15% adenocarcinoma. The average age of patients with cervical carcinoma is 40 to 60 years, with a median of 52 years. Squamous cervical cancer is strongly linked to some serotypes of HPV (99.7% of all cancers have oncogenic HPV DNA detectable) and, like HPV itself, is associated with early sexual activity and multiple partners. Therapy is based on stage of disease. Radical surgery is used for selected patients with stage I and stage II disease. Radiation therapy (brachytherapy, teletherapy) is used for stage IB and IIA disease or greater. Postoperative radiation therapy reduces the risk of recurrence by almost 50%. Chemotherapy does not produce long-term cures, but response rates of up to 50% have been obtained with multiagent combinations (cisplatin, doxorubicin, and etoposide; other combinations have also been successful).

In situ cancer shows histologically a complete lack of stratification through the whole epithelial thickness. It is a morphologic alteration of the cervical epithelium in which the full thickness of the epithelium is replaced with dysplastic cells (CIN III). Whereas the entire thickness of the epithelium is replaced with abnormal (dysplastic) cells, there is no invasion of the underlying stroma. This change is generally associated either spatially or temporally with invasive carcinoma. Although the basal layer is found intact, considerable leukocytic infiltration will be observed in the subjacent stroma, and a sharp, oblique dividing line between normal and abnormal cellular architecture has often been noted. These pathologic findings do not inevitably progress to invasive malignancy because untreated disease progresses to invasive carcinoma over the course of 12 to 86 months in only 15% to 40% of patients. Management of early disease is by cervical conization and endocervical curettage to confirm the absence of invasion or a more extensive lesion. In those wishing to preserve fertility, this may be curative; in others, standard hysterectomy may be considered. Ablative therapy can only be considered when the entire lesion is visible and invasion has been ruled out.

Early invasive carcinoma can also be indistinguishable at pelvic examination from benign granulations associated with lacerations or erosions of the cervix. Squamous carcinoma grows in the cervix, as elsewhere, in sheets of cells that may include the formation of epithelial pearls characteristic of the lesion. When advanced malignancy takes the form of a cauliflower growth, often covered with a dirty slough that breaks away with quick hemorrhage at the trauma of examination, the diagnosis of cancer is almost assured. It is in these advanced lesions, however, that cytologic tests may reveal only blood cells and necrotic epithelial elements. Some growths may reach a late stage of stromal invasion by submucous extension and yet be associated with only a minimal

Early carcinoma

Schiller's test demonstrating area of cells containing no glycogen

CERVICAL CANAL

Cancer

Very early squamous cell cancer starting at squamocolumnar junction

Cancer in situ showing oblique line of transition

Advanced carcinoma

Squamous cell cancer showing pearl formation

Adenocarcinoma (endocervical)

amount of surface involvement. This is especially true of lesions arising within the endocervical canal. Whenever clinical doubt exists, biopsy is the only definitive way of establishing the diagnosis.

The risk of nodal involvement in squamous cervical carcinoma is based on stage of disease, with only 15% pelvic node involvement in stage I disease, rising to 47% in stage III. Survival is similarly based on stage with 99% 5-year survival for stage IA and declining to

only 2% for stage IVB. One-third of patients develop recurrences, half within 3 years after primary therapy, with the best prognosis for later recurrences. Short-term serious complications will occur in 1% to 5% of surgical cases.

Adenocarcinoma of the cervix arises from the endocervical glands and exhibits under the microscope the typical pattern of a well-differentiated malignancy of epithelial glands.

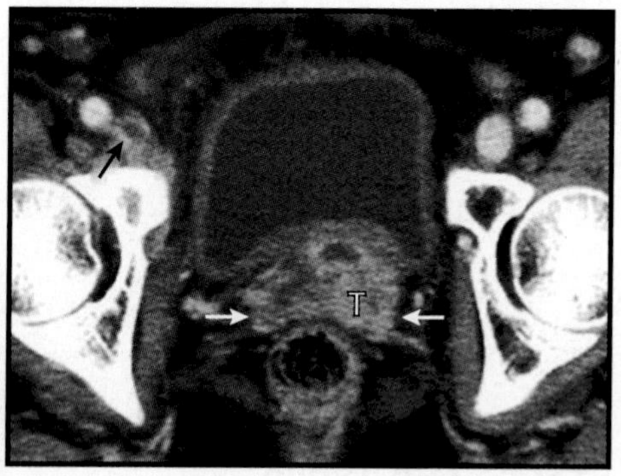

Plate 8.23

Reproductive System: VOLUME 1

CANCER OF CERVIX: EXTENSION AND METASTASES

Carcinoma of the cervix is initially a locally infiltrating cancer that spreads from the cervix to the vagina and paracervical and parametrial areas following a well-defined pattern of extension: spread of the disease occurs primarily either through local lymphatic channels or by direct invasion of adjacent organs.

First involved are the lymphatics in the broad ligaments followed by nodes deep in the pelvis. Rarely the inguinal nodes are involved; however, if the lower third of the vagina is involved, then the median inguinal nodes should be considered a primary node. From the original site, the malignancy may invade and spread directly through the whole thickness of the cervix, the upper vagina, the posterior wall of the bladder, or the anterior wall of the rectum. Death results more frequently from the uremic complications of extensive disease resulting in ureteral obstruction, either locally or in the node-bearing areas described above, than from late metastases to the liver, lungs, and bones.

Cervical cancer is characterized in two ways: histologically, according to the degree of differentiation from Grade I to Grade IV denoting increasingly more malignant and more rapidly growing cell types and, clinically, according to stages that indicate the demonstrable preoperative extension of the growth. From the prognostic point of view, the histologic grading bears little statistical relationship to 5-year survival rates after adequate therapy. Prompt institution of treatment early in the disease is the key to a good prognosis, and for this reason the clinical staging at time of first examination has a direct bearing on chances of survival. The staging of cervical cancer is as follows: stage I is tumor confined to the cervix; stage IA is microinvasion (preclinical), and stage IB is all other cases confined to the cervix; in stage IIA the tumor spreads to the upper two-thirds of the vagina, and stage IIB is where the tumor spreads to paracervical tissue but not to the pelvic walls; stage IIIA denotes tumor spread to the lower third of the vagina, and in stage IIIB the tumor has spread to the pelvic wall or obstruction of either ureter by tumor; in stage IV, tumor spread is to the mucosa of the bladder or rectum or outside the pelvis.

Evaluation of these patients should include a chest radiograph, intravenous pyelogram, and computed tomographic or magnetic resonance imaging (MRI) scans to assess extent of disease and to assist in staging. (As experience grows, MRI is displacing other imaging modalities because of its ability to assess lymph nodes [72%–93% accuracy] and possible tumor spread.) Colposcopy and cervical biopsy (conization preferred) and biopsy of vaginal or paracervical tissues may be

Axial CT image shows a cervical cancer (T) which is contiguous with the adjacent parametrial fat, indicating parametrial invasion (*white arrows*). Note the presence of a filling defect within the right external femoral vein suggesting deep venous thrombosis (*black arrow*). *(From Adam A, Dixon A, Grainger R, Allison D. Grainger and Allison's Diagnostic Radiology: 2 Volume Set, 5th ed. Churchill Livingstone, 2007.)*

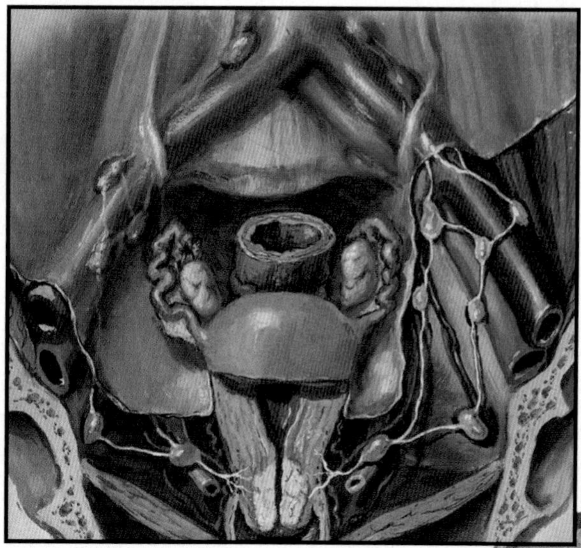

Routes of lymphatic extension

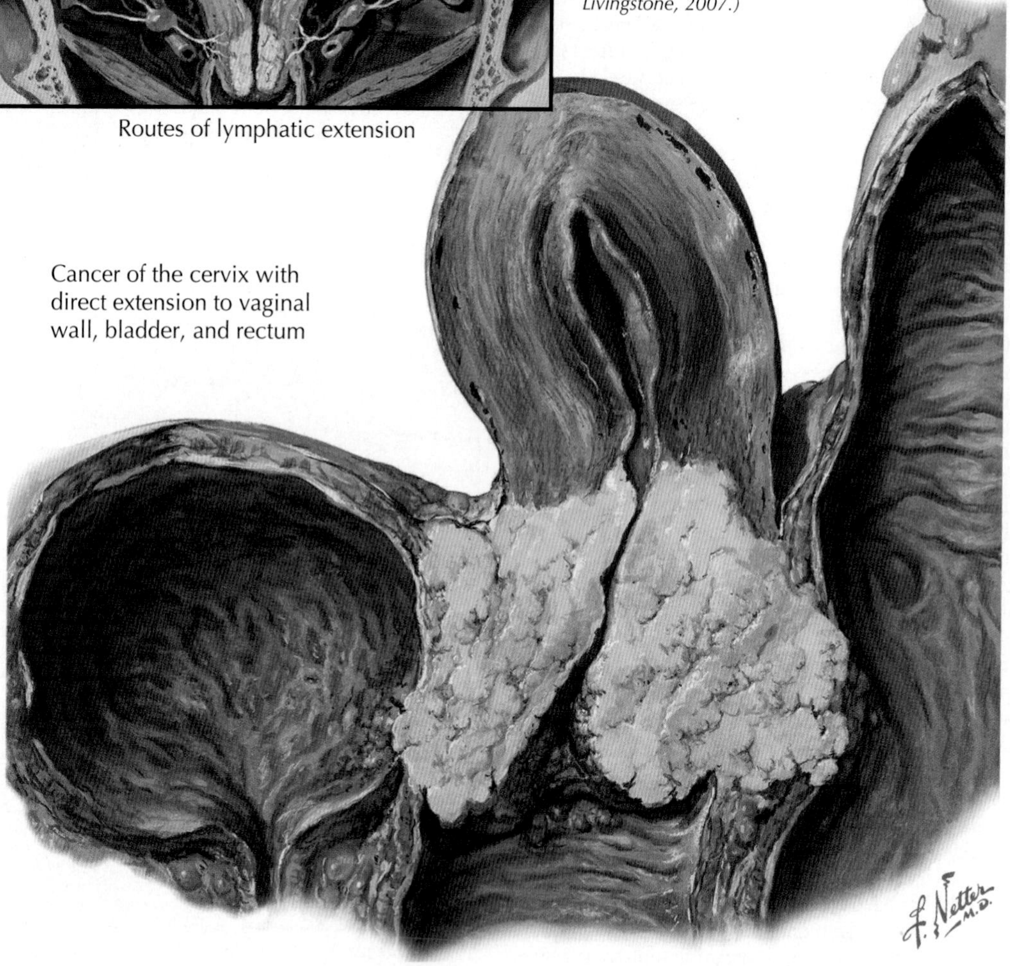

Cancer of the cervix with direct extension to vaginal wall, bladder, and rectum

required to assess extent of disease. Staging is currently clinical and relies primarily on clinical examination and the status of the ureters. For two major reasons, however, the most accurate preoperative clinical staging can never give more than an approximate prognosis in any individual case. First, it is clearly impossible to gauge accurately from the physical examination and other tests whether or not an apparently early, locally demarcated growth may not already have spread to lymphatic channels and nodes. Second, these

neoplasms show a marked individual variability in their response to radiation.

Therapy is based on stage of disease. Radical surgery is usually used for selected patients with stages I and II disease. Radiation therapy (brachytherapy, teletherapy) is used for stages IB and IIA disease or greater. Postoperative radiation therapy reduces the risk of recurrence by almost 50%. In situ carcinoma may be eradicated satisfactorily by surgery if an adequate margin of healthy tissue is excised.

Plate 8.24

Uterus and Cervix

ENDOMETRIAL HYPERPLASIA: EVOLUTION AND CLASSIFICATION

The cyclic changes of the endometrium are regulated and controlled, as described previously, by the hormonal secretions of the ovary. When ovulation fails to occur or an inadequate amount of progesterone is secreted, then endometrial changes recognized as the progestational or secretory phase of the cycle do not take place. Under the constant stimulus of estrogen, the proliferative phase persists, resulting in anaplastic or hyperplastic growth. The characteristic microscopic changes of such endometrial hyperplasia are recognizable in the epithelial glands, the endometrial stroma, and the vascular architecture. The glands often show irregular cystic dilation and are lined with low cuboidal epithelium. In long-standing cases, the size of the glands and their lumina varies to a great extent. This causes a characteristic pattern of tissue and holes, which has been called "Swiss cheese" type. The capillary network is prominent; venous lakes are evident and spiral arterioles are thick-walled and numerous. These adenomatous changes may, at times, be so extensive and may differ from the normal or hyperplastic endometrium by such enormous proliferation that it becomes difficult, if not impossible, to exclude the presence of an early adenocarcinoma. When nuclear atypia is present, more than 40% of patients will have a coexisting endometrial cancer.

Thus endometrial hyperplasia represents an abnormal proliferation of both the glandular and stromal elements of the endometrium with characteristic alteration in the histologic architecture of the tissues. (There is a greater gland-to-stroma ratio [>50%] than observed in normal proliferative endometrium.) It is this architectural change that differentiates hyperplasia from normal endometrial proliferation caused by estrogen stimulation early in the menstrual cycle. Simple hyperplasia represents the least significant form of alteration, whereas complex hyperplasia represents the most significant form of alteration. When cellular atypia is present, it is considered a precancerous condition. In 2014 the World Health Organization simplified the existing nomenclature into two types of endometrial hyperplasia: hyperplasia without atypia (nonneoplastic) and atypical hyperplasia (endometrial intraepithelial neoplasm).

The most common cause of endometrial hyperplasia is unopposed estrogen stimulation of the endometrium (such as chronic anovulation, estrogen therapy [four- to eightfold risk], or obesity [threefold risk]); other causes include nulliparity (two- to threefold risk), diabetes (two- to threefold risk), polycystic ovarian syndrome, and tamoxifen use. Five percent of patients with postmenopausal bleeding have endometrial hyperplasia.

Clinically, endometrial hyperplasia is most likely to present as abnormal uterine bleeding or menorrhagia, occurring in patients in their midforties to midfifties (perimenopausal). The increasing prevalence of obesity, polycystic ovarian syndrome, and chronic anovulation in this age group is thought to influence its age distribution. Because the clinical presentation is identical to that of endometrial cancer, further investigation to establish the diagnosis is imperative.

The most reliable means of detecting endometrial hyperplasia is by endometrial biopsy. Ultrasonography may detect thickening of the endometrial stripe, but no standard has emerged for a threshold of endometrial

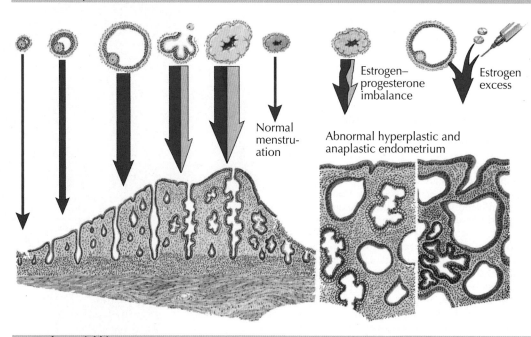

Normal cycle and hormonal imbalance

Estrogen–progesterone imbalance

Estrogen excess

Normal menstruation

Abnormal hyperplastic and anaplastic endometrium

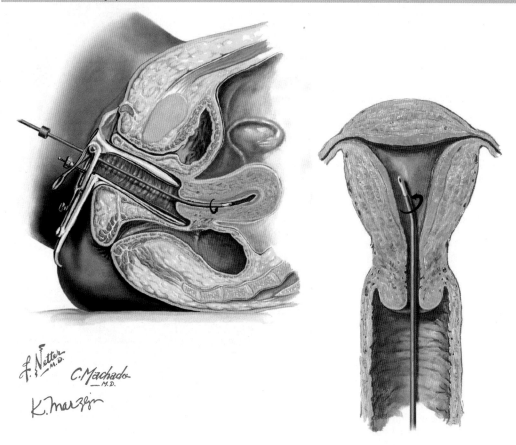

Endometrial biopsy

thickness that carries ideal positive and negative predictive values. Therefore it does not take the place of histologic evaluation of tissue obtained by office suction canula, blind curettage, or hysteroscopically directed biopsy. MRI may also diagnose endometrial thickening, but cost and low specificity argue against its use as a diagnostic tool.

In some cases, the histologic picture is mixed—some areas are typical of the proliferative phase and others show a characteristic secretory pattern, whereas still others may be necrotic and menstrual in type. The descriptive terms *dyssynchronous endometrium* or *disordered proliferative endometrium* have been applied to such findings, although the cause for this variation in endometrial development is not clear. Hormonal therapy, such as oral progestins or combined estrogens and progestins (oral contraceptives), is often the only therapy needed when simple hyperplasia is found.

Plate 8.25

Reproductive System: VOLUME 1

ENDOMETRIAL HYPERPLASIA: POLYPS AND TUBERCULOUS

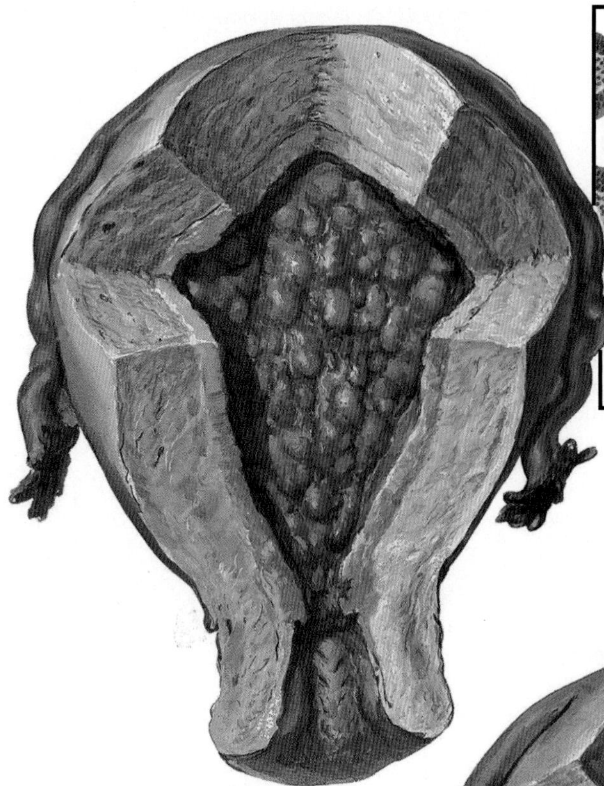

Endometrial polyps are one of the most common etiologies of abnormal genital bleeding. Under the prolonged influence of estrogen, the endometrial tissues become thickened and edematous. In other regions or cases, adenomatous buds or pockets with heaped-up epithelial lining may appear. The overgrowth in both glands and stroma and the mitotic activity in the hyperplastic endometrium are explainable by persistent estrogen stimulation. It is also thought that in polyps, as in normal endometrial tissue, progesterone may serve an antiproliferative function; absent this, proliferation occurs. Of some practical importance is the attractive concept that polypoid endometrial hyperplasia may originate from a step-like progression of abnormal changes, starting with simple polyps and proceeding either coincidentally or sequentially with cystic hyperplasia, adenomatous hyperplasia, anaplasia, carcinoma in situ, and, finally, adenocarcinoma. (Approximately 95% of endometrial polyps are benign.) Although no proof can be cited that even over a period of many years these pathologic changes will inevitably lead to a frank cancer, this theory constitutes a valid warning that these apparently benign conditions may not be wholly without serious consequences.

Macroscopically, in most endometrial hyperplasia one can observe little more than a diffuse swelling of the epithelial surface, which can sometimes be rather pale but is usually hyperemic. At times, isolated polyp-like efflorescences develop within the diffusely swollen endometrium; on other occasions, multiple polyps may be encountered, causing a rather uneven aspect to the entire surface. These fleshy tumors arise as local overgrowths of endometrial glands and stroma and project beyond the surface of the endometrium. Most have a vascular core that forms a sessile or pedunculated projection from the surface of the endometrium. Most polyps are small, but they can range in diameter from a few millimeters to several centimeters. These are most common in the fundus of the uterus but may occur anywhere in the endometrial cavity. They are generally solitary but may be multiple, filling the entire cavity. Polyp formation is common, being found in up to 10% of females (autopsy studies), and 20% of uteri removed for cancer. These polyps—single or multiple—develop after, as well as before, the menopause and may be the source of abnormal bleeding. Because they may develop during the course of normal ovulatory cycles and may even show varying degrees of secretory change, it is probable that at times these growths result from some local irritant or other factor in the endometrium itself, rather than from hyperplasia due to an endocrine abnormality such as anovulation. However, the etiology of diffuse, multiple polyps that may fill the uterine cavity is probably the same as that of nonpolypoid endometrial hyperplasia.

Endometrial polyps may also form in up to a third of postmenopausal females treated with tamoxifen. Polyps in these females may be large (>2 cm), multiple, or show

Endometrial hyperplasia
(microscopic appearance)

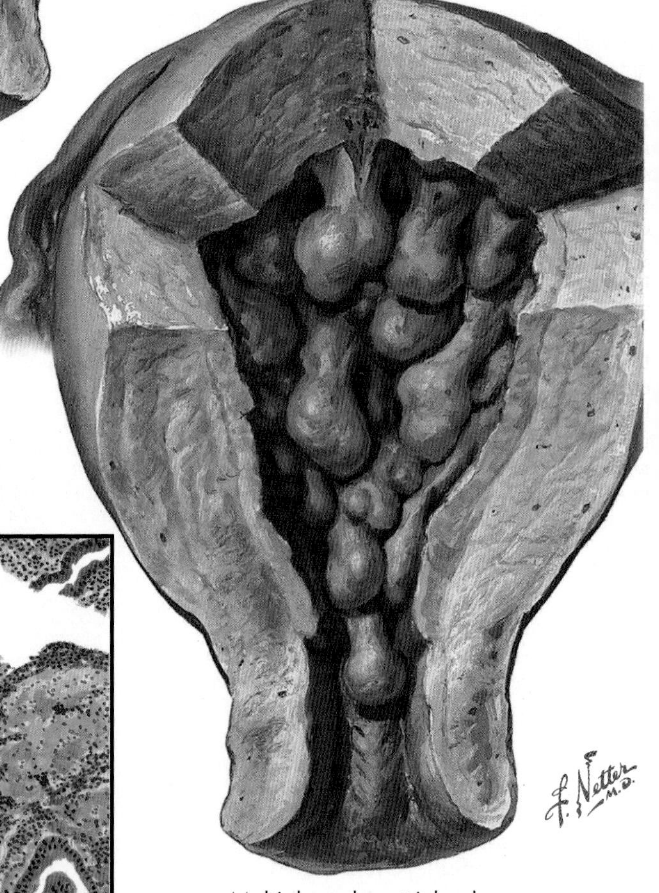

Extensive, diffuse
endometrial hyperplasia
with polypoid tendency

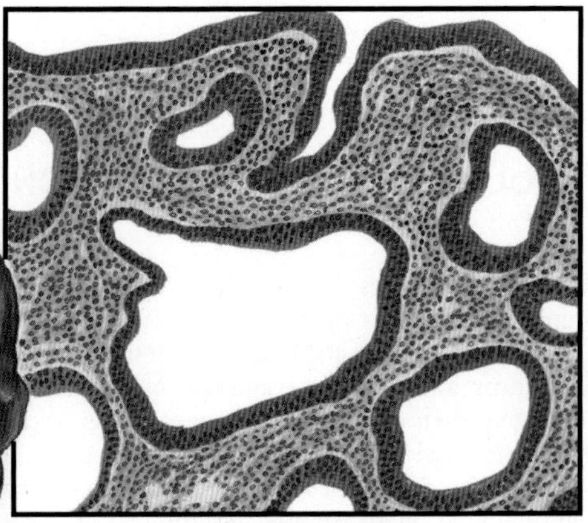

Multiple endometrial polyps

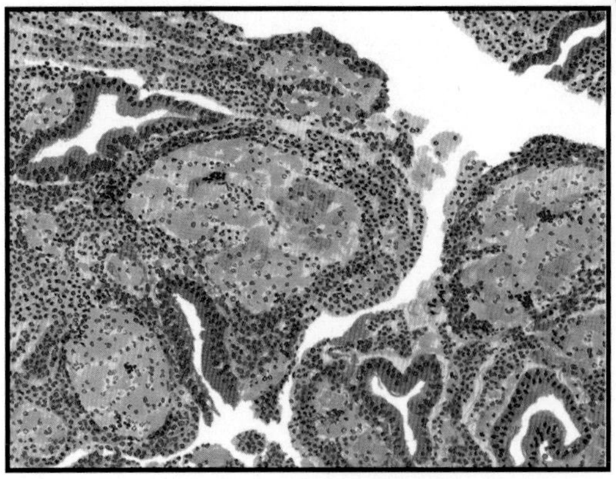

Tuberculous endometritis

molecular alterations. Characteristic cystic changes in the endometrium may be seen on ultrasonography in many of these females.

Tuberculous endometritis can cause local hyperplasia before devolving into scarring and atrophy. Tuberculous endometritis is frequently overlooked because it is uncommon in developed countries, and it causes no clear-cut unique symptomatology, being diagnosed only by microscopic section. With the rise in virally mediated and iatrogenic immunocompromise, the incidence is rising, making awareness of the possibility mandatory. Oligomenorrhea, or scanty flow, may not be an outstanding characteristic. It may be necessary to obtain ample endometrium by curettage to establish the diagnosis. The finding of characteristic centers of caseation in the endometrial stroma with giant cell formation is pathognomonic of the disease. In about half of the patients with genital tuberculosis, the uterus is involved, but, as a rule, this is secondary to a tuberculous infection of the tubes or pelvic peritoneum.

Plate 8.26

Uterus and Cervix

ADENOMYOSIS

Adenomyosis is a condition where endometrial glands and stroma are found within the uterine wall (myometrium). This is the intramural equivalent of extrauterine endometriosis. This is somewhat misleading because endometriosis and adenomyosis coexist in the same patient in about 15% of females although they are clinically different diseases. The only common feature is the presence of ectopic endometrial glands and stroma. Adenomyosis is thought to affect 20% to 35% of all females (on the histologic level) and may be as high as 60% in females 40 to 50 years old. The predominant age of patients with adenomyosis is between 35 and 50 years, and there appears to be a mild familial predisposition (polygenic or multifactorial inheritance) pattern.

Although no true cause is known, adenomyosis is derived from aberrant glands of the basalis layer of the endometrium. These grow by direct extension into the myometrium, or may arise de novo from müllerian rests. The resultant islands of glands rarely undergo the same cyclic changes as does the normal uterine endometrium. Histologically, the glands exhibit an inactive or proliferative pattern. Surrounding most foci of glands and stroma are localized areas of hypertrophy of the smooth muscle of the uterus, resulting in the typical globular enlargement of the organ noted clinically.

The pathogenesis of adenomyosis is unknown, but it is theorized that a disruption of the barrier between the endometrium and myometrium is an initiating step. It has been postulated that high levels of estrogen, high parity, or a history of postpartum endometritis constitute risk factors for the development of adenomyosis, but these remain speculative. Local endometrial invasion may be seen after cesarean delivery, myomectomy, or curettage.

Many cases of adenomyosis are asymptomatic, but up to one-half of patients report menorrhagia or dysmenorrhea, often with increasing severity. On physical examination, a symmetric "woody" enlargement of the uterus (up to 2–3 times normal) may be found, and uterine tenderness that varies with the cycle (worst just before menstruation) may be present. Because of the similarity of symptoms, adenomyosis must be differentiated from uterine leiomyomata (most often resulting in asymmetric uterine changes), endometriosis, or intrauterine pathology (polyps, hyperplasia, or cancer).

The presumptive diagnosis of adenomyosis is generally established on the basis of history and physical examination with imaging (ultrasonography or MRI) reserved to rule out other possible pathologic conditions. Either transvaginal ultrasonography or MRI may demonstrate abnormalities. (On ultrasonography, the uterus will have a heterogeneous echo pattern, without focal abnormalities.) MRI (T2-weighted or contrast-enhanced T1-weighted) will be more specific than ultrasonography and less subject to variation based on the observer, but neither is required to establish a clinical diagnosis. The characteristic history of painful, heavy periods, accompanied by a generous, symmetric, firm, or "woody" uterus suggests, but does not confirm, the diagnosis. Only histologic examination can confirm the diagnosis. (Diagnostic criteria require

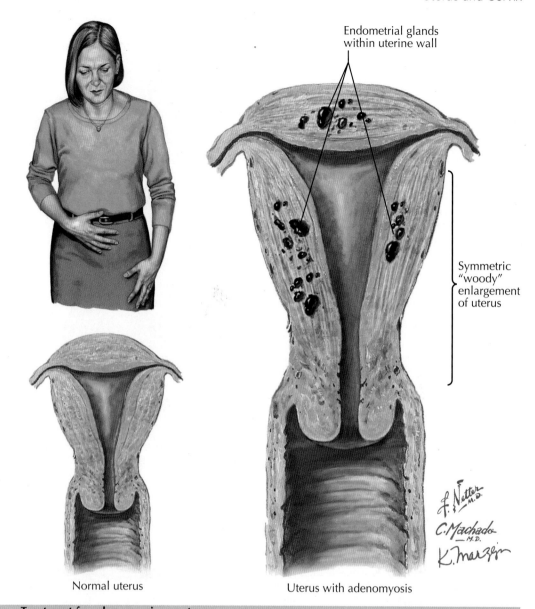

Endometrial glands within uterine wall

Symmetric "woody" enlargement of uterus

Normal uterus

Uterus with adenomyosis

Treatment for adenomyosis symptoms

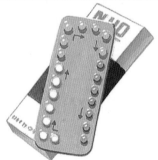
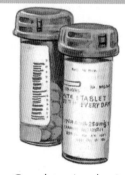

NSAIDs

Cyclic hormone therapy

Gonadotropin-releasing hormone agonists

glands to be identified more than 2.5 mm below the basalis layer of the endometrium.) An endometrial biopsy is seldom of help in establishing the diagnosis of adenomyosis, although it may be useful to rule out a possible endometrial cancer when that is a consideration. Adenomyosis is most often diagnosed incidentally by the pathologist examining histologic sections of surgical specimens.

Analgesics (NSAIDs), cyclic hormone therapy, or GnRH agonists may all be used as therapy for the

symptoms of adenomyosis. There is no satisfactory medical cure for adenomyosis. All medical therapy is aimed at ameliorating the symptoms or delaying the progression of the condition. Symptoms generally resolve with the loss of menstrual function at menopause. Hysterectomy is the definitive treatment for adenomyosis and unless associated with endometriosis, surgical therapy is curative. Uterine artery embolization to control symptoms has been suggested but remains little used for this purpose.

Plate 8.27

Reproductive System: VOLUME 1

ASHERMAN SYNDROME

Asherman syndrome (uterine synechia, IUA) is scarring or occlusion of the uterine cavity after curettage, especially when surgery is performed after septic abortion or in the immediate postpartum period. (Although the same changes occur after therapeutic endometrial ablation, the term is generally not applied in that setting.) This scarring generally results from endometrial damage involving the basal layers (normal curettage, excessive curettage, curettage when infection is present, or in the immediate postpartum period—some intrauterine adhesions form in 30% of patients treated by curettage for missed abortion) or endometrial infection (tuberculosis or schistosomiasis). More than 90% of the cases occur after pregnancy-related curettage. A severe pelvic infection unrelated to surgery, including endometrial tuberculosis infections, may also lead to Asherman syndrome. (Chronic endometritis from genital tuberculosis is a significant cause of severe intrauterine scarring in the developing world, often resulting in total obliteration of the uterine cavity.) A less common cause of IUA is severe endometritis or fibrosis after a myomectomy, metroplasty, or cesarean delivery. In some cases, the whole cavity may be scarred and occluded, resulting in secondary amenorrhea. Even with relatively few scars, the endometrium may fail to respond to estrogens, which means that there is a poor correlation between symptoms and the severity of scarring found.

The true prevalence of Asherman syndrome is unclear because of a lack of awareness of the symptoms or diagnosis and the nonspecific nature of those symptoms. Intrauterine scarring is estimated to affect 1.5% of females undergoing hysterosalpingography, between 5% and 39% of females with recurrent miscarriage, and >20% of patients who have undergone curettage for retained products of conception (incomplete abortion or postpartum).

Patients with uterine synechia generally present with amenorrhea, hypomenorrhea, recurrent early pregnancy loss, or infertility depending on the extent and intrauterine location of adhesions. Pain during menstruation and ovulation is also sometimes experienced and can be attributed to menstrual sequestration and obstruction. Most often the patient will have a history of one or more risk factors such as curettage or infection, and the temporal relation between these events and the onset of symptoms should be suggestive of intrauterine scarring. Hysteroscopy, sonohysterography, or hysterosalpingography may all be used to confirm the diagnosis. Ultrasonography, without the use of saline infusion, is not a reliable method of diagnosing intrauterine scarring. It has been suggested that sequential administration of estrogen followed by progestogen can be used as the initial diagnostic procedure when intrauterine scarring is suspected. Unfortunately, withdrawal bleeding occurs after administration of the steroids in most females with intrauterine adhesions, resulting in a lack of specificity of this approach. If left untreated, retrograde menstruation (if present) caused by outflow obstruction may result in the development of endometriosis.

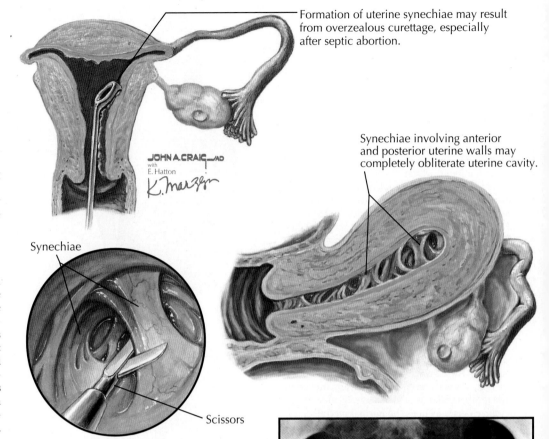

Formation of uterine synechiae may result from overzealous curettage, especially after septic abortion.

Synechiae involving anterior and posterior uterine walls may completely obliterate uterine cavity.

Synechiae

Scissors

Hysteroscopic lysis of synechiae may be required to return patency to uterine cavity.

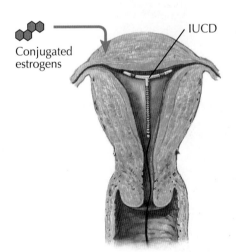

Conjugated estrogens

IUCD

IUCD is placed in uterine cavity postoperatively and patient is maintained on conjugated estrogens.

X-ray film of patient with Asherman syndrome. Patient (33 years, gravida 3, para 0, abortus 3) had been amenorrheic for 6 months after dilation and curettage for most recent therapeutic abortion. Filling of endocervical canal and nonvisualization of endometrial cavity are consistent with complete obliteration of cavity by adhesions or with obstruction at internal os level by adhesions in lower endometrial cavity. This appearance may also be seen with advanced endometrial tuberculosis. *(From Richmond JA: Hysterosalpingography. In Mishell DR Jr, Davajan V. Infertility, Contraception and Reproductive Endocrinology, 4th ed. Blackwell Scientific Publications, 1997.)*

When uterine synechiae are diagnosed, resection of intrauterine scars under hysteroscopic control (sometimes with laparoscopy used as a protective measure against uterine perforation), followed by IUCD insertion and estrogen therapy may be curative, providing a return of normal menstrual function and fertility. Repeated scarring may occur in up to 50% of cases, necessitating postoperative follow-up or repeated treatment. For this reason, follow-up tests, including a hysterosalpingogram, hysteroscopy, or sonohysterography, are necessary to ensure that scars have not reformed. Patients who have undergone resection of intrauterine adhesions who subsequently become pregnant are at greater risk for having abnormal placentation, including placenta accreta.

The prognosis for these patients is a function of the initial severity: small scars can usually be treated with success; extensive obliteration of the uterine cavity or fallopian tube ostia may require several surgical interventions or even be uncorrectable. In these cases, surrogacy, in vitro fertilization, or adoption may be the only alternatives.

Plate 8.28

Uterus and Cervix

MYOMA (FIBROID): LOCATIONS

Uterine myomata are the most frequent tumors found in the female pelvis, with a reported incidence of 4% to 11%. Fibroids are found in 30% of all females and in 40% to 50% of females older than 50 (one study has demonstrated a rate of more than 80% in African Americans older than 50). Leiomyomata account for approximately 30% of all hysterectomies. They are a benign monoclonal connective tissue tumor found in or around the uterus, which may be disseminated in rare cases. They are commonly called *fibroids*, although these tumors derive not from fibrous tissue components but from vascular smooth muscle cells. From the point of view of the pathologist, the tumors under discussion should be classified as leiomyomata (from *leios*, meaning smooth).

Historically, it was thought that these fibromuscular tumors were produced by some imbalance or excess of ovarian hormone secretion. In almost all instances they remain static or even shrink considerably in size after the menopause, implying that estrogen provides the stimulus for their growth. It is now thought that these tumors arise from a single smooth muscle cell (of vascular origin) resulting in tumors that are each monoclonal. Estrogen, progesterone, and epidermal growth factor are all thought to stimulate growth. In general, fibroids are multiple.

Leiomyomata generally arise within the interstitial substance of the uterine wall. As they expand, they may remain as intramural fibroids, or they may progress toward either surface of the uterus to become subserous or submucous tumors. Seventy percent to 80% of uterine fibroids are found within the wall of the uterus, with 5% to 10% lying below the endometrium and less than 5% arising in or near the cervix. Leiomyomata may become pedunculated either within the uterine cavity or on the surface of the uterus. Multiple fibroids are found in up to 85% of patients. Growth is generally slow. However, it is progressive until the menopause, when production of estrogen ceases. Uterine fibroids may be considered analogous to adenomata of the prostate; however, it is important to point out that malignancy frequently develops in the latter but appears very rarely in association with leiomyomata.

The most common symptom—that of profuse or prolonged bleeding—occurs in approximately 50% of reported cases. The tremendous variety in size, location, and position of these tumors brings out the importance of recognizing that in many cases the basic cause of the bleeding may not be the fibroid itself. Obviously, in such instances removal of the tumor alone will not guarantee freedom from subsequent hemorrhages. Symptoms of pain and pressure are not common complaints, except in the presence of massive fibroids; dysmenorrhea, menorrhagia, or intermenstrual bleeding occurs in 30% to 40% of patients. Pelvic examination is generally sufficient to establish the diagnosis, although this may be augmented by ultrasonography, but is generally not required.

A fibroid uterus is enlarged and irregular. The tumors have a rubbery, firm consistency and, when cut open, they show a typical whorled arrangement of tough,

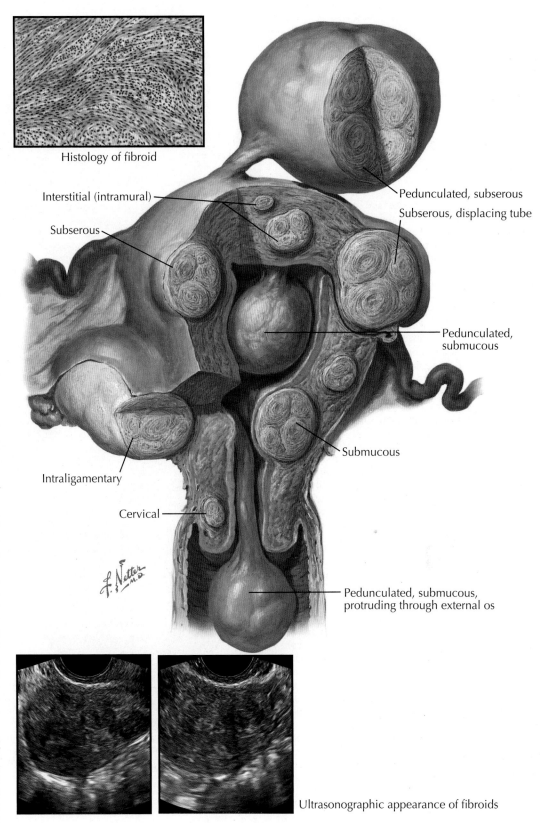

Histology of fibroid

Interstitial (intramural)

Subserous

Intraligamentary

Cervical

Pedunculated, subserous

Subserous, displacing tube

Pedunculated, submucous

Submucous

Pedunculated, submucous, protruding through external os

Ultrasonographic appearance of fibroids

pinkish-white muscular bundles. The cut surface protrudes outward owing to release of the constriction caused by the well-demarcated pseudocapsule. Leiomyomata do not have a true capsule but are well circumscribed, which facilitates surgical removal. In microscopic section, myomata are dense and cellular, showing strands and bundles of characteristic spindle cells devoid of mitotic activity.

Fibroids may grow laterally into the broad ligament (intraligamentary). When large, they may grossly distort the anatomy of ureters and uterine vessels. Those that arise near the cornua may impinge upon the patency of the intramural portion of the fallopian tube. The blood supply of fibroids that have become pedunculated is in constant jeopardy owing to the possibility of torsion of the pedicle, resulting in acute symptoms.

Plate 8.29

Reproductive System: VOLUME 1

Myoma (Fibroid): Secondary Changes

Fibroids vary greatly in size and position. Proper management therefore demands a consideration of the biologic life cycle of such tumors and an individual evaluation of each patient's age, physiologic status, and procreative ambitions.

The diagnosis of a fibroid uterus is not in itself a justification for either myomectomy or hysterectomy. Historically, the indications for surgery were undue bleeding, increasing pressure on bladder or bowel, a rapid increase in size or change in consistency of the tumor, or some degenerative change causing pain. With improved imaging and more effective medical therapies available, the need for surgical intervention has been more limited: symptoms unresponsive to therapy and acute pain. There has also been a limited role for myomectomy when a few large fibroids are present and there has been recurrent pregnancy loss.

When a leiomyoma is diagnosed in the absence of any of the indications just listed, a policy of watchful waiting is justified. If none of these signs or symptoms is present in younger females with fibroids, the problem may be complicated by the question of infertility. Small subserous or interstitial fibroids are unlikely to be etiologically responsible for subfecundity unless one or both uterine cornua are grossly distorted thereby. On the other hand, submucous fibroids are more likely to become a factor, because they are commonly considered to be the cause of prolonged or profuse menses and also may interfere with implantation. Without a suspicious history of recurrent early loss, ascribing a role in the infertility to these myoma may be difficult.

Intraligamentary tumors, although rare, may be considered for removal because if they are left to grow to large size, surgery in this area may become quite complicated. Pedunculated submucous fibroids may undergo torsion of the pedicle, cutting off the blood supply and causing slough and necrosis. Occasionally, a myoma on a long pedicle is gradually forced through the external os and may prolapse to such a degree as to cause complete inversion of the uterus.

Large tumors sometimes outstrip their blood supply, and cystic degeneration may occur centrally. In such cases, the characteristic tough, rubbery consistency is lost, and the differential diagnosis from sarcomatous change may have to await removal and gross sectioning. Cystic degeneration is typified by amorphous, jellylike material in contrast to the friable, red, solid appearance of a sarcoma.

Occasionally, a fibroid growing downward from the posterior aspect of the fundus becomes incarcerated in the cavity of the sacrum. It is surprising that even under these circumstances, lower bowel or ureteral obstruction is rare, whereas gross anatomic distortions, such as lateral displacement of the ureters and rectosigmoid, may occur.

Calcification in a fibroid is not unusual. The deposition of calcium may throw a characteristic shadow on x-ray examination, and this is sometimes a valuable aid in the differential diagnosis of a rocky, hard pelvic mass in older females.

The relation of fibroids to the successful culmination of pregnancy is affected by the situation in the individual case. The location of the tumor may be more important than its size. Those arising from the cervix or the lower segment may be so large as to cause obstruction of the passage of the fetal head through the birth canal.

Although small subserous or interstitial fibroids may not interfere in any way with gestation, during the course of pregnancy (probably owing to pressure), the vascular supply to an interstitial fibromyoma is sometimes sufficiently embarrassed so that hemorrhage into the stroma of the tumor results. This "red degeneration" of the tumor may lead to necrosis and become a serious complication of the pregnancy.

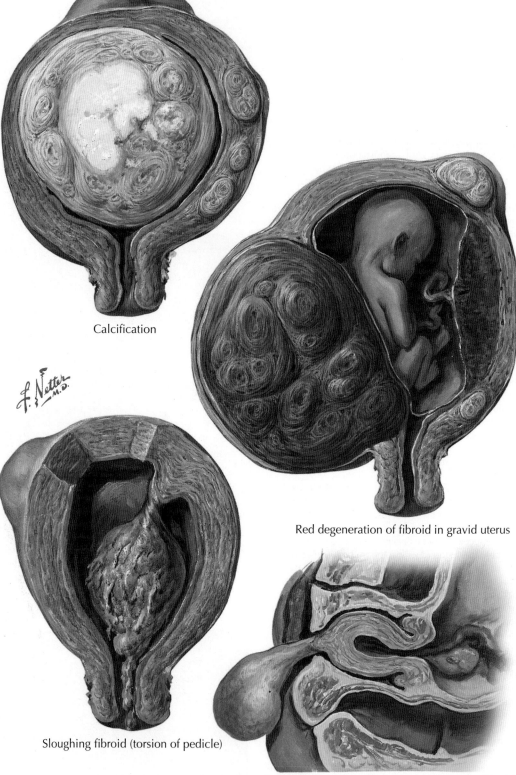

Calcification

Red degeneration of fibroid in gravid uterus

Sloughing fibroid (torsion of pedicle)

Inversion of uterus due to prolapse of submucous fibroid

Plate 8.30

Uterus and Cervix

Myoma (Fibroid): Degeneration, Obstruction

Although the diagnosis of fibroids is generally a clinical one, it must be remembered that it is impossible to prove, without surgery, either the suspected diagnosis of a fibroid uterus or the assumption that such a tumor may be the cause for symptoms; ovarian neoplasms occasionally adhere to and invade the fundus posteriorly and present a mass with misleading characteristics; and bleeding may be caused by an endocrine dysfunction. After the menopause, such bleeding from a benign endometrial hyperplasia may be a telltale sign of a functioning ovarian tumor that might be overlooked unless it is recalled that fibroids almost never initiate bleeding in the postmenopausal period and certainly never cause endometrial proliferation.

Many factors play a role in each patient's decision of management. Justification for multiple myomectomy is found in those desiring to preserve the chance of pregnancy. In those with abnormal bleeding and small fibroids at the climacteric, after the possibility of cancer has been investigated by endometrial biopsy or curettage, the diagnosis of anovulatory cycles may suggest hormonal therapy, with the hope that the complaint may be controlled until ovarian function ceases. Uterine artery embolization may be used for patients who are not surgical candidates or those who wish to preserve fertility. (Successful pregnancy is possible, but because uterine embolization has been associated with a number of both short- and long-term complications, it is considered experimental in females who desire fertility.) If the cervix has been the site of persistent atypia, or if cystocele, rectocele, or uterine prolapse is present, then in those females beyond an interest in childbearing, it is wise to remove a fibroid uterus as a part of the reconstruction of a firm pelvic floor. Occasionally and unfortunately, a patient may be told that she has a tumor, and she may become so concerned with undue anxiety with regard to cancer that no choice is left to set her mind at rest but operative removal of the fibroids.

At times, a large fibroid may outgrow its blood supply, with resultant cystic degeneration. The arterial supply of myomas is significantly less than that of a similarly sized area of normal myometrium. As a result, degeneration occurs when the tumor outgrows its blood supply. The severity of the discrepancy between the myoma's growth and its blood supply determines the type of degeneration: hyaline, myxomatous, calcific, cystic, fatty, or red degeneration and necrosis. The mildest form of degeneration of a myoma is hyaline degeneration. Grossly, in this condition the surface of the myoma is homogeneous with loss of the whorled pattern. Histologically, with hyaline degeneration, cellular detail is lost as the smooth muscle cells are replaced by fibrous connective tissue.

A large fibroid originating from a sharply retroverted fundus may become incarcerated in the hollow of the

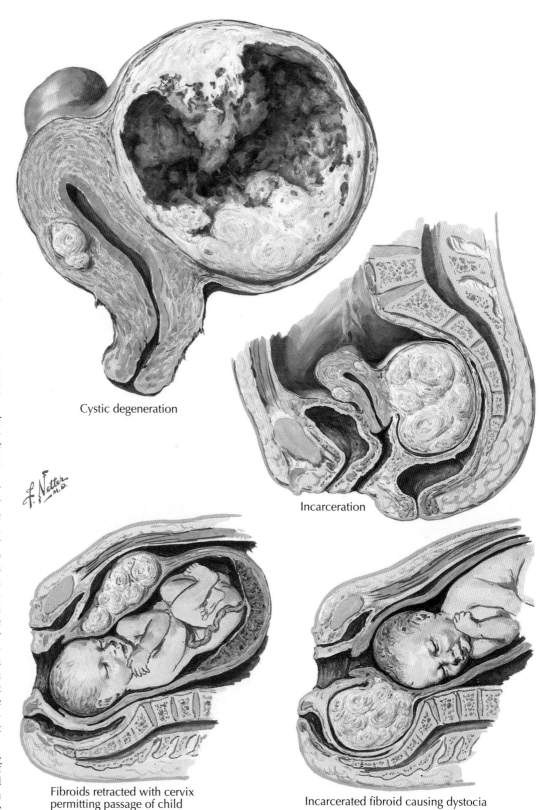

Cystic degeneration

Incarceration

Fibroids retracted with cervix permitting passage of child

Incarcerated fibroid causing dystocia

sacrum, pressing on the rectum, causing obstipation, although obstruction from this cause is probably rare. A similar situation is pictured as resulting from a fibroid arising posteriorly from the endocervical region.

Cervical fibroids in the uterus at term may retract upward as cervical dilation proceeds, allowing for an uncomplicated delivery, or they may be forced downward, causing dystocia and making delivery impossible.

Rarely, the high levels of both growth and ovarian hormones can stimulate existing fibroids to grow rapidly during mid- to late pregnancy, resulting in problems for the pregnancy. This rapid growth may be associated with pain, especially when the growth outstrips the available blood supply and degeneration or necrosis ensues. This form of degeneration occurs in approximately 5% to 10% of gravid females with myomas.

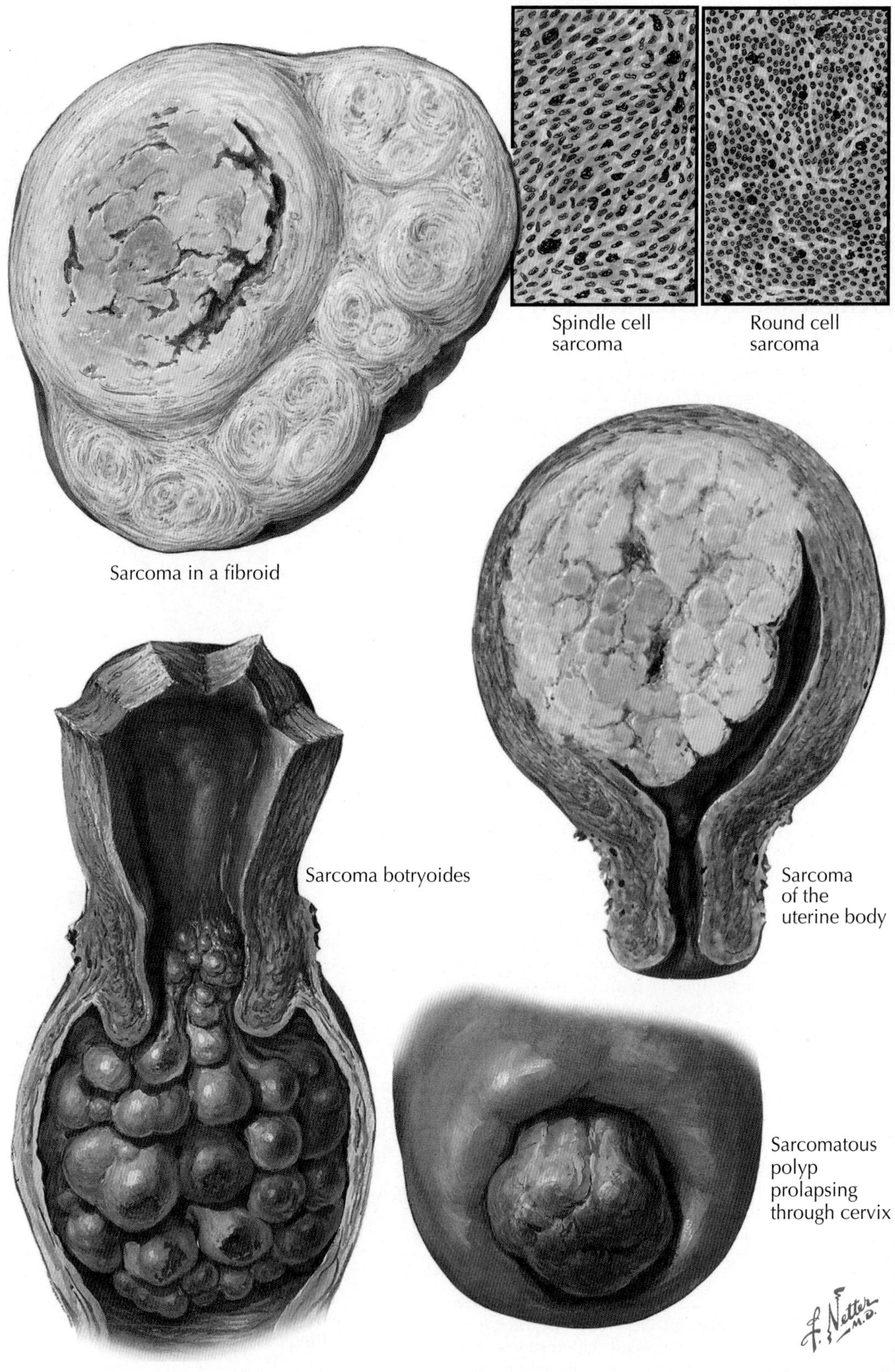

Plate 8.31

Reproductive System: VOLUME 1

SARCOMA

Sarcomatous change can occur in the tissues of the müllerian system, including the endometrial stroma and myometrium. Mixed müllerian sarcomas may include elements not native to the genital tract such as cartilage or bone (heterologous type). Sarcoma of the uterus, whether primary or occurring secondary to a preexisting fibroid, is a relatively rare disease. Of all malignancies of the female genital tract, sarcomas represent less than 5% of uterine malignancies, or roughly 1 of 800 smooth muscle tumors, with a prevalence of 0.67 per 100,000 females older than 20 years. The incidence of sarcomatous degeneration of a myoma is less than 1%. It has been found in ages from childhood to many years after menopause, although most uterine sarcomas occur in patients over age 40. (The mean age at diagnosis is approximately 60 years old.) There appears to be no genetic pattern, and although sarcomas are reported more often in Black females (twofold), there is no racial predisposition. Leiomyomas have been proposed as risk factors for these tumors, as have estrogen and obesity, although evidence is lacking. The use of oral contraceptives is associated with a reduced risk.

These tumors grow with surprising rapidity. Even in children, tumors have been observed that were larger than a pregnant uterus at term. The grave prognosis of such a tumor, even when treated with radical surgery, makes it advisable to cut open all leiomyomas at the time of their removal and submit all surgical specimens for histologic evaluation. A sarcoma is most apt to appear at the center of the larger tumors. It is easily recognized on cross sections, as it is soft and meaty and lacks the firm, characteristic whorled appearance of a myoma. Inadequate blood supply is often responsible for a central necrosis or hemorrhage.

Sarcomas may originate in any part of the uterus that contains mesodermal tissue, but whether the tumor is a mural or endometrial sarcoma, whether it derives from connective tissue of the endometrium, endocervix, or blood vessels or develops from muscle cells of the myometrium or myoma cells, and whether it may be classified as spindle cell or round cell or mixed cell sarcoma, its invasive and metastatic tendencies are seemingly the same. Size and extent of the tumor are more important, as far as the prognosis is concerned, than is its location or its histologic classifications.

The diagnosis may be difficult in many cases and is not necessarily final until the pathologist has rendered the verdict after extensive examination of the tumor postoperatively. Because of technical difficulties, biopsy specimens examined by the frozen-section technique are seldom helpful.

A primary sarcoma arising directly from the uterine body may easily be mistaken for a benign submucous fibroid. At times, it may be impossible to differentiate

Spindle cell sarcoma

Round cell sarcoma

Sarcoma in a fibroid

Sarcoma botryoides

Sarcoma of the uterine body

Sarcomatous polyp prolapsing through cervix

the spindle cell sarcoma from a benign cellular fibroid without resorting to microscopic examination, which will reveal the presence of numerous mitoses in the case of the former.

Occasionally, uterine polyps show sarcomatous degeneration. When this has occurred, the only treatment is that of radical panhysterectomy.

The "grape" sarcoma or sarcoma botryoides is very rare. It consists of multiple, soft, berrylike formations, varying in size from that of a pea to that of an olive. This

tumor carries a grave prognosis and occurs almost exclusively in young children. Clusters of tumor masses arising from the cervix or the vagina may present themselves at the introitus, or they may be extruded by hemorrhage. In view of the rapid growth of the neoplasm, a very early and radical hysterectomy with extensive pelvic node dissection offers the only hope of survival. On the occurrence of vaginal bleeding in any young child, the possibility of this serious neoplasm must not be overlooked.

Plate 8.32

Uterus and Cervix

CANCER OF CORPUS: VARIOUS STAGES AND TYPES

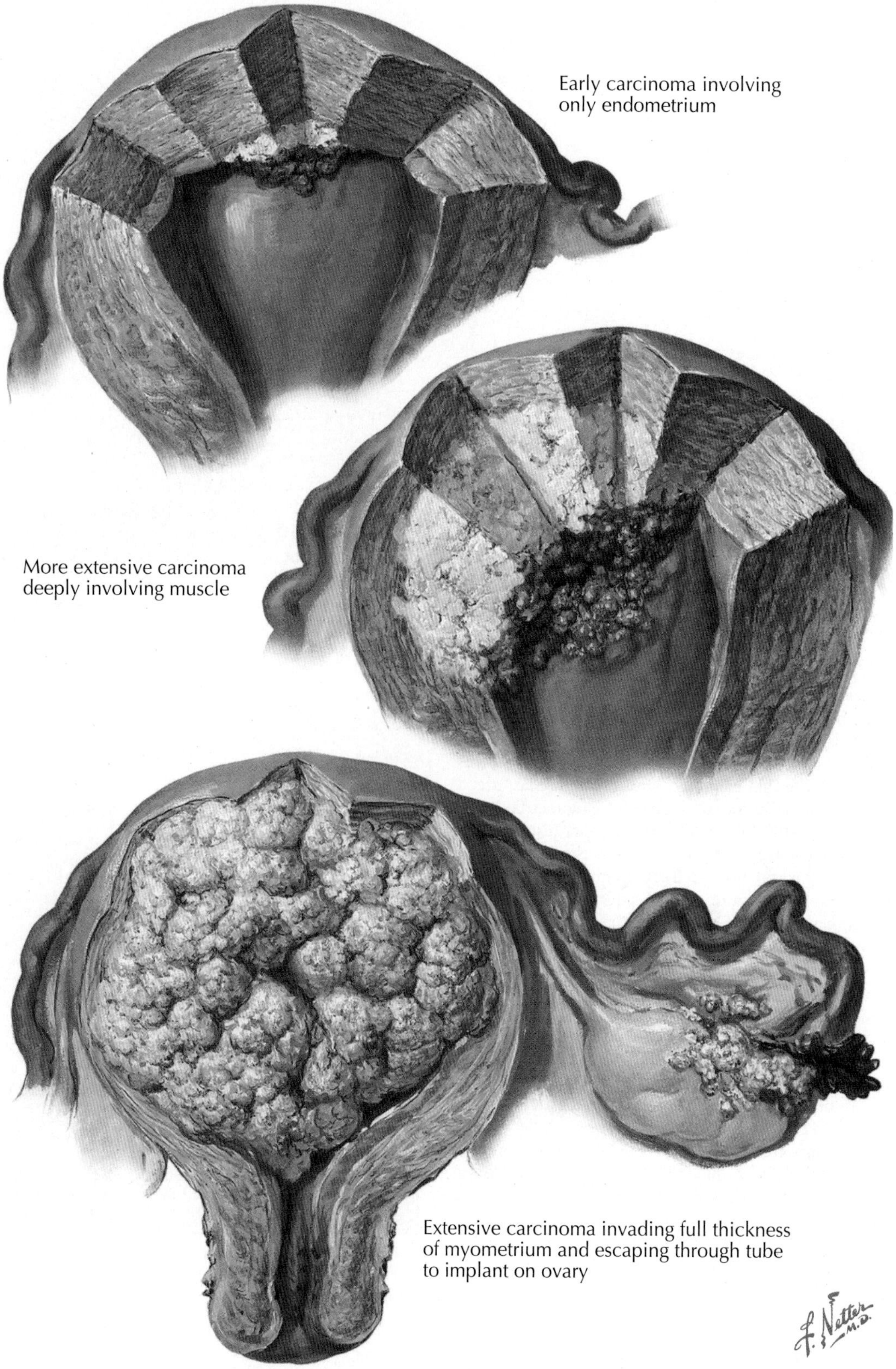

Cancer of the uterine corpus usually involves malignant change of the endometrial tissues. These are generally of the adenocarcinoma, adenosquamous, clear-cell, or papillary serous cell types. These cancers are the most frequent malignancy of the female reproductive tract, representing the eighth leading site of cancer-related deaths among American females.

Although the possibility of adenocarcinoma must be considered in patients with abnormal bleeding during preclimacteric years, cancer of the uterine body must always be suspected with the appearance of abnormal spotting or staining from the fifth decade on. Any discharge from a normal cervix occurring in the post-menopausal age group should be regarded as highly suspicious of fundal malignancy. The discharge may at times be watery rather than frankly bloody. Pain, except in the presence of pyometrium, is not an early sign. When present, it may signify extension to other organs.

Risk factors for the development of endometrial cancer include unopposed (without progestins) estrogen stimulation (such as in polycystic ovary syndrome, obesity, chronic anovulation, and estrogen replacement therapy without concomitant progestin). This may be a factor in up to 90% of cases. Selective estrogen receptor modulators with uterine activity (such as tamoxifen) may also place the patient at increased risk. Oral contraceptives reduce the risk of endometrial cancer.

If exfoliated malignant endometrial cells are found in the vaginal smear, the diagnosis may be considered definite. (Cervical cytologic tests detect only about 20% of known endometrial carcinomas.) Transvaginal ultrasonography or sonohysterography may be useful (although some have raised concerns about the possibility of extrauterine spread induced by tubal spill of fluid during sonohysterography). The final diagnosis, however, depends inevitably upon tissue sampling and histologic evaluation. Endometrial biopsy is approximately 90% accurate.

The current surgical staging classification relies on an operative evaluation with particular emphasis on myometrial invasion in stage I. In stage IA the tumor is limited to the endometrium; IB invasion is to less than half of the myometrium; and IC invasion is to more than half of the myometrium. In stage IIA there is endocervical glandular involvement only; in IIB there is cervical stromal invasion. In stage IIIA the tumor invades the serosa and/or adnexa and/or there is positive peritoneal cytology; in stage IIIB there are vaginal metastases; and in stage IIIC metastases to pelvic and/or paraaortic lymph nodes have occurred. Stage IVA includes tumor invasion of the bladder and/or bowel mucosa, whereas stage IVB consists of those with distant metastases, including intraabdominal and/or inguinal lymph nodes. Pelvic washings are no longer required for surgical staging; however, the presence of cancer cells in the peritoneal cavity is a poor prognostic factor. Most cases are diagnosed in stage I because of the prompt evaluation of postmenopausal bleeding, improving the overall prognosis, which is strongly dependent on the stage of the disease: stage I disease has an approximate 90% 5-year survival, whereas stage IV disease has a survival of less than 20%. The histologic type is also related to prognosis, with the best prognosis associated with typical adenocarcinomas as well as better differentiated tumors with or without squamous elements and secretory carcinomas. Approximately 80% of all endometrial carcinomas fall into the favorable category. Poor prognostic histologic types are papillary serous carcinomas, clear-cell carcinomas, and poorly differentiated carcinomas with or without squamous elements.

Tumor grade and stage both affect the risk of lymph node spread in endometrial cancer. There are differences in the proportion of positive nodes between stages IB and IA cases as well as tumor grade. The frequency of nodal involvement becomes much greater with higher grade tumors and with greater depth of myometrial invasion: the risk of lymph node involvement appears to be negligible for endometrial carcinoma involving only the endometrium and for lower-grade tumors with a depth of invasion involving only the inner third of the myometrium.

Early carcinoma involving only endometrium

More extensive carcinoma deeply involving muscle

Extensive carcinoma invading full thickness of myometrium and escaping through tube to implant on ovary

Plate 8.33

Reproductive System: VOLUME 1

Cancer of Corpus: Histology and Extension

The majority of uterine cancers have a relatively well-differentiated glandular architecture. In general, of course, the more anaplastic tumors may be expected to grow more rapidly and to metastasize earlier than do the more mature adenocarcinomas. The differentiation between well-differentiated uterine adenocarcinoma and atypical, adenomatous hyperplasia of the endometrium is not simple, and often fixed and stained rather than frozen sections must be obtained before submitting the patient to the treatment established for an ascertained malignancy.

Squamous epithelium commonly coexists with the glandular elements of endometrial carcinoma. Historically, the term *adenoacanthoma* was used to describe a well-differentiated tumor and *adenosquamous carcinoma* to describe a more anaplastic carcinoma with squamous elements. The term *adenocarcinoma with squamous elements* is now used with a description of the degree of differentiation of both the glandular and squamous components. Uterine papillary serous carcinomas are a highly virulent histologic subtype of endometrial carcinomas (5%–10% of cases). These tumors histologically resemble papillary serous carcinoma elsewhere in the body (e.g., ovary). Clear-cell carcinomas of the endometrium are less common (<5%), and histologically they are similar to clear-cell adenocarcinomas of the ovary, cervix, and vagina. Clear-cell tumors tend to develop in postmenopausal females and carry a worse prognosis. Survival rates of 39% to 55% have been reported, versus 65% or better for endometrial carcinoma.

Successful therapy primarily depends on the surgical extirpation of the disease while it is confined to the uterus. Unfortunately, many of these patients are not good surgical risks owing to chronic or intercurrent afflictions common to the sixth and seventh decades of life. Primary treatment consists of surgical exploration with hysterectomy, bilateral salpingo-oophorectomy, and paraaortic node sampling. (Intraabdominal cytology is no longer required for surgical staging; however, the presence of cancer cells in the peritoneal cavity is a poor prognostic factor.) For patients with significant medical comorbidities, radiation therapy alone can be used, although at a cost in efficacy. Postoperative radiation to the vaginal cuff reduces local recurrence. Distant metastatic disease is treated with high-dose progestins, cisplatin, and doxorubicin. The use of adjuvant radiation therapy in females with disease limited to the uterus based on systematic surgical staging is controversial. For patients with stage I, grade 1 tumors, postoperative radiation (vaginal brachytherapy and/or external beam irradiation) may be considered if there is deep myometrial invasion to the outer third or if there is any invasion and the surgical staging was limited.

The treatment of stage II disease is less well defined. Three therapeutic options have been employed: primary operation (radical hysterectomy and pelvic node dissection), primary radiation (intrauterine and vaginal implant and external irradiation) followed by an operation (extrafascial hysterectomy), and simple hysterectomy followed by external beam irradiation. Most patients with stage II disease are treated with a combination of radiation and extrafascial hysterectomy, resulting in 5-year survival rates that approach 75%.

Patients with stage III and IV endometrial cancer have a high risk of hematogenous and lymphatic spread of their cancer outside of the pelvis. Therefore systemic therapy plays a key role in the management of these patients. Both hormonal and cytotoxic agents have activity in patients with advanced endometrial cancer. In addition, there continues to be a role for radiation therapy to gain local control or to treat pelvic disease.

After treatment, patients should be monitored by follow-up Pap smears from the vaginal cuff every 3 months for 2 years, then every 6 months for 3 years, and then yearly. A chest radiograph should be obtained annually. Ten percent of recurrences will occur more than 5 years after initial diagnosis.

Death results from distant metastases to vital organs more commonly in endometrial carcinoma than in cervical neoplasms. These distant metastases are unquestionably bloodborne. Local obstruction of the ureters is rare.

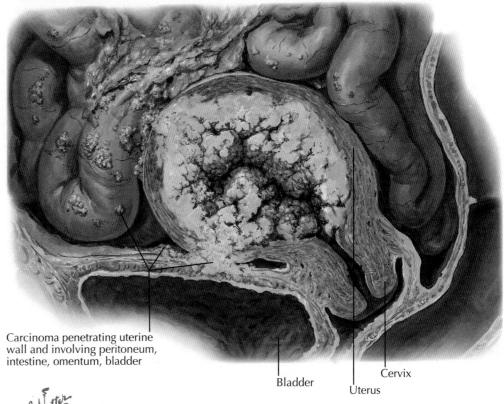

Extensive carcinoma

Carcinoma penetrating uterine wall and involving peritoneum, intestine, omentum, bladder

Bladder
Uterus
Cervix

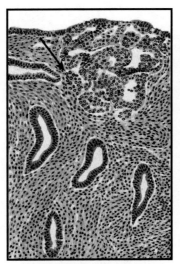

Carcinoma in situ (stage 0). Focus of crowded glands with atypical cells (*arrow*)

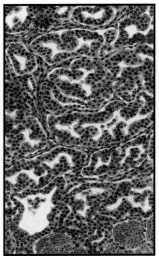

Adenocarcinoma. Large cluster of abnormal glands with atypical cells

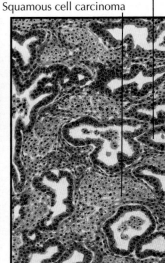

Malignant gland
Squamous cell carcinoma

Adenoacanthoma. Sheets of squamous cell carcinoma mixed with malignant glands

FALLOPIAN TUBES

Plate 9.1

Reproductive System: VOLUME 1

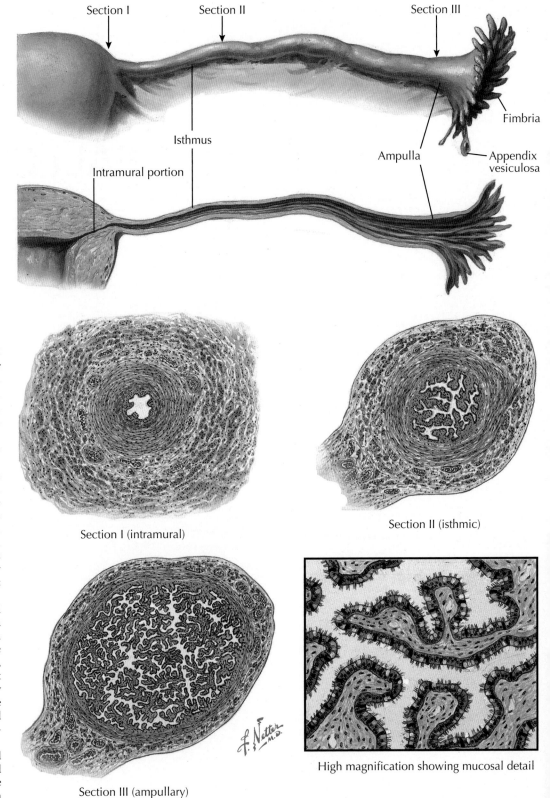

Section I   Section II   Section III

Fimbria

Isthmus

Ampulla — Appendix vesiculosa

Intramural portion

Section I (intramural)

Section II (isthmic)

Section III (ampullary)

High magnification showing mucosal detail

FALLOPIAN TUBES

The fallopian tubes are musculomembranous structures, each about 12 cm in length, commonly divided into the intramural, isthmic, and ampullary sections.

The intramural (interstitial) portion traverses the uterine wall in a more or less straight fashion. It has an ampulla-like dilation just before it communicates with the uterine cavity. On hysterosalpingography, this tiny tubal antrum either is connected with the shadow of the uterine cavity by a threadlike communication or is separated from it by a narrow, empty zone. This constriction of the tubal shadow, usually designated as the tubal sphincter, is caused by an annular fold of the uterine mucosa at the junction of both organs.

The isthmic portion is not quite so narrow as the intramural part. Its course is slightly wavy. The ampullary portion is tortuous and gradually widens toward its outer end. It terminates in a fimbriated infundibulum, which resembles a ruffled petunia or sea anemone. One of the fimbriae, the fimbria ovarica, is grooved and runs along the lateral border of the mesosalpinx to the ovary. Frequently, one or more small vesicles filled with clear, serous fluid, called appendices vesiculosae or hydatids of Morgagni, are attached to the fringes of the tube by a thin pedicle. They are remnants of mesonephric tubules.

The wall of the tube consists of three layers—a serosal coat, a muscular layer, and a mucosal lining. The tunica muscularis is composed of an inner circular and an outer longitudinal layer of smooth muscle fibers. The interstitial portion is equipped with an additional, innermost, longitudinal muscle layer. The muscular coat is thicker in the medial section than in the ampullary portion, where the longitudinal muscle bundles are more widely separated. Contraction of the longitudinal muscle fibers of the ovarian fimbria brings the infundibulum in close contact with the surface of the ovary.

The abundant blood supply of the tubes is derived from the ovarian and uterine blood vessels. The blood vessels are strikingly abundant, particularly in the infundibulum and the fimbriae, where they form with interspersed muscle bundles a kind of erectile tissue, which, if engorged, enables the tube to sweep over the surface of the ovary.

The mucosa (endosalpinx) is thrown into longitudinal folds that are sparse, low, and broad in the inner portions but numerous, branched, and slender in the ampullary portion. The simple mucosal arrangement of the inner sections contrasts strikingly with the complicated, labyrinth-like appearance of the arborescent mucosa in the ampulla.

The mucosa rests on a thin basement membrane, is connected with the muscularis by a thin layer of loose, vascular connective tissue, and can undergo moderate decidual reaction if a fertilized ovum becomes implanted in the tube.

The tubal mucosa consists of a single layer of columnar cells, some of which are ciliated, whereas others are secretory. A third group of peg-shaped cells with dark nuclei is intercalated between the ciliated and secretory cells and represents apparently worn-out cells, which are gradually cast out into the lumen of the tube. The numerical relationship between ciliated and secretory cells changes during the menstrual cycle. The number of secretory cells that secrete nutrient material to sustain the ovum during its stay in the tube is greater in the luteal phase. The height of the tubal epithelium reaches its peak during the period of ovulation and is lowest during menstruation.

The motion of the tubal cilia is directed toward the uterus, causing a current that can sweep small particles into the uterus, but peristaltic action and not the ciliary motion drives the ovum toward the uterus.

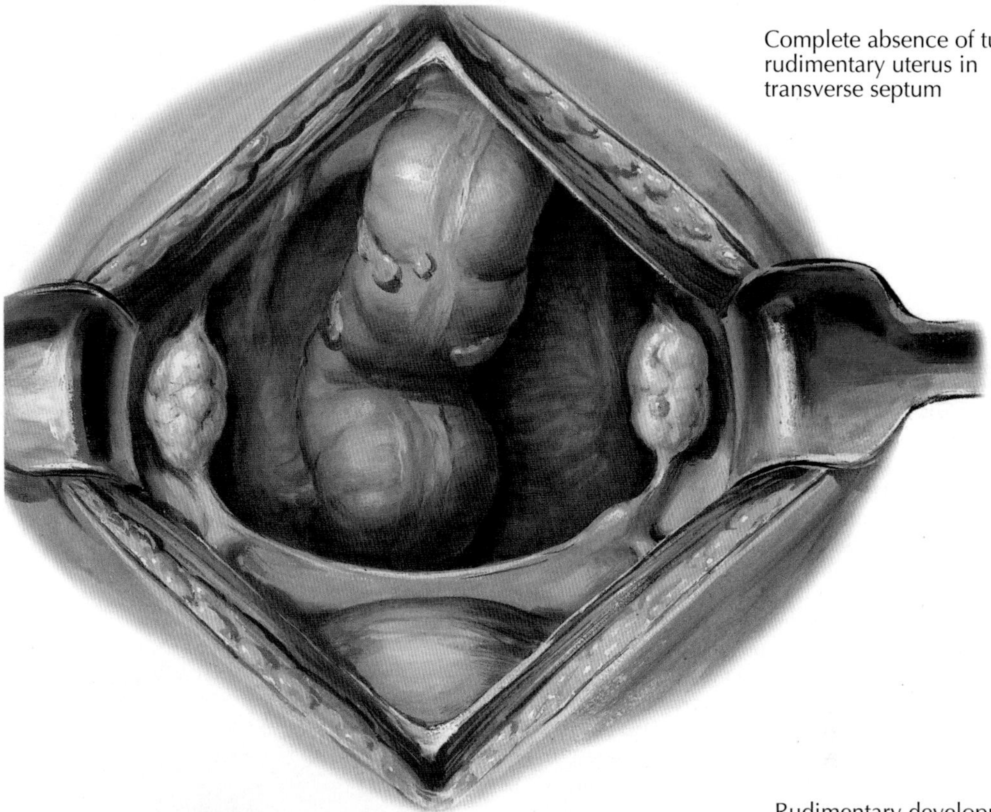

Plate 9.2   Fallopian Tubes

Complete absence of tubes; rudimentary uterus in transverse septum

CONGENITAL ANOMALIES: ABSENCE, RUDIMENTS

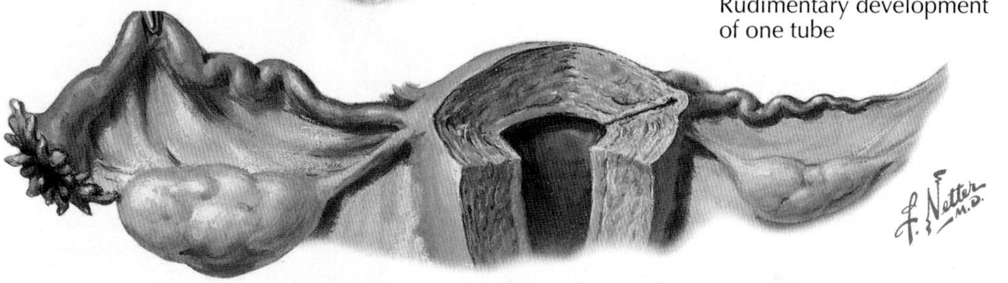

The fallopian tubes arise from the unfused cranial portions of the müllerian (paramesonephric) ducts. The origin of these ducts is first indicated in embryos of 8.5 to 10 mm in length by grooves in the thickened epithelium of the urogenital ridge lateral to the wolffian ducts, which were formed in an earlier stage of development. Soon these grooves become deeper and advance caudad as tubes until they meet the epithelium of the urogenital sinus in a prominence, the müllerian tubercle.

The development and growth of the müllerian ducts depend on the presence of the wolffian ducts. As a rule, the müllerian duct fails to develop when the ipsilateral wolffian duct is lacking. In the absence of müllerian inhibiting factor made by the Sertoli cells of the developing testes, the mesonephric ducts regress, and the paramesonephric ducts develop into the female genital tract. The more cephalad portions of the paramesonephric ducts, which open directly into the peritoneal cavity, form the fallopian tubes.

The paramesonephric ducts, and similarly the wolffian duct, grow more slowly than the fetal trunk as a whole. As a result, the location of the coelomic ostia of the ducts gradually slides caudally to the fourth lumbar segment. Originally, the urogenital fold, which contains the mesonephros and the wolffian and müllerian ducts, has a sagittal course parallel to the spine. The development and growth of the adrenals and kidneys cephalad to these structures change the direction of the urogenital fold, bending it laterally in its upper section. With progressive descent of the ovary and the fallopian tube, the direction of the tube becomes more transverse, whereas the lower parts of the müllerian ducts, which give rise to the uterus, retain their original longitudinal course and fuse in the midline.

The muscular and connective tissues of the tubes are first apparent in the third month of fetal life and may be clearly demonstrated in the fifth month. However, the ampullary portion does not take on its characteristic appearance until the last month of gestation.

Congenital anomalies of the fallopian tubes may be due to developmental error or injury, such as torsion or inflammation. Complete absence of both tubes is sometimes observed in combination with aplasia of the uterus. In such cases, a transverse pelvic septum, corresponding to the broad ligament, connects the ovaries and may contain muscular nodules in the lateral sections of its upper margin that represent rudiments of the müllerian ducts. The round ligaments, which have a separate origin, may be well developed. In these cases, aplasia of the vagina is common but not the rule.

Absence of the ampullary portion of the tube is probably caused by twisting and subsequent necrosis with

Rudimentary development of one tube

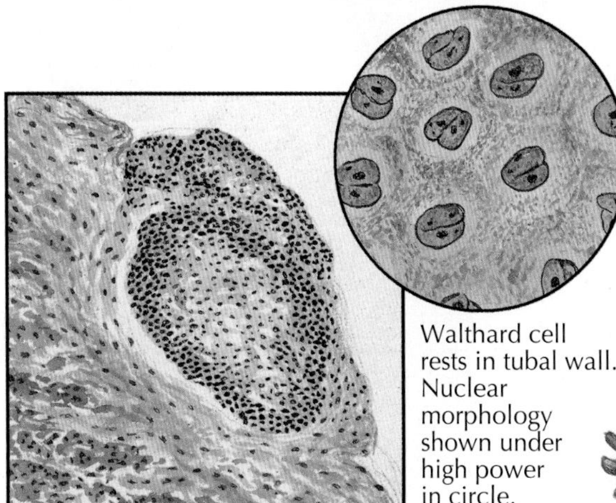

Walthard cell rests in tubal wall. Nuclear morphology shown under high power in circle.

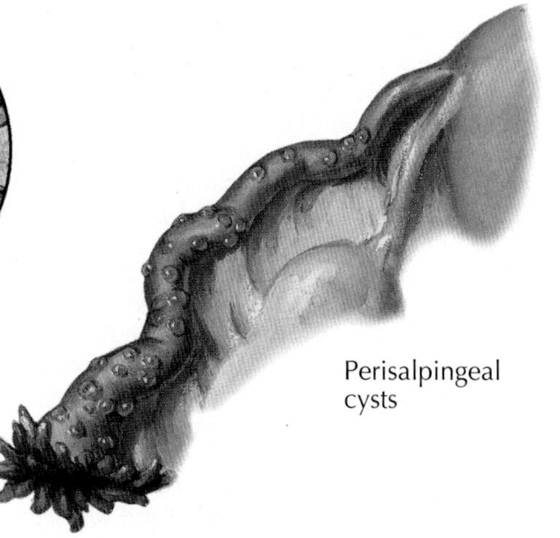

Perisalpingeal cysts

resorption of the ampullary portion of the tube rather than a result of developmental failure. A congenital defect of the wolffian duct is, as a rule, followed by a defect of the homolateral müllerian duct. The resulting anomaly is characterized by the absence of the fallopian tube, the uterine horn, the ipsilateral kidney, and the ureter.

Small, solid, or cystic nodules of a type first described by Walthard and thus called "Walthard cell rests" are commonly found in the subserosal tissue of the fallopian

tube. The nuclei of these Walthard cells show a median groove or fold, which is a fundamental characteristic of these cells.

Frequently found on the surface of otherwise normal fallopian tubes are tiny multiple serosal (perisalpingeal) cysts. They apparently originate from an invagination and occlusion of the serosal epithelium and do not have any practical significance. The supposition of some authors that these cysts are caused by chronic inflammation is not generally accepted.

Plate 9.3

Reproductive System: VOLUME 1

CONGENITAL ANOMALIES: ATRESIA, DEFECTS

Unilateral complete or partial defects of one müllerian duct are more common than aplasia of both ducts. Many variations of this anomaly are encountered, such as uterus unicornis, with or without rudimentary contralateral horn; unilateral atresia; or total, partial, or regional defect of the fallopian tube. The genesis of partial defects of the fallopian tubes is very hard to explain. But the same holds true for similar congenital defects occurring in other hollow organs, for example, the esophagus, the small intestine, and the vas deferens. The nature of the temporarily inhibiting factor responsible for the defects in the lumen or the continuity of these organs is unknown, and all attempts to explain these lesions have failed hitherto.

More frequent than defects due to inadequate tubal development are excess anomalies such as accessory tubal ostia, accessory tubes, and supernumerary tubes. Nevertheless, a supernumerary tube (tuba supernumeraria or tertia) is a great rarity. Such a tube runs parallel to the main tube and has the same structure. It can occur with or without a supernumerary ovary.

In contrast to the rarity of supernumerary tubes, accessory tubes and accessory tubal ostia are very frequent. The accessory tubes arise either from the main tube or from the mesosalpinx and consist of a more or less well-developed wreath of fimbriae with a pedicle, which is usually thin and may be either hollow or solid. Even if hollow, it does not communicate with the cavity of the main tube. If the lumen of the accessory tube is closed at both ends, it becomes transformed into a small pedunculated vesicle. Production of tubal fluids within this blind segment can result in cystic dilation, mimicking a hydrosalpinx or ovarian cyst.

Although accessory tubes may arise from any part of the ampullary portion of the tube and even from the isthmic section, accessory tubal ostia are always situated near the main ostium. The accessory ostia have the same appearance and structure as the main ostium. They always communicate with the tubal cavity. There has even been a single case report in which laparotomy demonstrated that the proximal portion of one fallopian tube was absent and that the distal end was separated into three portions.

Hypoplasia of the fallopian tube is frequently seen. The hypoplastic tube is thin and ischemic, its musculature weak, and its ampulla poorly developed. A special type, commonly designated as "infantile tube," is characterized by tight windings that are bridged by peritoneal folds and, therefore, cannot be straightened. It may be that the peritoneal bridges between the tubal windings interfere with the tubal peristalsis in the same way as do adhesions and predispose to retention of the fertilized ovum in the tube and thereby to the occurrence of ectopic pregnancy.

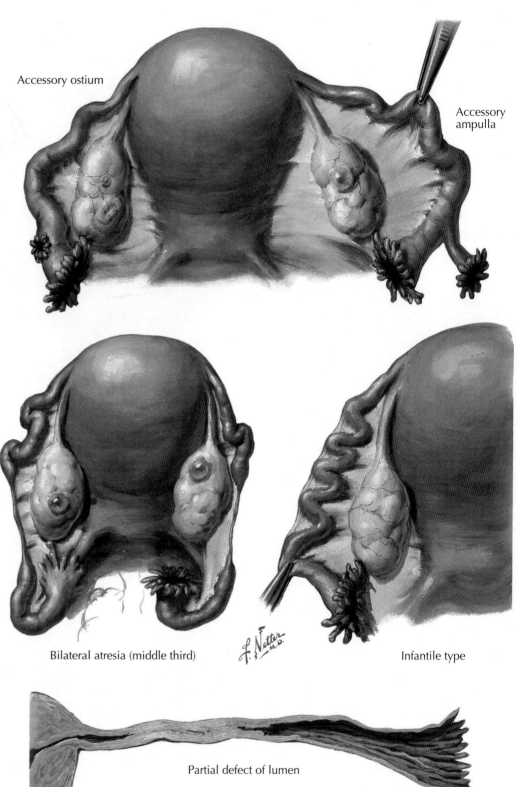

Accessory ostium

Accessory ampulla

Bilateral atresia (middle third)

Infantile type

Partial defect of lumen

In utero exposure to diethylstilbestrol has been associated with fallopian tubes notable for pinpoint ostia, constricted fimbriae, and a short or a sacculated or convoluted course. These changes may be a cause of female infertility and are generally not detected by hysterosalpingography. It has also been postulated that salpingitis isthmica nodosa may follow diethylstilbestrol exposure during gestation.

Incomplete descent and steep course of the tube are other forms of developmental arrest. Excessive descent and dislocation of the tubes and ovaries in inguinal hernias may occasionally be seen, especially in intersexual individuals. Incomplete union of the müllerian ducts in their uterine sections and lateral flexion of the uterine horn favor the dislocation of the tube and ovary into inguinal hernias.

Conventional therapy consisted of surgical correction, where possible, but the availability and success of oocyte harvesting, in vitro fertilization, and embryo transfer have generally supplanted surgical therapy.

Plate 9.4

Fallopian Tubes

ACUTE SALPINGITIS: BACTERIAL ROUTES, PARAMETRITIS

Inflammatory diseases are not only frequent but also potentially serious—with both immediate and long-term consequences. The open communication of the fallopian tube with the peritoneal cavity exposes the tube to any peritoneal infection and vice versa. Appendicitis is a frequent source of infection of the right or of both tubes; sigmoiditis and diverticulitis often migrate to the left tube. Sometimes the hematogenous route infects the tubes. This is the rule in tuberculous salpingitis.

Inflammatory disorders of the uterus frequently extend to the fallopian tubes. The ciliary current of the tube is a very weak protective apparatus, and the narrow communication between tube and uterus is an ineffective barrier. Besides, the narrow lumen proves to be a serious handicap when the tube is inflamed. Swelling of the mucous membrane may cause complete occlusion of the uterotubal junction, thereby preventing drainage of inflammatory secretions into the uterine cavity and potentially forcing infected material further toward the fimbrial end and the peritoneal cavity.

The uterus, because of its free drainage and periodic menstrual shedding, may appear healed, whereas the inflammation in the occluded tubes persists. On the other hand, the occurrence of tubal inflammatory disease is favored by the tendency of the uterus to react to abnormal stimuli, such as bacteria or chemicals, by spasm of the internal cervical os and severe contractions, which drive these noxious agents into the tubes. Lipid imaging solutions, which are occasionally used for hysterosalpingography, may cause serious damage to the tubes.

Bacteria may invade the tubes from the uterus or from the bloodstream. The latter holds true for *Mycobacterium tuberculosis,* whereas gonococci, *Chlamydia,* and most other bacteria reach the tube by way of the mucous membranes. Gonococci settle mainly in the mucosa and have little tendency to invade deeper tissues, though they do tend to cause a transluminal inflammatory response. In contrast, chlamydial infections tend to engender a much milder but longer-lived inflammatory response, accounting for their often indolent course and greater degree of long-term tubal damage.

Streptococci and staphylococci also propagate in the mucosa but rapidly penetrate the deeper structures and invade the lymphatics and blood vessels of the uterine and tubal walls and adjacent connective tissue. The most conspicuous changes, which occur in streptococcic and staphylococcic infections, take place in the pelvic connective tissue.

The parametral lymphatics and veins are filled with pus and partly solid, partly liquefied thrombi, whereas the surrounding tissue is distended by serous and seropurulent exudate. These changes constitute parametritis, which is mainly a lymphangitis and thrombophlebitis. Because the blood and lymph vessels are contained in the condensed zones of the pelvic connective tissue, the inflammatory infiltrate assumes the shape of these zones. It is wedge-shaped, with the base directed toward the pelvic wall and the blunt apex at the uterus. According to

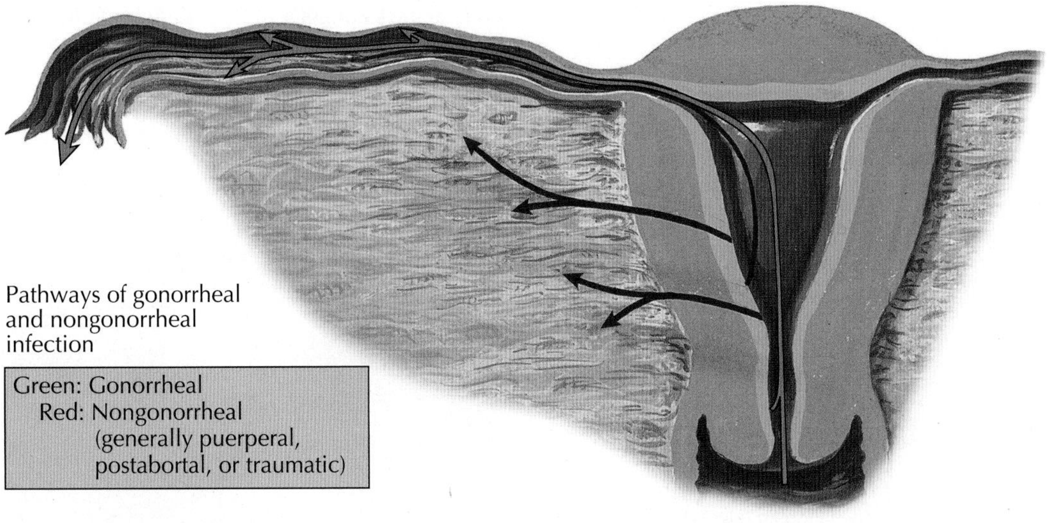

Pathways of gonorrheal and nongonorrheal infection

Green: Gonorrheal
   Red: Nongonorrheal
      (generally puerperal, postabortal, or traumatic)

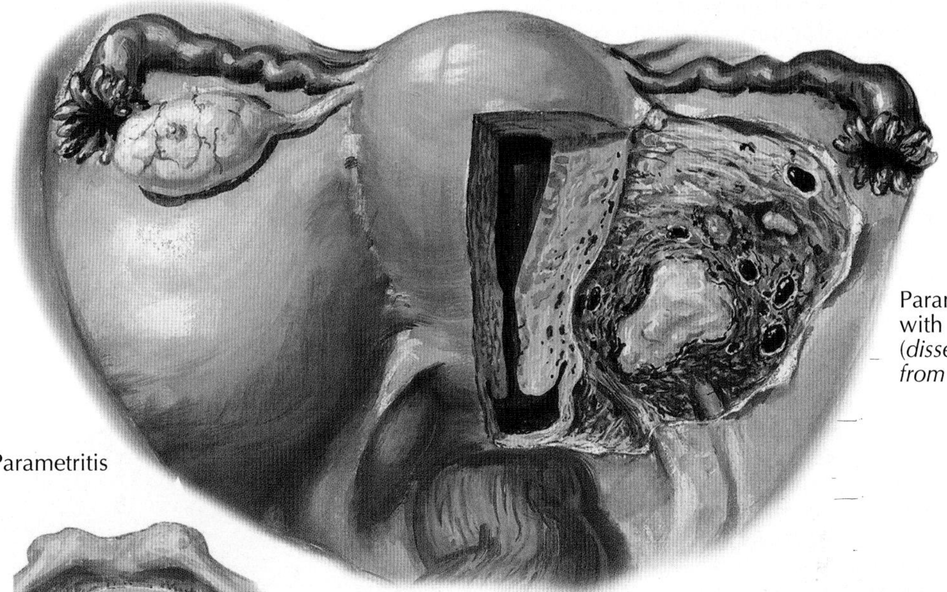

Parametritis

Parametritis with abscess (*dissection from behind*)

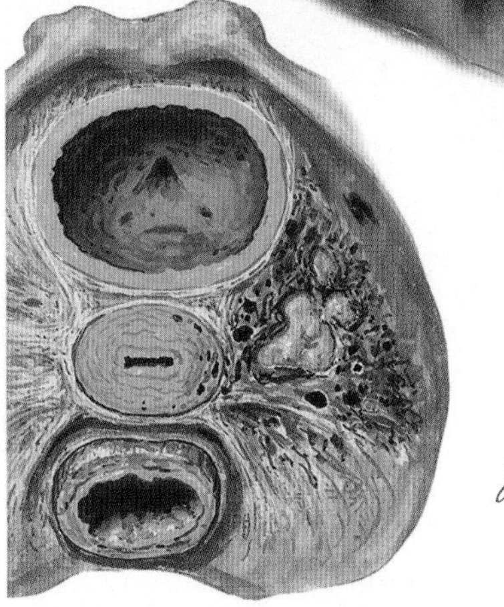

Parametritis with abscess (*dissection from above*) showing extension laterally, forward, and backward

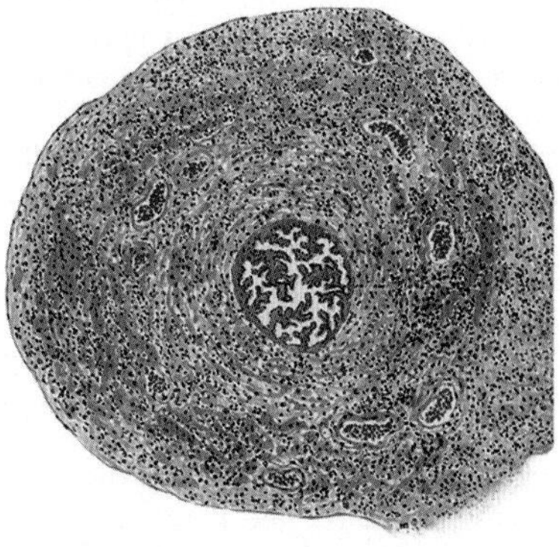

Nongonorrheal salpingitis; infiltration chiefly in tubal wall

the arrangement of the zones of condensed connective tissue, an anterior, posterior, and median parametritis can be distinguished. In severe infections, all three zones are affected. Sometimes the purulent infection destroys the parametrial structures, causing a parametrial abscess, which may break into the zones of loose connective tissue and rapidly spread within these zones and the connected areas. The rounded shape of a large parametrial abscess can modify somewhat the wedge shape of the unliquefied, rigid parametrial infiltrate.

Risk factors for salpingitis include early (age) sexual activity and multiple sexual partners. These and related risk factors primarily affect the likelihood of acquiring gonococcal and chlamydial infections of the cervix, which, in turn, ascend into the upper genital tract, causing salpingitis. Uterine instrumentation (hysterosalpingography, intrauterine contraceptive device placement, endometrial biopsy, dilation and curettage) can also cause salpingitis, but this occurs infrequently in the absence of sexually transmitted infections.

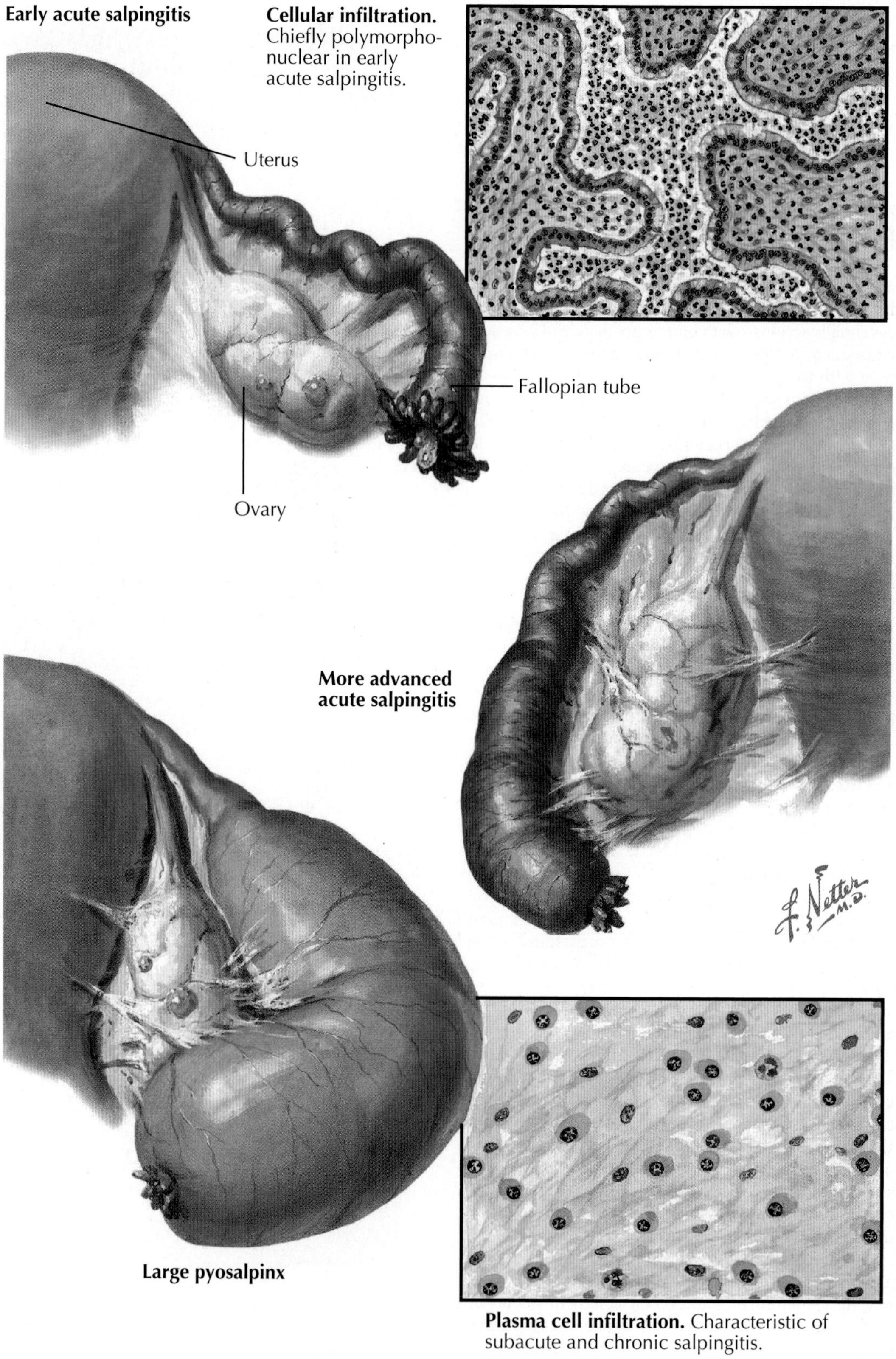

Plate 9.5

Reproductive System: VOLUME 1

ACUTE SALPINGITIS: PYOSALPINX

In acute salpingitis the fallopian tube is swollen and reddened, its tortuosity is more pronounced, the mucosal folds are thickened and hyperemic, and its lumen is filled with pus. The serosa loses its luster and may be covered with fibrinous or fibropurulent exudate (perisalpingitis).

In nongonorrheal salpingitis, all layers share about equally in the inflammatory changes. The lymphatics and blood vessels are dilated and filled with polynuclear leukocytes and thrombi. In gonorrheal salpingitis, the infiltrate is located chiefly in the mucosa. The epithelium of the edematous folds is destroyed in wide areas, and the denuded edges of the folds become adherent.

The course of any salpingitis may be very slow and indolent. In exceptional cases, the acutely inflamed tube may heal with complete restoration of structure and function. Usually, however, the acute stage is followed by a subacute and eventually by a chronic inflammatory stage, with various anatomic and functional sequelae. The polynuclear leukocytes gradually diminish in number and are replaced by plasma cells, which are particularly numerous in gonorrheal salpingitis but are not pathognomonic of this infection. The ampullary ostium, sometimes unilaterally, sometimes bilaterally, may close early by inversion and conglutination of the fimbriae. The inflammatory processes may also cause a closure of the uterine end of the tubes, and in other instances both the uterine and ampullary sections may become partially or completely occluded. When this closure occurs, the tube becomes more and more distended. It loses its normal windings and changes into a sausage- or retort-shaped structure called a pyosalpinx. Usually, the causative bacteria disappear in the purulent contents, whereas they may survive for a long time in the depth of the tubal wall, maintaining a chronic inflammatory condition. With gradual dilation of the tube, its folds become lower and can be destroyed. The tubal wall is usually thickened, and the musculature is replaced by connective tissue in some areas. The serosa is deprived of its endothelium in many places and becomes adherent to neighboring organs. The content of a pyosalpinx may be liquid and show fibrinopurulent flakes suspended in a serous exudate, or it may contain thick, greenish-yellow pus or mucopurulent fluid. Old pyosalpinges frequently contain cholesterol crystals or, sometimes, aggregated cholesterol concrements.

Under favorable circumstances, the immunologic system eliminates the offending organisms and the inflammatory processes halt, but they often leave a thickened, closed fallopian tube densely adherent to the ovary and the posterior leaf of the broad ligament. In other cases, the inflammatory changes progress, and the pyosalpinx perforates into the rectum, into the peritoneal cavity, or, less frequently, into the bladder. Whereas

the perforation into the rectum brings about temporary relief, the perforation into the bladder causes considerable dysuria, and the perforation into the peritoneal cavity results in serious peritonitis, which requires immediate surgical intervention. The danger of such an accident is highly increased in cases of pregnancy complicated by unilateral pyosalpinx. Loosening of protective adhesions, rupture of the pyosalpinx, and escape of pus into the higher regions of the abdomen have been repeatedly observed in such cases.

Very often an acute pyosalpinx combines, especially in puerperal sepsis, with a parametritis. Then the infection spreads along the lymphatics and veins as well as along the mucosal lining. When the parametritic exudate, thanks to its greater healing tendency, has been absorbed, the pyosalpinx may be palpated—in the subacute and chronic cases—as a tender, fixed, sausage-shaped, or ovoid tumor, usually situated in pouch of Douglas (cul-de-sac), which, if large enough, pushes the uterus anteriorly and toward the less affected side.

Early acute salpingitis

Cellular infiltration. Chiefly polymorphonuclear in early acute salpingitis.

Uterus

Fallopian tube

Ovary

More advanced acute salpingitis

Large pyosalpinx

Plasma cell infiltration. Characteristic of subacute and chronic salpingitis.

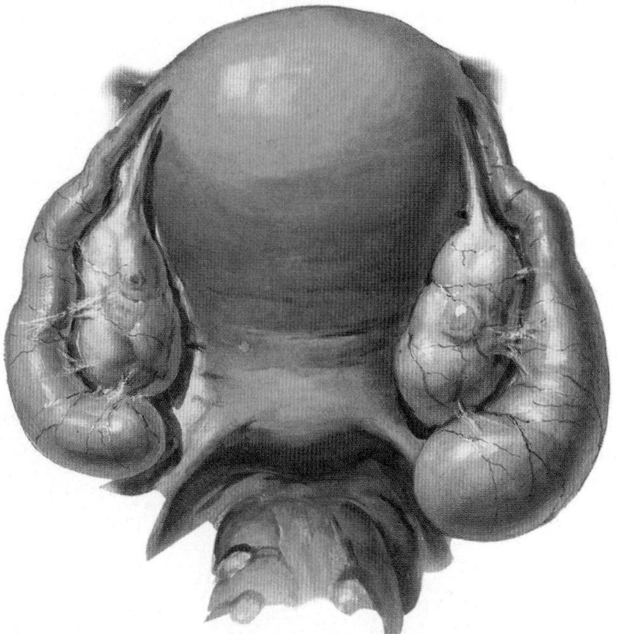

Plate 9.6

Fallopian Tubes

HYDROSALPINX

Recurrent or chronic adnexal infections may result in a cystic dilation of the fallopian tube (hydrosalpinx), which may present as an adnexal mass. The purulent contents of the pyosalpinx may thicken and gradually be replaced by granulation tissue, which is sometimes calcified and, in rare instances, even ossified. More often, however, the solid constituents of the tubal contents are gradually liquefied and changed into a sterile serous or serosanguineous fluid, thus transforming the pyosalpinx into a hydrosalpinx.

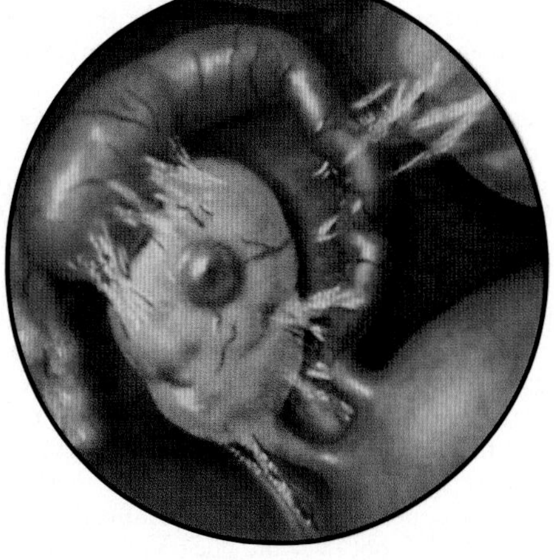

After resorption of the inflammatory infiltrate and the degenerated tissue, the tubal wall becomes thin and poor in muscle fibers and assumes a translucent appearance. The size of the hydrosalpinx can vary from twice that of a normal tube to that of a large sausage-like creation 3 cm or more in diameter, which, in form, has completely lost all resemblance to the tube from which it derived. The fimbriae in such a hydrosalpinx may have completely disappeared.

In cross sections, the mucosal folds are low and separated from each other by flat areas. Sometimes the folds are completely effaced and are indicated only by flat ridges or are not recognizable at all.

This form of hydrosalpinx (sometimes referred to as hydrosalpinx simplex) may develop over a period of many years without causing any symptoms that would prompt a patient to seek medical attention. This is understandable, because microscopically this thin-walled cavity may appear to have lost all evidence of the originally infectious and inflammatory process. In other instances, foci of a chronic inflammation can be found in the tubal wall. As a rule, however, microorganisms cannot be cultured from the cystic fluid.

The same holds true for the pseudofollicular hydrosalpinx, which differs from the simplex type only in its cross section. Here the tubal folds may have been preserved to a certain extent but have grown together at their opposing ridges and branches, forming a labyrinth of hollow spaces. This pseudofollicular hydrosalpinx is said to be most often the result of gonorrheal infection but may also be encountered in chronic salpingitis of other origin.

The occlusion of the tube on its uterine end is not always tight. In rare cases, the tubal lumen is blocked in this section only by valvelike folds and may open if the hydrosalpinx becomes distended. This condition, which is characterized by the periodic escape of tubal contents and accompanied by colicky pain, is called "hydrops tubae profluens."

In hydrosalpinx, the peritubal adhesions are often few and filmy, and hence torsion of an oviduct is no rare occurrence. Extravasation of blood into the twisted tube changes the hydrosalpinx into a hematosalpinx.

The diagnosis of hydrosalpinx, and incidentally also of pyosalpinx, is not always an easy one. They may be mistaken, particularly if they are very large, for ovarian cysts, although the latter are more movable and rounded. Laboratory pregnancy tests may prove useful in the differentiation from ectopic pregnancy. From a cooperative patient, one will always obtain a history of a past acute episode of pelvic infection, which, with the findings of the physical examination, will lead to the correct diagnosis. Although a patient may report a history of a past acute episode, the history of pelvic infection is usually not volunteered.

Surgical therapy for a hydrosalpinx (salpingectomy or salpingoophorectomy) is curative. Neosalpingostomy may be considered when fertility is to be maintained, but the success of this procedure is inversely proportional to the size of the hydrosalpinx and is generally less than 15%. More often, in vitro fertilization, bypassing the damaged tubes, is recommended, though the success rates are lower in these patients and pregnancy complications higher if the damaged tube is allowed to remain in place. Prior to in vitro fertilization, removal of the affected hydrosalpinx improves implantation and pregnancy rates.

Small and moderate-sized hydrosalpinx

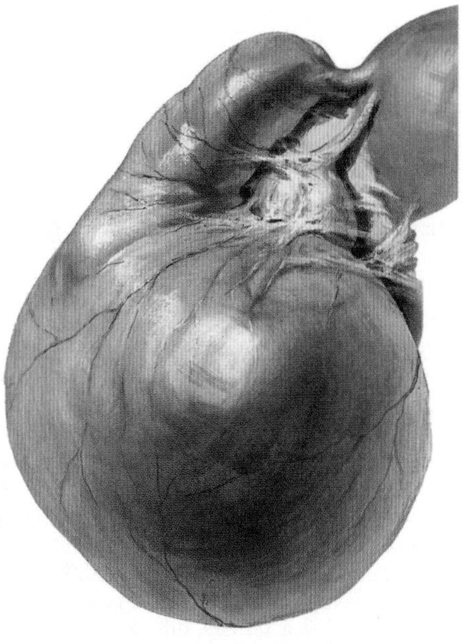

Large cystic hydrosalpinx

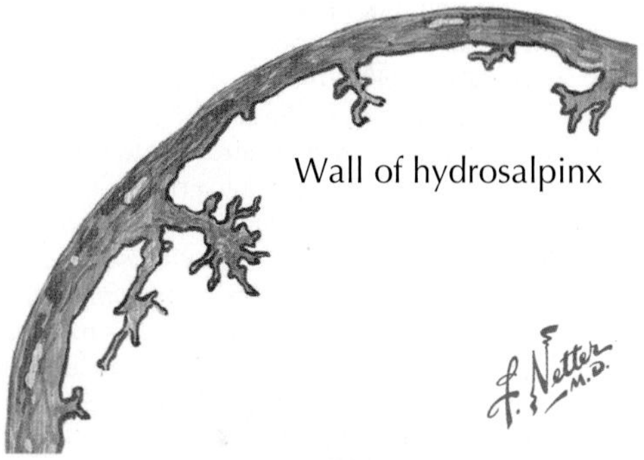

Wall of hydrosalpinx

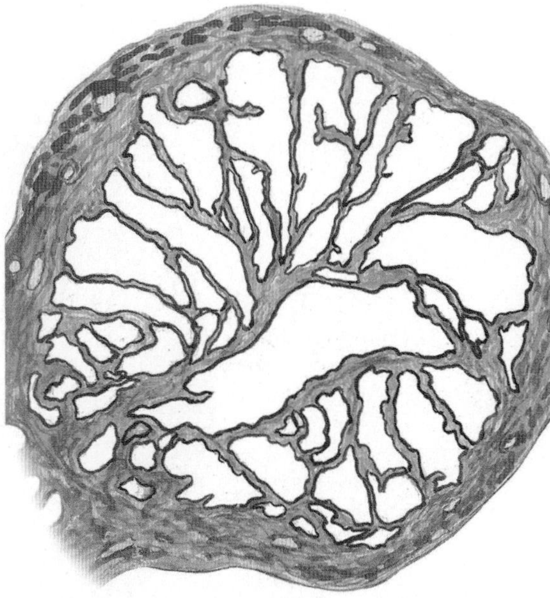

Pseudofollicular hydrosalpinx

Laparoscopic view

Plate 9.7

Reproductive System: VOLUME 1

PELVIC PERITONITIS, ABSCESS

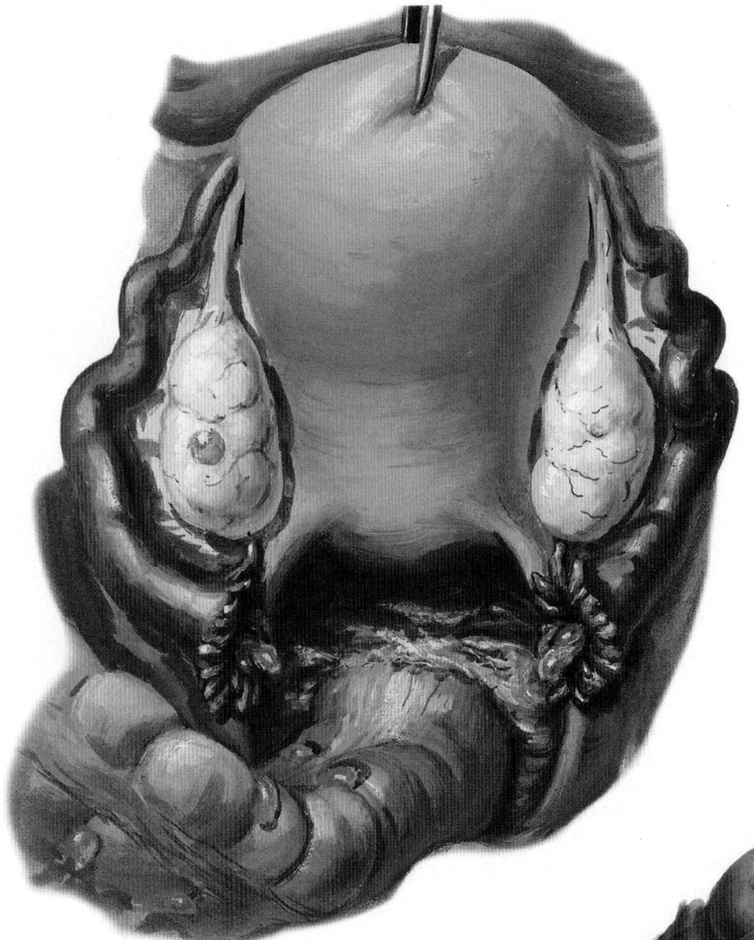

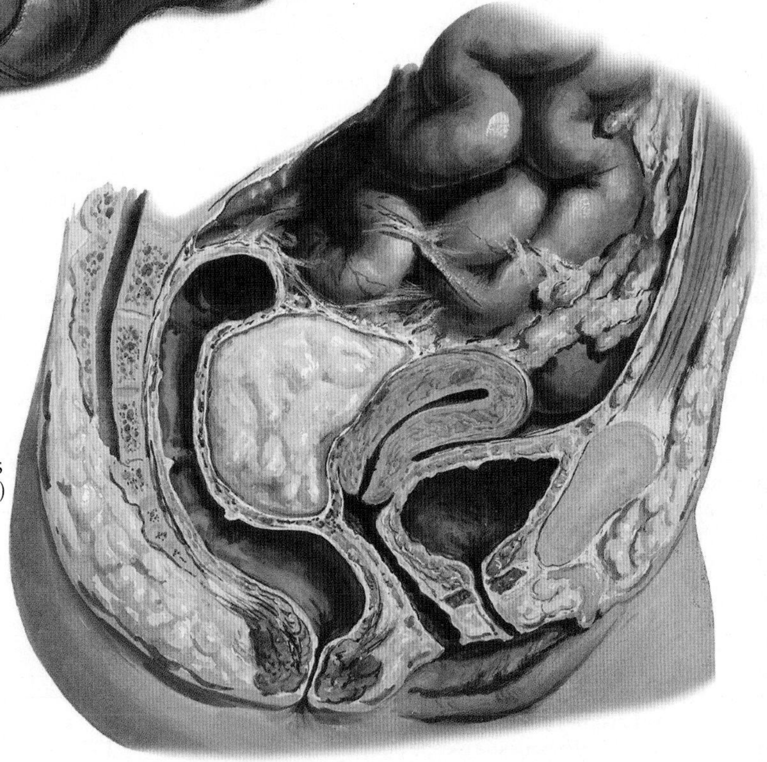

If the ampullary ostium is patent, the purulent contents of the infected fallopian tube escape into the peritoneal cavity, causing a peritonitis, which is at first diffuse but, in favorable cases, may become confined to the pelvic cavity. Even when the tubes have become blocked, widespread peritonitis may result from spread of perisalpingitis, tubal lymphangitis, or rupture of a tube. Whereas acute parametritis often leads to septicemia, if the loose or liquefied infected thrombi enter the general circulation, acute salpingitis causes a diffuse or circumscribed pelvic peritonitis. Thus pelvic inflammatory disease (PID) is a serious, diffuse, frequently multiorganism infection of the pelvic organs that results in significant morbidity.

The severity and extent of the peritonitis depend on the type of pathogenic bacteria, their virulence, the resistance of the patient, and the efficiency of treatment. In roughly one-third of cases, the causative organism is *Neisseria gonorrhoeae* alone. One-third of cases involve infection with *N. gonorrhoeae* and additional "mixed" infections with other organisms. The last third of infections are due to mixed aerobic and anaerobic bacteria, including respiratory pathogens such as *Haemophilus influenzae, Streptococcus pneumoniae,* and *Streptococcus pyogenes* found in up to 5% of patients. Polymicrobial infections are present in more than 40% of patients with laparoscopically proven salpingitis, with one study reporting an average of 6.8 bacterial types per patient. Only approximately 15% of females with cervical *N. gonorrhoeae* infections develop acute pelvic infections. Orgasmic uterine contractions, disruption of normally protective cervical mucus at ovulation or during menses, the attachment of *N. gonorrhoeae* to sperm or direct inoculation at the time of surgical procedures, like placement of an intrauterine device, may provide transportation to the upper genital tract. *Chlamydia* is involved in roughly 20% of patients, with this rate rising to roughly 40% among hospitalized patients. Infection of the upper genital tract by *Chlamydia* often causes an indolent course of salpingitis with more insidious symptoms.

During upper genital tract infections, purulent material accumulates in the cul-de-sac and may become sealed off from the rest of the peritoneal cavity by adhesions between the pelvic organs, omentum, and intestinal loops. Frequently, the sigmoid and the mesosigmoid become adherent to the uterine fundus and the upper border of the broad ligament, forming a protective roof over the pocket of pus. This pelvioperitonitic abscess, commonly called a tubo-ovarian abscess, is a protective mechanism to localize and contain the infectious process.

A tubo-ovarian abscess can be surgically opened and drained via the anterior abdominal wall, by laparotomy or laparoscopy, or by a transvaginal route. In some unique situations, interventional radiologists may drain a tubo-ovarian abscess by inserting an imaging guided catheter into the affected area. Pelvic peritonitis very seldom heals without leaving adhesions between the pelvic organs, the sigmoid, and the omentum. Very often, the uterus is pulled backward into a permanent state of retroflexion by adhesions with the rectum and

Pelvic peritonitis

Cul-de-sac abscess
(pouch of Douglas)

the pelvic wall. This fixed uterine retroflexion can cause troublesome symptoms such as backache, constipation, and pain during defecation and copulation. Surgical extirpation may be the only option when symptoms are significant and unresponsive to other therapies.

Roughly one in four females with acute PID experiences medical sequelae. Pelvic inflammatory disease leads to tubal factor infertility, ectopic pregnancy, and chronic abdominal pain in a high percentage of patients. The risk of infertility roughly doubles with

each subsequent episode, resulting in a 40% rate of infertility after only three episodes. One single episode of severe PID can cause infertility. Females with documented salpingitis have a fourfold increase in their rate of ectopic pregnancy, and 5% to 15% of females require surgery because of damage caused by pelvic inflammatory disease. Peritoneal involvement may spread to include perihepatitis (Fitz-Hugh-Curtis syndrome). Rupture of a tubo-ovarian abscess, with subsequent septic shock, may be life-threatening.

Plate 9.8

Fallopian Tubes

CHRONIC SALPINGITIS, ADHESIONS

In chronic salpingitis, the uterine tubal ostium is often obliterated, and the tube cannot be visualized by hysterosalpingography. This must be differentiated from spasms of the isthmic portion of the tube, which are frequently encountered and resist uterotubal insufflation. Spasms can be overcome using moderate pressure or at the time of laparoscopy under general anesthesia.

Peritoneal adhesions connecting the tube with the ovary and the posterior leaf of the broad ligament may kink the tube and thus cause infertility. They are recognizable on hysterosalpingography by a characteristic spill pattern. Frequently, these pelvioperitonitic adhesions involve all pelvic organs, including the omentum and low intestinal loops. The adhesions are richly vascular at first, but gradually they become poorly vascularized, frail, and spiderweb-like. Only in rare cases may they disappear entirely.

The most conspicuous symptom of chronic salpingitis is pain, which may be continuous or elicited by stress, defecation, and intercourse and may be aggravated by the hyperemia and swelling of the premenstrual phase. Dysmenorrhea may also occur, but more frequently the menstrual flow relieves the pain, and the patient feels better during and after menstruation. Dyspareunia is frequent, and intermenstrual pain (mittelschmerz) is occasionally observed.

Females with chronic adnexitis are usually sterile. If the tubes become finally patent again, ectopic pregnancy often occurs owing to impaired peristalsis, stenosis, loss of normal ciliary function, and kinks in the tubes. Assisted reproduction techniques that bypass the damaged tube can result in conception, but these patients tend to continue to have higher than normal pregnancy loss rates as long as the damaged tube is retained.

The differential diagnosis between an inflammatory adnexal tumor and a parametritic infiltrate is not always easy. The adnexal tumor has convex outlines, whereas the surfaces of the parametritic infiltrate are concave. In combined diseases of the adnexa and the parametrium, the palpable tumor is convex above and concave below, and its broad base is attached to the lateral pelvic wall. An adnexal tumor can be separated from the pelvic wall by the examining finger, whereas parametritic infiltrates are frequently in close contact with the wall structures. Ultrasonography may only demonstrate cystic loculations, making it difficult to differentiate between ovarian cysts, consolidated adnexal damage, and entrapped omentum and bowel.

Ectopic pregnancy may develop in a chronically diseased tube. The menstrual history in such instances is often not characteristic. Tenderness of the palpated tumor, increased erythrocyte sedimentation rate, and moderate leukocytosis are common for both ectopic pregnancy and adnexal tumor. A positive pregnancy test indicates pregnancy, but a negative test does not always disprove it. Rapid increase in the size of the tumor, despite normal temperature, and development of severe unilateral colicky pain or of sudden shock speak for ectopic pregnancy. Ultrasonography may demonstrate decidual changes in the uterine cavity but no gestational sac. A gestational sac may or may not be seen in the adnexa.

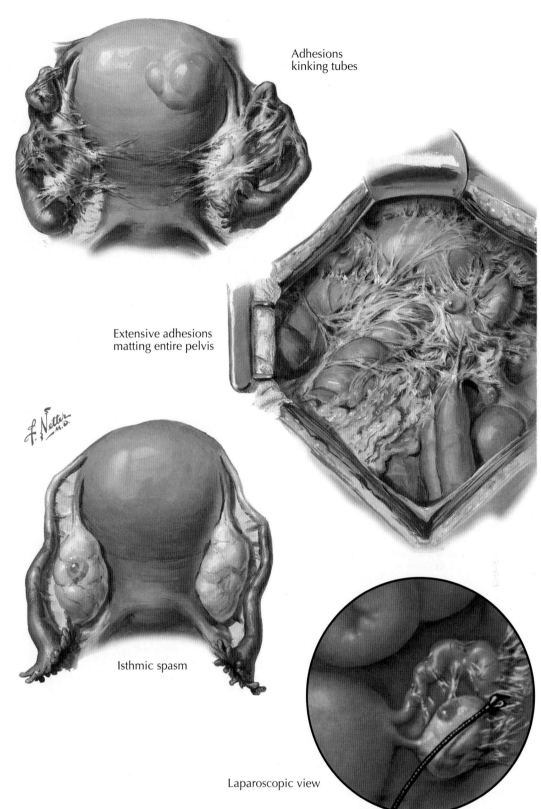

Adhesions kinking tubes

Extensive adhesions matting entire pelvis

Isthmic spasm

Laparoscopic view

Very difficult is the differentiation between a tubal carcinoma and an inflammatory adnexal tumor. With no history of inflammatory disease, the presence of tubal malignancy is probable. A blood-tinged or amber-colored serous discharge is suspicious for tubal carcinoma but may easily be mistaken for a hydrops tubae profluens. A definite diagnosis is usually possible only after microscopic examination following surgery.

History, bilaterality, and the demonstration of gonococci facilitate the differentiation between salpingitis during a gonorrheal or puerperal infection and appendicitis. A tumor on the right side connected with the uterus does not disprove a primary appendicitis with secondary infection of the right tube. In the differential diagnosis between chronic appendicitis and chronic salpingitis, the exact localization of the most tender spot of the abdominal wall and visualization of the appendix on computed tomography or magnetic resonance imaging may prove to be helpful. Sometimes one must resort to laparoscopy or laparotomy.

Plate 9.9

Reproductive System: VOLUME 1

Obstruction Following Chronic Salpingitis

Recurrent or chronic adnexal infections may result in a cystic dilation of the fallopian tube (hydrosalpinx), which may present as an adnexal mass. The chronically inflamed tube, with the exception of the tuberculous tube, is usually closed. It often remains open at its ampullary end, but, owing to the changes in the tubal wall, it only rarely allows the fertilization of the ovum and its transportation into the uterus. Forty percent of female infertility is the result of tubal damage, including the most severe form, hydrosalpinx. Most hydrosalpinx are sterile and are the inactive end stage of tubal disease.

The occlusion of the tube may be located at the uterotubal junction, the isthmic section, or the fimbrial end of the tube. It may be restricted to a closely limited area or may involve large portions of the tube, especially in the narrow isthmic section. If only the interstitial portion is closed, or there is obliteration of the isthmic portion, the outer aspect of the tube may remain unchanged. Only rarely is there a nodular enlargement of the isthmic section of tube.

Following inflammation, the shape of the ampullary end shows many variations. The ampulla may still exhibit a small tuft of short fringes, or it may be clubbed, without any traces of fimbriae. Sometimes a central, shallow dimple may indicate the original tubal opening. In other cases, the inverted fimbriae and the tubal ostium are still recognizable. This latter condition has been called "phimosis" of the tube. Another, less frequent condition, "paraphimosis," consists of a tight constriction of the tube, just medial to its fimbriated end.

Sometimes one tube may be completely closed, whereas the tube on the other side still permits the introduction of a fine probe. As a rule, the tubes remain separated, but in rare cases they may adhere to each other and to the posterior wall of the uterus.

Various attempts to explain the mechanism of tubal closure at the fimbriated end have remained unsuccessful.

The site of tubal obstruction can be determined by laparoscopy or by hysterosalpingography. Sometimes the correct interpretation of hysterosalpingograms requires great experience, and the procedure is not harmless if a nonabsorbable contrast medium such as Lipiodol is used. The latter is usually retained in the closed tube for years, becomes inspissated and causes a foreign-body reaction, which may have a deleterious effect on the hitherto patent portion of the tube. Most contrast materials in use now are water soluble, reducing this risk. A water-soluble contrast medium also provides better visualization of the tubal mucosal folds than does an oil-based medium. It is important to be able to evaluate the appearance of the intratubal architecture to determine the extent of damage to the oviduct. If a hydrosalpinx is seen at hysterosalpingography, an antibiotic such as doxycycline should be continued for 1 week following the procedure. The diagnosis of the site of tubal obstruction is naturally simpler by means of laparoscopy.

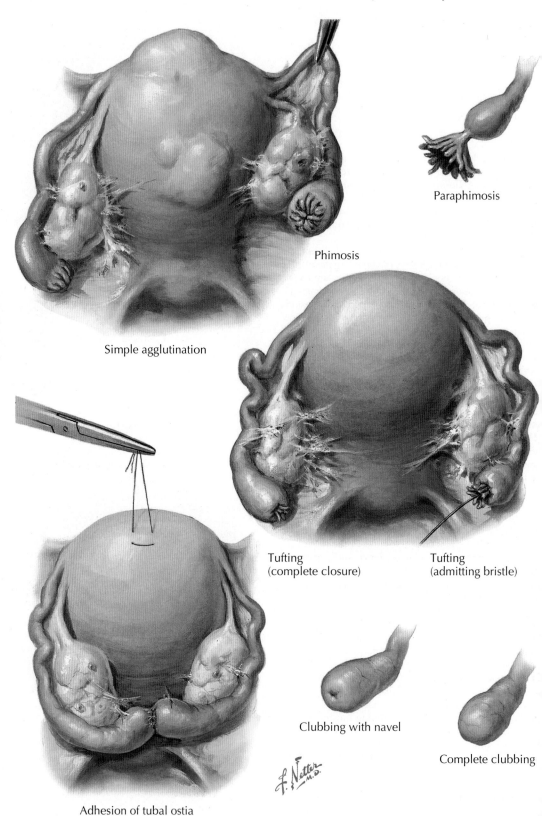

Paraphimosis

Phimosis

Simple agglutination

Tufting (complete closure)

Tufting (admitting bristle)

Clubbing with navel

Complete clubbing

Adhesion of tubal ostia

Surgical therapy (salpingectomy or salpingo-oophorectomy) is curative. Neosalpingostomy may be considered when fertility is to be maintained, but the success of this procedure is inversely proportional to the size of the hydrosalpinx and is generally less than 15%. More often, in vitro fertilization, bypassing the damaged tubes, is recommended, though the success rates are lower in these patients. If the hydrosalpinx is large and clearly visible on ultrasound, it is preferable to perform laparoscopic salpingectomy prior to in vitro fertilization.

When associated pelvic adhesions are symptomatic, they may be lysed during laparoscopy or laparotomy. The success of this is often variable or disappointing either because of reformation after the trauma of surgery or incorrect attribution of symptom causality to the adhesions.

Plate 9.10

Fallopian Tubes

TUBO-OVARIAN ABSCESS

Pathogenesis of tubo-ovarian abscess

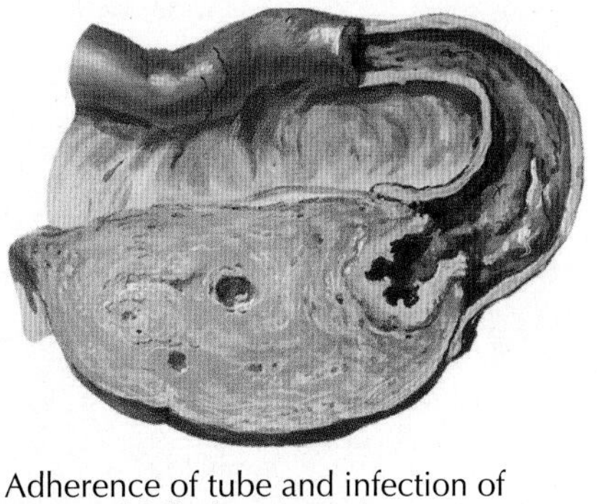

Adherence of tube and infection of ruptured follicle (corpus luteum)

Abscess has progressed, involving most of ovary

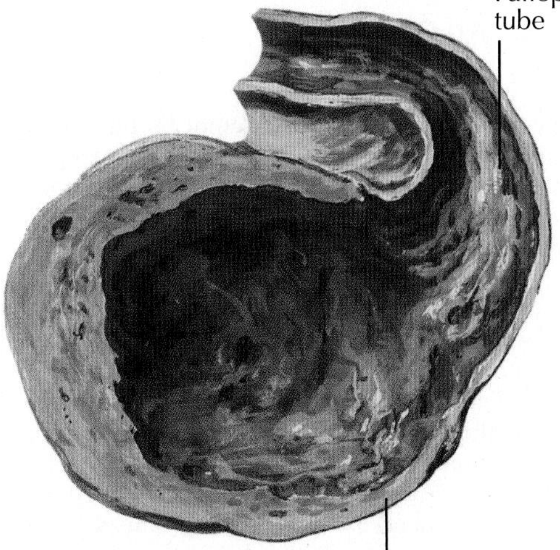

Fallopian tube

Ovary

Fully developed abscess

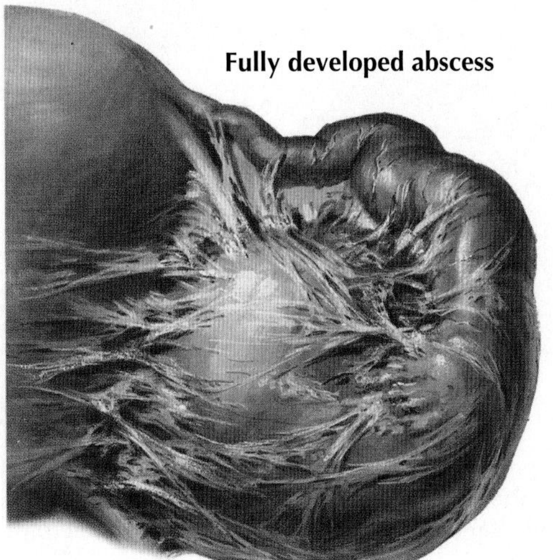

Large tubo-ovarian cyst

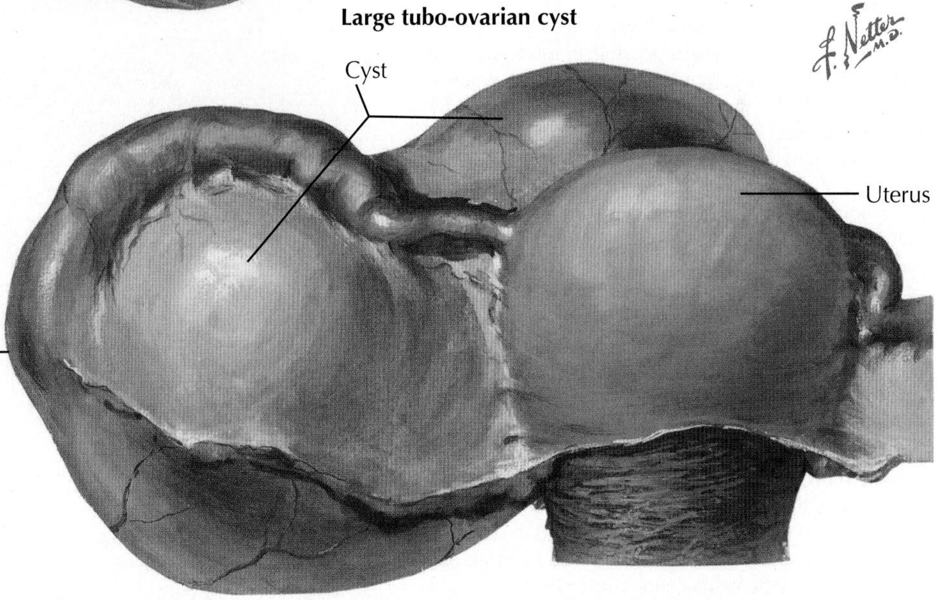

Cyst

Uterus

Fallopian tube

Occasionally, a pyosalpinx communicates with a ruptured follicle or a corpus luteum, leading to a tubo-ovarian abscess. Combined lesions of the fallopian tubes and the ovaries are, however, not limited to this formation, but they are the rule in all tubal inflammations. The ovary may be the site of true bacterial inflammation or may merely be involved in a circulatory disorder and degenerative changes arising from the inflammation of the neighboring tube. The latter changes consist of hyperemia, hemorrhages, and edema of the ovarian stroma; disintegration of the follicular apparatus; loss of surface epithelium; and formation of periovarian adhesions.

The bacterial inflammation may be slight and may heal in the course of time, with or without fibrosis of the ovarian parenchyma, or it may be severe and may result in the formation of abscesses, which may develop in ruptured follicles or in corpora lutea or within the ovarian connective tissue. The follicular and luteal abscesses occur usually when the infection takes place on the surface of the ovary, as is the case in purulent salpingitis or appendicitis. Abscesses in the ovarian stroma are often of hematogenic origin and may remain within the limits of the ovary, though they may reach a large size. Sometimes, however, they burst into the tube or into the peritoneal cavity or a neighboring organ, such as the rectum or the bladder.

Gradually, the follicular components and the specific ovarian stroma are completely destroyed in such ovaries, and the thick wall of the ovarian abscess consists merely of callous connective tissue which is poor in blood vessels and is infiltrated by leukocytes, lymphocytes, and plasma cells, which are accumulated in the inner, granulating lining of the abscess wall.

Follicular and corpus luteum abscesses more often perforate into the tube than do interstitial ovarian abscesses. They may heal after discharging their content into the tube or may be transformed into tubo-ovarian abscesses, with progressive destruction of the ovarian parenchyma. Ovarian and tubo-ovarian abscesses have little tendency to spontaneous healing because of the thickness of their walls. They are a serious and potentially life-threatening condition. However, intravenous administration of broad-spectrum antibiotics may result in resolution of the infection. When medical treatment fails, surgical management is required. They can be emptied either from the posterior vaginal fornix or from the abdomen if they are large and can be reached in this way without exposing the free peritoneal cavity to contamination with the purulent content of the abscess. A definite cure can, however, be achieved only by complete removal of the diseased adnexa, usually in connection with the uterus.

In rare instances, a tubo-ovarian abscess may finally change into a tubo-ovarian cyst. The latter is a retort-like formation consisting of the dilated tube, which communicates with a unilocular ovarian cyst. As a rule, the tubo-ovarian cyst contains clear serous fluid but at times also some red blood cells and leukocytes. On its inner surface, the transition between the tube and the ovary is often indicated by a sharp ring through which the flattened fimbriae pass into the ovarian cyst, spreading in the form of low ridges in its wall. In other cases, no demarcation between tubal and ovarian tissues is recognizable macroscopically. All, or almost all, tubo-ovarian cysts are of inflammatory origin, though a few result from true tubo-ovarian abscesses. In most cases, they originate from the union of a hydrosalpinx and a retention cyst or a seropapillary ovarian cyst. As a rule, the tubo-ovarian cyst is a benign structure, changing very little in the course of time. Only in rare cases does a cancer develop in a tubo-ovarian cyst. Because of the effect of both the tubo-ovarian cyst and the processes that lead to it, symptoms of pain, subfecundity, or recurrent infections may precipitate the need for surgical intervention.

Plate 9.11

Reproductive System: VOLUME 1

Tuberculosis of tubal serosa. As part of more widespread peritoneal tuberculosis.

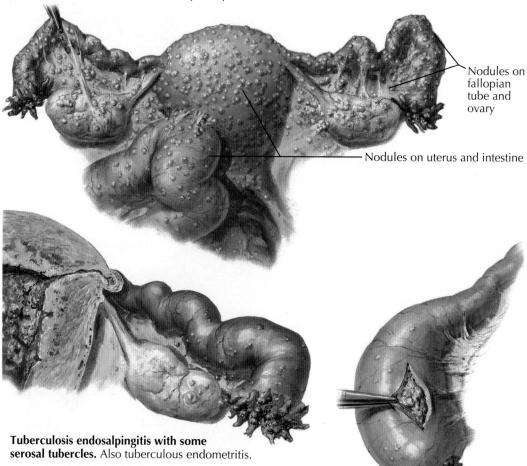

Nodules on fallopian tube and ovary

Nodules on uterus and intestine

TUBERCULOSIS

At one time, about 10% of all inflammatory disease of the tubes was tuberculous. Tuberculosis of the upper genital tract, primarily chronic salpingitis and chronic endometritis, is now a rare disease in the United States. However, pulmonary tuberculosis is steadily increasing in the United States, and with this rise it is likely that the incidence of pelvic tuberculosis also will increase. Tuberculosis is a frequent cause of chronic pelvic inflammatory disease and infertility in other parts of the world and may be encountered in immigrants, especially those from Asia, the Middle East, and Latin America. Genital tuberculosis may occur at any age but is most often encountered in females between 20 and 30 years old, though it will occur in postmenopausal females 10% of the time. Both tubes almost always are involved in the tuberculous disease, whereas the uterus is affected in slightly more than 50%. The other reproductive organs are only rarely involved.

As a rule, the infection is carried to the tubes by the hematogenous route from a primary focus in the lung or the hilar lymph nodes. Early in the course of pulmonary infection, the bacteria spread and the infection becomes located in the tubes, and from there the bacilli usually spread to the endometrium and less commonly to the ovaries. Despite these possible coinfections, the oviducts are the primary and predominant site of pelvic tuberculosis. Pelvic tuberculosis may be produced by either *Mycobacterium tuberculosis* or *Mycobacterium bovis*. The focus may be quite small and insignificant and may not cause any clinical symptoms. However, in the majority of cases, it is impossible to determine whether the infection has spread from the peritoneum to the tube or from the tube to the peritoneum. The possibility of an infection of the tubes by intracavitary or lymphatic ascent of tubercle bacilli introduced into the vagina by coitus with a tuberculous male cannot be denied. However, this mode of infection is extremely rare.

Changes in the fallopian tube as a result of an infection with tubercle varies to a great extent. In the initial stages, the tubal mucosa may be studded with miliary tubercles. In females with tuberculous peritonitis, the serosa of the tubes, as well as the surfaces of the uterus and the ovaries, is dotted with small tuberculous nodules. In more advanced cases of tuberculous endosalpingitis, the miliary nodules coalesce to form an exudate that also infiltrates the outer layers of the tube, causing marked thickening of the tubal wall. Because the tuberculous process occurs in separate foci and not diffusely, the tube appears nodular ("rosary" form), with increased sinuosity. The infiltrate may undergo caseous necrosis, producing a pyosalpinx filled with caseous purulent material. In more favorable cases, the granulation tissue may become fibrotic, shrunken, and calcified.

The diagnosis of genital tuberculosis is difficult in most cases. The patients quite frequently report in a rather vague fashion only about amenorrhea and a dull

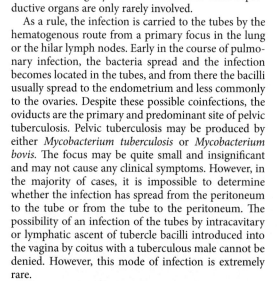

Tuberculosis endosalpingitis with some serosal tubercles. Also tuberculous endometritis.

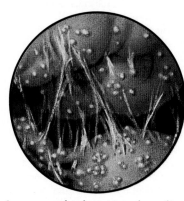

Tube with tuberculosis pus

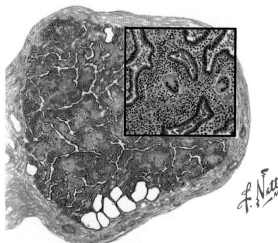

Caseated, occluded tube. Inset shows granulomatous inflammation with multinucleated giant cells.

Laparoscopic view. Note the miliary nodules and the fibrous adhesions.

pain in the lower abdomen (35% of cases); they sometimes request medical advice only because of sterility. Suspicious signs of genital tuberculosis are as follows: slow, insidious development of adnexal tumors; without any history, signs or symptoms of gonorrhea or operative infection; palpable nodules in the cul-de-sac; rosary-type thickening of the tubes; moderate deviations of temperature; and lymphocytosis. The findings at pelvic examination are normal in approximately 50% of

cases. An endometrial biopsy, probatory curettage, or the demonstration of tubercle bacilli in the uterine secretions gives evidence of tuberculous genital infection. Differentiation of tubercle bacilli requires culture.

The course of the disease becomes stormy if diffuse peritonitis intervenes or if a caseous pyosalpinx becomes secondarily infected by pyogenic bacteria. The course of the infection may be one of either an insidious or a rapidly progressing disease.

Plate 9.12

Fallopian Tubes

SALPINGITIS ISTHMICA NODOSA, CARCINOMA

The nodular enlargement of the innermost isthmic portion of the tube, called salpingitis isthmica nodosa, once was the subject of lively discussion among gynecologists and pathologists regarding its origin or pathogenesis. It consists of glandular ramified projections of the mucosa into the thickened tubal wall. Most authors assume that nodular isthmic salpingitis is of inflammatory origin. However, it may be, in some or even in most cases, the result of a noninflammatory endosalpingosis, a condition closely related in its nature to uterine adenomyosis or endometriosis. (Approximately two-thirds of females with adenomyosis have coexistent pelvic pathology, including salpingitis isthmica nodosa.) Some studies indicate that salpingitis isthmica nodosa can be documented histologically in more than 50% of patients with ectopic pregnancies. The diagnosis is best made radiographically at hysterosalpingography, where the characteristic finding consists of multiple nodular diverticular spaces in close approximation to the true tubal lumen. Visualization of nodular thickening of the tubes on laparoscopy also suggests the diagnosis.

Neoplasms of the uterine tubes are much rarer than those of the ovaries or the uterus. They may be epithelial in nature such as papillomas, adenomas, carcinomas, and chorioepitheliomas, or they may be mesenchymal tumors such as fibromas, myomas, lipomas, chondromas, osteomas, and angiomas. Mixed tumors may, in rare cases, also arise from the tubal walls. Endosalpingosis occupies an intermediary position between inflammatory and neoplastic diseases.

Foci of endometrial tissue are commonly found in the endosalpinx and are particularly frequent in the interstitial portion of the tube. In the interstitial and the adjoining isthmic region, they may produce a nodular thickening of the tube similar to that caused by chronic inflammatory irritation. In both cases, ramified glandular projections are the most conspicuous constituents of the nodules. However, the presence of cytogenic stroma characterizes the endometriotic nodules, whereas the absence of cytogenic stroma and the presence of scar tissue and round cell infiltration indicate the inflammatory origin of nodular isthmic salpingitis.

The most important tubal neoplasms are carcinomas, which may originate in the tubal mucosa or may be secondary to a primary carcinoma of the ovary, the uterus, or the gastrointestinal tract. In primary tubal carcinoma, the tube forms an elastic or firm, sausage- or pear-shaped tumor, which is usually adherent to its surroundings and filled with papillomatous, cauliflower-like or villous, friable masses of grayish-red or grayish-white neoplastic tissue. The tumor secretes a clear or turbid fluid, which may occasionally escape from the uterus, causing a rather conspicuous watery discharge. The cells of the tumor are arranged in single or multiple layers, and mitoses are frequent. Squamous cell carcinoma has, in rare cases, also been found in the tubes.

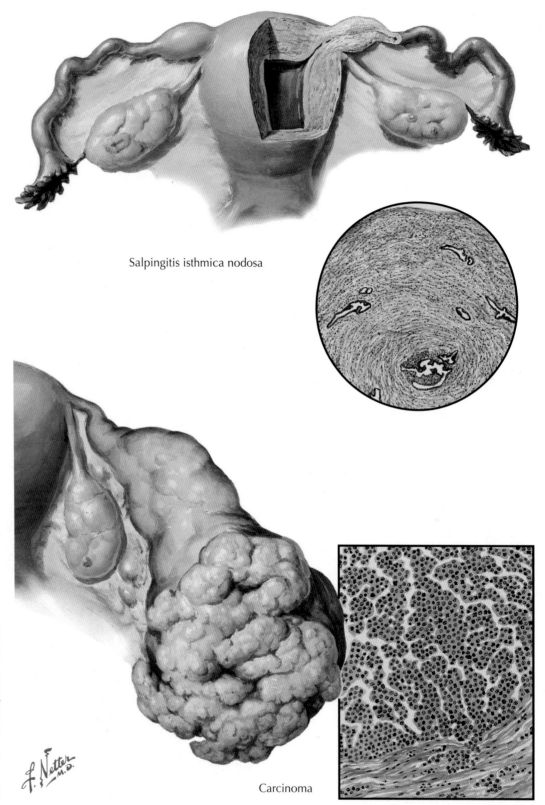

Salpingitis isthmica nodosa

Carcinoma

Extension of the carcinoma takes place via the lymph or bloodstream, along the peritoneal surface, or by contiguity. The ovaries and the uterus are frequently involved in the disease, and invasion of the iliac and lumbar lymph nodes is common.

The symptoms are minimal in the initial stage of the disease. Burning or darting pains in the lower abdomen, hemorrhages, and clear or turbid, serous or serosanguineous discharge may be present. Approximately 50% of patients with fallopian tube cancer present with vaginal bleeding. Ascites and progressive emaciation occur only in very advanced stages. Abnormal cervical cytology is occasionally present, with a reported range of 10% to 40%.

Owing to a lack of frank symptoms and signs, the diagnosis is difficult and in most cases is only tentative. Because the disease is rarely recognized at an early stage, the prognosis is poor, and permanent cures by operation and radiation are rare exceptions.

Retrospective studies have shown that 17% of females with tubal carcinoma harbor germline *BRCA* mutations. This suggests that the *BRCA1/BRCA2* mutations have a role in fallopian tube tumorigenesis.

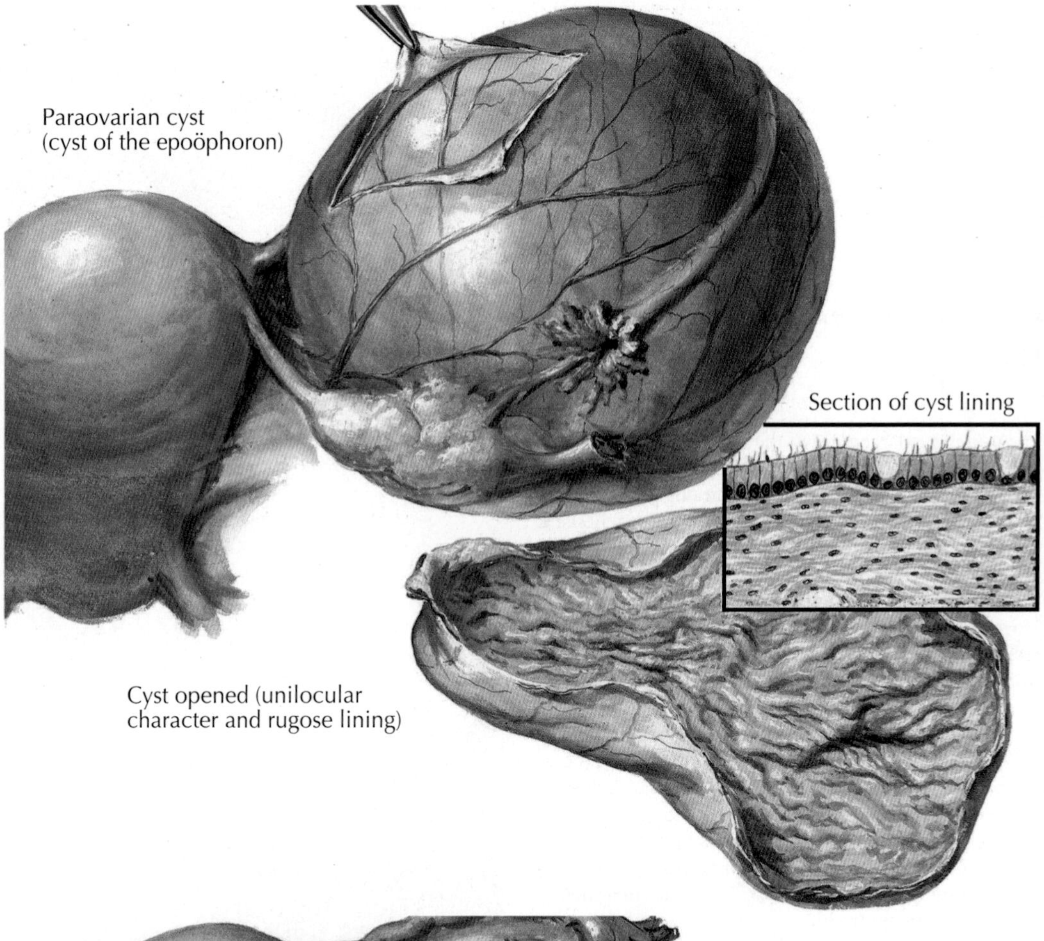

Plate 9.13

Reproductive System: VOLUME 1

PARAOVARIAN OR EPOÖPHORON CYST

Mesonephric cysts can develop from the permanent portion of the mesonephron, which is the paraovarian or epoöphoron, or from the inconstant residue of the wolffian (Gartner) duct. The former, called paraovarian or epoöphoron cysts, may be small and may represent simple retention cysts; some, however, are true blastomas, which grow continuously and may finally attain an enormous size. As a rule, even the giant cysts remain unilocular.

Owing to the intraligamentary location of the epoöphoron, the paraovarian cysts are always intraligamentary and are covered by the distended peritoneum of the broad ligament. Exceptionally, the cyst is fixed to its surroundings by dense inflammatory adhesions or, instead of expanding upward toward the peritoneal cavity, it may grow downward toward the pelvic floor or into the mesosigmoid.

The tube and the ovary are displaced and stretched out by the cyst. As a rule, the tube encircles the tumor by running around it from the anterior to the posterior surface of the cyst, where it reaches the flattened and elongated ovary with its fimbriated end.

Paraovarian cysts do not have true pedicles, but if they continue to project into the peritoneal cavity, some kind of pedicle develops; this consists of the tube, the proper ovarian ligament, and the suspensory ligaments. Torsion of this pedicle is by no means rare.

The wall of the epoöphoron cyst is usually thin and flaccid. It consists of a dense, lamellated outer and a loose, reticular inner layer of connective tissue and an innermost single-layered epithelial lining. The connective tissue is intermingled with elastic fibers and sparse smooth muscle fibers. The epithelium is low in some places and cylindrical and ciliated in others. In most cases the inner surface is smooth but often becomes corrugated when the cyst is opened and emptied. The rugose appearance of the cyst wall is due to the retractability of its elastic constituents. Sometimes the inner surface of the cyst is puckered, and in isolated cases even studded with papillary, cauliflower-like excrescences. As a rule, paraovarian cysts are benign. Malignant degeneration is exceedingly rare.

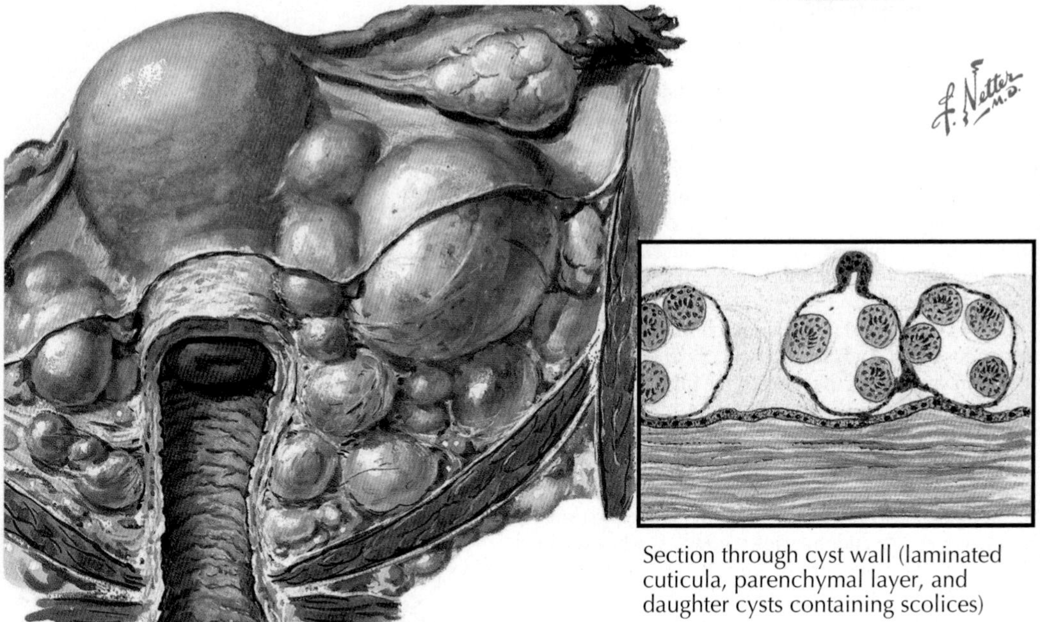

In all cases of cysts situated in the broad ligament or in the deeper pelvic connective tissue, the possibility of *Echinococcus* cysts should be taken into consideration. *Echinococcus* cysts represent a rare hydatid form of *Taenia echinococcus,* which is a tapeworm living in the intestine of various animals, notably dogs and sheep. The disease is sporadic in the United States but common in Australia, Iceland, Argentina, and some parts of Germany and Russia. Having arrived in the human intestine, the oncospheres lose their sheaths, pierce the intestinal wall with their hooklets, and penetrate into the bloodstream either directly or by way of the

Paraovarian cyst (cyst of the epoöphoron)

Section of cyst lining

Cyst opened (unilocular character and rugose lining)

Section through cyst wall (laminated cuticula, parenchymal layer, and daughter cysts containing scolices)

Hydatid (*Echinococcus*) cysts

lymphatics. They settle most commonly in the liver and lungs but occasionally also in the pelvic connective tissue, where the oncospheres develop into cherry- to head-sized cysts which are filled with clear fluid of low specific gravity (1.010–1.015). The wall of the cyst consists of an outer lamellar cuticle and an inner granular parenchymal layer. From the latter, daughter cysts develop, as well as budlike structures, the scolices, each provided with a crown of hooklets and two lateral suckers.

In the pelvic connective tissue, the cysts are usually multiple because of an exogenous proliferation of a single original cyst or because of a primary infection with multiple oncospheres. A membrane of inflammatory connective tissue containing lymphocytes and leukocytes, particularly numerous eosinophils, surrounds the cysts.

The treatment is surgical. Only complete removal of all cysts prevents recurrence. Opening the cysts and spilling their contents must be avoided.

OVARIES

Plate 10.1

Reproductive System: VOLUME 1

OVARIAN STRUCTURES AND DEVELOPMENT

The ovaries develop from a thickening of cells that form ridges medial to the müllerian and wolffian bodies. These germinal ridges appear at the sixth week. Primary oocytes, arising in the umbilical vesicle (yolk sac) and migrating along the mesentery of the hindgut, arrive in the embryonic gonads and are thought to provide the countless thousands of ova that crowd the ovary at birth.

By the third month of gestation, the ovaries descend toward the pelvis. The pull of the gubernaculum—an abdominal fold that grows more slowly than the rest of the fetus—exerts a downward traction on the gonadal ridges. Later, these folds fuse in their midportion with that part of each müllerian duct that develops into the uterine fundus. The lateral half and the medial portion of the folds become the round ligaments and the suspensory ligaments of the ovary, respectively.

The infant ovary is a sausage-shaped structure, with a pale and smooth surface. A gradual thickening and shortening occur throughout the first decade of life. The major gain in size and weight takes place after the menarche and during adolescence. Two layers, the germinal epithelium and the tunica albuginea, constitute the surface of the prepubertal ovary. They are crowded with primordial ova that are surrounded by dark-staining cells, the origin of the future granulosa cells. The granulosa cells are polygonal and rather uniform, round, with sharply outlined nuclei in a poorly stainable cytoplasm that contains, however, numerous granules, from which this layer derives its name.

As the primordial follicle develops, it sinks, with its single layer of epithelial cells, toward the center of the ovary. The attendant cells proliferate to form a many-layered coating of granulosa cells around the developing follicle. A crescentic cavity forms eccentrically, in which follicular fluid accumulates. From the surrounding ovarian stroma, a capsule of theca cells differentiates. The theca interna is rich in capillaries, upon which the avascular theca granulosa must depend for nourishment. Before menarche, while still little or no follicle-stimulating hormone is present, these follicles develop no further but degenerate and become atretic.

The mature gonad is an approximately almond-shaped structure, pitted and scarred by the stigmata of ovulation. Spiral arteries enter at the hilum and are involved in sequential changes during the cyclic ebb and sway of follicle growth and development of corpora lutea. In the hilum are also found cells with morphologic and histochemical properties, like the interstitial cells of the testis—vestiges from the fetal period, before sex differentiation took place. Proliferation of these cells or tumor formation may result in virilization.

In the ripening follicle, the oocyte is a spherical body composed of clear protoplasm. It contains a round, dark-staining nucleus, with a definite surrounding membrane and an eccentric nucleolus. A transparent membrane, the zona pellucida, encloses a fluid-filled perivitelline space in which the egg floats freely. A dense layer of granulosa cells, the cumulus oophorus, closely envelops the egg and attaches it to the follicular

wall. The cumulus cells immediately next to the zona arrange themselves radially outward to form the corona radiata.

The two-layered theca envelope coats the follicle. The theca interna is composed of large epithelioid cells interspersed in connective tissue and rich in blood and lymph vessels. The theca externa is thick and dense, consisting of circularly arranged connective tissue fibers.

In the follicles that do not mature but degenerate, the granulosa layer first becomes disorganized. The corona loses its radial arrangement. Thereafter, the follicular cavity shrinks, and soon the egg itself loses its characteristic features. Hyaline is deposited in a wavy, concentric band. Up to this point, the theca interna has continued to be a prominent layer of large, vesicular, nucleated cells. Degenerative changes rapidly progress until nothing is left except an amorphous hyaline scar.

Infant ovary

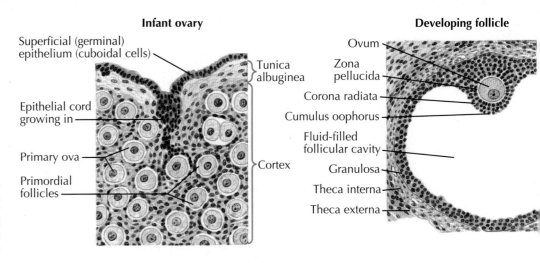

Developing follicle

Stages of ovum and follicle

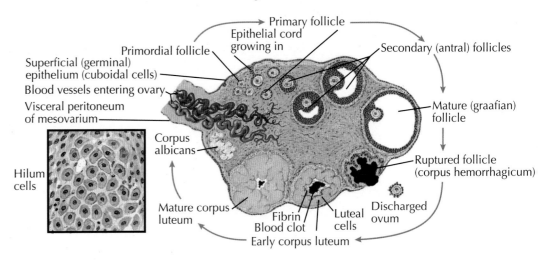

Aging ovary

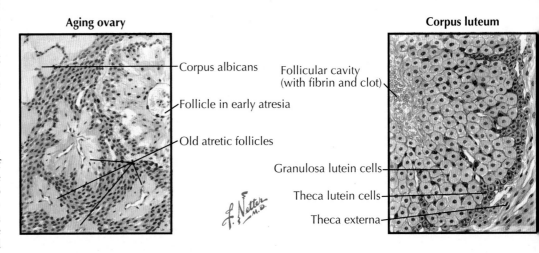

Corpus luteum

Plate 10.2

Ovaries

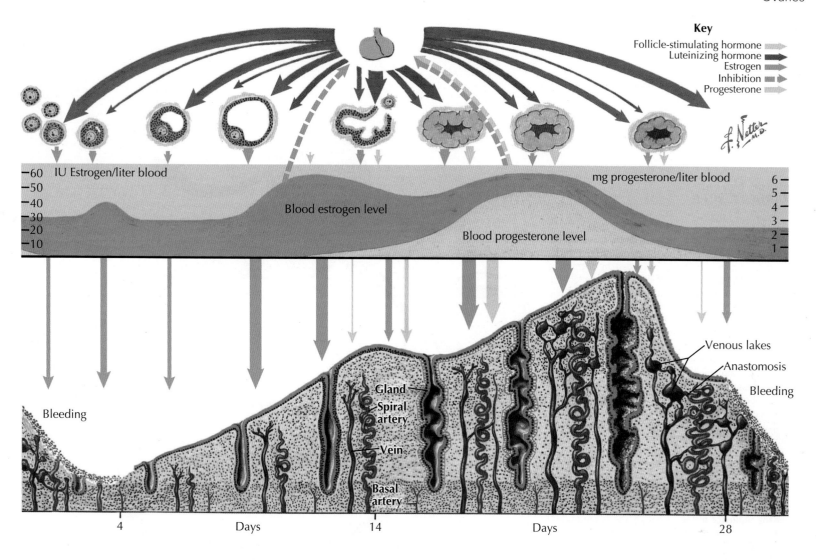

ENDOCRINE RELATIONS DURING CYCLE

Menarche, or the first menstrual cycle, heralds the onset of adult reproductive function, which continues until menopause, when the major part of ovarian function ceases. Between these events, the hormonal ballet of cyclic menstruation takes place.

Two anterior pituitary gonadotropins and two ovarian steroids are primarily involved in this periodic occurrence of menstruation: the pituitary contributes follicle-stimulating hormone (FSH) and luteinizing hormone (LH), whereas the ovary secretes β-estradiol and progesterone.

Up to puberty—even during fetal life—ovarian follicles are constantly developing to a stage in which an antrum has formed, regressing then to become atretic. Eventually, one or more follicles produce enough estrogen to cause a proliferation of the endometrium. It is unlikely that any of these early follicles, though producing estrogen, achieve ovulation; more likely, atresia sets in and the endometrium breaks down, with resultant bleeding. It is probable that the mature cycle will not become established for several months after this, the first menstruation.

At the onset of menstrual flow (day 1), production of estrogen is low, but FSH levels rise and initiate another round of folliculogenesis. A cohort consisting of several follicles begins the maturation process approximately 375 days prior to day 1 of the menstrual cycle. By the onset of menses, these have matured enough to respond with growth and an increase in estrogen. Most of the follicles, however, have a relatively short life. Their granulosa cells and ovum degenerate, leaving an atretic follicle. A few continue to enlarge, but in most cycles only one emerges as the mature graafian follicle that ruptures or ovulates about day 14.

Through about day 12 of the cycle, the secretion of FSH decreases with the increase of estrogen production. Although follicle growth beyond the stage of antrum formation must be initiated by the pituitary and continues to be dependent on this stimulus for the first week or so of the cycle, after about day 8 further development is autonomous. A surge of LH (and to a lesser extent FSH) at midcycle reflects this rising estrogenic tide and it provides the endocrine trigger for ovulation.

After ovulation the estrogen level drops slightly during a lag period between the functional peak of the mature follicle and that of the fully developed corpus luteum. Some uterine spotting or even bleeding for a day or two is not rare at this time ("midcycle bleeding").

Within a few hours after ovulation, the empty cavity of the ruptured follicle becomes filled with blood clots, and a network of capillary fingers stretches tentatively inward along fibrin strands from the theca interna. Theca cells containing a yellow lipochrome, named lutein, proliferate centripetally at a rapid rate along with the capillary mesh. Progesterone production is quickly accelerated, and its effect can be detected by secretory changes in the endometrium within 48 hours after ovulation.

Stimulation of the thermal center in the brainstem, by progesterone, causes a rise in basal body temperature, which is sustained as long as the corpus luteum functions. Cervical mucus becomes scanty and viscid and, when rapidly dried on a slide, no longer crystallizes in a "fernlike" pattern. By day 20, the estrogen level is usually as high as that just before ovulation, and the corpus luteum has also reached a peak of production of progesterone.

Under the influence of estrogen and progesterone, growth and the secretory activity of the endometrium progress continuously through day 25 or 26. Unless fertilization has occurred, degeneration of the corpus luteum is initiated. With the consequent decline of both estrogen and progesterone, changes occur in the endometrium that lead inevitably to slough and necrosis. By day 28, the pituitary, now released from the inhibitive levels of estrogen, starts again and rapidly reaches its peak of FSH output, which supports a new crop of primary follicles for the next cycle.

Plate 10.3

Reproductive System: VOLUME 1

OVARIAN CYCLE

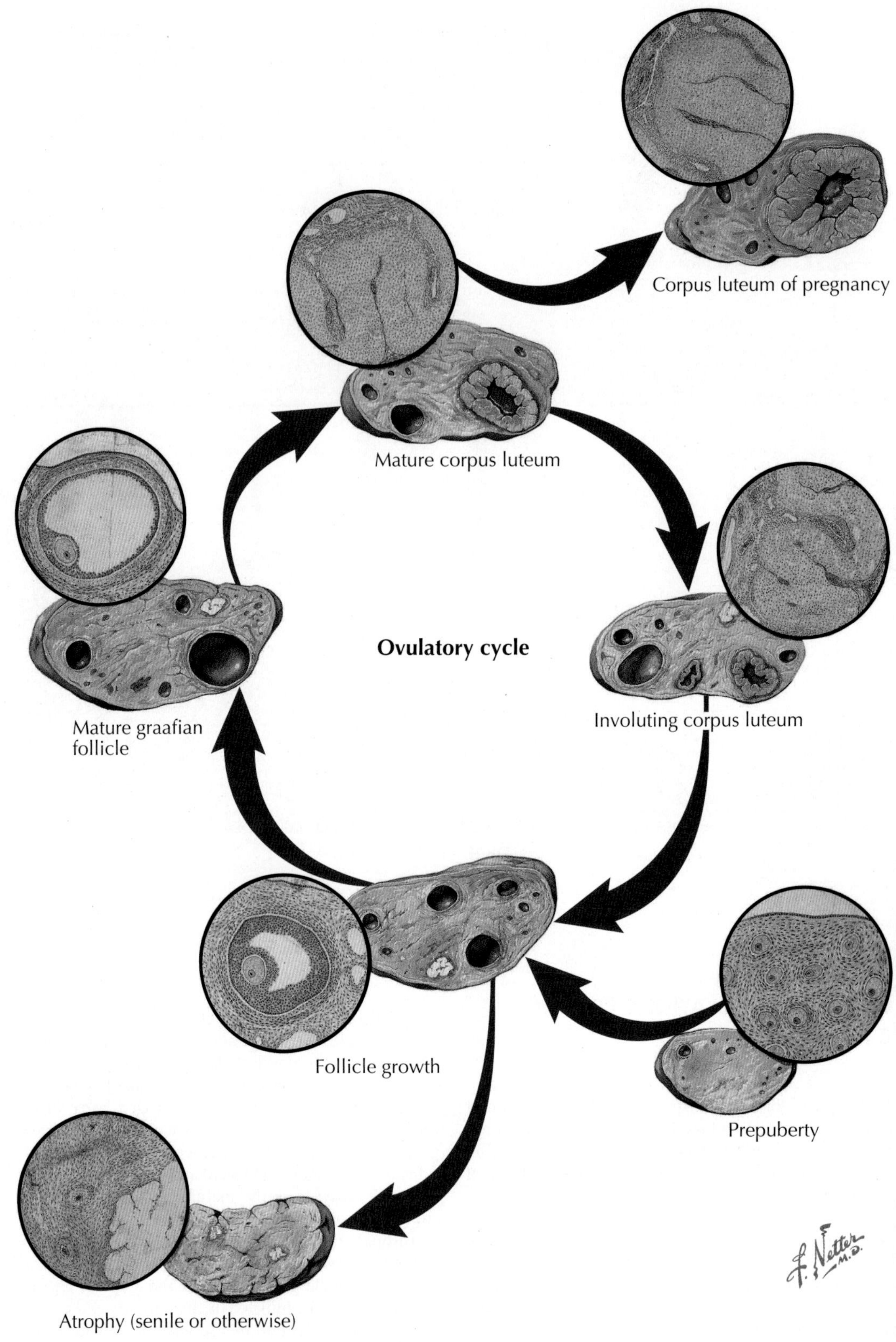

Although follicle growth is relatively even, it is slow for 10 to 12 days, during which time the granulosa layer thickens and the antrum becomes distended by increasing amounts of estrogen-rich liquor folliculi. After the follicles have reached a diameter of about 0.5 cm, they start their migration outward toward the ovarian surface, and about 12 days after the start of this cycle of growth, one follicle "gains ascendancy" in one of the ovaries, reaching a diameter of 1.5 to 2 cm in a short time. Simultaneously, it begins to protrude from the ovarian surface. This surge of development is accompanied by a similarly sudden wave of atretic processes, which wipes out all lesser developing follicles in both ovaries. Because the granulosa is the first layer to degenerate in this change leading to atresia, it is probable that the theca is responsible for transient continuing secretion.

Whether follicle migration is accomplished by hormonal or enzymatic reactions or merely by the physical forces involved in a rapidly expanding cystic structure enclosed in a tough, fibrous stroma by a relatively inelastic tunica, is not known. During this development under the influence of the LH surge, the ovum undergoes the first maturation division, and the first polar body is extruded, reducing the number of chromosomes from 46 to 23. The granulosa cells become widely separated by edema, thus loosening the egg and its surrounding cumulus for detachment from the inside of the follicle cavity. Finally, through compression of the capillary net at the weakest point of the follicle wall near the surface, a relatively avascular area is produced, and through this area a break occurs. Intrafollicular pressure forces the egg, cumulus, and some detached granulosa cells with the liquor folliculi out into the peritoneal cavity.

Bleeding to some degree from the break in the richly vascular theca interna always attends ovulation. Usually, the rupture point is rapidly sealed off, though in patients with compromised clotting ability, this can result in hemorrhage. The cavity of the follicle is filled with blood-containing fluid—the so-called *corpus hemorrhagicum*—and an immediate differentiation of cells sets in, which spreads inward from the granulosal remnants. These lipid- and pigment-containing cells—the lutein cells—grow on a network of capillaries from the theca interna. This process causes an appearance of infolding as the walls of the former follicle thicken and encroach more and more on the fibrin-containing, blood-filled cavity ultimately representing the mature corpus luteum. When pregnancy occurs, this development continues under the influence of human chorionic gonadotropin and increases until the bright-yellow body may make up as much as one half the total volume of the ovary—the corpus luteum of pregnancy. Sometime after the second month of gestation, a slow process of regression of the corpus luteum occurs and is accompanied by the luteal-placental shift, where the placenta becomes the

primary organ of hormonogenesis for the remainder of pregnancy.

If conception does not take place, the fate of the corpus luteum is involution. The crenated, yellow margin shrinks relatively rapidly, and the lutein cells degenerate into amorphous, hyaline masses held together by strands of connective tissue. The yellow color is in most part lost. The shrunken convolutions of hyalinized material are known as a *corpus albicans*. It is during this regressive phase that the decrease of estrogen and progesterone

production prompts a new output of pituitary gonadotropins, producing stimulation of a new crop of ovarian follicles, and a new ovulatory growth cycle is once more initiated.

The senile ovary is a shrunken and puckered organ, containing few if any follicles, and made up for the most part of old corpora albicantia and corpora atretica. In menopause, the senile ovary continues to produce hormones, albeit at lower levels and with a more androgenic profile.

Corpus luteum of pregnancy

Mature corpus luteum

Ovulatory cycle

Involuting corpus luteum

Mature graafian follicle

Follicle growth

Prepuberty

Atrophy (senile or otherwise)

Plate 10.4

Ovaries

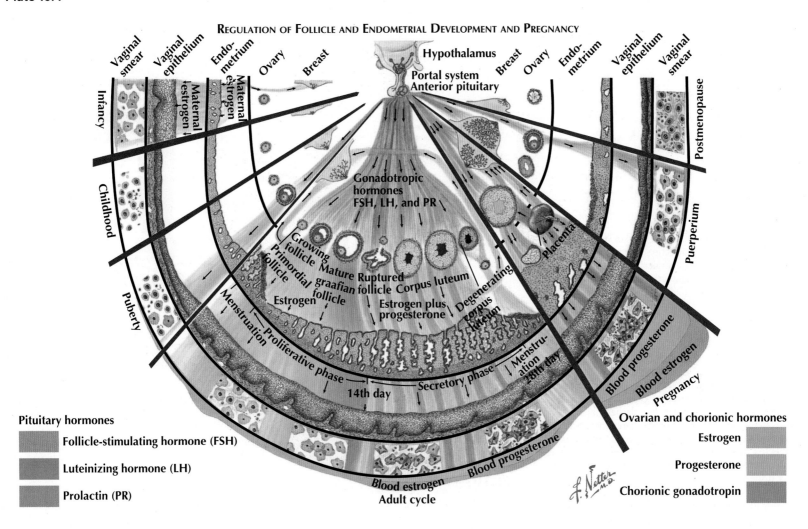

REGULATION OF FOLLICLE AND ENDOMETRIAL DEVELOPMENT AND PREGNANCY

HORMONAL INFLUENCE DURING LIFE

The placenta provides no barrier to the high concentration of maternal estrogens prior to parturition. As a result, the infant's breasts may show some enlargement, and milk can occasionally be expressed. The external genitalia are precociously developed, and the endometrium has been stimulated to proliferate. Within a week or so after birth, all the stigmata of estrogen stimulation recede.

From the postnatal recessional changes to the time of puberty, the ovaries gradually show a buildup of interstitial tissue from an accumulation of fibrous stroma, as a constant succession of primordial follicles degenerate in atresia.

Pituitary maturation and consequent secretion of gonadotropins results in the initiation of enhanced ovarian steroid production at the time of puberty. The uterus is the first to respond, and the endometrium proliferates with the development of straight, tubular glands. Next, the vaginal wall thickens and becomes stratified, with cornified superficial cells appearing. In the ovary, primordial follicles progress beyond the stage of a one- or two-layer granulosa with a tiny antrum and exhibit identifiable several-thickness granulosa and theca interna layers. In the breast, the areolae show

pigmentation along with a domelike change, becoming elevated as a conical protuberance. Fat is deposited about the shoulder girdle, hips, and buttocks, and the adult pelvic and, later, axillary hair patterns typical of the female begin to develop.

In the decade of adolescence, the skeletal system reacts to estrogen, first by an accelerated growth rate of the long bones and, second, by a hastening of epiphyseal closure, the balance affecting final height.

In the mature cycle, the endometrium undergoes cyclic changes (described elsewhere) under the stimulus of estrogen secreted by ovarian follicles in response to FSH. By day 12 in a typical 28-day cycle, one follicle attains dominance and exhibits a rapid growth toward maturity. The release of LH at midcycle on day 14 induces ovulation of the mature follicle and initiates progesterone excretion from the rapidly forming corpus luteum. Endometrial glands become saw-toothed and secretory. If fertilization and implantation do not occur, the corpus luteum degenerates on about day 26, and in consequence with the rapid withdrawal of its estrogen and progesterone secretion the endometrium shrinks, undergoes autolysis, and breaks away with bleeding on day 28.

When conception occurs, the early excretion of chorionic gonadotropin maintains the corpus luteum. In pregnancy, the peak production of chorionic hormone is seen by about day 90 after the last menstrual period, declining thereafter to a plateau. The corpus luteum is

responsible for increasing progesterone and estrogens throughout the first 3 months, after which the placenta takes over until the end of the pregnancy. The augmentation of both estrogen and progesterone is approximately linear throughout the 9 months of gestation. The breasts react to the increasing steroid stimulation with an extension of both ductile and alveolar growth, and there is congestion without actual lactation.

The withdrawal of estrogen and progesterone after placental delivery combined with the psychoneural mechanisms initiated by the suckling reflex bring about the release of prolactin. Breast tissues, already conditioned by growth, respond with milk production. Ovarian activity is often held in abeyance for approximately 6 months in females who are fully breastfeeding; it may well occur sooner in those who are partially breastfeeding. Reestablishment of the pituitary-ovarian cycle can, and often does, take place before weaning, so that another conception can occur before the advent of a menstrual flow.

In the United States, menopause occurs late in the fourth or early in the fifth decade (mean age 51 ± 2). The ovaries no longer contain any follicles capable of responding to pituitary stimulation and increasing amounts of FSH are released in response to lower estrogen and inhibin levels. Estrogen deficiency is reflected by senile changes in the breasts, uterus, and vagina and in the skin, bony skeleton, and vascular system.

Plate 10.5

Reproductive System: VOLUME 1

PITUITARY AND OVARIAN HORMONE CHANGES IN MENOPAUSE

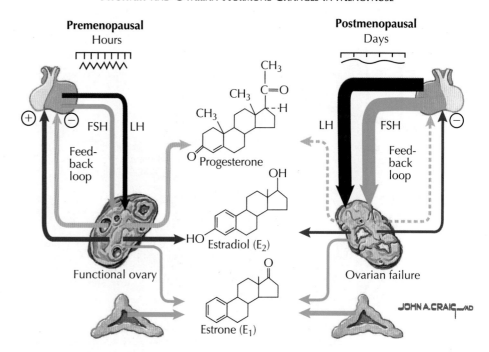

MENOPAUSE

Menopause is the loss of normal ovarian steroidogenesis because of age, genetic alteration, chemotherapy (alkylating agents), radiation, or surgical therapy. (Menopause may be viewed as an endocrinopathy: the loss of an endocrine function with adverse health consequences.) Menopause naturally occurs at a median age of 51.4, with 95% of females going through this transition between ages 44 and 55. Menopause may occur at a younger age in smokers, those with poor nutrition or chronic illness, or those who have a loss of genetic material from the long arm of the X chromosome.

When ovarian steroidogenesis is lost, menstrual function (if the uterus is present) ceases. Up to 85% of females will also experience hot flashes, flushes, and night sweats, with the most severe symptoms associated with the steepest or most abrupt declines in hormone levels (e.g., surgical menopause). Symptoms last a median of 4 to 10 years. Vaginal atrophy, vulvodynia, dysuria, urinary urgency, and urgency incontinence, urinary frequency, nocturia, and an increased incidence of stress urinary incontinence are also common with the loss of estrogen (genitourinary syndrome of menopause). For many females, there is a decrease in libido, independent of that caused by vaginal dryness and the attendant dyspareunia. Around the time of menopause, there is an estrogen-dependent accelerated loss of bone mass. There is a suggestion of an increased risk of cardiovascular disease associated with natural menopause and strong evidence of this in premature surgical menopause.

During the natural transition from ovulatory function to postmenopause ovarian activity (the "climacteric period"), many females will experience irregular vaginal bleeding and may experience the beginnings of hot flashes or flushes. Following menopause, the ovary is not truly quiescent: LH stimulation of theca cell islands in the ovarian stroma results in testosterone and androstenedione production. Although these are produced at a much lower level than before menopause, androgens become the primary hormonal product of the ovaries.

Although the timing and symptoms of menopause are sufficiently characteristic to allow a diagnosis to be made by history and physical findings alone, when the symptoms are atypical or the timing other than expected, alternative causes for the symptoms such as pregnancy, hypothyroidism, polycystic ovary syndrome (PCOS), a prolactin-secreting tumor, or hypothalamic dysfunction should all be considered. Measurement of serum FSH is not a reliable indicator of menopause. Similarly, serum estradiol levels may be determined (generally less than 15 pg/mL) but are less reliable as a marker of ovarian failure. A pregnancy test is always indicated in sexually active perimenopausal females who are not using contraception. (Up to 25% of cycles lasting longer than 50–60 days may be ovulatory; therefore females in the perimenopause stage still can become pregnant.) Bone densitometry may be indicated for those at special risk

Hormone levels increase and decrease cyclically during the menstrual cycle. Modulation occurs by pulsatile release of gonadotropins and positive and negative feedback loops.

In the postmenopausal period, gonadotropin levels increase and ovarian hormone levels decrease secondary to ovarian failure. Endogenous estrogen is primarily of adrenal origin, and E_1-to-E_2 ratio is reversed.

LH and FSH (mIU/mL)

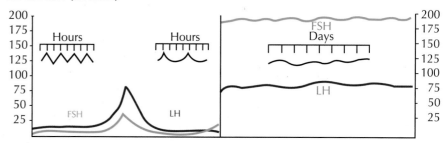

Estrogen (pg/mL) and progesterone (ng/mL)

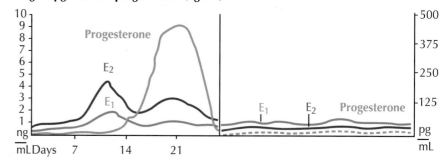

for bone loss. When noncyclic bleeding occurs in these patients, pelvic examination, Pap smear, and endometrial biopsy should be strongly considered. Females who have ovarian failure before age 30 should have a karyotype performed.

The management of menopause and its symptoms has become controversial in recent years. Estrogen replacement therapy is still indicated when symptoms such as vasomotor or urogenital symptoms warrant, but most suggest that this therapy should be time

limited. Hormone replacement therapy targeted primarily toward the prevention of bone loss or to reduce the risk of heart disease has generally been replaced by more specific osteoporosis therapies and cardiac risk reduction strategies. When estrogens are used, progestins are usually added to the regimen if the patient has a uterus present to reduce the risk of endometrial hyperplasia or cancer. (Continuous estrogen exposure without periodic or concomitant progestins increases the risk of endometrial carcinoma six- to eightfold.)

Plate 10.6

Ovaries

DEVELOPMENTAL ANOMALIES

Turner syndrome is the most common sex chromosome abnormality in females, and ovarian failure is one of the hallmarks. The typical picture involves not only ovarian agenesis but also coexisting congenital abnormalities of the skeletal, cardiovascular, and nervous systems. It is characterized by short stature, primary amenorrhea, sexual infantilism, high gonadotropin level, and multiple congenital abnormalities.

Following midgestation, there is a rapid increase in oocyte atresia compared with normal ovaries, often resulting in early ovarian failure. The rate of complete depletion varies; some have primary amenorrhea with no secondary sexual characteristics, whereas others have varying degrees of pubertal development. The depleted ovaries are usually represented by thin, elongated, firm, whitish thickenings on the posterior surface of each broad ligament. On section, they are usually composed of spindle-like cells, arranged in whorls, without evidence of germ cells or follicles. The internal genitalia are markedly hypoplastic, being smaller than those seen in the newborn infant.

The diagnosis is usually made after puberty, when a primary amenorrhea and the absence of secondary sex characteristics are noted in conjunction with other congenital defects. The estrogen deficiency is manifested by undeveloped genitalia and breasts, sparse pubic and axillary hair (due to low testosterone), short stature and delayed epiphyseal union, osteoporosis, and fine wrinkling of the skin (precocious senility).

The patients are short, averaging 52 in. and rarely attaining a height of more than 58 in. A variety of congenital anomalies have been associated with this syndrome, including cubitus valgus (increased carrying angle), webbing of the neck, and a shieldlike chest (broad, deep, stocky chest). Other abnormalities include spina bifida; syndactylism; malformation of the ribs, wrists, or toes; Klippel-Feil syndrome; coarctation of the aorta; deafness; mental deficiency; hypertension; and ocular disorders.

Laboratory abnormalities include a marked increase in gonadotropin levels, approximating titers found in sterilized females or those who are postmenopause, and 17-ketosteroids that are only slightly reduced. This minimal decrease in adrenocortical function is insufficient to prevent the growth of sparse pubic and axillary hair. Karyotyping will unequivocally establish the diagnosis.

Therapy is substitutional, because the ovaries are incapable of stimulation. Estrogens may be given daily for 2 to 6 months to start sexual development and then changed to cyclical administration. After 4 to 6 months of estrogen-only therapy, progesterone is usually added in a cyclical fashion to achieve a more natural endometrial shedding, reducing the risk of iatrogenic hyperplasia. Under this regimen the breasts develop, the axillary and pubic hair increase, the external and internal genitalia mature, and the vagina becomes more capacious.

Developmental anomalies of the ovary other than ovarian aplasia are rare. They include absence of one ovary, ectopic ovary, third ovary, accessory ovaries, and congenital displacements. The absence of one ovary is almost invariably associated with a failure in development of the corresponding tube, half the uterus, a kidney,

Ovarian agenesis

Rudimentary ovaries or primitive genital streaks

Microscopic section: complete absence of follicular elements

Short stature, absence of secondary sex characteristics, infantile genitalia, sparse pubic hair, high gonadotropin level, estrogen deficiency, and multiple congenital abnormalities (web neck, shieldlike chest, cubitus valgus)

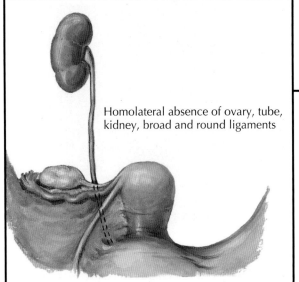

Homolateral absence of ovary, tube, kidney, broad and round ligaments

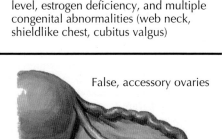

False, accessory ovaries

and the ureter. An ectopic ovary, usually with only the osteal end of the tube attached, may be present in the retroperitoneal lumbar region or inguinal area. A third ovary is exceedingly rare. It may conceivably arise from a duplication of the gonadal site. This diagnosis is unquestionable if an associated third fallopian tube is present. Such a true, supernumerary ovary may be intra- or extraperitoneal and is prone to the development of neoplastic cysts, teratomas, or sarcomas. False, accessory ovaries are separate segments of ovarian tissue, attached to a normally situated ovary by intervening bands of fibrous or attenuated ovarian tissue. The term *bipartite* or *succenturiate* ovary is sometimes applied to this splitting or partitioning effect.

Congenital displacements include herniation of the ovary within a peritoneal sac in the inguinal, femoral, sciatic, obturator, or perineal regions. Excessive degrees of prolapse into the cul-de-sac of Douglas may occur, sometimes leading to a true vaginal herniation of the ovary.

Plate 10.7

Reproductive System: VOLUME 1

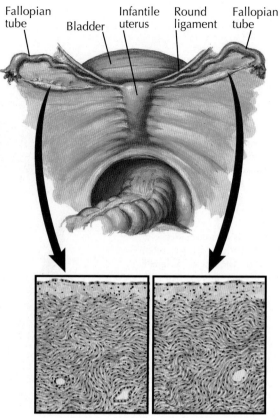

Primitive genital streaks in place of gonads,
wavy stroma with absence of germinal elements

GONADAL DYSGENESIS

Gonadal dysgenesis is a developmental abnormality of patients who do not carry the stigmata of Turner syndrome but still experience absent menarche because of chromosomal abnormalities and abnormal (streak) gonads. These patients are generally tall (>150 cm), are more normal in appearance, and are a chromosomally heterogeneous group: 46, XX, 46, XY, or mosaic X/XY karyotypes.

Gonadal dysgenesis occurs in 1 of 2500 female births, and Turner syndrome is estimated to occur in 1 of 2700 female births. Most patients with Turner syndrome have a sporadic loss of one X chromosome (45, XO, 60% of cases; others partial losses: amenorrhea with long-arm loss; short stature with short-arm loss). Ninety-eight percent of conceptuses with only one X chromosome abort in early pregnancy. Gonadal dysgenesis can occur with other chromosomal abnormalities including 46,XY gonadal dysgenesis (Swyer syndrome) and 46, XX q5 X chromosome long-arm deletion, and with mixed or mosaic states.

The symptoms and stigmata expressed by these individuals depend on the amount of chromatin that has been lost: primary amenorrhea and infertility (95%–98%) are the most common. (Gonadal dysgenesis is the most common cause of failure to begin menstruation and in approximately 60% of females with primary amenorrhea, an abnormality of gonadal differentiation or function has occurred during the fetal or neonatal period.) These patients have early and accelerated oocyte atresia resulting in few, if any, oocytes remaining in the ovarian cortex at the time of normal puberty. (Germ cell involution occurs soon after they migrate into the undifferentiated gonad. This results in fibrous streak gonads that are hormonally inactive.) Those with complete loss of the X chromosome generally are of short stature (<150 cm) and have a short neck, high palate, low hairline, and widely spaced, hypoplastic nipples (80%). Seventy percent to 75% have a broad (shield) chest, nail hypoplasia, lymphedema, cubitus valgus, prominent anomalous ears, multiple nevi, and hearing impairment. Two-thirds of these patients have webbing of the neck and a short fourth metacarpal. Renal and cardiac anomalies are also common. Gonadoblastomas or virilization may occur if the individual is mosaic for 45, X/46, XY.

The diagnosis of gonadal dysgenesis or Turner syndrome is usually established by karyotyping. (Forty percent of those thought to have Turner syndrome have a mosaic karyotype or have an abnormal X or Y chromosome.) FSH and LH levels are high in these individuals, but the elevation is nonspecific.

These individuals generally require hormone replacement therapy, and they may require growth hormone therapy if the diagnosis is established before age 10. When there is a mosaicism involving a Y chromosome, surgical extirpation of the gonads must be performed because of a 25% to 30% risk of malignant gonadal

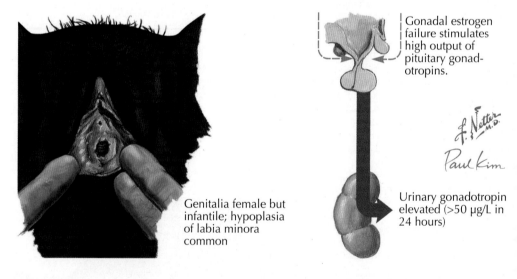

Genitalia female but infantile; hypoplasia of labia minora common

Gonadal estrogen failure stimulates high output of pituitary gonadotropins.

Urinary gonadotropin elevated (>50 µg/L in 24 hours)

80% of cases chromatin-negative; XO chromosomal pattern most common

20% of cases chromatin-positive; isochromosomes XX, translocation or deletion of X chromosomal fragment X^, mosaicism XO/XX/XY, or other

tumors. Timing of gonadal removal in patients with a Y chromosome is controversial: removal as soon as the diagnosis is made versus delaying removal until pubertal changes are complete. (The risk of cancer in XY gonadal dysgenesis is 3% at age 10, 10% at 13, and 75% at 26 years of age.) If hormonal replacement is undertaken, it must be done with care because adolescents are much more sensitive to the effects of estrogen than are females postmenopause, allowing doses in the range of

0.3 mg of conjugated estrogen, 0.5 mg of estradiol, or their equivalent daily. After 6 to 12 months of therapy at this level, the dose should be doubled and a progestin should be added or the patient's therapy should be switched to combination oral contraceptives. This generally results in regular menstruation, and normal pubertal development proceeds on its own when the patient reaches a bone age of 13. Growth hormone may be effective if given before age 10.

Plate 10.8

Ovaries

PHYSIOLOGIC VARIATIONS, NONNEOPLASTIC CYSTS

The preponderance of small cystic structures within the ovary represents physiologic variations of the normal ovulatory cycle. These follicle and corpus luteum derivatives are nonneoplastic, that is, they are incapable of autonomous growth. Their clinical recognition and differentiation from true ovarian cysts is most important. A small neoplastic ovarian cyst may be simulated by a single, large-follicle cyst; by multiple cystic follicles; or by a corpus luteum cyst. A large or cystic corpus luteum of pregnancy may be mistaken for an ectopic pregnancy or an ovarian cyst. A corpus luteum hematoma may present with signs comparable to those associated with torsion of a small cyst. A ruptured graafian follicle or ruptured hemorrhagic corpus luteum may be misdiagnosed as acute appendicitis or ruptured tubal pregnancy. It is not uncommon to find adnexal cysts during pelvic ultrasonography performed for other reasons, and these are generally not of any clinical significance.

Follicle cysts are distended atretic follicles more than 6 to 8 mm in diameter. They are usually not more than 1 to 2 cm in diameter, thin-walled, translucent, and filled with watery fluid. The cysts may project slightly above the surface of the ovary or may lie more deeply within the cortex. If pricked, the follicle fluid may spurt out under pressure. The inner lining appears smooth and glistening. Microscopically, the granulosa cell lining varies in thickness and may be well preserved or may show evidence of degeneration. On pelvic examination, a unilateral, smooth, cystic, slightly tender, movable, plum-sized ovary may be felt. Therapy is based on the principle that during the reproductive years a cystic ovary up to 6 cm in diameter is presumed, unless proved otherwise, to be a physiologic variation that will undergo subsequent resolution. The patient is reexamined at intervals. If the ovarian enlargement persists or increases in size, additional evaluation, including surgical intervention, may be indicated.

The mature corpus luteum presents a central core filled with blood. With resorption, the cavity may be distended with hemorrhagic or clear fluid or newly formed connective tissue. Variations in the size of the lumen occur normally. A corpus luteum hematoma is the result of excessive hemorrhage into the corpus cavity during the stage of vascularization. This increased accumulation of blood under pressure may result in local pain, ovarian enlargement, and tenderness. A corpus luteum cyst follows the resorption of a corpus luteum hematoma. It is usually 2 to 4 cm in diameter. Grossly, the yellowish hue of the cyst wall may be evident. A corpus albicans cyst is the sequel to a corpus luteum cyst in which the lutein cells are replaced by a dense, wavy band of fibrous or collagenous tissue.

A ruptured graafian follicle or hemorrhagic corpus luteum may be associated with varying degrees of intraabdominal bleeding. The former is likely to occur

between the 12th and the 16th days and the latter during the last week of an average menstrual cycle. Rupture may occur spontaneously or may follow trauma, pelvic examination, coitus, or exercise. Symptoms and signs include lower abdominal pain, nausea and vomiting, abdominal spasm, tenderness and rebound tenderness, an enlarged, tender ovary, fullness in one adnexal region or the posterior cul-de-sac, and tenderness on manipulation of the cervix. The temperature may be

slightly elevated and leukocytosis may be found, but the leukocyte sedimentation rate remains normal. Ultrasonography will demonstrate the cystic mass and free fluid in the cul-de-sac. Mild cases may be confused with acute appendicitis or torsion. With bed rest the symptoms and signs gradually abate. If rupture is associated with severe bleeding, it may simulate a ruptured ectopic pregnancy. The blood loss, at times, may exceed 1000 mL.

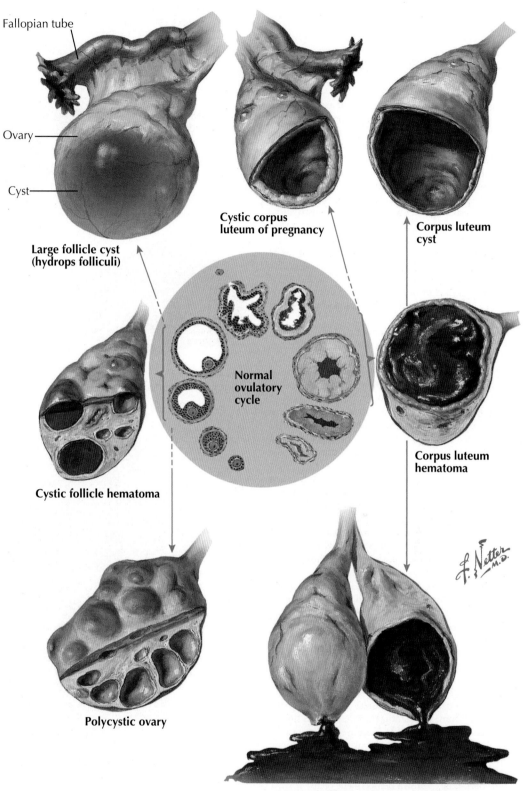

Fallopian tube

Ovary

Cyst

Large follicle cyst (hydrops folliculi)

Cystic corpus luteum of pregnancy

Corpus luteum cyst

Normal ovulatory cycle

Cystic follicle hematoma

Corpus luteum hematoma

Polycystic ovary

Ruptured hemorrhagic corpus luteum

Plate 10.9

Reproductive System: VOLUME 1

ENDOMETRIOSIS: PELVIS

Endometriosis refers to the growth of endometrium outside of its normal intrauterine location (ectopic) that retains the histologic characteristics and biologic response of the endometrium. It is nonneoplastic—that is, incapable of autonomous growth—but it is dependent on estrogenic and progesterone stimulation. Endometriosis may arise by one of several proposed mechanisms—lymphatic spread, metaplasia of coelomic epithelium or müllerian rests, seeding by retrograde menstruation, or direct hematogenous spread. Instances of presumed iatrogenic spread (surgical) have been reported. A role for an immunologic defect is debated but remains to be conclusively established. The greatest incidence occurs between 30 and 40 years of age and may be found in 5% to 15% of females, 20% of gynecologic laparotomies, 30% to 70% of patients with chronic pain, and 30% to 50% of patients with infertility.

Small lesions may be asymptomatic (30%). The diagnosis may be suggested by the presence of infertility, dysmenorrhea, sacral backache, deep thrust dyspareunia, and abnormal uterine bleeding. Pain caused by endometriosis characteristically begins premenstrually and ceases shortly after the menstrual flow is established. Involvement of the rectovaginal septum, cul-de-sac, or rectal wall may be responsible for rectal pain. If bowel endometriosis has penetrated the intestinal wall, the rectum may bleed cyclically. Bladder endometriosis may cause periodic hematuria and bladder irritability.

The presumptive diagnosis of pelvic endometriosis is based on the history, the absence of a previous pelvic infection, and characteristic findings of nodularity on bimanual vaginal and rectal examinations. A final diagnosis requires laparoscopy, laparotomy, or histologic confirmation. Pelvic examination may reveal the presence of small, firm, tender, fixed nodules in the region of the uterosacral ligaments, the posterior cul-de-sac, and the posterior surface of the uterus. The uterus is not infrequently retroverted, retroflexed, and fixed. Endometrial cysts are usually bilateral, rarely larger than a lemon or orange, cystic, and firmly fixed behind the uterus.

At laparotomy, endometriosis may be found incidentally to other pelvic lesions, particularly uterine fibroids and uterine retrodisplacements. Peritoneal implants may be seen as small, scattered, scarred puckerings or irregular, brown ("tobacco-stained") areas anywhere on the pelvic peritoneum. The peritoneum may be the site for atypical endometriosis, vesicles from clear, to red, to the classic dark-brown lesion. The ovarian or uterosacral ligaments may contain single or multiple discrete or confluent cicatrized nodules, with partially enveloped, minute, dark-blue or brown hemorrhagic blebs.

Endometriosis of the ovary may be manifested by minute surface "implants," small hemorrhagic cysts within the cortex, or by large cysts, which may practically replace the substance of the ovary. In surface endometriosis, tiny red, purple, or dark-brown hemorrhagic blebs are encompassed within puckered, cicatricial tissue. Endometrial cysts (chocolate cyst) vary in size but are rarely larger than 10 cm in diameter. They are frequently bilateral. The outer surface appears irregular, puckered, and adherent. Black or brown hemorrhagic areas may be evident. Along with its corresponding tube, the ovary is usually found adherent to the posterior surface of the broad ligament, uterus, lateral pelvic wall,

and rectosigmoid. An attempt to free the adnexa usually results in rupture of the cyst with escape of large quantities of thick, chocolate-colored fluid. The cyst wall appears thick, irregularly convoluted, and yellow-white in color. The inner lining has a dark, hemorrhagic stain. Microscopically, typical endometrial stroma and glands may line the cyst wall. Older lesions, presumably due to repeated desquamation and pressure of retained blood, may show little evidence of endometrial tissue. The cyst

may be lined by a broad zone of pseudoxanthoma cells, containing a hemoglobin derivative (hemosiderin). Hyalinization and fibrosis are seen in other areas.

Therapy depends on the age, parity, location, and extent of the lesions, severity of symptoms, the desire for children and the possibility of pregnancy, the patient's attitude toward loss of menstrual function or premature castration, and the coexistence of other pelvic pathology such as uterine fibroids.

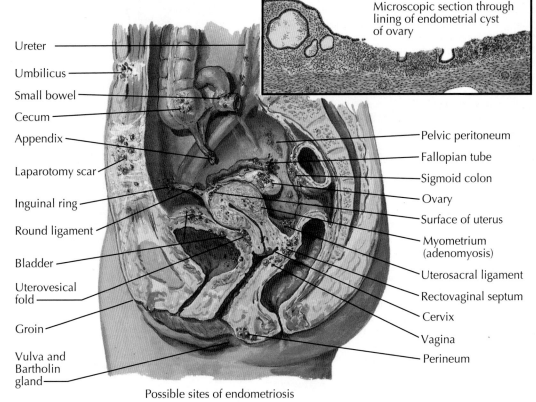

Diffuse pelvic endometriosis: ruptured endometrial (chocolate) cyst

Hemisection of ovary with endometrial cysts and corpus luteum

Microscopic section through lining of endometrial cyst of ovary

Ureter

Umbilicus

Small bowel

Cecum

Appendix

Laparotomy scar

Inguinal ring

Round ligament

Bladder

Uterovesical fold

Groin

Vulva and Bartholin gland

Pelvic peritoneum

Fallopian tube

Sigmoid colon

Ovary

Surface of uterus

Myometrium (adenomyosis)

Uterosacral ligament

Rectovaginal septum

Cervix

Vagina

Perineum

Possible sites of endometriosis

Plate 10.10

Ovaries

INFECTIONS

Infections of the ovaries are usually secondary, with most the result of cervical gonococcal or chlamydial infections that have ascended into the upper genital tract (pelvic inflammatory disease [PID]). Tubercular infections and infections in the gastrointestinal tract (particularly in association with appendicitis) also occur. Transmission may be through direct contact with infections of contiguous organs; lymphatic spread, particularly of streptococcal infections of the uterus to the ovarian hilum; and hematogenous extension from distant foci, as may occur in mumps, scarlatina, measles, diphtheria, tonsillitis, typhoid fever, and cholera. Most tubo-ovarian abscesses occur as a complication of PID.

Acute oophoritis due to surface invasion may be mild and superficial, resulting in thin, fibrinous periovarian adhesions. Chronic perioophoritis is evidenced in the residuals of PID, where dense, fibrous adhesions bind the ovary to the tube, posterior surface of the broad ligament, and lateral pelvic wall. Microscopically, a diffuse oophoritis may show hyperemia, edema, and leukocytic infiltration. The presence of multiple small abscesses indicates a lymphatic invasion. The open punctum of a ruptured graafian follicle or a thinly covered current hemorrhagic corpus luteum offers a favorable point of entry for contiguous infection. At times, an expanding ovarian abscess may replace the entire ovary. Fusion with the tube, or pyosalpinx, followed by a breakdown of intervening tissue, results in a tubo-ovarian abscess.

Streptococci and colon bacilli may secondarily infect a tubo-ovarian abscess of gonorrheal origin. Clinically, it is indistinguishable from a large pyosalpinx. Tubo-ovarian abscesses may gradually resolve, exacerbate intermittently, perforate locally to form a large pelvic abscess, or rupture into the rectum, bladder, vagina, or abdominal cavity. A chronic tubo-ovarian abscess may be relatively quiescent or asymptomatic. In the more acute state, it may give rise to low abdominal pain, nausea, vomiting, abdominal distension, evidence of pressure upon the bladder and rectum, fever, lower abdominal spasm and tenderness, leukocytosis, and a rapid sedimentation rate. Pelvic examination may reveal a fixed retrodisplaced uterus and bilateral, soft, irregular, fixed, tender masses laterally and behind the uterus. With subsidence of the infection and resorption, a tubo-ovarian cyst may result. These are large, retort-shaped, thin-walled, cystic structures, densely adherent to the pelvic peritoneum, broad ligament, and uterus. Tubo-ovarian abscesses must be differentiated from ovarian neoplasms with infarction, secondary infection, or rupture; appendicitis with pelvic abscess; diverticulitis; ovarian, tubal, or sigmoidal carcinoma; endometriosis; and ruptured tubal pregnancy with hematocele.

Streptococcal infections of the ovary and contiguous structures may follow postoperative or puerperal infections, instrumentation or cauterization of the cervix, insertion of a radium "tandem," and cervical stenosis with pyometra. Parametritis and pelvic cellulitis may progress until a firm, brawny, fixed, tender mass fills the posterior cul-de-sac and extends across the pelvis to the lateral pelvic walls. The ovaries are secondarily involved by lymphatic spread and contact. Large abscesses may

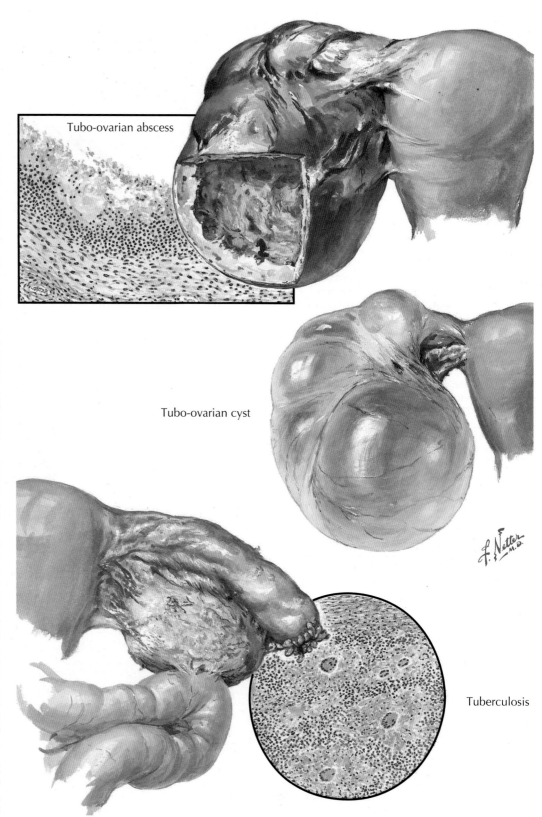

Tubo-ovarian abscess

Tubo-ovarian cyst

Tuberculosis

be formed that may be drained, may perforate, resolve, and recur.

Pelvic tuberculosis is almost invariably secondary to an old or recent acid-fast infection elsewhere, particularly of the lungs. The hematogenous route first involves the tubal endosalpinx, usually bilaterally, followed by direct invasion of the myosalpinx, perisalpinx, and pelvic peritoneum. This is often followed by perioophoritis, with penetration into the ovarian cortex. Thus tuberculosis of the ovary is secondary to a tuberculous salpingitis by contiguity. The ovary may appear grossly normal or slightly enlarged, studded with tubercles and covered by dense adhesions. In advanced cases caseation and an ovarian abscess with thick, ragged walls may be seen, sometimes eventuating into a pelvic abscess. Microscopically, only a few tubercles or marked infiltration with caseation may be noted. If resolution does not occur with standard tuberculosis antibiosis, total hysterectomy and bilateral salpingo-oophorectomy offers the best chance for cure.

Plate 10.11

Reproductive System: VOLUME 1

Large cyst

Smaller cysts containing yellowish fluid

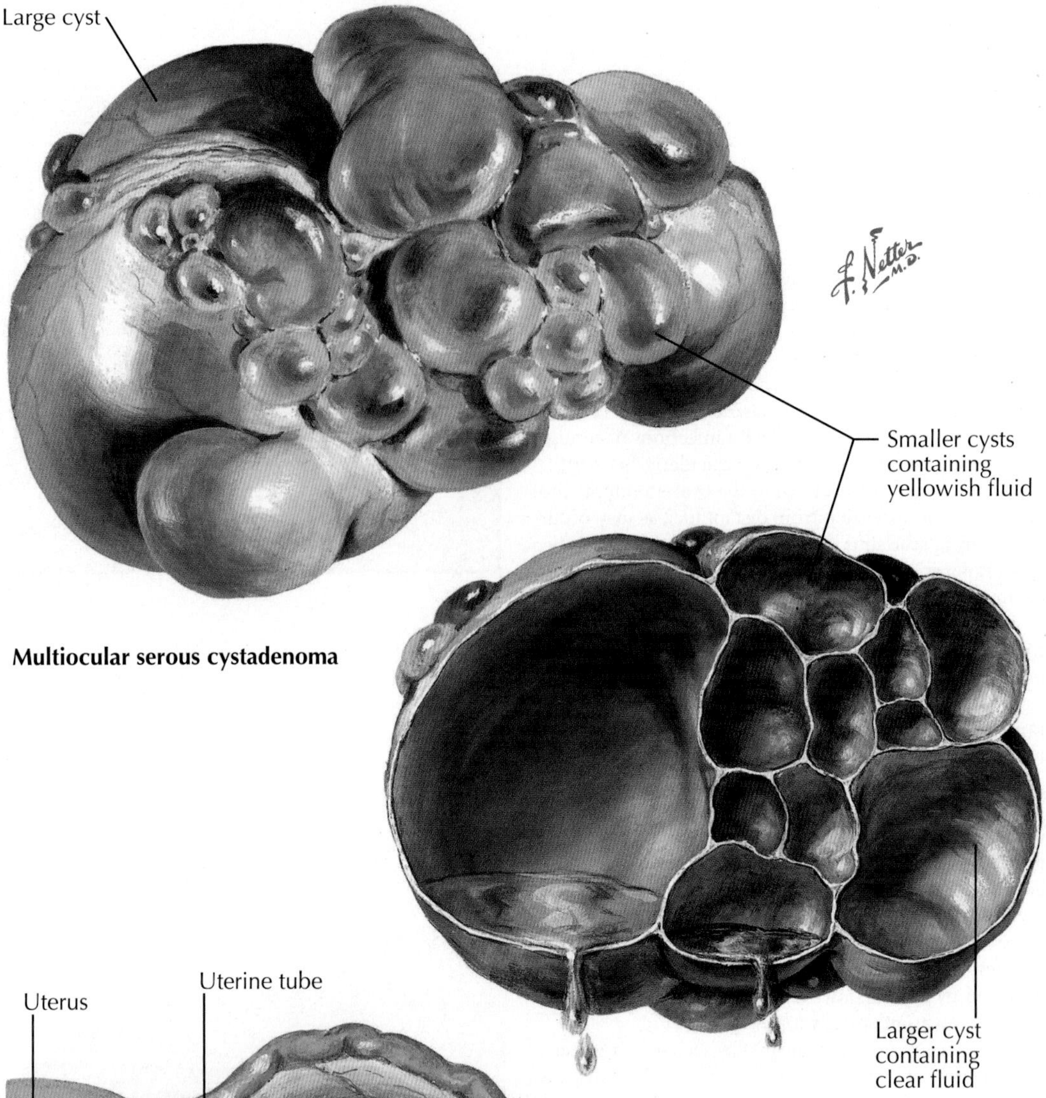

Multiocular serous cystadenoma

Larger cyst containing clear fluid

Uterine tube

Uterus

Simple serous cyst (serous cystoma)

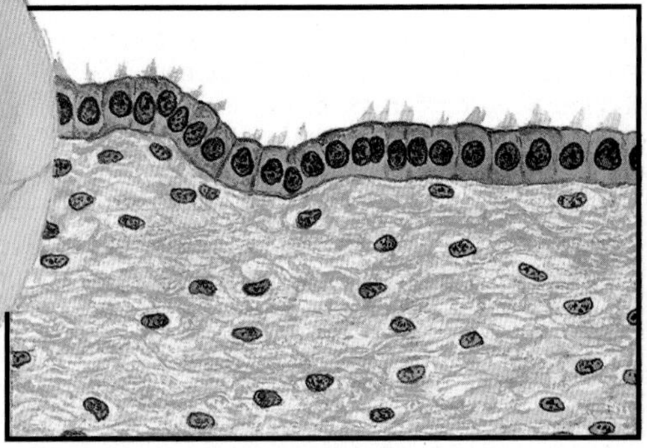

Serous epithelial lining

SEROUS CYSTOMA AND CYSTADENOMA

Cystadenomas are the most common ovarian neoplasms. Benign ovarian tumors are most frequently diagnosed at the time of routine examination and are asymptomatic. They are divisible, according to their lining epithelium, into serous and mucinous varieties. Approximately 90% of ovarian tumors encountered in younger females are benign and metabolically inactive. More than 75% of the benign adnexal masses are functional. Functional cysts are not true neoplasms but rather are anatomic variants resulting from the normal function of the ovary.

The proliferating elements in serous cysts include a connective tissue as well as an epithelial component. Depending on the rate of growth and predominance of each of these constituents, a variety of neoplastic patterns have evolved. These present gross and microscopic differences of sufficient degree to warrant division into subgroups. The simplest form is the serous cystoma, in which a single layer of cuboidal epithelium lines a fibrous cyst wall. In serous cystadenomas, the epithelium shows increased adenomatous proliferation. Papillary serous cystadenomas manifest an additional tendency toward papillary epithelioid growths. In surface papillomas, a single layer of "serous" epithelium covers numerous fibromatous excrescences. When fibrous tissue proliferation is accentuated and the "serous" epithelium retains an adenomatous tendency, the term *fibroadenoma,* or *adenofibroma,* is applied. If this variant includes cystic dilations of conspicuous size, it may be designated as a serous cystadenofibroma.

The simple serous cyst (serous cystoma) is a unilocular ovarian cyst lined by "serous" epithelium. Although a large size may be attained, it rarely exceeds that of an orange. It is usually unilateral, oval, or spherical in shape, thin-walled, smooth-surfaced, and grayish-white or translucent amber in color. On section, the thin walls collapse, with the escape of a clear, serous, watery, or straw-colored fluid. The latter is rich in serum proteins and lacks the viscid quality of mucinous fluid. The inner lining appears smooth and glistening. Microscopically, the characteristic "serous" epithelium is composed of a single layer of cuboidal or low cylindrical cells, with central, dark-staining nuclei. Cilia may be demonstrable. The lamellated, fibromatous tissue comprising the rest of the cyst wall is devoid of adenomatous structures. Occasionally, flattened, verrucous papillae may be found on the inner surface, made up of connective tissue cores covered by cuboidal epithelium like that lining the cyst.

The serous cystadenoma is a uni- or multilocular serous cyst of the ovary with glandlike, adenomatous, epithelial proliferations in its wall. It is generally smaller than the mucinous variety but may reach the size of a child's head. On rare occasions, it may be huge. Bilateral ovarian involvement is frequent. When multilocular, the cystadenomas are irregular in shape, with a bossed, smooth surface, traversed by many fine vessels. The color may vary in individual locules. A thickened, fibrous wall may appear grayish-white. Depending on the degree of

hemorrhagic discoloration, the component cysts may appear amber, brown, red, blue, or purple. Hemisection of a multilocular serous cystadenoma reveals chambers of varying size. The intervening septa may be thin, thick, partial, or complete. Communications between locules are established as a result of pressure necrosis. In the more solid portions of the intercystic septa, small daughter cysts may be evident. Histologically, a typical single layer of cuboidal or low columnar ciliated epithelium lines the acini and cyst walls.

The grapelike cystadenoma is a variation of the serous cystadenoma. Multiple, individual pedunculated cysts that project from the surface of the ovary characterize it. The tumor is multicystic rather than multilocular. The term is derived from its resemblance to a bunch of grapes of varying size. The histologic features are like those of the cystadenoma.

Simple cysts and serous cystadenomas are benign neoplasms. Cystectomy or a partial ovarian resection may suffice as therapy.

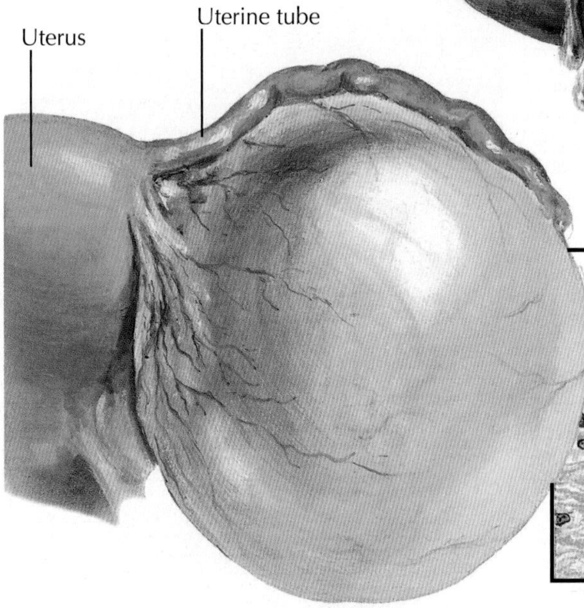

Plate 10.12

Ovaries

PAPILLARY SEROUS CYSTADENOMA

Papillary serous cystadenomas are serous cysts that manifest intra- or extracystic papillary growths in addition to adenomatous proliferations. Papillary serous cystadenomas are commonly multilocular, spherical, and lobulated. When papillations are confined to the inner wall, the cyst is apt to be unilateral and may attain a large size. When external and internal papillary masses are present, they are usually smaller and more frequently bilateral. Aside from their papillary structures, these neoplasms grossly resemble the serous cystadenomas. They are irregular in contour, with variations in the size of the component cysts, the color of the serous contents, and the thickness and completeness of the intervening septa. The papillary excrescences are the most striking feature of these tumors. They may involve isolated segments of one or more locules or the entire inner surface. They may be flat, warty, nodular, or villous. Fine, pedunculated, branching papillae may coalesce and form large cauliflower masses. Increased congestion may impart a red or raspberry color. Edema and myxomatous changes may induce a dead-white, swollen, translucent appearance. Necrosis and fatty changes may result in a grayish-yellow hue. Calcium deposits in the form of psammoma bodies render the papillations sandy to the touch.

On microscopic examination the cyst wall is composed of fibrous tissue of varying thickness and density, with an inner lining of "serous" epithelium. The latter is one cell in thickness, though tangential sections may give the appearance of pseudostratification. The cells, in general, are low columnar or cuboidal, with a dark-staining central vesicular nucleus. Cilia are frequently demonstrable. Variations in cell structure, including the presence of pear-shaped and intercalary or "peg" cells, suggest a similarity to tubal epithelium. Glandlike alveolar proliferations of the lining epithelium into the cyst wall give an adenomatous appearance. At times, local squamous cell metaplasia may be seen. The adenomatous spaces, when distended with serous secretion, are transformed into cystic cavities. The papillae may present a varying architecture, including an arborescent pattern. They are composed of a central core of connective tissue covered by a single layer of "serous" epithelium. The central core may be broad or narrow, coarse or fibrillar, dense or edematous. As a consequence of local degeneration, small deposits of calcium or psammoma bodies are not infrequently seen.

About two-thirds of papillary serous cystadenomas are encountered during the reproductive years (20–50). The cysts may be asymptomatic or may give rise to local discomfort, enlargement of the abdomen, or pressure symptoms, with urinary or bowel dysfunction. A twisted pedicle with infarction is not uncommon. Rupture of the cyst may occur following trauma or torsion. Pelvic examination may reveal moderate-sized, irregular, movable ovarian neoplasms. Peritoneal surface implantations, associated with papillary cystadenomas, may regress spontaneously following removal of the ovarian neoplasms. On the other hand, recurrences have been described after extirpation of an apparently benign papillary serous cystadenoma. Prognosis must be guarded, because the tumor may be grossly and histologically

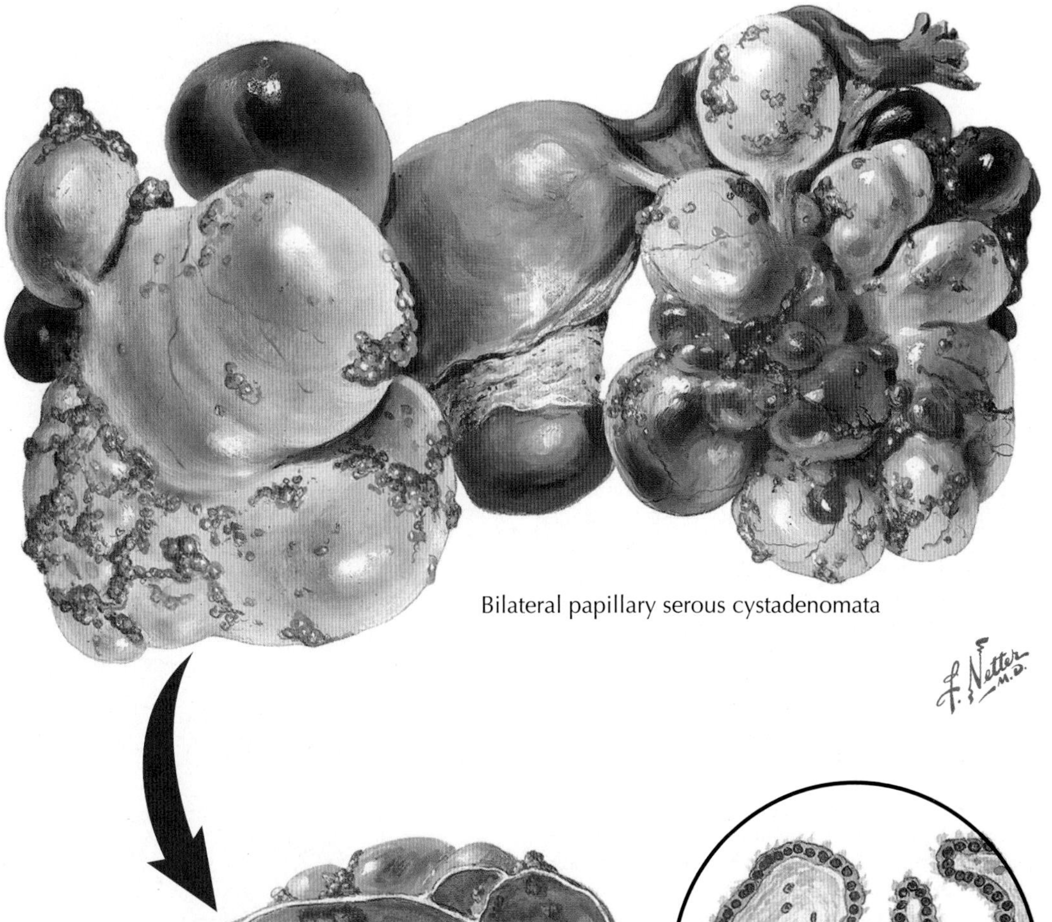

Bilateral papillary serous cystadenomata

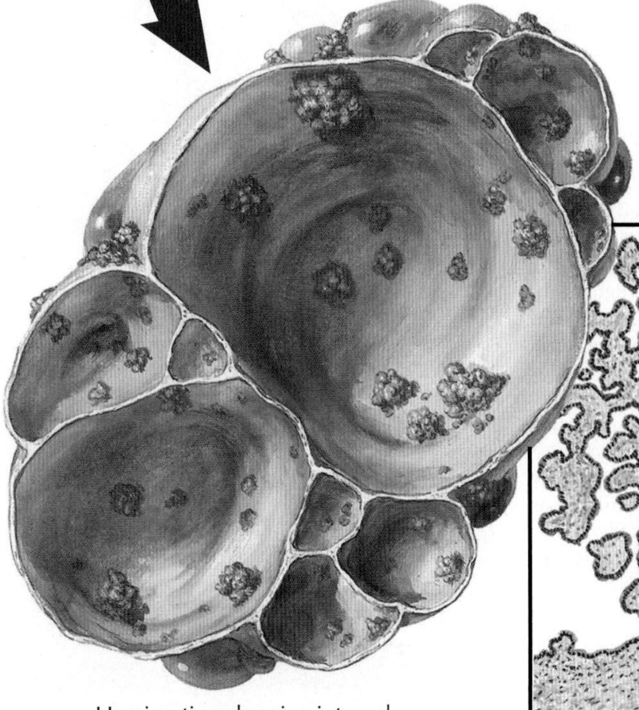

Hemisection showing internal papillary excrescences

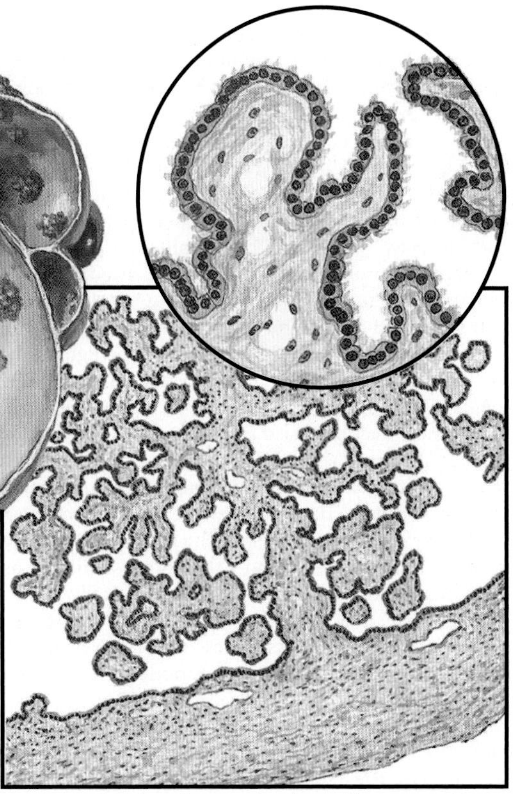

Branching architecture of papillary growth

benign but may manifest malignant tendencies. For this reason, a careful selection of representative areas and multiple microscopic sections is always indicated with papillary serous cystadenomas. In general, the presence of external papillations or peritoneal implants is considered evidence of malignancy unless proved otherwise. Ascites is not infrequent. At times, a pleural effusion may be associated with a papillary cystadenoma, as in Meigs syndrome.

Therapy may depend on a number of factors. A conservative attitude may be adopted in the presence of youth, slow growth, unilateral involvement, intact capsule, and sparse papillae. A total hysterectomy and bilateral salpingo-oophorectomy are indicated in females in their 40s or in the presence of bilateral involvement, peritoneal implants, external excrescences, and ascites. Aspiration or rupture of the cyst should be avoided to prevent dissemination and implantation.

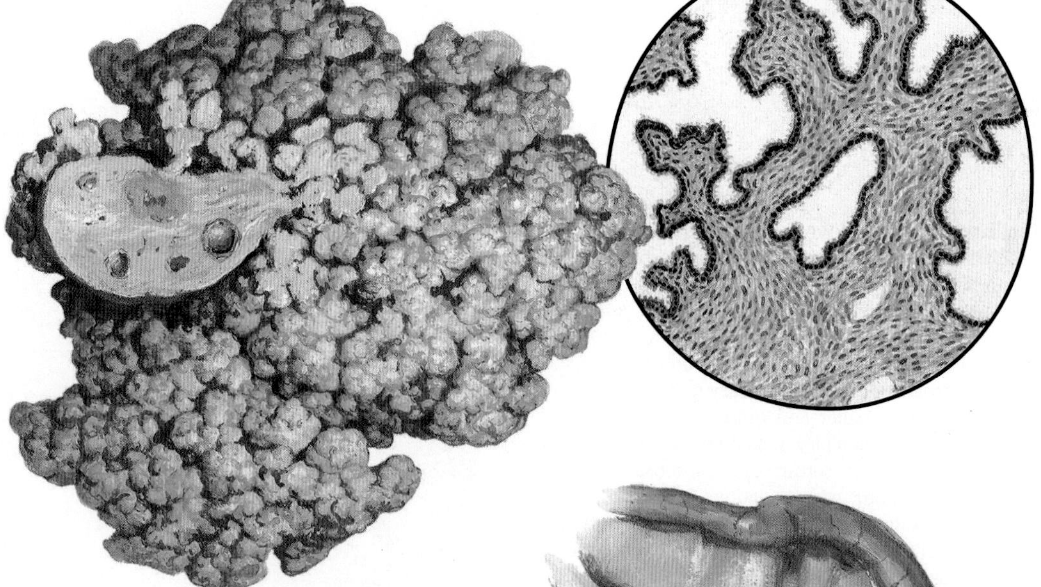

Plate 10.13

Reproductive System: VOLUME 1

Benign surface papilloma

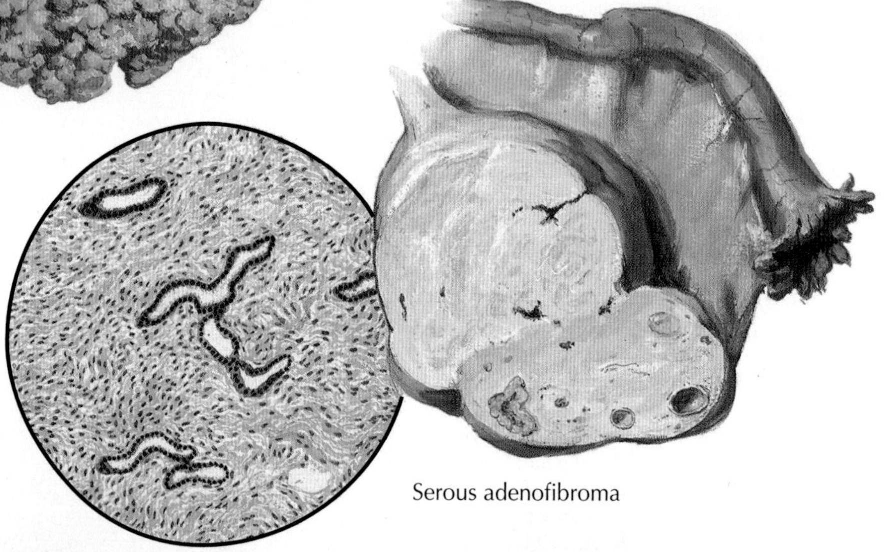

Papilloma, Serous Adenofibroma, and Cystadenofibroma

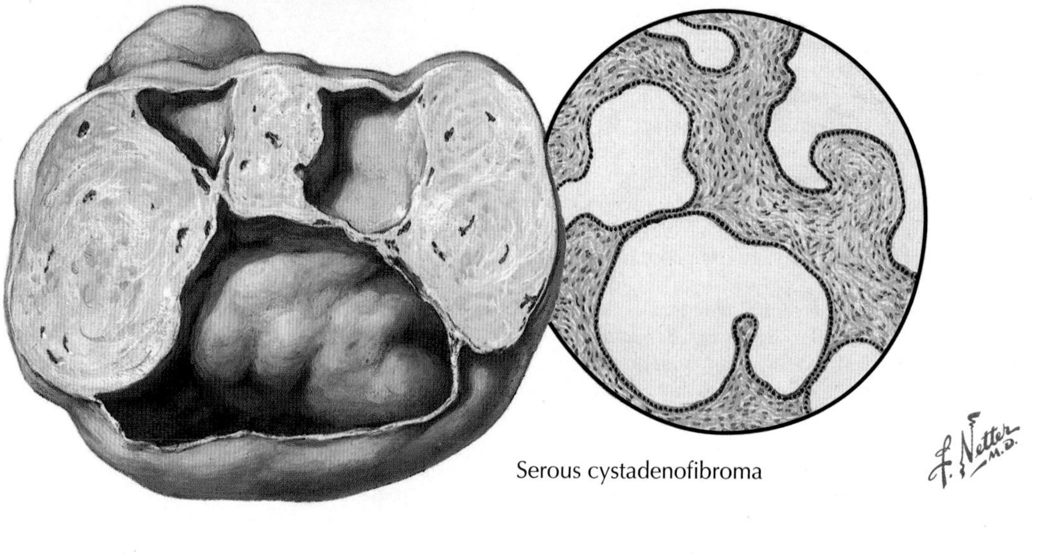

The serous epithelial tumors of the ovary include three subgroups in which the fibromatous elements overshadow the proliferation of "serous" epithelium. Although histogenetically similar, they present gross and microscopic differences. These variants may be classified as surface papillomas, adenofibromas, and cystadenofibromas. Adenofibromas are most commonly found as ovarian masses but may also occur in the cervix or uterine body. Adenofibromas are also closely related to cystadenofibromas that contain cystic areas but still contain more than 25% fibrous connective tissue.

Surface papillomas are solid fibromatous papillomas covered by "serous" epithelium. They may appear as a localized accumulation of minute, fine, warty excrescences; as conspicuous, multiple, finger-like, polypoid projections; or as large cauliflower growths, completely enveloping the ovary and filling the pelvis. Microscopically, the papillae are composed of fibrous tissue with varying degrees of cellularity and hyalinization, covered by a single layer of mesothelial or cuboidal cells. Surface papillomas may occur singly or in conjunction with other forms of serous epithelial tumors. They are benign and, usually, of no clinical significance. However, the marked proliferative activity, evidenced in large exophytic papillary growths, makes a gross decision as to their benign or malignant character most difficult.

Serous adenofibromas of the ovary are benign, fibromatous tumors containing serous adenomatous elements. They represent a variation of serous epithelial neoplasms. They have also been referred to as *fibroadenomas*, *fibromas with inclusion cysts*, *cystic fibromas*, *serous cystadenomas*, *solid adenomas*, and *adenocystic ovarian fibromas*. The lesion is rare and occurs most often after the age of 40 years. The tumors are usually encountered accidentally on pelvic examination or as incidental findings at laparotomy. Occasionally, if sufficiently large, they may give rise to local discomfort or pressure symptoms. Grossly, these neoplasms are solid, slightly irregular in contour, smooth-surfaced, and firm. On section, they are composed of gray-white, compact, interlacing bundles of connective tissue. Minute cystic spaces may be visible. The tumors vary considerably in size. They may be unilateral or bilateral (15%), single or multiple. An early lesion may appear as a tiny, firm, white, flat, oval, or serrated structure on the surface of the ovary or as a small nodule in the ovarian cortex. Growing, the tumor may replace most of the ovary. Grossly, the serous cystadenofibroma resembles the Brenner tumor, fibroma, fibromyoma, or theca cell tumor. Histologically, the neoplasm is composed of a dense connective tissue matrix in which are embedded numerous small cystic spaces. The latter are lined by compact, single-layered, cuboidal or low-columnar, often ciliated epithelium. The fibromatous tissue is predominant. It manifests a whorl-like arrangement of spindle cells, with varying degrees of hyalinization.

Serous adenofibroma

Serous cystadenofibroma

The epithelial glands are round, oval, irregular, or slit-like. Psammoma bodies are frequently found.

Serous cystadenofibromas are adenofibromas in which the cystic spaces are conspicuously enlarged. They may also be regarded as cystadenomas in which at least one quarter of the tumor mass is solid and fibromatous. The neoplasms possess all the gross and microscopic features of adenofibromas, except that they are usually larger, more irregular, and semicystic. Within the cystic spaces, papillations may occur.

Serous adenofibroma and cystadenofibroma are benign. Malignancy has not been observed, despite the fact that such potentialities would be expected to be similar to those of serous cystadenomas. Therapy consists of surgical excision. This is in contrast to pure serous tumors, which are more likely to be found with poorer differentiation. Papillary surface carcinomas of the ovary are most likely to be serous in type. A frozen section histologic evaluation should be considered for any ovarian mass that appears suspicious for malignancy.

Plate 10.14

Ovaries

Mucinous Cystadenoma

Mucinous (pseudomucinous) cystadenomas are cystic neoplasms of the ovary in which the lining epithelium is mucus-producing. Compared with serous cystadenomas, mucinous cystadenomas occur less frequently, are more likely to be multiloculated, are larger, and are less often bilateral (less than 5% versus 20%–25%). They are usually smooth-surfaced, tensely cystic, pedunculated, and benign. Usually, they are encountered during the reproductive years (20–50 years), rarely before puberty or after the menopause. In contrast to serous epithelial growths, they are less likely to be papillary (10%) and are rarely malignant (5%–15%). Mucinous cystadenomas may be minute in size or may fill the abdomen: mammoth ovarian cysts are apt to be of the mucinous type. Generally, they are recognized and are removed before reaching a diameter of 15 to 30 cm. Torsion of the pedicle is common (20%). Ascites is rare but may occur. Hydrothorax and hydroperitoneum, as encountered in Meigs syndrome, have been described. Intracystic hemorrhage, secondary suppuration, and spontaneous rupture are rare. Penetration of the capsule, with implantation and growth of mucinous epithelium in the peritoneal cavity, may cause pseudomyxoma peritonei. The rate of growth is generally slow. Rupture of a cyst by trocar, aspiration, or handling should be avoided. Unilateral removal of ovary and tube is the therapy of choice, at which time the specimen must be carefully examined for evidence of localized, firm infiltrations in the cyst wall.

Grossly, the outer surface of mucinous cysts appears smooth, lobulated, glistening, and grayish-white or whitish-blue in color. The cut surface may present a variety of architectural patterns, including a unilocular cyst with internal, sickle-shaped ridges representing the remnants of previous interlocular septa; a multilocular, semisolid neoplasm, with chambers of varying size and honeycombed cystic aggregates projecting into the lumen; or a more solid tumor composed of numerous minute compartments that present a spongelike appearance. Internal papillary excrescences are uncommon (10%). The cyst wall is fibrous and of varying thickness. Septa are firm, fibrous or adenomatous, complete or incomplete. The characteristic fluid is mucoid, viscid, and transparent or cloudy. As a result of bleeding, the fluid contents may assume a red, tan, brown, or black color.

Microscopically, the connective tissue capsule is composed of an outer layer of dense, fibrous tissue and an inner zone, which is looser and more cellular. Evidence of localized degeneration may be noted, including edema, inflammation, necrosis, fatty acid deposits, and calcification. The dividing septa are extensions from the inner zone of connective tissue. A well-differentiated, single-layered epithelium lines the cyst walls and trabeculae. It invaginates into the connective tissue stroma to give an adenomatous appearance. The epithelial lining is composed of tall columnar cells, with deeply staining basal nuclei and abundant acidophilic, finely granular cytoplasms. Actively secreting goblet cells are scattered irregularly between the columnar cells.

Pseudomyxoma peritonei refers to the secondary implantation on the peritoneum of mucinous tissue, with subsequent local invasion, proliferation, and overproduction of thick, gelatinous, mucinous material, which may fill the pelvis, abdomen, and subphrenic spaces. Pseudomyxoma peritonei may follow rupture of a mucinous cystadenoma of the ovary or a mucocele of the appendix. Recent histologic studies suggest that in most patients the appendix is the primary tumor source. In rare cases, metaplasia by the cells of the peritoneal surface may account for this tumor. Clinically, pseudomyxoma peritonei may give rise to a progressive enlargement of the abdomen, evidence of increased abdominal pressure, interference with bladder and bowel function, and cachexia. The condition is progressive and, though histologically benign, may cause a fatal outcome owing to mechanical interference. The rate of growth may be rapid, or the progress may be drawn out over many years.

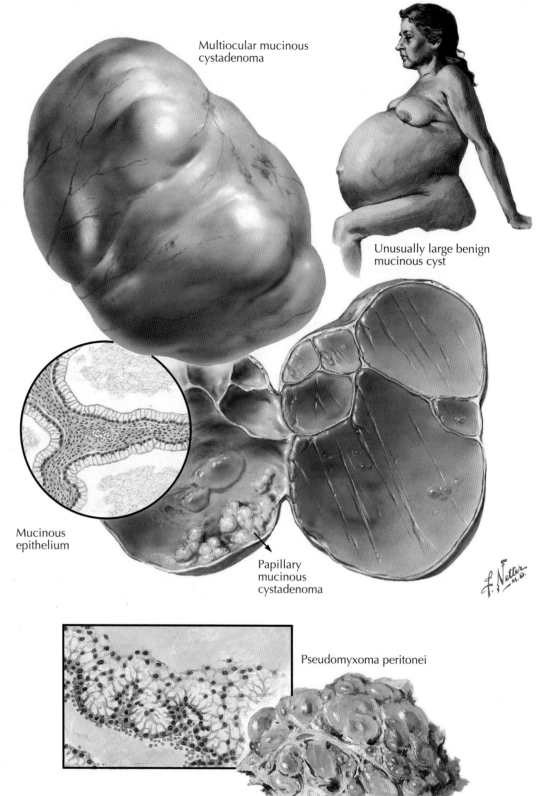

Multiocular mucinous cystadenoma

Unusually large benign mucinous cyst

Mucinous epithelium

Papillary mucinous cystadenoma

Pseudomyxoma peritonei

Plate 10.15

Reproductive System: VOLUME 1

TERATOMA

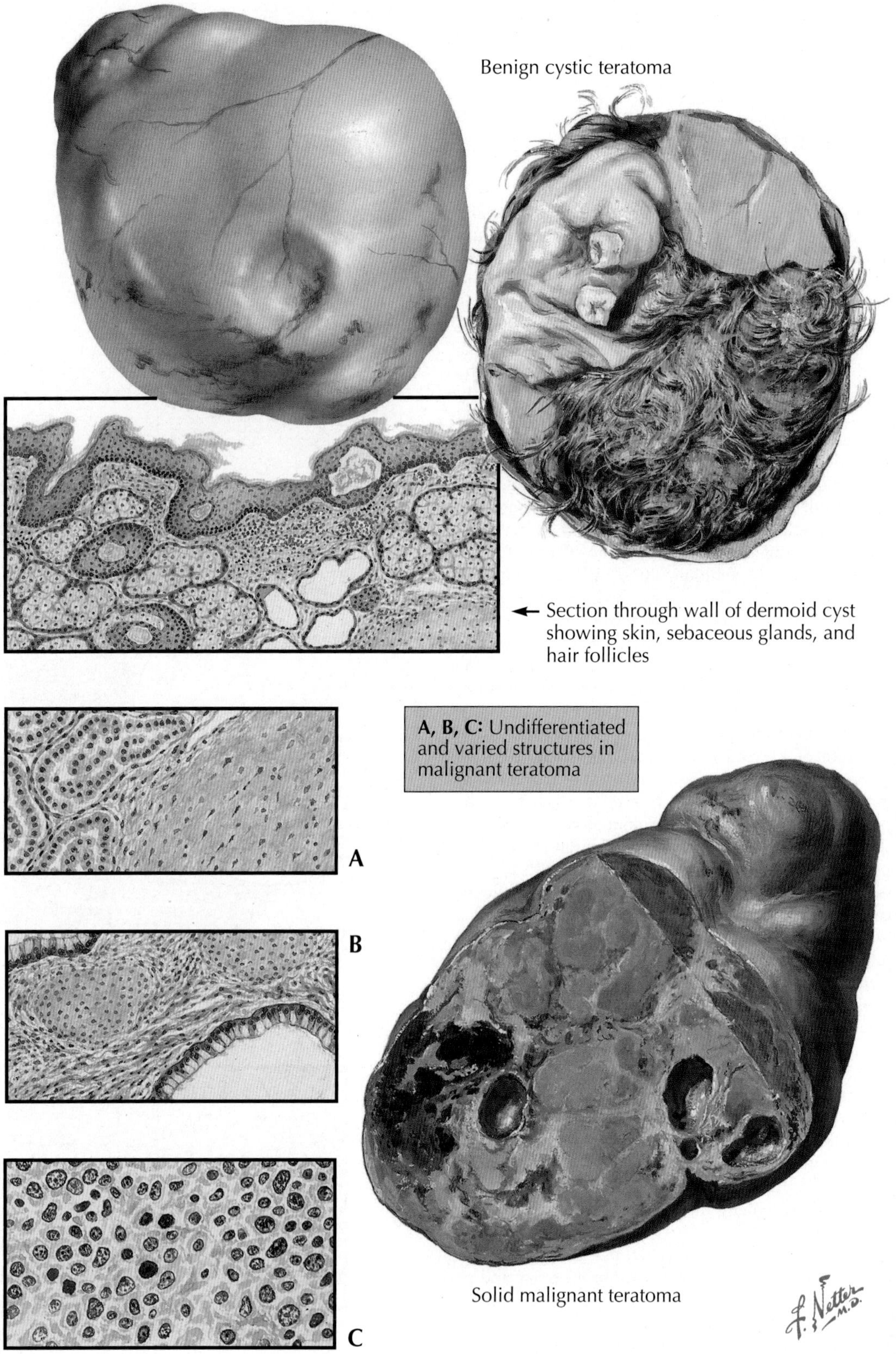

The most common ovarian tumor in young, reproductive-age females is the cystic teratoma, or dermoid, which originates from a germ cell and contains elements from all three germ cell layers. They are the most common ovarian neoplasm in the second and third decades of life. These tumors may be benign or malignant (1%–2% malignant, usually in females older than 40 years). They account for 20% to 25% of all ovarian tumors and one-third of all benign tumors. A dermoid cyst may be microscopic in size or may reach proportions up to 40 cm. Bilateral involvement occurs in 10% to 25% of cases. The tumors are usually round or oval, doughy and rather heavy, with a smooth, opaque, gray-white, or yellow surface. The open specimen reveals fatty, sebaceous material, strands of long hair and an intracystic plug, covered by scalplike skin. The tufts of hair originate mostly in this skin-lined area. The color of the hair bears no relation to that of the host. The remainder of the cyst lining appears smooth and glistening or rough and granular. Cartilage, bone, and teeth are found in two-thirds of the cases.

Histologically, almost any well-differentiated tissue of ectodermal, mesodermal, or endodermal origin may be found. The skin and its appendages predominate. Section through the dermoid plug, which corresponds to the embryonic area, may reveal the presence of stratified squamous epithelium, sebaceous glands, sweat glands, and hair follicles. Mesodermal elements, occasionally found, include plaques of cartilage, tracheal, thyroid, and adipose tissue. Development of specific tissues may give rise to a struma ovarii (functional thyroid tissue), pseudomucinous cyst, fibroma, chondrofibroma, or osteofibroma. Portions of the cyst wall, other than the dermoid plug, may be lined by flattened or cuboidal epithelium, or granulation tissue containing phagocytic, pseudoxanthoma cells and foreign-body giant cells.

Clinically, dermoid cysts may be asymptomatic or associated with lower abdominal pain, abdominal enlargement, or pressure symptoms. A position anterior to the uterus is common. Palpation of a doughy, cystic, heavy ovarian tumor is suggestive. X-ray demonstration of teeth is pathognomonic. Ultrasonography usually reveals a unilocular cystic mass, which can contain hyperechoic contents, and areas of acoustic shadowing, reflective of the varied architecture of these tumors. Because dermoids are almost always pedunculated, torsion is common. Leakage or rupture gives rise to an irritative, chemical peritonitis and dense adhesions; adhesions around dermoids are common. Therapy includes cystectomy or oophorectomy. Because of the frequent bilateral involvement, the opposite ovary should be carefully inspected. It must be kept in mind that dermoids may be multiple in a single ovary.

The solid or embryonal teratomas are malignant tumors composed of poorly differentiated, highly proliferative elements derived from all three germ layers. They constitute less than 1% of all dermoid growths. These neoplasms are usually unilateral, round or oval, smooth or lobulated. Most often they are small or moderate in size but may reach large proportions. Though generally solid and firm, necrosis and cystic degeneration may impart a softer consistency. The capsule may be intact or perforated by the highly malignant, proliferating tissue, with adherence to surrounding structures. On section, a variegated consistency and coloration are apparent, depending on the predominance of different

tissues and the degree of degeneration, hemorrhage, and cavitation. Microscopically, well-differentiated areas may exist side by side with young embryonal, undifferentiated portions as well as unidentifiable sarcomatous or carcinomatous tissues. Mesodermal structures are frequently more abundant and include connective tissue, cartilage, bone, lymphoid tissue, and smooth or striated muscle. Ectoderm may be represented by nervous system tissue. Skin and appendages are rare.

The diagnosis is usually not made until laparotomy or laparoscopy is performed. The presence of a solid, heavy, rapidly growing neoplasm in a young individual is suggestive. Perforation of the capsule, local extension, dissemination throughout the abdomen, retroperitoneal lymph node involvement, and distant metastases may occur. Metastatic extension may involve only a sarcomatous or adenocarcinomatous portion of the neoplasm. The prognosis is poor.

Benign cystic teratoma

← Section through wall of dermoid cyst showing skin, sebaceous glands, and hair follicles

A, B, C: Undifferentiated and varied structures in malignant teratoma

A

B

C

Solid malignant teratoma

Plate 10.16

Ovaries

ADNEXAL TORSION

Adnexal torsion is the twisting of part or all of the adnexa on its mesentery, resulting in tissue ischemia and frank infarction. This usually involves the ovary but may include the fallopian tube as well. Although this accounts for only 2% to 3% of all gynecologic operative emergencies, it is nonetheless a significant event that often results in the loss of the ovary. Torsion of the adnexa is usually associated with the presence of an ovarian, tubal, or a paratubal mass (50%–60% have an ovarian tumor or cyst, >5 cm in diameter). The risk of torsion is higher during pregnancy (20% of cases) or after ovulation induction. The average age of patients experiencing adnexal torsion is between the mid-20s and mid-30s.

Torsion in prepubertal females may be caused by a pelvic mass or due to mechanical factors unique to children. In early puberty the ovaries drop from their prepubertal position at the pelvic brim into the pelvis. This is driven by the pubertal surge of gonadotropins. Some young females may have longer supportive ligaments, predisposing them to torsion at this time. Approximately 60% of the time ovarian torsion occurs on the right side and is often confused with appendicitis. The sigmoid colon in the left lower quadrant helps prevent the left ovary from twisting.

The first indication of torsion is generally abrupt, intense, and unilateral abdominal pain. This occurs with swelling and inflammation due to venous obstruction, which generally occurs before arterial obstruction. The pain of adnexal torsion is generally intermittent, with a periodicity that varies from hours to days or longer; this is in contrast to the variable pain caused by obstruction of the bowel, ureter, or common bile duct, which is more regular and frequent. The pain is often accompanied by nausea and vomiting (60%–70% of cases), and physical examination most often can demonstrate a unilateral tender mass (90% of cases). Because these symptoms and findings can be nonspecific, the possibility of other causes such as an ectopic pregnancy, rupture or bleeding into a cyst, abscesses, or small bowel obstruction must all be considered.

Ultrasonography may demonstrate a cystic adnexal mass, but the acute character and intensity of symptoms usually encountered means that the diagnosis is most often made at the time of surgery. Doppler-flow studies to demonstrate the presence or absence of blood flow to the ovary may be helpful but the absence of flow is not diagnostic of an adnexal torsion: however, normal Doppler findings are seen in 45% to 61% of torsion cases. On computed tomography, a whirl sign is characterized by the appearance of a twisted ovarian pedicle and has a positive predictive value of 75% to 80%.

Patients with confirmed adnexal torsion (and those with a high degree of suspicion) are generally treated by surgical exploration. Conservative operative management may be possible in more than 75% of patients. It is thought that irreversible ischemia may not occur for as long as 72 hours after the initial obstruction. This allows the ovary to be conserved by "detorsion" of the ovary. Most authors suggest removing an ovarian or

Clinical findings

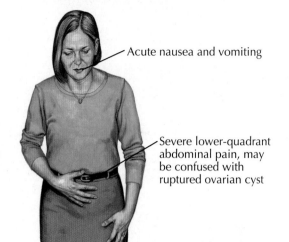

Acute nausea and vomiting

Severe lower-quadrant abdominal pain, may be confused with ruptured ovarian cyst

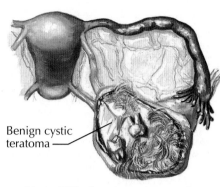

Benign cystic teratoma

Up to 50% of torsion cases may be associated with a medium-sized (10–12 cm) mass

Mechanism of torsion

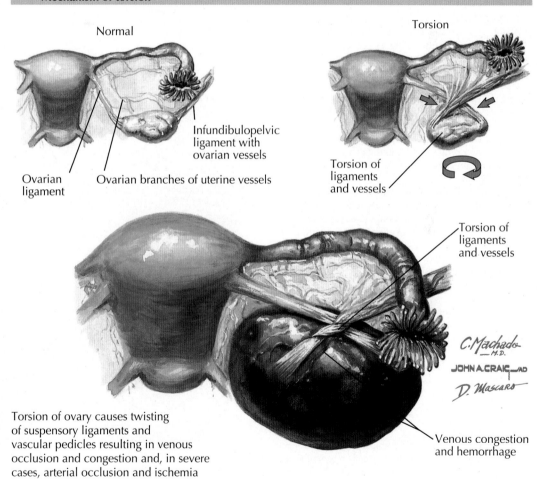

Normal

Ovarian ligament

Ovarian branches of uterine vessels

Infundibulopelvic ligament with ovarian vessels

Torsion

Torsion of ligaments and vessels

Torsion of ligaments and vessels

Venous congestion and hemorrhage

Torsion of ovary causes twisting of suspensory ligaments and vascular pedicles resulting in venous occlusion and congestion and, in severe cases, arterial occlusion and ischemia

tubal mass following "detorsion" to reduce the risk of recurrence. Part or the entire ovary may thus be salvaged if intervention takes place early enough in the process. Unfortunately, when significant ischemia or underlying pathology is present, removal of part or all of the ovary may be required. There are insufficient data to resolve the value or need for oophoropexy following detorsion.

Concerns about the possibility of freeing a thrombus from the obstructed venous supply of the adnexa have been raised. If such a thrombus were present, the possibility that this could embolize to the heart and lungs would militate against untwisting the adnexa. Although a theoretical risk, this has not been demonstrated to occur clinically, making conservative management of these cases more acceptable.

Plate 10.17

Reproductive System: VOLUME 1

FEMINIZING NEOPLASMS

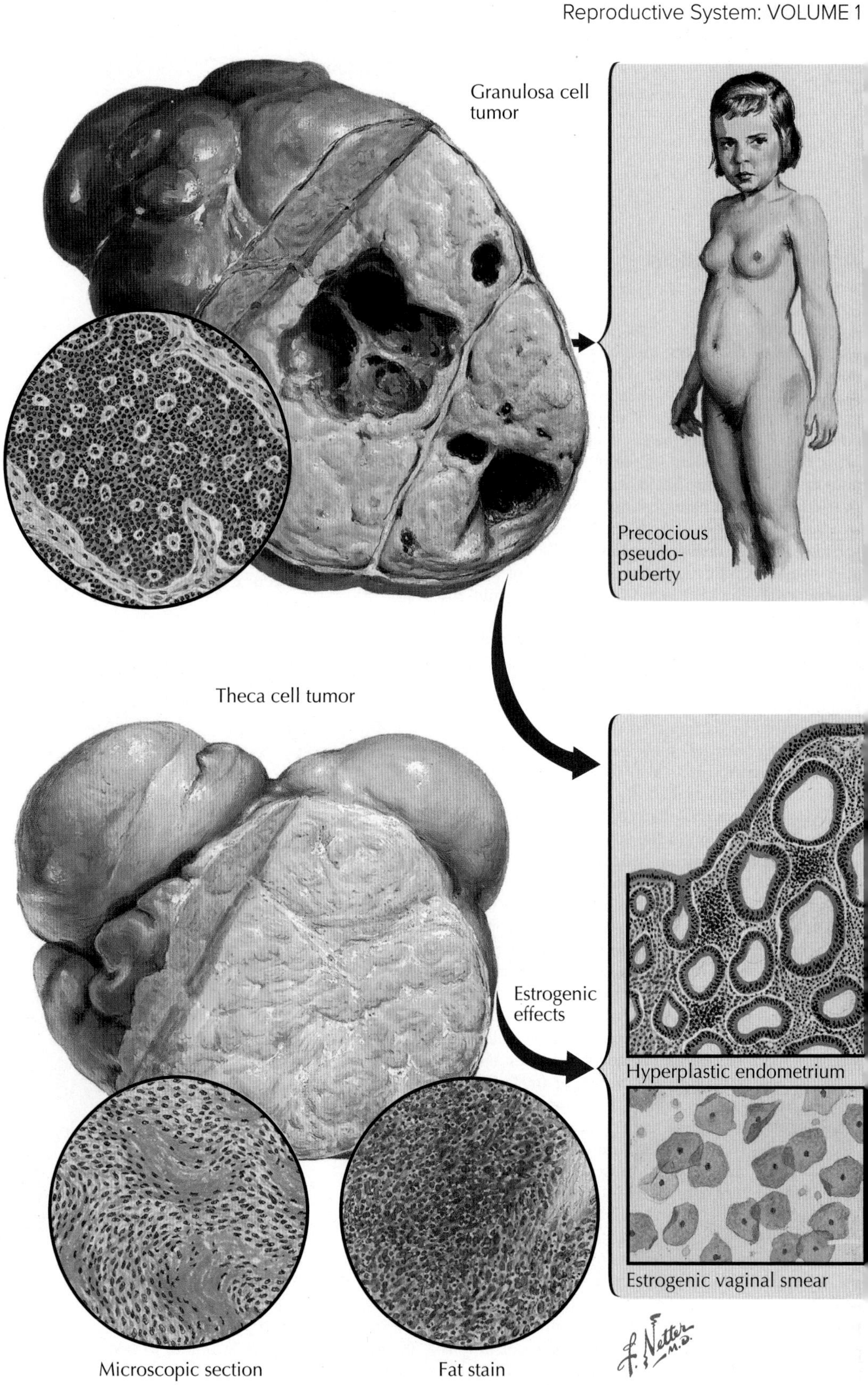

The granulosa cell tumor is a feminizing neoplasm composed of cells that resemble, in appearance and arrangement, the granulosa cells of the graafian follicle. It is the most common of the hormonal tumors of the ovary, comprising 6% of all ovarian tumors, and is the most common type of potentially malignant ovarian sex cord stromal tumor. Unlike theca cell tumors, it may be found in the prepubertal years (5%). The degree of hormonal activity is variable. The clinical characteristics depend on age: in childhood, hyperestrogenism is responsible for the syndrome of precocious pseudopuberty manifested by the premature development of secondary sex characteristics (feminine contour, breast growth, pubic and axillary hair, enlargement of the genitalia, anovulatory menses, acyclic uterine bleeding, hyperplastic endometrium, and estrogenic vaginal epithelium); during sexual maturity, the granulosa cell tumor may induce irregular vaginal bleeding; postmenopausally, irregular uterine bleeding, a marked estrogenic vaginal epithelium, and endometrial proliferation or hyperplasia may occur. Breast enlargement, growth of uterine fibroids, endometrial hyperplasia with polyps, and a concomitant endometrial carcinoma may develop. The tumor, by virtue of its size and weight, may give rise to abdominal pain, pressure symptoms, and torsion of the pedicle with infarction, hemorrhage, rupture, ascites (10%), and Meigs syndrome. Most granulosa cell tumors have an indolent growth pattern. Prognosis does not correlate with the histologic pattern of the tumor: 90% of tumors found are stage I and the prognosis is good (90% 10-year survival); a poorer prognosis is found with tumors >15 cm that have ruptured or have a high mitotic rate or aneuploidy.

Granulosa cell tumors are usually unilateral (98%), solid, movable, round to oval, encapsulated neoplasms, with a smooth, lobulated, yellow-tan surface. Their consistency is moderately firm or soft, depending on the degree of necrosis and cystic degeneration. They vary in size from a few millimeters to 40 cm in diameter. Section reveals solid or partially cystic, cellular, granular, slightly trabeculoid tumors, with large areas of grayish-white to yellow or tan-brown color, scattered necrotic foci, hemorrhage, and liquefaction.

Derived from the sex cords of the ovary and the stroma of the developing gonad, these tumors have a predominance of granulosa cells. Classically, these tumors contain eosinophilic bodies surrounded by granulosa cells (Call-Exner bodies). Poorly differentiated tumors may be confused with adenocarcinomas (especially small cell carcinoma). Somatic mutations in FOXL2 have been identified in 97% of adult subtype granulosa cell tumors.

Theca cell tumors are benign, unilateral, solid, estrogen-producing neoplasms composed of cells resembling the theca interna. They are histogenetically and biologically like the granulosa cell tumors, which may coexist to a greater or lesser degree. The majority occur during the menopausal and postmenopausal years (70%), are rarely seen before 30 years of age, and do not occur before puberty. Their hormonal effects are like those of the granulosa cell neoplasms.

Theca cell tumors are solid, round to oval, slightly irregular, firm, encapsulated, yellowish and fibromatous, varying from a few millimeters to 20 cm or more in diameter. The surface is smooth, free of adhesions, and grayish-yellow. On section, interlacing strands and whorls of tissue suggest a fibroma-like appearance.

Granulosa cell tumor

Precocious pseudo-puberty

Theca cell tumor

Estrogenic effects

Hyperplastic endometrium

Estrogenic vaginal smear

Microscopic section

Fat stain

The essential difference from the granulosa cell tumor, however, is the presence of areas of yellowish hue, which may, at times, be more orange, tan, or brown. Foci of necrosis, cystic degeneration, and calcification may occur.

Histologically, the tumor is composed of interlacing, broad sheets of cells, showing varying degrees of cellularity. Bands of collagenous, fibrous tissue may separate bundles of typical thecoma cells. The characteristic theca cells have an epithelioid appearance, are elongated and ovoid, with plump, oval nuclei, indistinct borders, and moderate fibrillar, reticulated, and occasionally vacuolated cytoplasm. Clusters of more spherical, luteinized cells may also be seen. Hyaline plaques and collagenous strands are irregularly distributed throughout the tumor. The ovarian parenchyma in the involved and uninvolved ovaries may show evidence of stromal hyperplasia and thecomatosis.

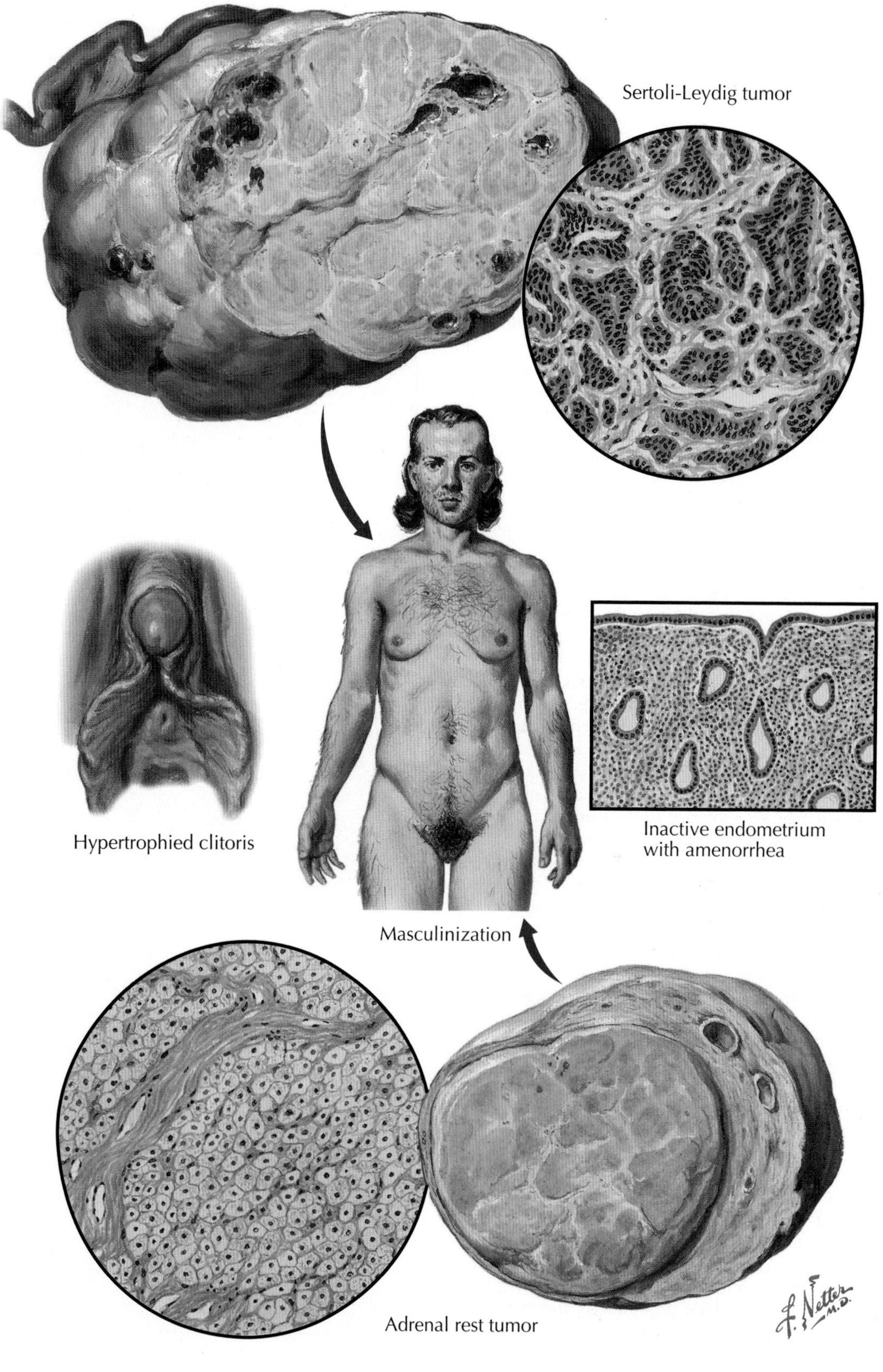

Plate 10.18

Ovaries

MASCULINIZING NEOPLASMS

Masculinizing tumors are rare sex cord tumors of the ovary (<0.5% of ovarian tumors) that carry male elements and may be associated with virilization. Tumors vary in size but generally are 5 to 15 cm in diameter. For the sake of simplicity, they may be divided into two categories: the Sertoli-Leydig cell tumor (formerly arrhenoblastoma) and the adrenal rest tumor. The picture of virilization associated with these neoplasms is the result of defeminization and masculinization. Defeminization is manifested by amenorrhea, infertility, loss of feminine contour, decrease in size of the breasts, genital hypoplasia, and coarse skin texture. Masculinization is evident in hirsutism, male escutcheon, enlargement of the clitoris, increased muscular development, acne, and hoarseness of the voice. Metabolic disturbances, including hypertension and disorders of carbohydrate metabolism, are relatively uncommon with adrenal rest tumors but may occur with Sertoli-Leydig cell tumors. Plasma levels of testosterone, androstenedione, and other androgens may be elevated; urinary 17-ketosteroid values are usually normal. (Androgen secretion by the tumor may result in erythrocytosis.) Laboratory studies cannot reliably differentiate between virilization caused by adrenal tumors and virilization caused by ovarian sources. Symptoms referable to the presence of a pelvic mass, torsion of a pedicle, necrosis, hemorrhage, and ascites may occur.

Therapy includes a surgical exploration and resection. Young patients with stage 1A disease (80%) may be treated with unilateral salpingo-oophorectomy. Undifferentiated tumors or advanced-stage disease requires more aggressive surgical resection and may be treated with adjunctive chemotherapy (vincristine, actinomycin D, and cyclophosphamide) or radiation.

The Sertoli-Leydig cell tumor is believed to be derived from originally male-directed cells of the indifferent bisexual, embryonal gonads. The tumors represent varying degrees of similarity to testicular structures. Although rare, Sertoli-Leydig cell tumors are the most common of the masculinizing tumors. The predominant age is older than 30 (70%), with less than 10% older than 50. The tumors are unilateral (95%), solid, smooth, lobulated, encapsulated, gray-yellow neoplasms. The size is generally between 5 and 15 cm. The cut surface is firm and grayish-yellow. Numerous necroses, hemorrhages, and cystic changes can be recognized. Sex cord (Sertoli) cells and stromal (Leydig) cells are present in varying proportions, but tubular patterns predominate. Individual cells may appear immature. Lipochrome pigments (crystalloids of Reinke) are present in 20% of tumors. These tumors may be hard to differentiate from granulosa cell tumors and may mimic endometrioid or Krukenberg tumors.

Most Sertoli-Leydig cell tumors are stage I at diagnosis. The tumors tend to behave as low-grade malignancies, and the 5-year survival rate is reported to vary from 70% to 90%. Survival is poorer for higher stage and poorly differentiated tumors. Excessive hair often regresses but does not disappear; clitoral enlargement and voice changes (if present) are unlikely to reverse. Pregnancy is unlikely in the presence of these tumors because of anovulation induced by the hyperandrogenism, although there is no direct effect on the pregnancy,

should they coexist. (Hormonal effects on the fetus could be postulated; however, usually placental aromatase can convert androgens into estrogens except in cases of extreme hyperandrogenism.)

Adrenal rest tumors have also been referred to as *luteoma, hypernephroid tumor, adrenal adenoma,* and *adrenocorticoid tumor.* It is suggested that they may arise from aberrant adrenal rests. They are extremely rare, unilateral, solid, small, round or oval, encapsulated tumors, which may replace only part of the ovary.

The surface is yellow-orange to brown, rubbery or moderately firm, and divided into lobules by fibrous septa. Necrosis, hemorrhage, and cystic degeneration are frequent. Histologically, they may show irregular masses of large, polyhedral, sharply defined cells, with prominent, irregular nuclei and abundant, finely granular, vacuolated cytoplasm. Other areas may reveal nests or syncytial groups of small polygonal cells with uniform, round nuclei and solid, granular cytoplasm, resembling the peripheral cells of the adrenal cortex.

Sertoli-Leydig tumor

Hypertrophied clitoris

Masculinization

Inactive endometrium with amenorrhea

Adrenal rest tumor

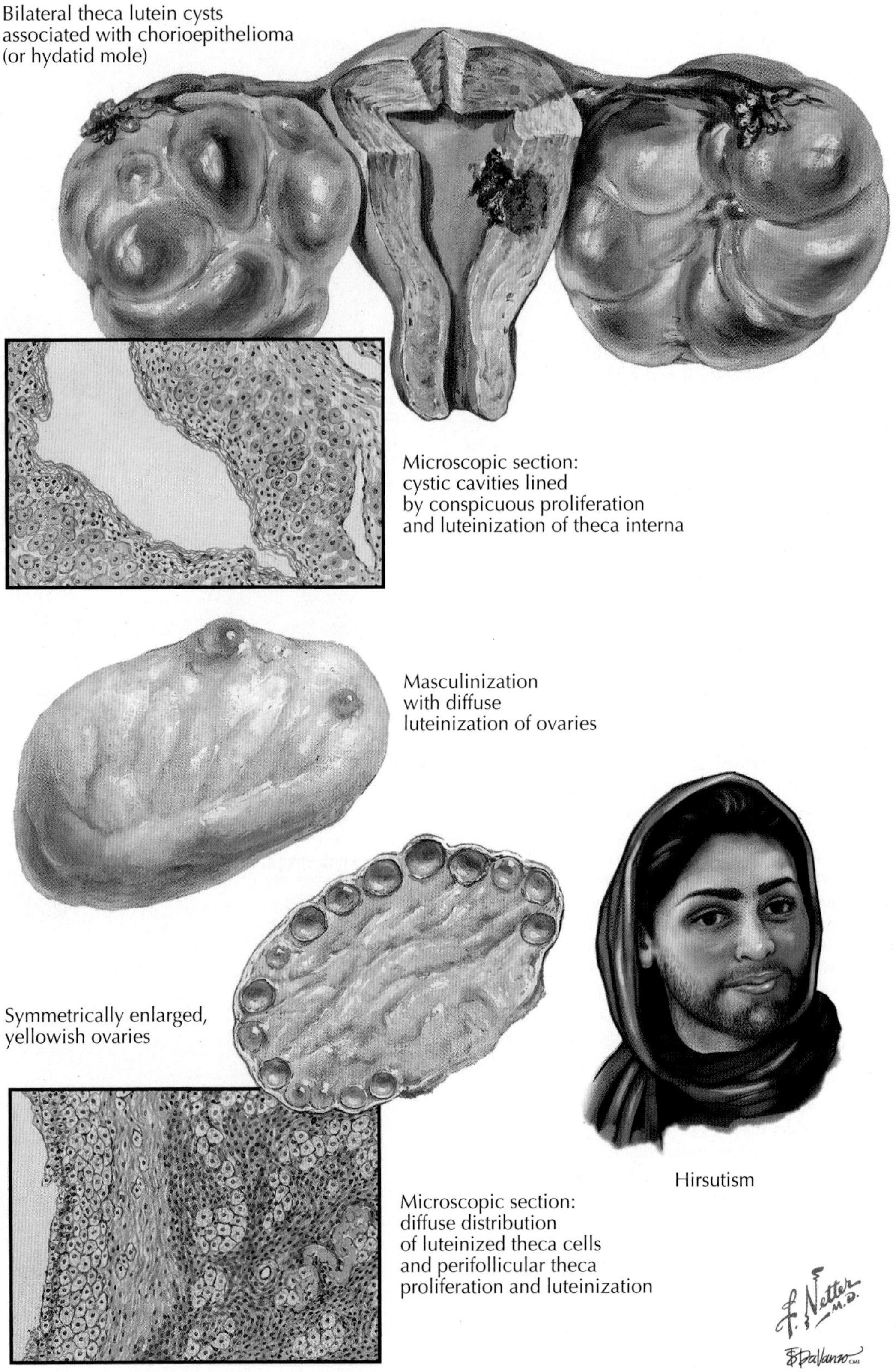

Plate 10.19

Reproductive System: VOLUME 1

Bilateral theca lutein cysts
associated with chorioepithelioma
(or hydatid mole)

Microscopic section:
cystic cavities lined
by conspicuous proliferation
and luteinization of theca interna

Masculinization
with diffuse
luteinization of ovaries

Symmetrically enlarged,
yellowish ovaries

Microscopic section:
diffuse distribution
of luteinized theca cells
and perifollicular theca
proliferation and luteinization

Hirsutism

ENDOCRINOPATHIES: LUTEINIZATION

In the presence of a hydatidiform mole or chorioepithelioma, the ovarian response to the elevated gonadotropin level may be markedly exaggerated and give rise to multiple theca lutein cysts (hyperreactio luteinalis). A palpable enlargement of the ovary due to theca lutein cysts occurs in about 60% of hydatidiform moles and 10% of choriocarcinomas. The lesions may be small or may reach proportions up to 20 to 30 cm in diameter. Smaller theca lutein cysts may be found in multiple gestations. Bilateral involvement is usual, though often asymmetric. The ovaries are polycystic and irregularly oval in shape, with a lobulated, smooth surface. The individual cysts are of variable size, thin-walled, gray or translucent, and often tinged with yellow. On section, a multilocular or honeycombed appearance is noted. The contained fluid may be clear, amber, or blood-tinged. The more solid portions of ovarian tissue may be edematous, with minute cystic cavities. Microscopically, the theca interna cells are strikingly hyperplastic and luteinized. The wall of a theca lutein cyst includes an inner lining of cicatricial tissue and an outer, thickened layer of luteinized theca cells. On occasion, areas of granulosa cells may be seen internal to the theca layer, with evidence of proliferation and luteinization. Isolated islands of luteinized theca cells may be scattered through the ovarian parenchyma. Multicystic ovaries may be asymptomatic or may manifest symptoms related to their increased size and weight. Following termination of the pathologic pregnancy, they gradually regress and disappear within a few to several weeks.

Masculinizing changes in the female occur, with hyperplasia, adenoma, or carcinoma of the adrenal cortex, pituitary basophilic adenoma, pituitary basophilism (Cushing syndrome), and thymic tumors, but they may also be produced by a variety of ovarian tumors, including the Sertoli-Leydig cell tumor, adrenal rest tumor, and hyperplasia of the Leydig cells of the ovarian hilum.

An additional masculinizing syndrome is that associated with diffuse luteinization of the ovaries, often known as *hyperthecosis* (thought to be a variant of PCOS). In contrast to the primary, defeminizing ovarian tumors, the gonadal changes in this endocrinopathy are probably secondary. The clinical symptoms manifested by patients with diffuse luteinization of the ovaries include pronounced and progressive hirsutism of the face, trunk, and extremities; male escutcheon; hypertrophy of the clitoris; occasional voice and breast changes; obesity; oligo- or amenorrhea, preceded by irregular menses or menometrorrhagia; and sterility.

The ovaries are two to five times larger than normal, firm, smooth, and grayish-white in color, with irregular areas of yellowish hue. On section, numerous small, cystic follicles rim the periphery of the cortex. The medullary portion of the ovary appears hyperplastic, with scattered orange-yellow areas. The essential features, on microscopic examination, include parenchymal hyperplasia, diffusely distributed accumulations of luteinized

cells, and perifollicular theca cell proliferation and luteinization. Cystic atretic follicles are conspicuously distended. Scattered throughout the ovary, in both cortex and medulla, are irregular clusters or groups of large, round, or oval cells, with granular, light-staining, vacuolated cytoplasm and vesicular nuclei with distinct nucleoli. They resemble well-developed, luteinized theca cells. Sudan III stain shows them to be filled with lipid material. Although corpora albicantia are present,

recent corpora lutea are usually not found. The ovarian parenchyma suggests hyperplasia, not only because of its increased thickness but also because of the obviously increased cellularity. Many of the parenchymal cells appear epithelioid. The essential features of this entity are strikingly similar to those of polycystic ovary syndrome, except for the more conspicuous masculinization and exaggerated diffuse distribution of luteinized cells within the parenchyma.

Plate 10.20

Ovaries

ENDOCRINOPATHIES: POLYCYSTIC OVARY SYNDROME

In 1935, Stein and Leventhal described a group of patients in whom the symptoms of amenorrhea, sterility, slight hirsutism, and occasional obesity were associated with the presence of bilaterally enlarged, polycystic ovaries. The syndrome is now known as *PCOS*. The exact pathophysiology of PCOS is not well established, but increased amplitude of gonadotropin-releasing hormone pulsation and abnormal secretion of FSH and LH during puberty are thought to result in androgen excess. Elevated levels of LH persist and may be used to help establish the diagnosis. Insulin resistance is a prominent aspect of this syndrome (40% of patients). There is a genetic predisposition to PCOS; however, it is likely that several genes are involved.

The syndrome is not infrequent, affecting up to 10% of all females and 30% of secondary amenorrhea cases. It is the most common hormonal disorder among females of reproductive age. Although other criteria to make the diagnosis exist, the most accepted (Rotterdam) criteria requires two of the following three: Oligo- and/or anovulation, clinical or biochemical evidence of hyperandrogenism, and polycystic appearing ovaries on ultrasonography. The patient usually presents because of infertility or secondary amenorrhea. Some degree of virilism is evident in 70% of cases. Hirsutism may be minimal or conspicuous, involving the face, chest, breasts, and extremities, with male escutcheon. Generalized obesity has been noted in 50% of cases. On pelvic examination, the ovaries are symmetrically enlarged to the size of golf balls. The uterus may be hypoplastic. Endometrial biopsy will usually reveal a proliferative phase endometrium. Elevated levels of LH may be used to help establish the diagnosis. (A 2:1 ratio of LH to FSH is considered diagnostic.) Patients suspected of having adrenal sources of hyperandrogenism can be screened for adrenal hyperactivity by measuring 24-hour urinary free cortisol, an adrenocorticotropic hormone stimulation test, or an overnight dexamethasone suppression test. Serum testosterone (total) is generally 70 to 120 ng/mL and androstenedione is 3 to 5 ng/mL. Dehydroepiandrosterone sulfate is elevated in roughly 50% of patients. Ultrasonography (abdominal or transvaginal) may identify ovarian enlargement or the presence of multiple small follicles. Magnetic resonance imaging or computed tomography may be used to evaluate the adrenal glands.

Grossly, the ovaries are conspicuously and symmetrically enlarged. They may be two to five times normal in size, round or oval in shape, and gray-white or pearly white in color. The ovarian surface is smooth, with occasional slight elevations, suggesting the presence of underlying cystic follicles. At times, the gonads may be slightly flattened ("oyster" ovaries), or one may be slightly larger than the other. On section, the tunica albuginea usually appears thickened. Beneath it, numerous cystic follicles, 2 to 15 mm in diameter, ring the cortex. The ovarian parenchyma is conspicuously hypertrophied and may contain occasional yellow flecks. Microscopically, the important features relate to the presence of a hyperthecosis. Around many of the atretic cystic follicles, the theca interna layer shows marked proliferation and luteinization. The ovarian parenchyma appears hyperplastic, with evidence of increased cellularity. Many of the cells are more

Bilaterally enlarged, pale white, egg-sized polycystic ovaries

Uterus

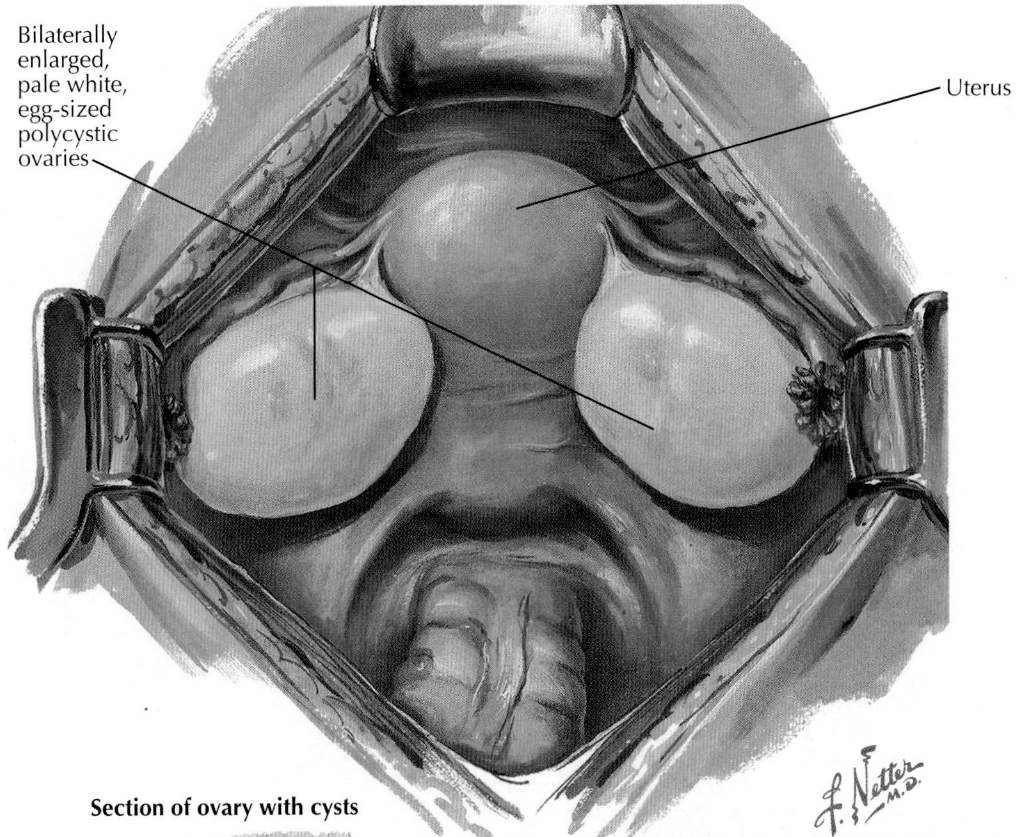

Section of ovary with cysts

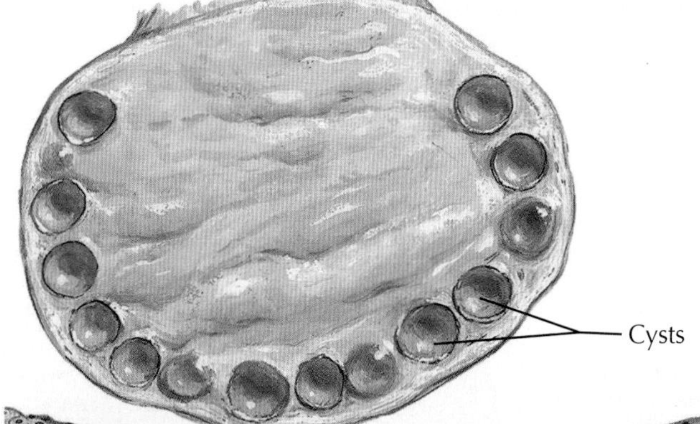

Cysts

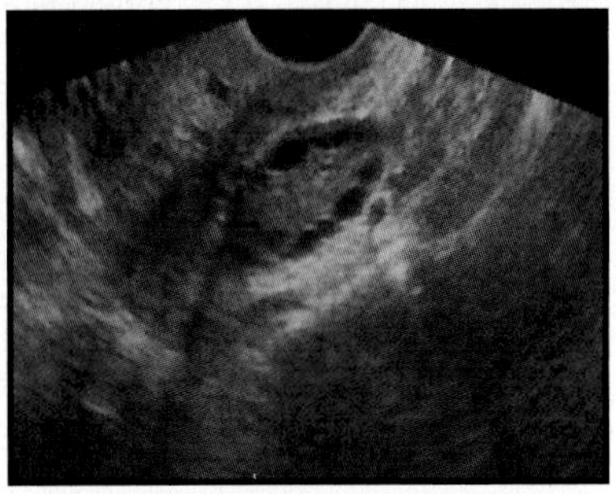

▲ Ultrasonographic appearance of polycystic ovaries

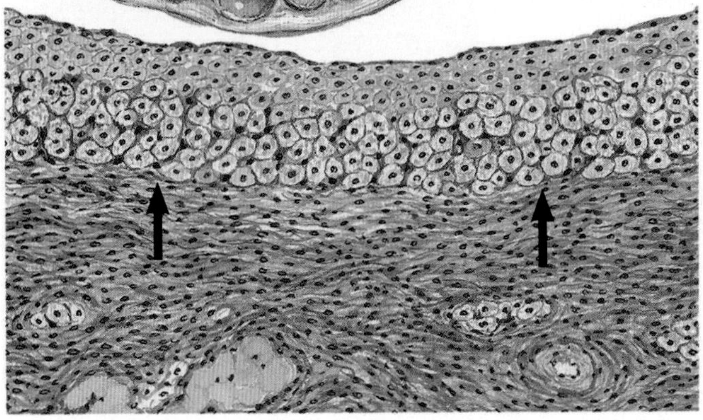

◄ Perifollicular theca interna proliferation and luteinization, microscopic section

epithelioid in appearance. Small groups of luteinized cells may be seen scattered throughout the parenchyma.

Medical therapy has replaced surgical treatment. Treatment depends on the desire for pregnancy; if pregnancy is desired then ovulation induction may be required. Weight loss is often associated with resolution of symptoms and a return of menstrual function in patients with mild or early polycystic ovary disease. Combination oral contraceptives (<50 μg formulation and a progestin

other than norgestrel) may reduce further hair growth. If dehydroepiandrosterone sulfate is elevated, dexamethasone may be added to oral contraceptives. Metformin (1500 mg/day) is often used as an adjunctive treatment for ovulation induction and is now considered as first-line therapy for PCOS.

There is an increased risk of diabetes, endometrial hyperplasia, and endometrial carcinoma in patients with polycystic ovaries and chronic anovulation.

Plate 10.21

Reproductive System: VOLUME 1

Dysgerminoma

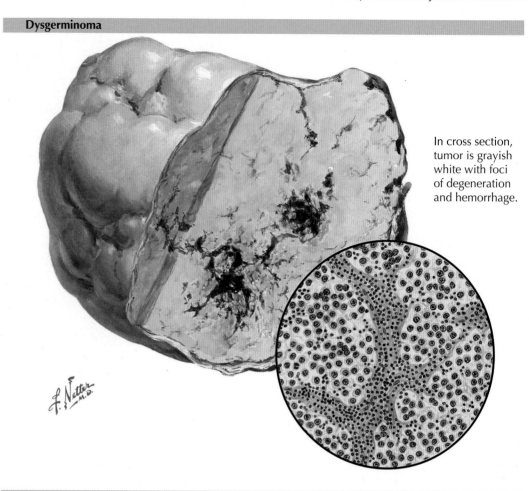

In cross section, tumor is grayish white with foci of degeneration and hemorrhage.

DYSGERMINOMA, BRENNER TUMOR

The dysgerminoma is an ovarian tumor made up of germ cells and stroma that appear analogous in structure to the seminomas found in the male testes. Although rare (2% of ovarian tumors), these tumors are the most common malignant germ cell tumors (>30% of ovarian germ cell malignancies). At times, they may be associated with evidence of sexual underdevelopment or pseudohermaphroditism. Although found at all ages, at least 75% of cases occur in young individuals between 10 and 30 years of age. Unilateral involvement is usual (>90%).

The clinical manifestations of dysgerminoma are those associated with any rapidly growing pelvic neoplasm. Tumor degeneration may induce a low-grade fever, leukocytosis, and a rapid sedimentation rate. Ascites is not infrequent. Torsion with infarction may occur (5%). Dysgerminomas usually grow rapidly. Extension takes place by perforation of the capsule with direct infiltration, by peritoneal spread, and by lymphatic and hematogenous routes. These tumors tend to spread by lymphatic channels. Recurrence of tumor is found in 20% of patients, but recurrent disease generally responds well to additional surgery, chemotherapy, or radiation. The prognosis is good for patients with pure dysgerminomas less than 15 cm in size. With limited disease and no indication of spread at the time of surgery (stage I, 75% of cases), there is a >95% 5-year survival rate.

Grossly, the dysgerminoma is a solid, round, oval, or irregular tumor, which may vary in diameter from 3 to 5 cm or may fill the entire pelvis. It may be firm and rubbery or soft and pliable. The cut surface is grayish, cellular, and, at times, brainlike. Usually, there is degeneration, necrosis, hemorrhage, and cavitation. Histologically, columns or nests of the characteristic cells are separated by strands or trabeculae of loose, edematous, vascularized, connective tissue that shows hyalinization and infiltration with lymphocytes. The dysgerminal cells are large, sharply defined, round or polygonal, with centrally placed, round, uniform nuclei. The cytoplasm is abundant, clear, or finely granular. The nuclei are fine and diffuse, with prominent nucleoli. Mitoses may be present. Foci of degeneration and necrosis, with foreign-body giant cells, are common.

The transitional cell (Brenner) tumor is an epithelial tumor that is made up of cells that resemble urothelium and Walthard cell nests, intermixed with the ovarian stroma. Most are benign. It is relatively uncommon, comprising about 1% to 3% of all ovarian neoplasms. The majority are encountered after 40 years of age or postmenopausally. At times, a small Brenner tumor may be found incidentally in the wall of an ovarian cyst, usually of the mucinous variety. Clinically, there are no characteristic features. Rarely, it is associated with Meigs syndrome. At laparotomy, it may be difficult to differentiate a Brenner tumor from an ovarian fibroma, fibromyoma, theca cell tumor, or adenofibroma.

Brenner tumors may be microscopic in size or may vary from a few to 13 cm in diameter. They are unilateral, solid, round or oval, irregularly bossed, smooth,

Brenner tumor

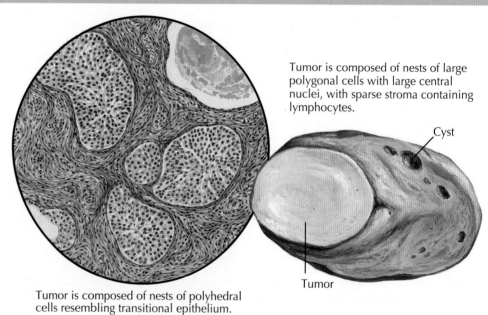

Tumor is composed of nests of large polygonal cells with large central nuclei, with sparse stroma containing lymphocytes.

Cyst

Tumor

Tumor is composed of nests of polyhedral cells resembling transitional epithelium.

firm, and grayish-white in color. On section, the tumor appears well demarcated, resembling a fibroma. Multiple, minute cystic spaces may be evident, containing viscid, opaque, yellow-brown fluid.

Histologically, irregular masses or columns of polyhedral cells are surrounded by rather dense, fibrous tissue. The epithelial cells are large, irregular, polyhedral, or oval in shape, with distinct cell membranes. The cytoplasm is abundant, granular, and vacuolated. The nuclei are oval

or slightly irregular, with distinct chromatin granules. Longitudinal nuclear grooving, representing a linear deposit of chromatin, may be seen. Microscopic cysts in the cell masses may be solitary or multiple. These are lined by flattened or cuboidal cells or by columnar epithelium containing glycogen and secretory granules that take a mucicarmine stain. The connective tissue about the epithelial strands is cellular, hyalinized, and avascular. Irregular, calcified deposits may be present.

Plate 10.22

Ovaries

STROMATOGENOUS NEOPLASMS

Ovarian fibromas are benign stromatogenous tumors. The most common benign ovarian tumor, this tumor is composed of stromal cells (fibroblasts). Although benign, these tumors are sometimes associated with ascites and hydrothorax (Meigs syndrome, 1% of patients). They may be minute or may reach a diameter of more than 27 cm. Unilateral involvement is usual (90%). Multiple fibromas of a single ovary occur occasionally (10%). Though encountered at any age, the majority are found postmenopausally. Because of its weight, torsion of the pedicle is apt to occur.

Fibromas are well-encapsulated, solid, heavy, oval, grayish-white tumors with an irregularly bossed, smooth surface. Adhesions may be present. The cut surface discloses dense, white, interlacing bundles of connective tissue. The larger neoplasms may show focal or diffuse areas of edema, hemorrhage, degeneration, and cyst formation. The cystic cavities result from tissue necrosis and may be irregular or ragged and filled with clear or blood-tinged fluid. Isolated or diffuse calcification occurs in 10% of cases. Microscopically, the tumor is composed of interlacing strands or whorls of spindle-shaped cells. The individual cell presents an indistinct border, a moderate amount of finely granular cytoplasm, and an elongated, deeply stained nucleus. In the larger fibromas, circulatory deprivation may result in edema, hemorrhage, infarction, degeneration, necrosis, and calcification. In edematous areas, the cells are widely separated and stellate in appearance. Dilated lymphatic channels may be conspicuous. Hyalinization is evidenced by the deposition of pink-staining homogeneous collagenous material. Phagocytic cells containing fatty material may be seen in areas of necrosis. Infarction may be manifested by a diffuse infiltration with erythrocytes, degeneration, and necrosis. Calcification is indicated by the deposition of granules or masses of darkly stained basophilic material.

If small, an ovarian fibroma may be asymptomatic. Those of larger size may give rise to localized discomfort or pain, pressure symptoms, and abdominal enlargement. The presence of a unilateral, hard, movable ovarian tumor with ascites, or ascites and hydrothorax, is most suggestive. Therapy for ovarian fibroma is surgical extirpation.

Meigs syndrome refers to the association of ascites and hydrothorax with a pelvic neoplasm, particularly ovarian fibromas. The syndrome has also been encountered with fibroadenomas, fibrosarcomas, Brenner tumors, theca cell tumors, teratomas, serous cystadenomas, multilocular pseudomucinous cystadenomas, adenocarcinomas, papillary cystadenocarcinomas, and even fibromyomas of the uterus. Ascites is present with the majority of ovarian fibromas of moderate or large size (40% if the tumor is >10 cm). The right side of the chest is involved in 75% of cases, the left in 10%, and both in 15%. No relationship between the side of the ovarian tumor and the side of the hydrothorax seems to be apparent. Varying amounts of fluid may accumulate rapidly in the peritoneal and pleural cavities. Fluid accumulation is likely related to substances such as vascular endothelial growth factor that increases capillary permeability. The hydrothorax and hydroperitoneum disappear completely with removal of

Fibroma

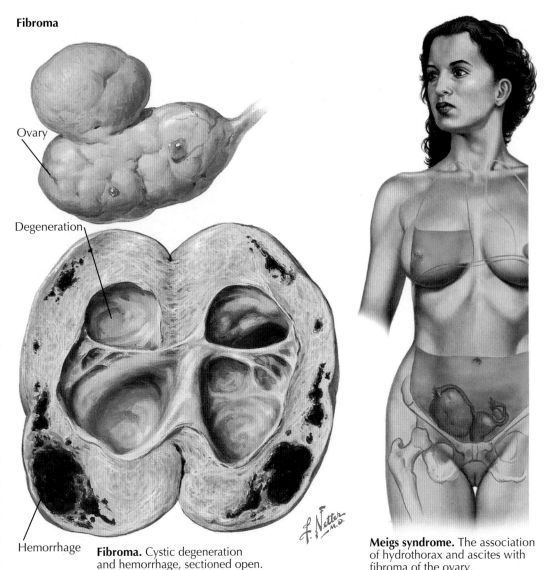

Ovary

Degeneration

Hemorrhage

Fibroma. Cystic degeneration and hemorrhage, sectioned open.

Meigs syndrome. The association of hydrothorax and ascites with fibroma of the ovary.

Fibroma

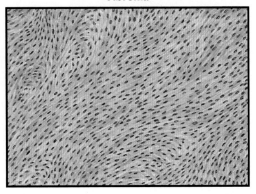

Spindle cell sarcoma

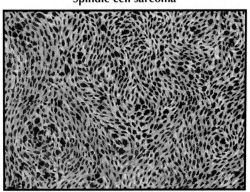

the pelvic tumor. Differentiation must be made from a malignant tumor with pulmonary metastases, cardiac or renal disease, hepatic cirrhosis, and tuberculous peritonitis.

Fibrosarcoma of the ovary is extremely rare. It is usually unilateral, solid, irregular, pedunculated, and of variable size. The cut surface may present a variegated appearance, depending on its cellularity and the tendency to hemorrhage, necrosis, and cystic degeneration. Areas may be gray-white or pink-tan in color,

sometimes suggesting raw pork. Histologically, it may resemble a cellular fibroma or a solid, anaplastic carcinoma. It includes spindle, mixed, or round cell varieties, with irregular hyperchromatic nuclei and giant cells. The symptomatology is not distinctive. Torsion and ascites may occur. Extension may be by direct invasion or through vascular channels. If unilateral, encapsulated, and of low-grade malignancy, the prognosis following surgery is relatively good; otherwise it is poor.

Plate 10.23

Reproductive System: VOLUME 1

PRIMARY CYSTIC CARCINOMA

Ovarian cancer represents the second most common malignancy of the genital tract (after endometrial cancer) but is the most common fatal gynecologic cancer. The lifetime risk of developing ovarian cancer is approximately 1 in 70. Papillary serous cystadenocarcinomas make up a high proportion of most reported series of ovarian carcinomas. Roughly half of all ovarian cystic cancers occur after menopause, with an average age of 59 years, and the highest rate between 60 and 64 years (70% of patients are age 55 years or older). Despite this, only one-quarter to one-third of ovarian tumors in females postmenopause are malignant. A family pattern is recognized in a small percentage of cases. There is an association with abnormalities of the breast cancer (*BRCA1* and *BRCA2*) gene. Hereditary ovarian cancers are rare but usually fatal; 95% of ovarian cancers are sporadic. More than 95% of patients with ovarian cancer have no risk factor other than age. Oral contraception, high parity, tubal ligation, hysterectomy, and breastfeeding reduce risk.

Serum testing for tumor markers, such as CA-125, lipid-associated sialic acid, carcinoembryonic antigen, α-fetoprotein, human epididymis protein 4, lactate dehydrogenase, and others should be reserved for following the progress of patients with known malignancies and not for prognostic evaluation. Ultrasonography, magnetic resonance imaging, and computed tomography are helpful in evaluating patients suspected of having ovarian cancer. (The normal postmenopausal ovary is typically 1.5–2 cm in size.) Asymptomatic simple cysts of less than 5 cm diameter can generally be followed conservatively. (Routine screening using transvaginal ultrasonography or serum markers has not been shown to be cost-effective without the presence of significant risk factors or symptoms.)

Symptoms may be vague or absent until the malignancy is well advanced. Lower abdominal pain and progressive enlargement of the abdomen occur in most instances. Loss of weight, debilitation, anemia, anorexia, early satiety, dyspepsia, nausea, and vomiting may be present. Local pressure or infiltration may give rise to urinary frequency and urgency, rectal pain, and backache. Ascites is found in about one-third of the cases. At the time of examination, the majority of ovarian carcinomas are relatively large (>5 cm), and bilateral ovarian involvement may be expected in more than one-half of cases. Most are diagnosed at stage III or IV. Metastatic extension may be evident in local peritoneal implantations, omental involvement, lumbar, abdominal and pelvic lymphadenopathy, and distant metastases to liver, lungs, and bones. Lymphatic spread occurs in roughly 20% of tumors that appear grossly confined to the ovary.

Ovarian cancer is a disease that requires surgical exploration, staging, and extirpation (generally including the uterus and contralateral ovary). Adjunctive chemotherapy (platinum-based and paclitaxel [Taxol]) or radiation therapy is often included based on the location and stage of the disease.

As yet, there are no effective screening tools for the early detection of primary ovarian cancer. Ultrasonography, magnetic resonance imaging, computed tomography, and biochemical markers such as CA-125, which are useful for evaluating a suspicious mass or following the progress of treatment, are not of value for mass screening. In those suspected of having recurrent disease and other selected patients, second-look surgery may be desirable to assess progress and discover occult disease. (When second-look surgery is negative, the associated 5-year survival is approximately 50%.) For those few patients at truly high risk (familial cancer syndromes), prophylactic salpingo-oophorectomy after childbearing is completed is preferable to any attempt at prolonged surveillance with current technology. Even this aggressive step does not preclude the development of "ovarian" cancer; up to 10% of ovarian cancers are found in females who have had bilateral oophorectomies.

If discovered early in the process and treated with aggressive surgical resection and adjunctive therapy, disease-free survival is possible. Survival is affected by stage, grade, cell type, and residual tumor after surgical resection. Survival (5-year) by stage: stage I, 80%; stage II, 70%; stage III, 45%; and stage IV, 15%. Serous adenocarcinoma has the poorest prognosis of the epithelial types.

Papillary serous cystadenocarcinoma

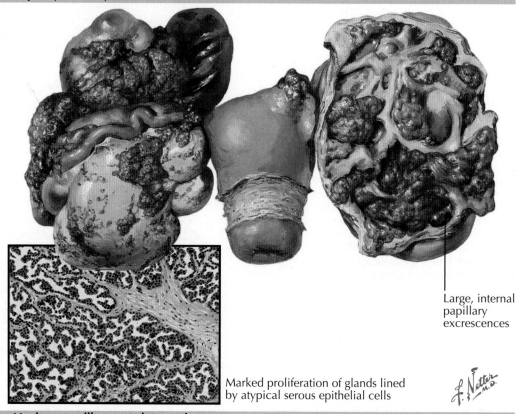

Large, internal papillary excrescences

Marked proliferation of glands lined by atypical serous epithelial cells

f. Netter

Mucinous papillary cystadenocarcinoma

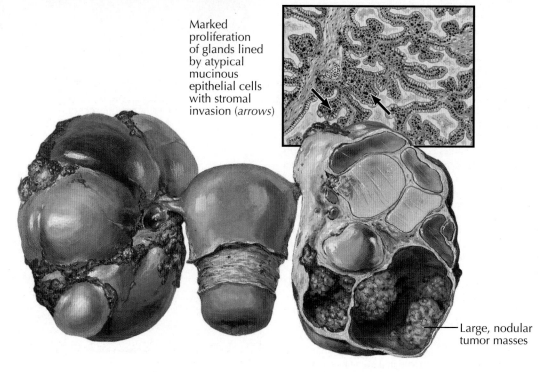

Marked proliferation of glands lined by atypical mucinous epithelial cells with stromal invasion (*arrows*)

Large, nodular tumor masses

Plate 10.24

Ovaries

Primary solid carcinoma

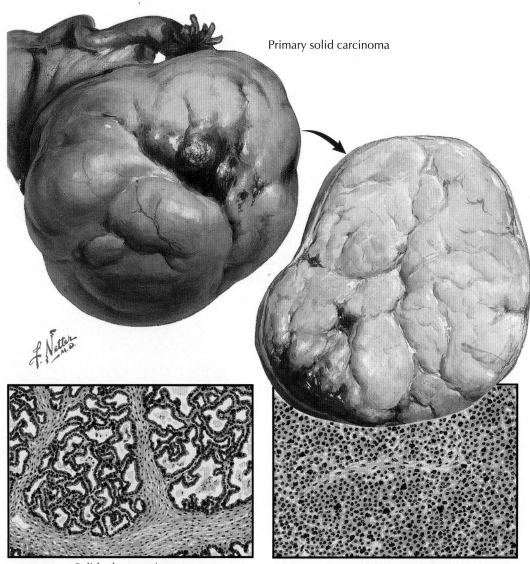

PRIMARY SOLID CARCINOMA

Primary solid ovarian carcinomas, also designated as the undifferentiated or unclassified group, may be arbitrarily divided on the basis of the architectural pattern of the epithelial and connective tissue elements into solid adenocarcinoma, medullary carcinoma, scirrhous carcinoma, alveolar carcinoma, plexiform carcinoma, clear cell, endometrioid, and adenocarcinoma with squamous cell metaplasia (adenoacanthoma). Primary solid carcinomas of the ovary are less common than the cystic variety. They may be unilateral or bilateral, small or large, ovoid or round, smooth or nodular, grayish-pink in color and solid. The consistency and color are dependent on the proportionate amounts of epithelial and connective tissue elements. If very cellular, they are apt to be relatively soft, meaty, and pink, often with areas of degeneration. If less cellular, they may be firm and whitish-gray. Focal necrosis, hemorrhage, cavitation, deposition of calcium, and psammoma bodies are not infrequent. In advanced cases, penetration of the capsule, infiltration, extension, and metastases occur.

Clear cell carcinoma is an ovarian tumor made up of cells containing large amounts of glycogen that gives them a clear or "hobnailed" appearance. These tumors may also arise in the endocervix, endometrium, and vagina. Cervical and vaginal tumors have been linked to in utero exposure to diethylstilbestrol. Despite the presence of hobnail cells that are similar to those seen in the endometrium, cervix, and vagina of females exposed to diethylstilbestrol in utero, there is no evidence that diethylstilbestrol has a role in clear cell ovarian tumors. These tumors represent 5% to 11% of ovarian cancers. They present as a pelvic mass (up to 30 cm)—partially cystic with yellow, gray, and hemorrhagic areas with papillary projections generally present, giving the mass a velvety appearance; 40% of tumors are bilateral. These tumors are usually found as a malignant tumor and require surgical exploration and extirpation, including the uterus and contralateral ovary. Adjunctive chemotherapy or radiation therapy is often included based on the location and stage of the disease. In those suspected of having recurrent disease and other selected patients, second-look surgery may be desirable to assess progress and discover occult disease.

Endometrioid tumors consist of epithelial cells resembling those of the endometrium. In the ovary, these neoplasms are less frequent (approximately 5%) than either the serous or mucinous tumors, but the malignant variety accounts for approximately 20% of ovarian carcinomas. Endometrioid carcinomas usually occur in females in their 40s and 50s. They may be seen in conjunction with endometriosis and ovarian endometriomas, although an origin from endometriosis is rarely demonstrated. Most endometrioid carcinomas arise directly from the surface epithelium of the ovary, as do the other epithelial tumors. Patients with clear cell or endometrioid cancer should be offered testing for DNA mismatch repair deficiency.

Medullary carcinoma is rich in epithelial elements, with very little connective tissue. It is a virulent type of ovarian malignancy that occurs in young females,

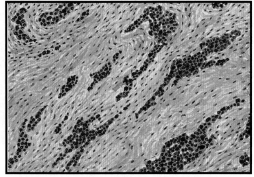

Solid adenocarcinoma

Medullary carcinoma

Scirrhous carcinoma

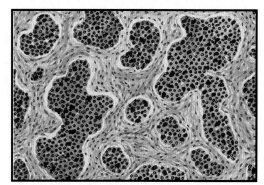

Alveolar carcinoma

usually between the ages of 15 and 30 years. Because of its histologic appearance, it has been designated a small cell carcinoma. The tumor is often, but not always, accompanied by hypercalcemia. Even when found with early-stage disease, this is an aggressive almost uniformly fatal malignancy that has been refractory to surgery, chemotherapy, or radiation.

In scirrhous carcinoma, the fibrous tissue predominates, whereas the epithelium is distributed in narrow columns or nests. Alveolar carcinoma is evidenced

by irregular groups of epithelial cells, separated by connective tissue.

Carcinoma simplex refers to a fairly equal division between the cellular and fibrous tissues. Plexiform carcinoma resembles scirrhous carcinoma, except that the epithelium is arranged in narrow anastomosing columns. Adenoacanthoma of the ovary refers to squamous cell metaplasia in adenocarcinoma. The squamous cells are large, polyhedral prickle cells. Keratinization and pearl formation may be observed.

Plate 10.25

Reproductive System: VOLUME 1

SECONDARY OVARIAN CARCINOMA

Metastatic cancer of the ovary accounts for only about 5% of ovarian cancer. The ovary is particularly prone to metastatic invasion by carcinoma. The primary sites include the breast, stomach, small and large intestine, appendix, liver, gallbladder, bile ducts, pancreas, uterus, tubes, opposite ovary, bladder and ureters, lungs, and meninges. Frequently, metastases are from primary tumors that originate elsewhere in the female reproductive tract, particularly from the endometrium and fallopian tube. Secondary ovarian carcinoma is most frequently seen from the fourth to the sixth decades of life. The ovaries are bilaterally involved in 66% to 75% of cases. Ascites is often evident (50%). The ovarian neoplasms may be asymptomatic or may manifest symptoms and signs similar to those produced by primary ovarian carcinoma. In the presence of a known primary lesion and palpable enlargement of the ovaries, the diagnosis of secondary carcinoma may reasonably be suspected. Similarly, the discovery of bilateral, solid ovarian growths on pelvic examination is an indication for a thorough search for a primary source elsewhere. Esophagoscopy, gastroscopy, sigmoidoscopy, or colonoscopy should be considered as a part of the evaluation when a gastrointestinal source is being sought.

In fully half of cases, the ovarian lesion may not be detectable grossly. The tumors may be minute or enlarged to diameters of 20 to 30 cm. The general contour of the ovary is usually retained. The typical secondary ovarian carcinoma is of moderate size, oval or kidney shaped, smooth or lobulated, firm, grayish-white in color, with a well-developed capsule and little tendency toward adhesions. Depending on the presence of necrosis, cystic degeneration, hemorrhage, myxomatous changes, and the degree of connective tissue proliferation, the cut surface may be firm, spongy, partly cystic, or gelatinous and grayish-white or yellow in color, with hemorrhagic areas of red or brown.

The histologic picture is generally similar to that of the primary lesion. The anaplastic, epithelial elements may appear as clusters of acini, cords, masses, or sheets, with varying degrees of mucoid change. The stroma may be abundant or sparse, cellular, edematous, and myxomatous.

The Krukenberg tumor refers to a secondary ovarian carcinoma that manifests marked proliferation of the connective tissue elements, sarcoma-like areas, epithelial anaplasia, and mucoid epithelial and myxomatous changes. Krukenberg tumors are the third most common metastatic ovarian cancer (after epithelial and germ-cell tumors) and make up 6% to 22% of these cancers. Signet ring cells, in which the nucleus is flattened to one side by secretion distending the cell, are characteristic. The most common site of origin is the stomach or large intestine, though metastatic breast cancer may appear similar histologically. Metastatic tumors from the gastrointestinal tract to the ovary can be associated with sex hormone production, usually estrogen. A few cases of Krukenberg tumors have been described with no apparent distant primary malignancy, suggesting the rare possibility of a primary ovarian tumor with the histologic features of a Krukenberg tumor.

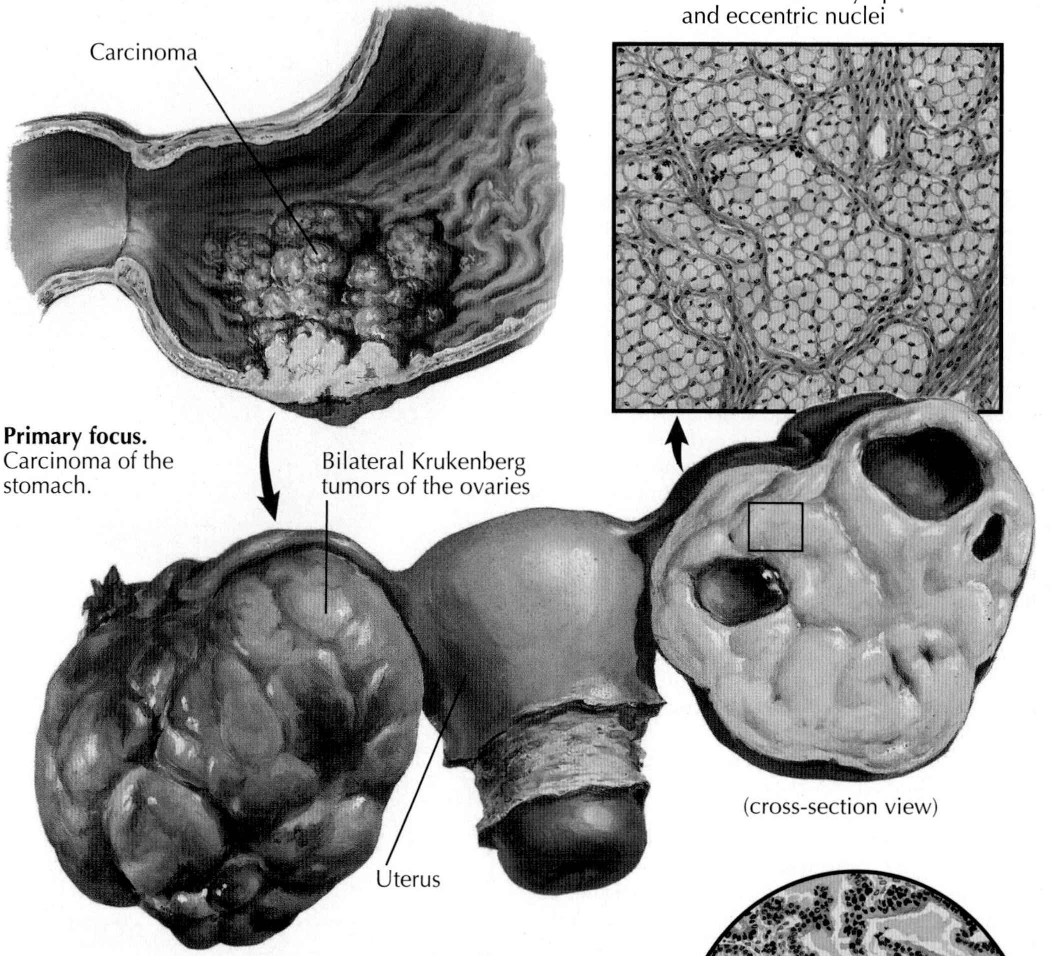

Debate exists over the exact mechanism of metastasis of the tumor cells from the gastrointestinal tract to the ovaries; classically, it was thought that direct seeding across the abdominal cavity accounted for the spread of this tumor, but some have suggested that lymphatic or hematogenous spread is more likely, because most of these tumors are found in the ovarian parenchyma and not the surface.

The prognosis in secondary ovarian carcinoma is extremely grave, with 5-year survival unlikely. Progression and spread of the primary tumor are generally well under way when the ovarian sites are discovered. If widespread metastases are evident, surgery is not indicated. If the diagnosis is confirmed on laparotomy, a total hysterectomy and bilateral salpingo-oophorectomy may make the patient temporarily more comfortable.

Carcinoma

Characteristic signet ring cells with clear cytoplasm and eccentric nuclei

Primary focus. Carcinoma of the stomach.

Bilateral Krukenberg tumors of the ovaries

(cross-section view)

Uterus

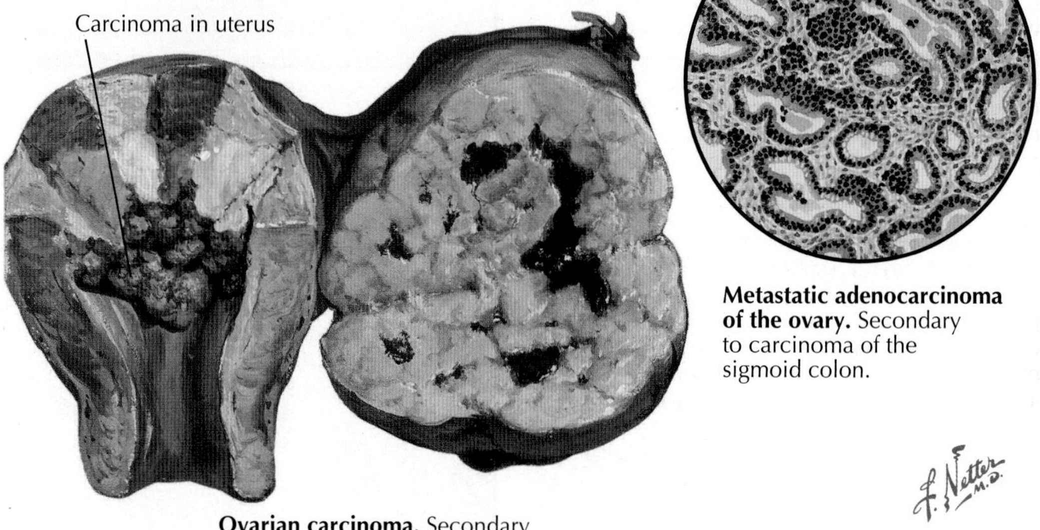

Carcinoma in uterus

Metastatic adenocarcinoma of the ovary. Secondary to carcinoma of the sigmoid colon.

Ovarian carcinoma. Secondary to carcinoma of the uterus.

Plate 10.26

Ovaries

DIAGNOSIS OF OVARIAN NEOPLASMS

Ovarian neoplasms may be found at any age. The majority occur during the reproductive years, though about 4% are present in children less than 10 years old. Of these, about half are malignant (dysgerminoma, solid teratoma, carcinoma, granulosa cell tumor) and the remainder benign (dermoid and epithelial cysts). Malignancy may be expected in about 15% of all ovarian tumors. The highest incidence of ovarian malignancy occurs between 40 and 60 years of age.

The most important objective of the management of an ovarian mass is the timely diagnosis of its type and origin. Subsequent therapy and assessment of risk are based on the correct diagnosis. For acutely symptomatic masses, rapid evaluation and intervention may be necessary.

The symptomatology presented by an ovarian tumor is dependent on its size, location, and type as well as on the presence of such complications as torsion, hemorrhage, infection, or rupture. Benign ovarian tumors are most frequently diagnosed at the time of routine examination and are asymptomatic. An insidious growth to large proportions may occur, with an increase in girth as the only subjective symptom. When symptoms do occur, they generally are either catastrophic (as when bleeding, rupture, or torsion occur) or indolent and nonspecific (such as a vague sense of pressure or fullness). Pain, if present, may be mild, intermittent, and localized in the hypogastrium or either lower quadrant. It may radiate to the anterior or lateral thigh. Severe pain usually attends an acute accident. Generally, the menses are not affected. The biologically active tumors manifest distinctive endocrinologic features. Solid, fixed, and infiltrating neoplasms may give rise to pressure symptoms related to impingement upon the bladder, rectosigmoid, or ureter.

History and physical examination are generally sufficient to establish the presence of the mass. There are no laboratory tests that are of specific help in the global diagnosis of ovarian masses. Laboratory investigations may support specific diagnoses. Ultrasonography, computed tomography, and magnetic resonance imaging are of limited value in evaluating small asymptomatic masses in young patients. Exceptions to this are patients in whom clinical assessment is impractical or inadequate (e.g., massive obesity) or those in whom malignancy is suspected. Serum testing for tumor markers, such as CA-125, lipid-associated sialic acid, carcinoembryonic antigen, α-fetoprotein, lactate dehydrogenase, human epididymis protein 4, and others should be reserved for following the progress of patients with known malignancies and not for prognostic evaluation.

Some authors favor giving young patients with small, presumably benign, cystic masses ovulation suppression therapy, such as oral contraceptives, to hasten the process of regression. Regression rates of 65% to 75% are often cited for this approach, but this strategy is largely a matter of personal choice because definitive studies are lacking and most evidence suggests that oral contraceptives are more likely to prevent the growth of new or existing cysts than to hasten regression. Physiologic ovarian enlargements, including follicular or corpus luteum cysts, should not be present if a patient is using oral contraceptives. For this reason, patients who are already using oral contraceptives and develop adnexal masses are more likely to have pathologic conditions that will not regress, increasing the possibility that eventual surgical exploration may be required. Patients in perimenopause and postmenopause may still have benign processes as a cause of an adnexal mass, but the likelihood of a malignant process is much increased (up to one-third of cases), altering management. In these patients, masses larger than 6 cm generally prompt surgical exploration and excision. The use of transvaginal ultrasonography to measure and track masses has allowed smaller masses that once would have required exploration to be followed conservatively. As in younger patients, the size, shape, mobility, and consistency of the mass should be estimated. Irregular, immobile, or mixed character masses (solid and cystic) are more likely to be malignant and deserve immediate consultation with a surgeon for exploration. The final diagnosis of ovarian cancer must be made surgically.

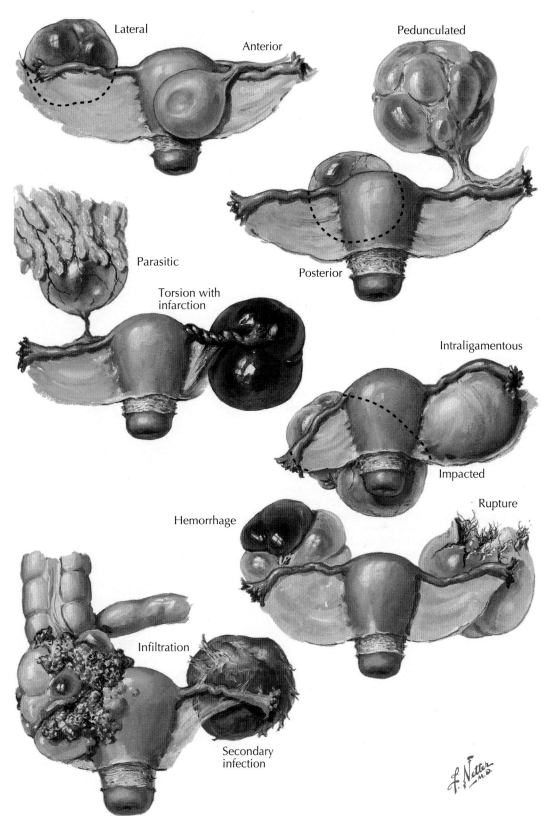

Lateral

Anterior

Pedunculated

Parasitic

Posterior

Torsion with infarction

Intraligamentous

Impacted

Rupture

Hemorrhage

Infiltration

Secondary infection

Plate 10.27

Reproductive System: VOLUME 1

Conditions Simulating Ovarian Neoplasms

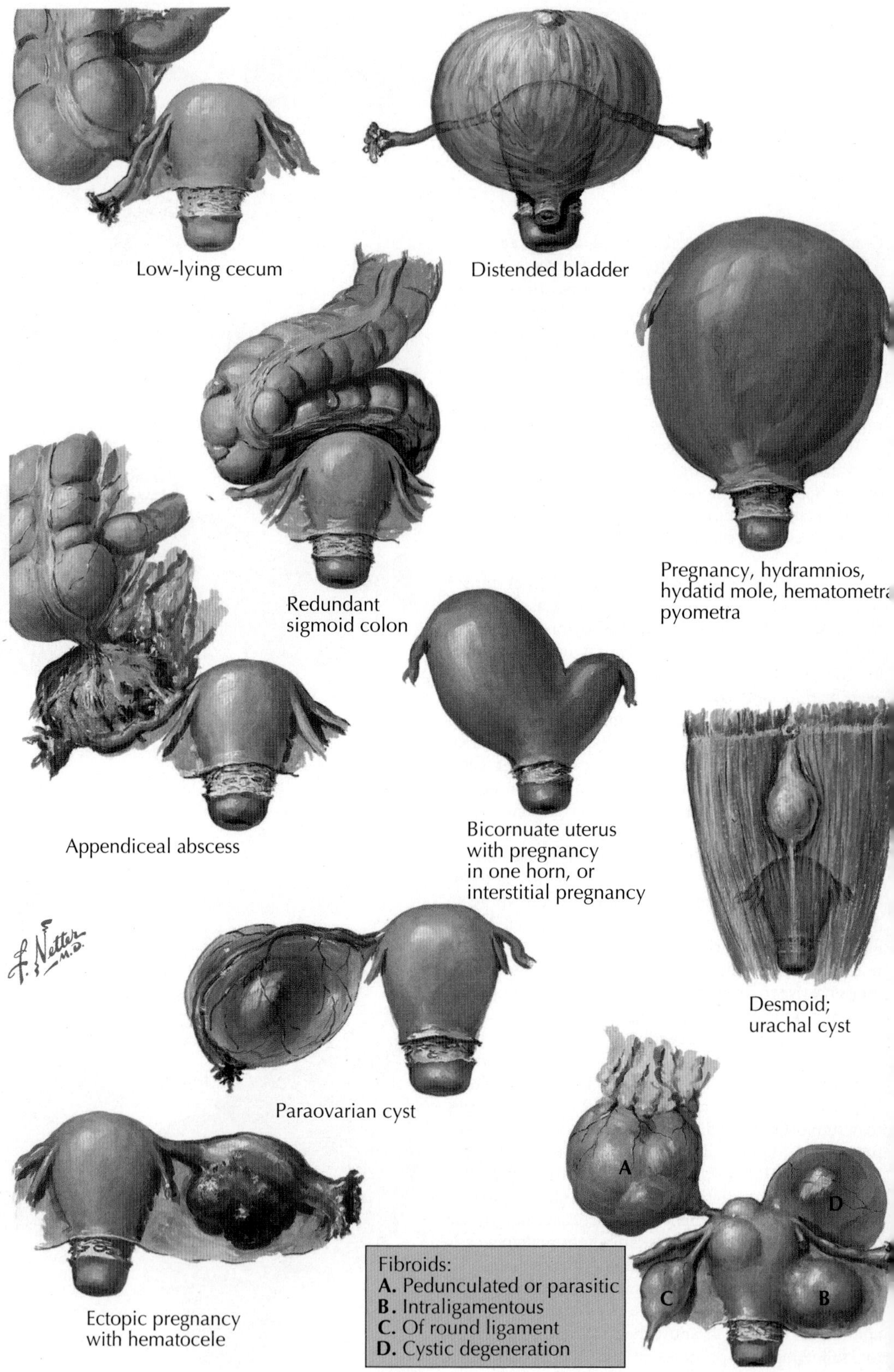

Low-lying distended cecum. Normally, the cecum lies in the right iliac fossa upon the iliopsoas muscle, with its apex or lowest point a little to the mesial side of the middle of the inguinal ligament. In some cases, however, the cecum hangs over the pelvic brim or is lodged entirely within the pelvic cavity. It may be mistaken for an ovarian cyst.

Redundant sigmoid colon. The sigmoid lies in close relationship to the uterine fundus within the true pelvis. When the redundant loop is filled with fecal material or gas, it may suggest the possibility of ovarian neoplasm.

Appendiceal abscess. When the cecum is low or the appendix is long, the latter may lie within the right pelvis. Should an acute appendix rupture, the resultant localized abscess may be situated in the region of the right adnexa. The pelvic findings may suggest the possibility of a hemorrhage, rupture, tubo-ovarian abscess, or torsion of an ovarian neoplasm. A low-lying, acutely inflamed appendix with adherent omentum may also simulate an accident involving an ovarian neoplasm.

Paraovarian cysts, derived from the vestigial remnants of the wolffian body within the broad ligament, are intraligamentous. They may be small, incidental findings at operation or may grow to a large size. A paraovarian cyst should be kept in mind if a unilateral, ovoid, fixed, thin-walled cyst is palpated.

Ruptured ectopic pregnancy with hematocele may, at times, be confused with an acute accident in an ovarian tumor, an enlarged cystic corpus luteum with incomplete abortion, a rupture of a graafian follicle or hemorrhagic corpus luteum, an acute appendicitis with adherent omentum, or an exacerbation of a predominantly unilateral chronic adnexitis.

Distended urinary bladder. A partially filled bladder may simulate a soft, thin-walled, anteriorly located neoplasm. If tensely distended, it may suggest a large cyst or uterine pregnancy. A catheter or bedside ultrasonography will resolve the question.

Intrauterine pregnancy. The corpus of a gravid uterus is oval, smooth, soft, cystic, and movable from side to side. When the isthmic portion of the uterus is particularly soft (Hegar sign), it is easily compressed between the examining fingers in the vagina and on the abdomen, suggesting the possibility of a cystic mass separate from the cervix. The body of a pregnant uterus in marked retroversion and retroflexion may similarly be mistaken for a cyst in the posterior cul-de-sac.

Pregnancy in one horn of a bicornuate uterus is associated with slight hypertrophy of the other horn. Pelvic examination during the first half of pregnancy may suggest the presence of a cystic mass contiguous to a slightly enlarged uterus. If a double vagina or a double cervix is found, a uterus bicornis or didelphys may be suspected.

Desmoid tumor. Situated in the hypogastric portion of the anterior abdominal wall, this tumor may, on examination, suggest a possible origin in the pelvis. Desmoids are solid, fibrous, benign tumors, oval in shape, and sometimes quite large. Sarcomatous changes may occur.

Urachal cyst. As a result of the incomplete obliteration of the urachus at birth, a cystic dilation may, at times, be found in the hypogastrium. Its location in the midline between the parietal peritoneum and the anterior abdominal wall aids in the diagnosis.

Uterine fibromyomas. The presence of other multiple fibromyomas is helpful but not conclusive proof of origin. A pedunculated fibroid is freely movable, as are most ovarian neoplasms. Its broad attachment, however, may be traced to a portion of the uterus other than the ovarian ligament. A pedunculated fibroid may undergo torsion of its pedicle with infarction and peritoneal irritation, similar to twisted ovarian cysts. Ultrasonography, computed tomography, or magnetic resonance imaging may be helpful but may not always provide an unambiguous diagnosis.

Low-lying cecum

Distended bladder

Redundant sigmoid colon

Pregnancy, hydramnios, hydatid mole, hematometra, pyometra

Appendiceal abscess

Bicornuate uterus with pregnancy in one horn, or interstitial pregnancy

Desmoid; urachal cyst

Paraovarian cyst

Ectopic pregnancy with hematocele

Fibroids:
A. Pedunculated or parasitic
B. Intraligamentous
C. Of round ligament
D. Cystic degeneration

Plate 10.28

Ovaries

CONDITIONS SIMULATING OVARIAN NEOPLASMS (CONTINUED)

Mesenteric cyst. Rarely, a cyst of the mesentery of the transverse colon or small bowel or of the omentum may reach large proportions and simulate a pedunculated, freely movable, extrapelvic ovarian cyst.

Polycystic kidney. The multilocular cystic replacement of the renal cortex and medulla may reach a huge size. On abdominal palpation the possibility of a large, adherent ovarian cyst may be suggested. Intravenous pyelography may demonstrate the bilateral renal involvement and characteristic elongation and spreading apart of the calyces. Abdominal ultrasonography will demonstrate the classic cystic nature of the kidneys and cysts, if present in the liver.

Pelvic kidney. An ectopic kidney may lie low in the lumbar region, in the iliac fossa, or in the true pelvis. It may be symptomless or may give rise to sacroiliac backache and pain in the lower abdomen, radiating to the hips and thighs. Pelvic examination may reveal the lower end of a smooth, oval, retroperitoneal, fixed mass with a distinctive rubbery consistency.

Retroperitoneal pelvic neoplasms. A variety of retroperitoneal tumors may be present in the pelvis and be mistaken for adherent ovarian neoplasms. They may be symptomless or associated with local or referred pain due to renal compression. On rectal or rectovaginal examination, a fixed, retroperitoneal tumor may be felt behind or lateral to the rectum. Sigmoidoscopy and barium enema may reveal external compression. Retroperitoneal pelvic tumors include lipoma, fibroma, sarcoma, dermoid, malignant teratoma, metastatic carcinoma, osteochondroma, and ganglioneuroma. Pyogenic infections of the sacroiliac joint, osteomyelitis of the pelvis, dissecting abscesses originating with tuberculosis of the spine, perivesical infections, and psoas abscesses must be taken into consideration.

Hematoma of the rectus muscle. As a result of direct trauma or unusual strain upon the recti muscles of the abdominal wall, rupture of the muscle fibers, with a hematoma, may occur. If localized over the right or left lower quadrants, the tender tumescence and voluntary spasm may suggest an acute accident in an ovarian tumor. An ecchymosis may or may not be apparent. Its superficial location may be demonstrated by tensing the abdominal muscles. The absence of palpable tumors, upon rectal or vaginal examination, will further clarify the issue.

Adherent bowel or omentum. Following pelvic surgery or as an aftermath of pelvic infections, the omentum, sigmoid colon, or small bowel may become adherent to one adnexa or the other. An irregular, matted mass may result and give the impression of a pelvic tumor.

Carcinoma of the sigmoid colon. The irregular, rather firm and often fixed mass felt with carcinoma of the sigmoid may suggest a carcinoma of the ovary and vice versa. Whichever site of origin is suspected, further differentiation is indicated. Altered bowel habits, diarrhea, constipation, colicky pain, ribbon stools, and melena point to possible intestinal difficulty. Rectal

examination, sigmoidoscopy, barium enema, and biopsy will demonstrate the presence of a lesion or filling defect.

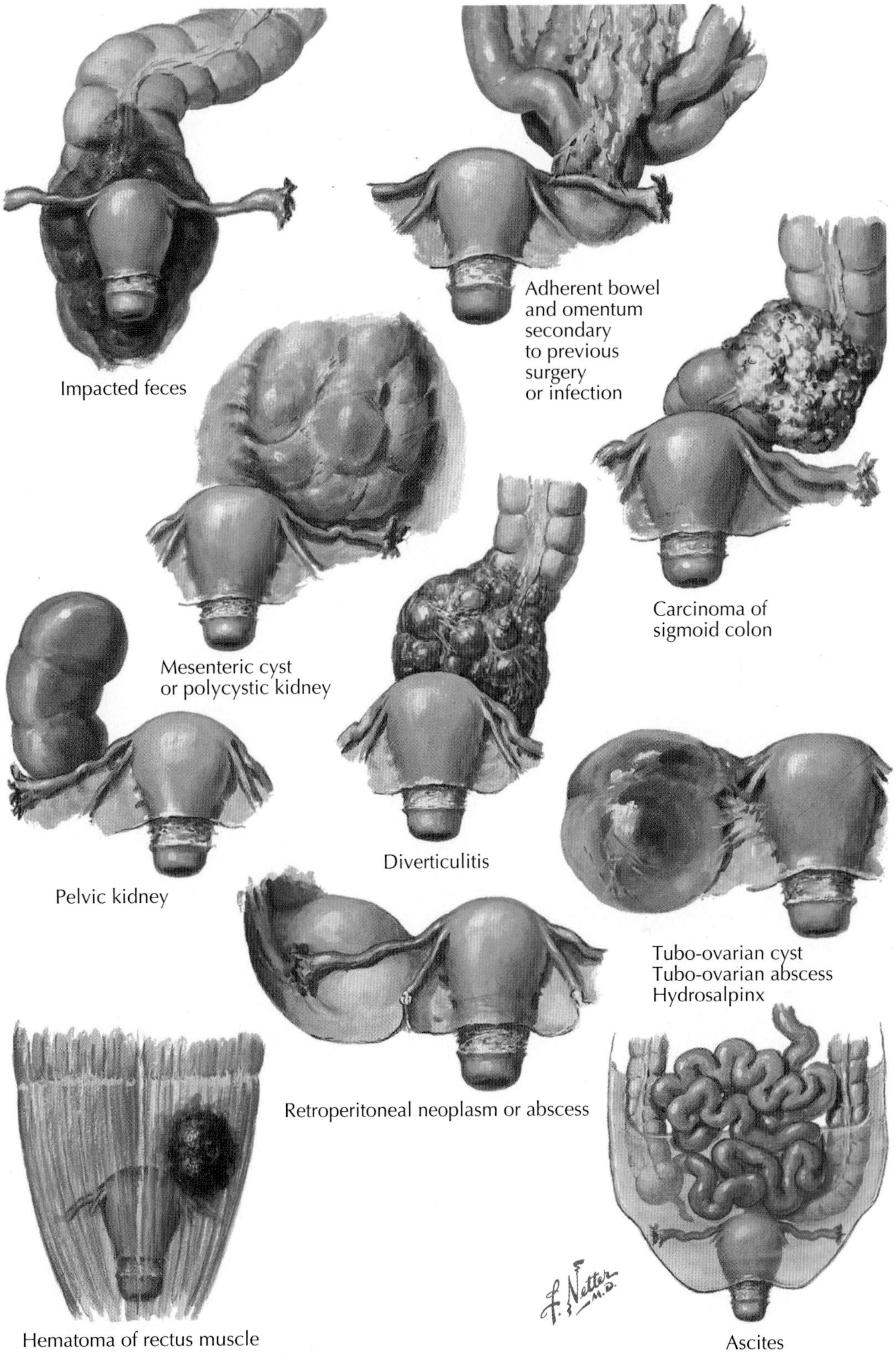

Diverticulitis. Uncomplicated diverticulosis of the descending and sigmoid colon is frequently asymptomatic. Perforation may result in a localized abscess, the adherence of bowel, omentum, and adjacent viscera, fistulous communications, granulomas, and stenosis of the bowel. A diverticulitis of the sigmoid may simulate a carcinoma of the sigmoid or ovary as well as pelvic infection.

Tubo-ovarian inflammatory masses. A large hydrosalpinx or tubo-ovarian cyst may be palpated as a thin-walled, retort-shaped, cystic structure, adherent to the uterus, broad ligament, and pelvic peritoneum.

Ascites. Ascitic fluid may give the impression of a large, flaccid cyst. The percussion note over an ovarian cyst is flat, with tympany in the flanks. On bimanual examination, fluctuation may be elicited. In the presence of ascites, tympany may emanate centrally and shifting dullness may be registered in the flanks. A fluid wave may be transmitted.

Impacted feces

Adherent bowel and omentum secondary to previous surgery or infection

Carcinoma of sigmoid colon

Mesenteric cyst or polycystic kidney

Diverticulitis

Pelvic kidney

Tubo-ovarian cyst
Tubo-ovarian abscess
Hydrosalpinx

Retroperitoneal neoplasm or abscess

Hematoma of rectus muscle

Ascites

OVUM AND REPRODUCTION

Plate 11.1

Reproductive System: VOLUME 1

Developing follicle

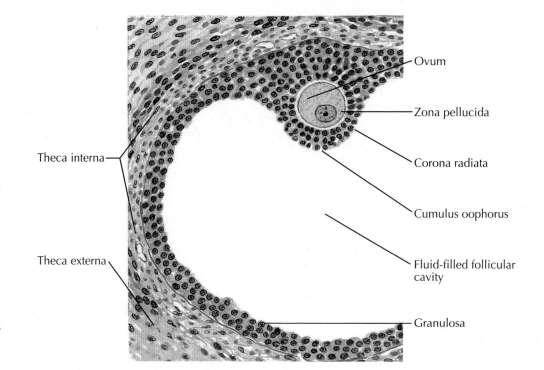

Ovum

Zona pellucida

Theca interna

Corona radiata

Cumulus oophorus

Theca externa

Fluid-filled follicular cavity

Granulosa

OOCYTE AND OVULATION

The completion of the final steps of meiosis I and the release of the oocyte from the parenchyma of the ovary constitute the process of ovulation. Through a process that takes approximately 375 days (13 menstrual cycles) a number of dormant, undeveloped primordial follicles begin to grow. These develop in a complex process of bidirectional hormonal feedback that results in the selection of one (or occasionally more than one) dominant follicle. (Advancing maternal age is associated with a higher frequency of multiple egg release with ovulation.) The preovulatory follicle (mature graafian follicle) contains an oocyte arrested in prophase of meiosis I. This is surrounded by a layer (corona radiata) of granulosa cells, a layer of mural granulosa cells, a protective basal lamina, and a network of blood-carrying capillary vessels sandwiched between a layer of theca interna and theca externa cells. A large collection of fluid, occupying the antrum, predominates in the follicle. These growing follicles are surrounded by granulosa cells, which engage in bidirectional messaging with the theca cells and the oocyte to facilitate follicular function. A dominant follicle is established by days 5 to 7 of the cycle.

Just prior to ovulation, the oocyte resumes meiosis, approaching completion of its reduction division. (Meiosis will not be completed until after a sperm has entered the egg and the second polar body is expelled.) During the preovulation phase, the granulosa cells of the follicle enlarge and acquire lipid inclusions, and the theca layer develops a rich vascular supply while the cells undergo vacuolization. There is also a transfer of inhibin production to luteinizing hormone (LH) control, ensuring continued function as follicle-stimulating hormone (FSH) levels drop.

Ovulation occurs because of a rapid increase in the follicular fluid and the direct action of proteolytic enzymes and prostaglandins. Follicular fluid accumulates gradually as the follicle grows but rapidly increases to 1 to 3 mL in response to the LH surge and a change in follicular wall elasticity. In addition, the theca cells surrounding the follicle begin to erode through the overlying epithelial covering of the ovary with the help of proteases, collagenase, plasmin, and prostaglandins E2, F2a, and other eicosanoids. These weaken the capsule and stimulate smooth muscle contractions in the cortex of the ovary, facilitating rupture of the follicle and the expulsion of the egg. The LH surge, by itself, is inadequate to induce ovulation in a follicle that has not undergone sufficient maturation. Once the oocyte has been released from the follicle, it is picked up by the fimbria of the fallopian tube for transport to the uterus, whether it becomes fertilized or not.

The remnant of the follicle, with its LH sensitized (luteinized) granulosa cells, is the corpus luteum, and is responsible for continued hormone production. There is a proliferation of the luteinized granulosa cells to fill

Stages of oocyte development and ovulation

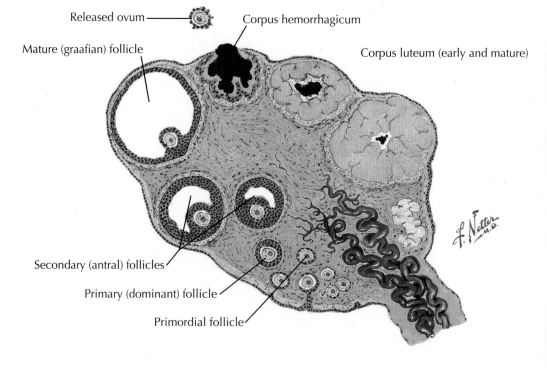

Released ovum

Corpus hemorrhagicum

Mature (graafian) follicle

Corpus luteum (early and mature)

Secondary (antral) follicles

Primary (dominant) follicle

Primordial follicle

the cavity. The corpus luteum reaches maximum production of estrogen and progesterone at about 10 days after ovulation. If conception has not occurred, the corpus luteum begins to regress, ending its function by about 14 to 15 days after ovulation. The exact reason for this involution is unknown, but only rescue by human chorionic gonadotropin can prevent its occurrence.

It is the continued production of estrogen, progesterone, and inhibin that suppresses the hypothalamus, decreasing its gonadotropin-releasing hormone production. This, in turn, decreases the release of FSH and LH from the pituitary, further preventing other follicles from maturing and releasing their eggs. This self-limiting process generally ensures that there is only one egg, which can be fertilized each month. Failure of this system to inhibit additional follicles, or the near-simultaneous rupture of more than one follicle, can set the stage for fraternal twinning.

Plate 11.2

Ovum and Reproduction

First polar body
Cumulus of granulosa cells
Zona pellucida
Egg (cytoplasm of egg)
Chromosomes in egg's nucleus

With the capacitation of the sperms and binding of progesterone to their heads in the female tract, sperms are then attracted to the egg by chemotaxis.

Increased motility and presence of hyaluronidase released from the acrosome through openings in the spermatic plasma membrane help the sperm to pass through the cumulus and reach the zona pellucida.

Coronal granules
Plasma membrane of egg
Zona pellucida
Perivitelline space

Acrosomal reaction comprises the fusion of the outer acrosome membrane and the cell membrane of the sperm, forming vesicles that are dispersed and exposing acrosomal enzymes (such as neuraminidase and acrosin) that help the sperm to pass the zona pellucida.

1. Sperm fuses with egg's membrane and its nucleus enters the cytoplasm of the egg.

2. Exocytosis of the content of the coronal granules promotes changes to the zona pellucida that becomes impervious to sperms, preventing polyspermy.

3. The sperm head swells and gives rise to the male pronucleus. The membrane of the pronuclei, which contain the haploid sets of chromosomes, disappears, and the chromosomes arrange themselves on the developing spindle for the first mitotic division.

C. Machado
M.D.

FERTILIZATION

The union of sperm and egg to form a zygote constitutes fertilization. The apparent simplicity and frequency of this phenomenon belie the complexity of the process. For fertilization to be accomplished, appropriate maturation of an oocyte in a dominant follicle must occur, ovulation must successfully release the egg, and sperm capable of fertilization must be present in adequate numbers. Even all of these events are not sufficient to accomplish either fertilization or pregnancy.

Following ovulation, the egg is picked up by the fimbrial end of the fallopian tube for transport to the uterine cavity. When the egg enters the fallopian tube, it is surrounded by a cumulus of granulosa cells and intimately surrounded by a clear zona pellucida. Within the zona pellucida are both the egg (in metaphase II stage) and the first polar body. Meanwhile, spermatozoa are transported through the cervical mucus and the uterus and into the fallopian tubes. Sperm are chemotactically directed toward the ovulated egg by sensing 1 part per billion of follicular fluid, acquiring the capacity to "smell" this fluid during their maturation within the epididymis. During this transport period, the sperm also undergo two changes: capacitation and acrosome reaction. These changes activate enzyme systems within the sperm head and make it possible for the sperm to cross the cumulus and the zona pellucida.

Once sperm and egg encounter each other (generally in the ampulla of the fallopian tube), capacitation leads to an increase in sperm motility, termed *hyperactivity*, and characterized by a high amplitude, asymmetric beating pattern of the sperm tail. This important change in sperm motility aids in sperm penetration of the cumulus and zona pellucida. ultimately leading sperm to attach to the cell membrane of the egg and enter the cytoplasm. When the sperm enters the cytoplasm, intracytoplasmic structures, the coronal granules, arrange themselves in an orderly fashion around the outermost portion of the cytoplasm just beneath the cytoplasmic membrane, and the sperm head swells and gives rise to the male pronucleus. Under this stimulus, the egg completes its second meiotic division, casting off the second polar body to a position also beneath the zona pellucida. The pronuclei, which contain the haploid sets of chromosomes of maternal and paternal origin, do not fuse, but the nuclear membranes surrounding them disappear, and the chromosomes arrange themselves on the developing spindle for the first mitotic division. In this way, the diploid complement of chromosomes is reestablished, completing the process of fertilization. The formation of this diploid cell, known as a *zygote*, constitutes fertilization.

Over the course of 20 hours following the attachment of the chromosomes to the spindle, cell division

(cleavage) occurs, giving rise to the two-cell embryo. A significant number of fertilized ova do not complete cleavage for a number of reasons, including failure of chromosome arrangement on the spindle, specific gene defects that prevent the formation of the spindle, and environmental factors.

Over the course of 3 to 4 days, the dividing cell mass passes down the fallopian tube toward the endometrial cavity. Early trophoblastic cells formed during the blastula

stage of development digest away the zona pellucida to allow the embryo to burrow into the thickened endometrium. Implantation of the embryo generally takes place about 3 days after the embryo enters the uterine cavity. Through most of this process, exposure to toxic agents (teratogens or radiation) is usually either completely destructive or causes little or no effect. Twinning may occur at any time from the two-cell stage until the formation of the blastula just prior to implantation.

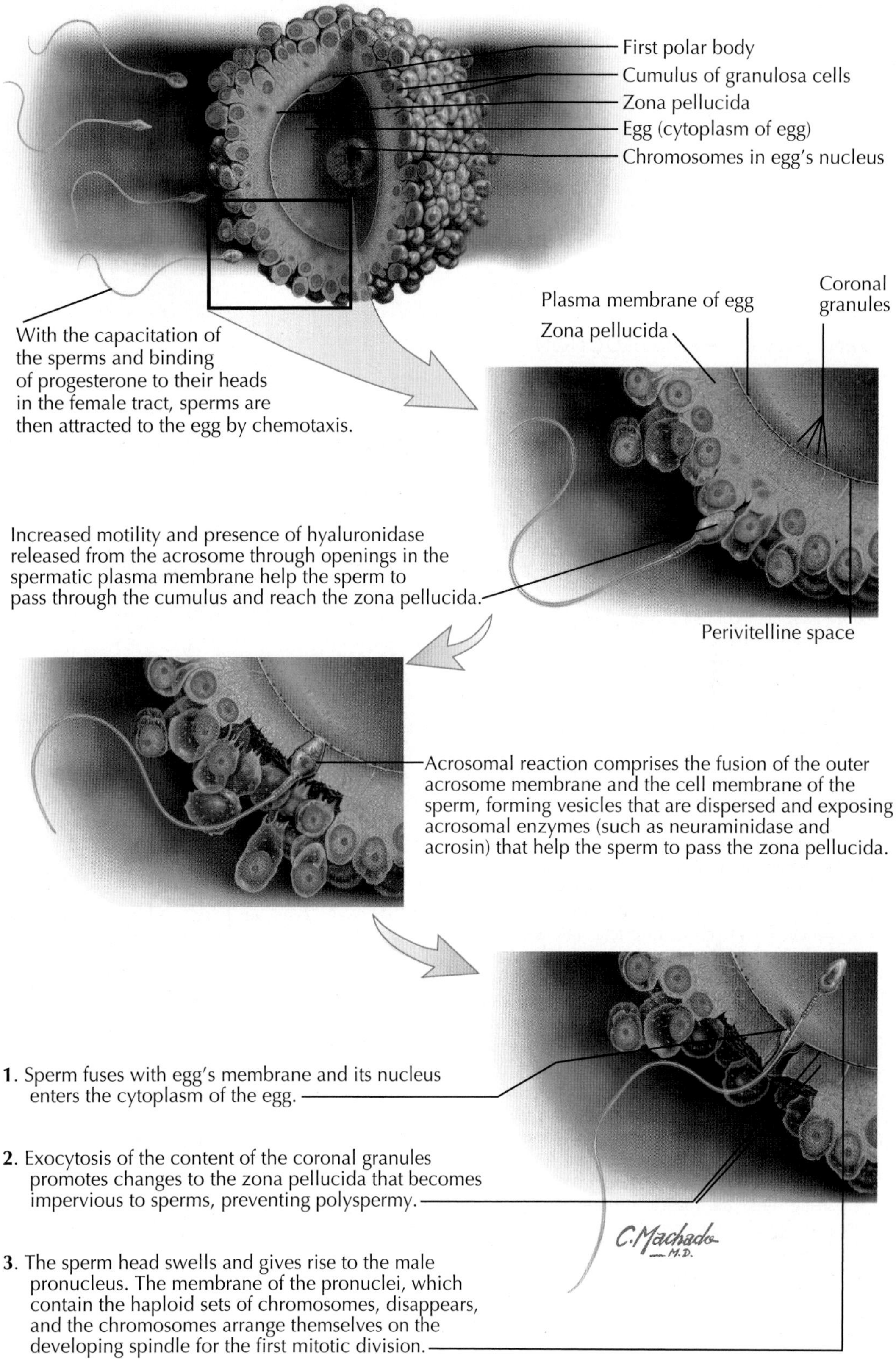

Plate 11.3

Reproductive System: VOLUME 1

Spermatogenesis

Oogenesis

Spermatogonium (*2n*)

Oogonium (*2n*)

Primary spermatocyte (*2n*)

Primary oocyte arrested in Prophase I (*2n*)

Meiosis I

------- *Puberty*

Secondary spermatocytes (*1n*)

First polar body

Early spermatids (*1n*)

Meiosis II

Secondary oocyte arrested in Metaphase II (*1n*)

------- *Fertilization*

First polar body may divide

Second polar body

Ovum (*1n*)

Maturation

Spermatozoa (*1n*)

J. Perkins
MS, MFA

GENETICS OF REPRODUCTION

The passage of genetic material, and thus information, across generations is one of the prime functions, if not necessities, of reproduction. In sexual reproduction the union of haploid gametes allows both parents to contribute to the genetic makeup of the new individual but also allows opportunities for new combinations and permutations, ensuring genetic diversity and the acquisition of new genetic traits.

To achieve the final haploid state, the gamete must reduce its genetic content through meiosis. Two meiotic cell divisions are required to accomplish this goal (meiosis I and II). In the male, meiosis generates four haploid gametes of equal reproductive potential, whereas in the female, the process generates only one oocyte and two to three polar bodies which eventually degenerate. Sperm production involving meiosis I and II begins at puberty and continues throughout life, with millions of sperm produced daily. In the female, meiosis begins during fetal life but arrests in prophase I until the oocyte begins maturation at puberty. (Oocytes in the early stage [prophase] of meiosis may be seen in the female fetus at 10 to 12 weeks gestation.) Of the five stages of meiosis necessary to form the oocyte, prophase I lasts the longest, occurs exclusively during fetal life, and sets the stage for genetic exchange that ensures genetic variation. Reentry into meiosis from the quiescence of childhood is signaled by the endocrine changes of puberty. Following maturation of the pituitary-hypothalamic-ovarian axis during puberty, one oocyte each month (generally) will complete meiosis I and be released by the process of ovulation. Meiosis II proceeds if fertilization occurs.

Genetic variation during meiosis is ensured as a result of crossing over between homologous chromosomes during prophase I and the independent segregation of homologous chromosomes. During prophase I, synapsis (or pairing) links the replicated homologous chromosomes. The resulting material (a tetrad) is composed of two chromatids from each homologous chromosome, forming a thick (four-strand) structure. Crossing over, or the exchange of genetic material, occurs when a chromatid breaks and reattaches to its homologue. This rearrangement of genetic material is responsible for the unexpected variation of various linked genetic traits. This unlinking of various characteristics, even when carried on the same chromosome, is responsible for the ability to get a mixture of traits from each parent. Although classic mendelian inheritance describes how each offspring of a pairing might inherit given traits, it is the exchange in genetic material between homologous chromosomes in prophase I that allows genes located on the same chromosome to be inherited independently of each other. The extent of this independence is a function of the distance between a pair of genes: those on separate chromosomes have the greatest independence,

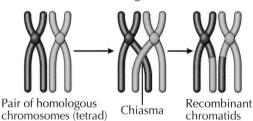

Crossing over

Pair of homologous chromosomes (tetrad)   Chiasma   Recombinant chromatids

Mendelian inheritance

Parental generation   F1 generation

F2 generation 3:1 red to white

those located on the same chromosomes but distant from each other have less independence, and those located nearby on the same chromosome the least.

In simple mendelian terms, genes that show phenotypic expression of their given trait, regardless of the allele they are paired with, are known as *dominant*, whereas those that are not expressed except when paired with another similar gene are termed *recessive*. This distinction is based on phenotypic expression, not the gene's ability to direct protein synthesis. In the case of a

"defective" gene, the presence of a healthy gene donated by the other parent may provide sufficient quantities of the needed protein that the cell, and thus the individual, is phenotypically normal. This distinction also ignores nuances such as selective gene inactivation and downregulation through epigenetics or small RNAs, and other newer insights into the complexity of gene function. This is still a useful construct clinically and when counseling patients about the risk of inheritable diseases or conditions.

Plate 11.4

Ovum and Reproduction

INFERTILITY: CAUSES

Under ordinary circumstances, 80% to 90% of healthy couples conceive during 1 year of attempting pregnancy, and 92% to 95% will conceive within 2 years.

Infertility is defined as the inability to conceive despite more than 1 year of unprotected intercourse. This interval is reduced to 6 months of contraceptive-free intercourse if the female is older than 35 years. Infertility is subdivided into primary and secondary types based on the patient's past reproductive history: nulligravida females and males who have not fathered a child, are in the primary infertility group; those who have become pregnant or fathered a child, regardless of the outcome of that pregnancy, are in the secondary infertility group. (Infertility affects two individuals, but the classification is generally based on the female's history, with less emphasis on the male partner's reproductive history.) Slightly more than one-half of patients with infertility fall into the primary group. It is estimated that infertility affects 6.1 million couples in the United States. The prevalence of infertility increases with the age of the female, and age-related infertility is becoming more common because about 20% of American females delay their attempts at pregnancy until after age 35. The effect of age upon male fertility is less obvious and more age-attenuated but real nevertheless.

Multiple factors can contribute to the inability to conceive and deliver a child. Conception requires the presence of competent gametes brought together at an appropriate time to allow fertilization. Once fertilization occurs, the fertilized ovum must be transported to an appropriately prepared uterine cavity where it must be able to implant and grow. This growth must be supported by a functioning corpus luteum until the placenta can take over hormonal support of the pregnancy. To deliver a child, the developing embryo must still successfully grow, differentiate, and transition to fetal state and grow to viability. The failure of any of these steps may result in infertility (or recurrent pregnancy loss). Most authors attribute the failure to conceive equally to the female, the male, and the couple (combined factors).

The male partner of a couple attempting pregnancy must bring to the union competent sperm. Approximately 35% to 50% of infertility is due to a male factor, such as azoospermia (no spermatozoa), asthenospermia (low sperm motility), or oligospermia (low sperm count). Problems with production, delivery, or quality of produced sperm can arise from genetic, inflammatory, anatomic, lifestyle, or other acquired causes. Female factors, such as ovulation disorders (20%–25%), tubal disease (10%–20%), endometriosis (15%), and cervical factors (5%), contribute to roughly 50% to 60% of female causes. The remaining 20% to 30% of couples have no identifiable cause for their infertility. If the female and male partners' evaluations are both deemed "normal," yet they remain infertile, this is termed *unexplained infertility*. If the male partner has an abnormal semen analysis but the cause is not known, this is termed *idiopathic infertility*. Couples experiencing primary infertility are more likely to have idiopathic or chromosomal causes than are couples who have conceived previously. Factors that increase the risk of anovulation (obesity, athletic overtraining, exposure to drugs or toxins), the risk of pelvic adhesive disease (infection, surgery, endometriosis), impaired sperm

production (mumps, varicocele, undescended testis), or sperm delivery (ejaculatory dysfunction or erectile dysfunction) all may increase the risk of infertility. In many cases, processes that impede fertility may not have an obvious clinical antecedent: half of all females found to have tubal factor infertility have no history of antecedent infections or surgery.

The evaluation of infertility is discussed further subsequently, but it is important to recognize that the

process of evaluation can be intrusive and may not yield a satisfactory resolution to the situation. Although the evaluation of infertility proceeds, couples should be instructed to continue attempting pregnancy through intercourse timed to the most fertile days of the cycle. Less than 40% of couples with primary infertility conceive after 6 years of therapy compared with more than 50% of secondary infertility couples who conceive by 3 years.

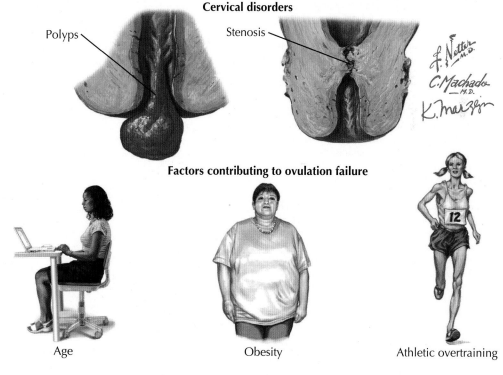

FEMALE FACTORS OF INFERTILITY

Uterine disorders

Cancer (or sarcoma) of uterine body

Fibroids

Cancer of cervix or endocervix

Trauma

Erosion

Chancre

Scarring

Blockage

Tubal disorders

Endometrial polyps

Adenomyosis

Narrowed or blocked fallopian tube

Ovulation disorders

Ovulation failure	
Flat pituitary hormone levels	■ Follicle-stimulating hormone
	■ Luteinizing hormone

Days 7 14 21 28

Corresponding ovarian activity

Cervical disorders

Polyps

Stenosis

Factors contributing to ovulation failure

Age

Obesity

Athletic overtraining

Plate 11.5

Reproductive System: VOLUME 1

INFERTILITY: EVALUATION OF FEMALE

Before any counseling or intervention for an infertile couple, the impediment to conception must be identified. Because 50% to 60% or more of identifiable causes of infertility are attributable to the female partner, individually or as part of the diad, much of the evaluation is focused on the female. However, it is strongly recommended that the male evaluation proceed concurrently with, or even precede, the female's. Beyond providing gametes to the union, the female must also provide patent conduits to allow the gametes to meet and to transport the fertilized egg and a readied chamber for the embryo to implant, develop, and grow to viability.

In females, the most common cause of infertility (20%–30%) is a disorder of ovulation. Failure of ovulation can arise owing to central or peripheral sources. If the ovary is incapable of responding to the hormonal signals coming from the pituitary (as in gonadal dysgenesis or following alkylating chemotherapy), ovulation cannot take place. Similarly, if the hypothalamic-pituitary-ovarian axis has been disrupted, the appropriate hormonal signaling may not be generated to result in the maturation and release of an oocyte. The use of basal body temperature measurements to detect the increase in temperature due to the postovulation surge in progestins has generally been replaced by the use of urinary LH surge monitoring kits even though an LH surge does not guarantee ovulation. An endometrial biopsy obtained after presumed ovulation can supply evidence of ovulation, but this method of documenting ovulation has also been replaced by less-invasive measures. Similarly, vaginal cytology as a marker of hormonal status is no longer used in the evaluation of infertility. When pituitary or ovarian failures are considered possible, direct measurement of serum FSH and/or LH may be made to assess their status.

The second most common cause for female infertility (10%–15%) is damage to the fallopian tubes interfering with proper transport of sperm or the fertilized ovum. Half of all females found to have tubal factor infertility lack a history of antecedent infections or surgery, supporting the need to evaluate tubal patency in patients regardless of their history. Hysterosalpingography, or alternately the flushing of the fallopian tubes with sterile saline colored with dye at the time of laparoscopy, has replaced less precise archaic methods such as the Rubin test in which carbon dioxide was used to assess tubal patency. Hysterosalpingography allows the size and shape of the uterine cavity to be assessed (important if recurrent pregnancy loss is an issue) and laparoscopy allows a more direct view of the fallopian tubes, ovaries, and surrounding areas (if pelvic adhesive disease or endometriosis are possibilities). Each is invasive to a degree and each offers advantages and disadvantages over the other, making the choice of procedure based on the patient's history and other clinical factors.

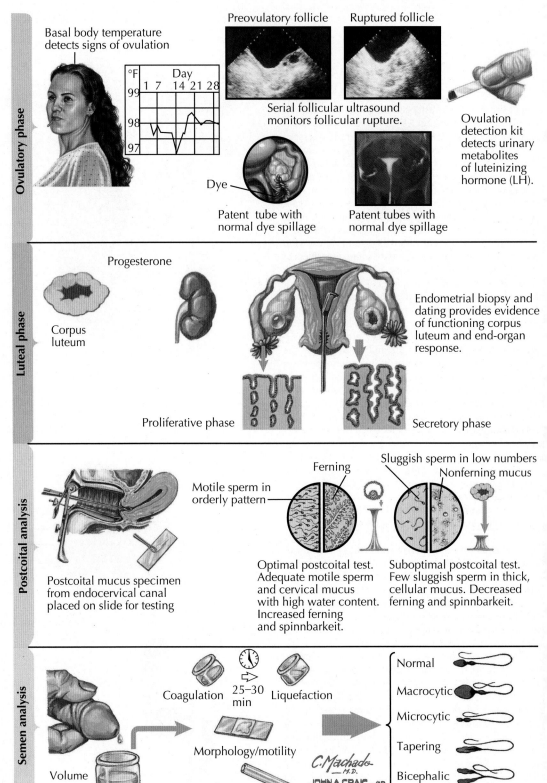

Although cervical factors are generally credited with about 5% of causes of infertility, the ability to bypass the effects of hostile or inadequate cervical mucus by assisted reproductive technologies has meant a decline in the importance of cervical mucus testing for infertility assessment. Although the cervical mucus can be evaluated for signs of ovulation (ferning or spinnbarkeit), like endometrial biopsy for the same purpose, these have been displaced by other methods.

Laparoscopy for the evaluation of tubal patency and the possibility of conditions such as endometriosis or pelvic adhesive disease can play an important role in the evaluation of the infertile. Hysteroscopy to evaluate the endometrial cavity can be useful, especially in couples in whom recurrent pregnancy loss has played a role in their childlessness. Chromosomal evaluations of infertile couples are seldom warranted except for selected infertility cases where a high degree of suspicion exists.

Plate 11.6

Ovum and Reproduction

INFERTILITY: EVALUATION OF MALE

Among infertile couples, 50% have causal or associated male factors. In addition, 1% to 5% of male factor infertility is a result of an underlying, often treatable but possibly life-threatening medical condition. For these reasons, the male evaluation is conducted systematically along with the female assessment. The evaluation includes a history, physical examination, semen analysis, and hormone assessment. Treatments include nonsurgical, surgical, and assisted reproductive options.

The history reviews past and current attempts at paternity. Important medical problems to elucidate include fevers and systemic illnesses such as diabetes, cystic fibrosis, cancer, and infections. Prior surgery, including orchidopexy and herniorrhaphy; trauma; and retroperitoneal, pelvic, bladder, or prostate procedures may impair infertility. A family history of cryptorchidism, midline defects, or hypogonadism is also important. A developmental history of hypospadias, congenital anomalies, and medication use may be revealing. A social history may elucidate the habitual use of the gonadotoxins such as alcohol, tobacco, recreational drugs, and anabolic steroids. Spermicidal lubricants and incorrect patterns of timing intercourse may be noted from a sexual history. Lastly, an occupational history determines exposure to ionizing radiation, chronic heat, benzene-based solvents, dyes, pesticides, herbicides, and heavy minerals.

The physical examination assesses body habitus, including obesity, gynecomastia, and secondary sex characteristics. The phallus may reveal hypospadias, chordee, plaques, or venereal lesions. The testes should be evaluated for size, consistency, and contour irregularities suggestive of a mass. Recall that 80% of testis volume is determined by spermatogenesis; hence, testis atrophy is likely associated with decreased sperm production. Palpation of the epididymides might reveal induration, fullness, or nodules indicative of infections or obstruction. Careful delineation of each vas deferens may reveal agenesis, atresia, or injury. The spermatic cords should be examined for asymmetry suggestive of a lipoma or varicocele, lesions differentiated by an examination in both the standing and supine positions. Meaningful varicoceles are diagnosed exclusively by physical examination. Lastly, a rectal examination is important in identifying large cysts or dilated seminal vesicles, which can be associated with infertility.

Although not a true measure of fertility, the semen analysis, if abnormal, suggests that the probability of achieving fertility is lower than normal. Two semen analyses, performed with 2 to 3 days of sexual abstinence, are sought because of the large biologic variability in semen quality. Lubricants should be avoided and the specimen kept at body temperature during transport. Recall that spermatogenesis takes 70 to 80 days to complete, so that an individual semen analysis reflects biologic influences occurring 2 to 3 months prior.

If the sperm concentration is low or there are signs of an endocrinopathy, then a hormonal evaluation should also be performed. This should include an assessment of the pituitary-gonadal axis with testosterone and FSH

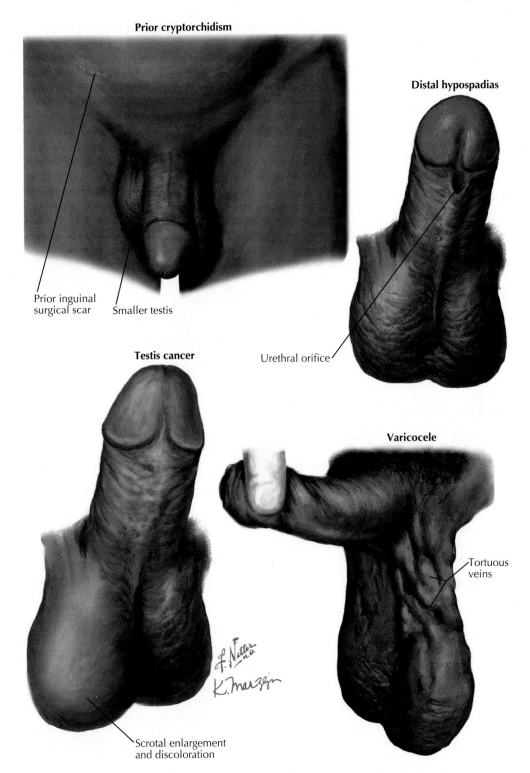

Prior cryptorchidism

Prior inguinal surgical scar

Smaller testis

Distal hypospadias

Urethral orifice

Testis cancer

Scrotal enlargement and discoloration

Varicocele

Tortuous veins

levels. The chance of a clinically significant endocrinopathy exists that presents as infertility is 2%.

The initial male evaluation may be normal or abnormal. If normal, further consideration should be given to female factor evaluation, including a more thorough assessment of ovulation, pelvic anatomy, and age-related fertility issues. If the initial male assessment reveals abnormalities, then further male evaluation or treatment is indicated. Adjunctive testing is undertaken depending on the findings but may include transrectal or scrotal ultrasound to evaluation ejaculatory duct obstruction or varicocele, semen testing for antisperm antibodies or leukocytes, postejaculate urinalysis, urine or semen cultures, semen fructose, or genetic testing. Correctable

abnormalities in the male should be treated before couples consider assisted reproduction.

Among infertile couples with unexplained infertility, further evaluation of male factor infertility is warranted, yet a precise algorithm to follow has not been defined. Antisperm antibodies; poor quality sperm chromatin structure, the latter reflective of increased levels of denatured sperm DNA; and disrupted sperm epigenetics can each be found in 10% to 20% of cases. Tests of sperm function include sperm DNA fragmentation, sperm epigenetics, and sperm acrosome reactivity and capacitation score, among others. Finally, many couples proceed to assisted reproduction with intrauterine insemination if the infertility remains unexplained.

Plate 11.7

Reproductive System: VOLUME 1

RECURRENT ABORTION

Recurrent abortion is the spontaneous loss of two consecutive, or three total, first-trimester pregnancies regardless of the outcome of other pregnancies. (Some definitions restrict this definition to three consecutive losses, which are not required to be intrauterine.) This is estimated to affect between 0.4% and 1% of reproductive-age females. There are few evidence-based diagnostic and treatment strategies and in only about one half of cases can a cause be found. Despite this, a number of obvious possible causes can still be addressed. Problems with the chromosomal makeup of the embryo, the hormonal environment of the pregnancy, or physical attributes of the uterus or endometrium may play a role in these losses. Risk factors for recurrent pregnancy loss are the same as those associated with single spontaneous abortion, including increasing maternal and paternal age, certain medical illnesses like uncontrolled diabetes mellitus and thrombophilias, and autoimmune disorders. In 50% of cases, no risk factor or cause will be identified. In general, about 70% of these patients will have a subsequent normal pregnancy without intervention.

When pregnancy losses occur early in gestation, there is a greater likelihood that a chromosomal abnormality is the cause (approximately 50%), whereas for later losses, a maternal cause such as a uterine anomaly is more likely. Although most chromosomal abnormalities result from disorders of meiosis in gamete formation or in mitosis after fertilization, up to 5% of couples that experience recurrent abortion have a detectable parental chromosomal balanced abnormality. For this reason, karyotyping of both parents is recommended when recurrent early abortions have occurred. When available, karyotyping of the abortus may be helpful but requires fresh tissue, specialized transport media, and appropriate laboratory capabilities. Those with parental chromosomal anomalies may be offered donor oocytes or artificial insemination with donor sperm to overcome the problem.

Two-thirds of recurrent abortions occur after 12 weeks gestation, which suggests that maternal or environmental factors play a larger role in this process than do genetic conditions. Surgically correctable uterine abnormalities, an incompetent cervix, or intrauterine septa or synechiae are the most common uterine abnormalities associated with early pregnancy loss. Indeed, uterine anomalies are found in 10% to 15% of females with recurrent abortion. When uterine anomalies are suspected, hysteroscopy is preferred for both diagnosis and therapy. Uterine anomalies or submucous fibroids may be treated in this way, although care must be taken to recognize the possibility of continued failure for other reasons and the possible effect on future delivery options made by such treatment.

The possibility of systemic factors such as hypothyroidism, coagulopathy, or thrombophilia or immunologic factors (e.g., lupus anticoagulant) as a cause of recurrent losses should be evaluated when there is reason for clinical suspicion or other evaluations have proven inconclusive. Without clinical suspicion, most societies recommend against routine testing for thrombophilia.

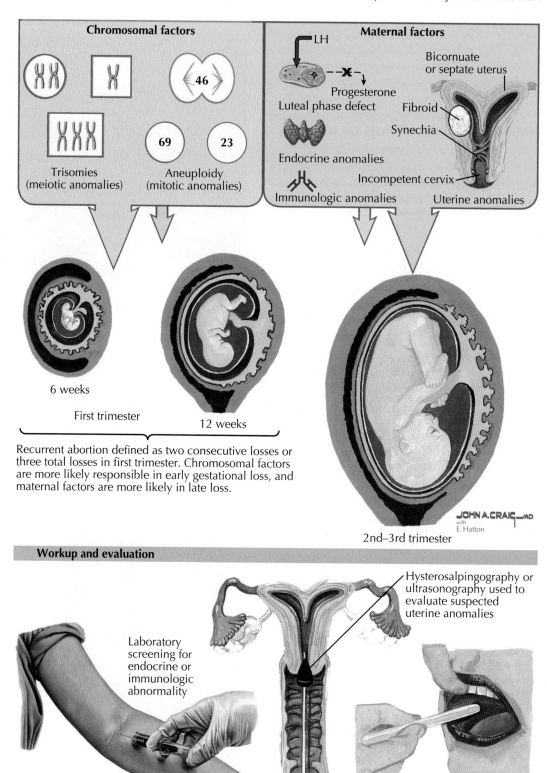

Recurrent abortion defined as two consecutive losses or three total losses in first trimester. Chromosomal factors are more likely responsible in early gestational loss, and maternal factors are more likely in late loss.

JOHN A. CRAIG—AD
with E. Hatton

Hysterosalpingography or ultrasonography used to evaluate suspected uterine anomalies

Laboratory screening for endocrine or immunologic abnormality

Karyotyping of parents recommended in cases of recurrent early abortions

When immunologic factors are present, the use of low-dose aspirin and subcutaneous heparin (5000 units twice daily) has reduced the rate of subsequent loss.

The evaluation of patients with recurrent pregnancy losses starts with a history and physical examination with an eye toward cervical incompetence, drug or chemical exposures, gastrointestinal diseases, a family history of miscarriages, birth defects, or thrombosis. The history and physical examination often direct the appropriate laboratory evaluation, including studies of thyroid-stimulating hormone and antithyroid antibodies. If all of these tests are normal, an evaluation of the uterine cavity by sonohysterography or hysteroscopy should be considered. It is not necessary to obtain endometrial bacteriologic cultures or perform human leukocyte antigen typing of the female or partner.

Therapeutic intervention for recurrent pregnancy loss is always based on the underlying cause. Progesterone and thyroid supplements have not been shown to reduce the risk of pregnancy loss.

Plate 11.8

Ovum and Reproduction

ASSISTED REPRODUCTION: IUI, IVF, IVF-ICSI

The success of infertility treatment depends to a great extent on the identified cause. Success is also a function of the age of the female partner: success declines and the rate of spontaneous pregnancy loss increases rapidly after age 35, adversely affecting the couple's ability to achieve a successful outcome.

A number of techniques are available to medically assist with conception. Among infertile couples seeking treatment, 85% to 90% can be treated with conventional medical and surgical procedures and do not require advanced assisted reproductive technologies such as in vitro fertilization. Sometimes the solution is as simple as improved timing of intercourse: when couples have intercourse four or more times per week, more than 80% achieve pregnancy in the first 6 months of trying. By contrast, only about 15% of couples conceive when intercourse happens less than once a week. Intercourse should be maintained on an every-other-day cycle from 3 to 4 days before the presumed ovulation until 2 to 3 days after that time. The use of ovulation detection kits (which detect urinary evidence of the LH surge) can facilitate this process.

Approximately 20% of females with infertility have ovulatory disorders. For this population, ovulation induction or control may be used to enhance the likelihood of pregnancy. With ovulation induction, couples achieve pregnancy at a rate nearly equivalent to that of normal couples (15%–25% probability in one menstrual cycle). The cause of anovulation will guide the selection of an appropriate treatment plan; some will need indirect therapies such as weight loss or metformin (polycystic ovary syndrome), others more direct hormonal manipulations such as afforded by clomiphene citrate, tamoxifen, aromatase inhibitors, or gonadotropins. All types of assisted reproductive technologies involving ovarian stimulation are associated with an increased incidence of multiple gestations (up to 40%): the majority of these pregnancies are twins (25%), and 5% are higher order gestations.

Tubal factor infertility may be addressed by either surgical repair of the damage or by bypassing the tubes completely through in vitro fertilization and embryo transfer (IVF/ET). Assisted reproduction techniques account for about 1% to 3% of live births and is associated with a roughly 40% live birth rate for females under the age of 35. Success rates for surgical repair, including the reversal of previous sterilization procedures are highly variable.

When male factors such as oligospermia are present, technologies such as intrauterine insemination (IUI) with donor sperm increase the chance of fertilization. In males with azoospermia, sperm may be able to be retrieved from the testicle and may result in successful fertility using IVF/ET along with intracytoplasmic sperm injection (ICSI), or single sperm injection into the egg. With this technology, developed in 1992, a single sperm is required for an egg to achieve fertilization, unlike the 500,000 sperm needed per egg with IVF alone. When either partner is incapable of supplying the necessary gametes, donor sperm or oocytes may be used to accomplish a pregnancy. In vitro fertilization and embryo transfer have allowed unprecedented access to gametes and the early developing embryo.

Basic options

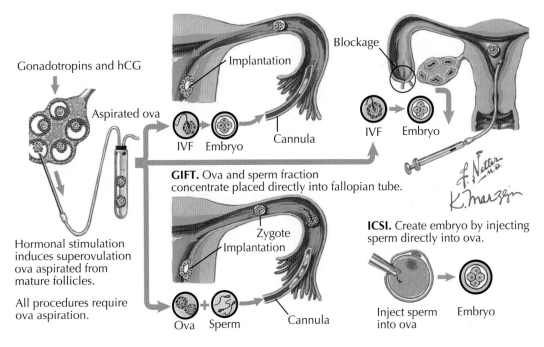

Gonadotropins and hCG by injection

Sperm fraction concentrate

Superovulating ovary with mature follicles

hCG triggers superovulation, providing numerous ova for potential fertilization.

Transcervical insemination bypasses interactive factor.

Timed intrauterine insemination with sperm fraction concentrate within 24 hours after ovulation increases potential for fertilization.

Advanced options

ZIFT. Ova fertilized in vitro; resulting embryos placed directly into fallopian tube.

IVF. Ova fertilized in vitro with sperm fraction concentrate. Embryo transferred directly into uterus, bypassing tubal occlusion.

Gonadotropins and hCG

Aspirated ova

Implantation

Blockage

IVF   Embryo   Cannula

IVF   Embryo

GIFT. Ova and sperm fraction concentrate placed directly into fallopian tube.

Hormonal stimulation induces superovulation; ova aspirated from mature follicles.

Zygote Implantation

ICSI. Create embryo by injecting sperm directly into ova.

All procedures require ova aspiration.

Ova   Sperm   Cannula

Inject sperm into ova   Embryo

Genetic developments, including the human genome project, the ability to amplify and comprehensively screen the genomic DNA from a single cell, and new diagnostic tests, in combination with micromanipulation in IVF (biopsy of a single or two blastomeres), have allowed for preimplantation genetic diagnosis (PGD) of embryos in vitro. PGD allows one to evaluate the embryo for single gene mutations and chromosomal abnormalities as it develops in vitro. Current indications for PGD "add on" technology include screening embryos in high-risk couples for the presence of mutated genes and associated deleterious syndromes in offspring, selecting unaffected embryos for uterine transfer, and screening developing embryos for chromosomal issues to prevent miscarriage or syndromic pregnancies that would normally be detected during pregnancy by amniocentesis. Currently 2% of all live births in the United States are IVF conceived.

Plate 11.9

Reproductive System: VOLUME 1

Human anatomy

Oocyte Layers

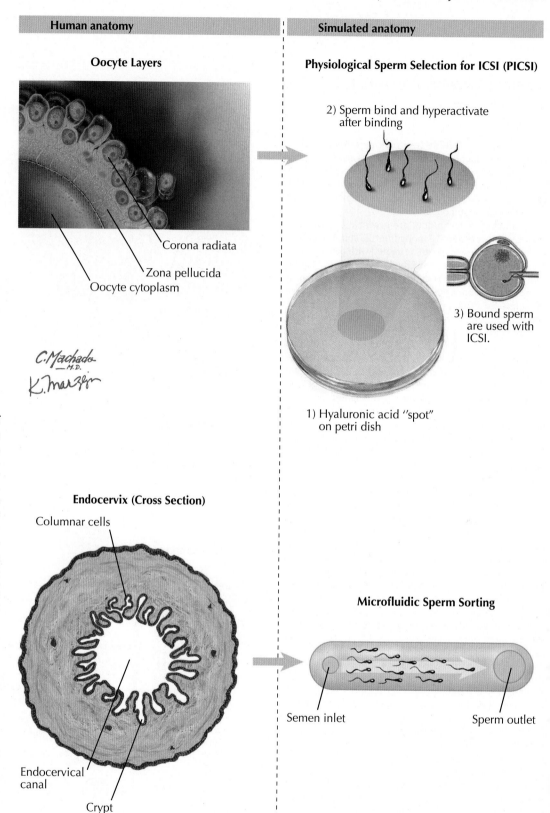

Corona radiata

Zona pellucida

Oocyte cytoplasm

C. Machado
M.D.

K. Marzen

Simulated anatomy

Physiological Sperm Selection for ICSI (PICSI)

2) Sperm bind and hyperactivate after binding

3) Bound sperm are used with ICSI.

1) Hyaluronic acid "spot" on petri dish

Endocervix (Cross Section)

Columnar cells

Endocervical canal

Crypt

Microfluidic Sperm Sorting

Semen inlet

Sperm outlet

ASSISTED REPRODUCTION: ADVANCED SPERM SELECTION TECHNIQUES

Although highly evolved over millions of years of evolution, it is not clear exactly what sperm selection criteria natural selection employs during intercourse, IUI, or IVF to reliably achieve a successful conception. However, in cases of IVF-ICSI in which an embryologist chooses the sperm to inject into the egg in vitro, sperm morphology or shape and motility are the governing criteria. One concern here is that we now recognize that (a) the standard descriptive semen analysis correlates poorly with fertility in general; (b) sperm functional assays such as those that assess sperm DNA fragmentation, epigenetic integrity or capacitation/acrosome reactivity correlate better with fertility; and (c) sperm function assays correlate poorly with the standard semen analysis. Hence, there is no doubt that natural selection is altered in such cases of assisted reproduction in which sperm are hand-picked for ICSI.

For the past half century, sperm have been processed by either centrifugation or "swim up" techniques for use with IUI or IVF and ICSI. These techniques can concentrate sperm and select for motile sperm, but they may also induce mechanical or chemical harm that adversely affects sperm quality. Currently, there are several emerging technologies, termed *advanced sperm selection techniques*, that noninvasively seek to restore or simulate the natural selection process during sperm preparation. The single most important consideration regarding sperm selection technology is that the sperm cannot be stained, lasered, or otherwise chemically or mechanically altered as this negates any qualitative benefits that are sought in the process. The first of these is physiologic ICSI or PICSI, which takes advantage of the natural inclination of mature sperm to bind to the zona pellucida and then become hyperactivated as part of the egg fertilization process. When sperm are placed on a dish coated with hyaluronic acid, the main constituent of the zona pellucida surrounding the egg, they either bind to the coating or not. Bound and hyperactivated sperm have been shown to have lower sperm DNA fragmentation, improved morphology and less aneuploidy than unbound sperm. As such, the bound sperm are preferentially chosen for ICSI.

Another advanced sperm selection approach takes advantage of the work that sperm naturally do in traversing the cervical canal during natural conception. Anatomically, the endocervical canal consists of columnar cells arranged in multiple crypts and folds which serve as constrained microchannel pathways that sperm must traverse to enter the uterus. Microfluidic technology has been developed that simulates this cervical anatomy. Ejaculated sperm are "loaded" onto the microfluidic chamber or chip and, after incubating for 20 minutes, the sperm that complete the journey within the chip are retrieved at the channel end. The quality of the sperm that complete the journey through the chip is far superior to the starting population in terms of DNA integrity, nuclear maturity, morphology and motility and these sperm are then chosen for ICSI. Although these technologies make sense biologically and have shown demonstrable improvements in key metrics of sperm function, the indications for their use, whether routine or selective, have yet to be precisely determined.

Plate 11.10

Ovum and Reproduction

CONTRACEPTION

Few capabilities have had the wide-reaching social implications than that of the ability to control fertility. Changing patterns of sexual expression, new technologies, increased consumerism, and heightened cost pressures all affect the choices made in the search for fertility control.

In the United States, about half (49%) of all pregnancies are unplanned, despite the fact that 90% of individuals at risk (genetic females who are fertile, sexually active, and neither pregnant nor seeking pregnancy) are using some form of contraception. The 10% or so of females not using contraception account for more than half of these unintended pregnancies. The remaining unplanned pregnancies occur as a result of either failure of the contraceptive method used or the improper or inconsistent use of the method.

There is no "ideal" contraceptive method. Although efficacy and an acceptable risk of side effects are important in the choice of contraceptive methods, these are often not the factors upon which the final choice is made. Motivation to use, or continuing to use, a contraceptive method is based on education, cultural background, cost, and individual needs, preferences, and prejudices. Factors such as availability, cost, coital dependence, personal acceptability, and the patient's perception of the risk all have a role in the final choice of methods. For a couple to use a method, it must be accessible, immediately available (especially in coitally dependent or "use-oriented" methods), and of reasonable cost. The effect of a method on spontaneity or the modes of sexual expression preferred by the patient and her partner may also be important considerations.

Currently available contraceptive methods seek to prevent pregnancy primarily by preventing the sperm and egg from uniting or by preventing implantation of the embryo that results from the fertilized egg. Most contraceptive methods have multiple possible mechanisms of action. For example, hormonal contraceptives, including postcoital contraceptives, work primarily by preventing the development and release of the egg but, if ovulation occurs, may affect the likelihood of either the sperm and egg uniting or reducing the likelihood of implantation. Copper intrauterine devices, by contrast, work primarily through a toxic effect on sperm and egg; in the event of fertilization, however, the likelihood of implantation is decreased. By contrast, barrier contraceptives, including mechanical barriers such as male and female condoms; chemical barriers such as spermicides; and temporal barriers such as withdrawal and fertility awareness methods (e.g., rhythm method) work exclusively by preventing union of the sperm and egg.

Adolescent patients require reliable contraception, but often have problems with compliance. Careful counseling about options (including abstinence), the risks of pregnancy and sexually transmitted disease as well as the need for both contraception and disease protection must be provided. These patients may be better served by methods that rely less on the user for reliability (intrauterine contraceptive devices [IUCDs] or long-acting hormonal agents such as injections, ring, patches, and implants) than those that depend on consistent use (use-oriented methods and those that are very time sensitive such as progestin-only oral contraceptives).

Fertilization inhibitors

IUDs

Cervical barrier devices

Condoms

Sponges

(male)

(female)

Spermicides

Diaphragm

Ovulation and implantation inhibitors

Vaginal ring

Oral contraceptives

"Morning after" pill (levonorgestrel)

Contraceptive patch

Implantable rods

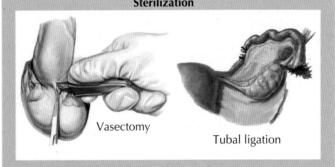

Sterilization

Vasectomy

Tubal ligation

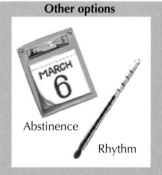

Other options

MARCH 6

Abstinence

Rhythm

Some adolescents will also benefit from the cycle control offered by long-cycle oral contraceptives and hormone-bearing IUCDs.

Patients over the age of 35 may continue to use low-dose oral contraceptives if they have no other risk factors and do not smoke. Compliance concerns are generally less in these patients, making use-oriented methods more acceptable and reliable. Long-term methods (IUCDs, long-acting progesterone contraception, or sterilization) may also be appropriate. Until menopause is confirmed by clinical or laboratory methods, contraception must be continued.

When unprotected intercourse occurs, pregnancy interdiction can often be achieved by the use of high-dose progestins (2–0.75 mg levonorgestrel tablets given up to 120 hours after intercourse) or the placement of a copper-bearing IUCD (up to 10 days after midcycle intercourse).

PREGNANCY

Plate 12.1

Reproductive System: VOLUME 1

IMPLANTATION AND EARLY DEVELOPMENT OF OVUM

Fertilization of the human ovum usually occurs in the ampullary portion of the oviduct, although in rare instances it may take place elsewhere in the genital tract or even in the ovary. Soon after the spermatozoon enters the ovum, the male and female pronuclei fuse to form the segmentation nucleus, which rapidly divides and redivides. Segmentation, thus initiated, continues until the original fertilized ovum is transformed into a mass of cells called the *morula*.

At this early stage, two types of cells can be distinguished; some proliferate more rapidly, forming a sphere that encloses the aggregate of more slowly dividing cells. A semifluid substance is excreted from the outer cells and is collected in a cavity, which forms simultaneously. The sphere-shaped structure is called the *blastodermic vesicle* or *blastocyst*. One layer of ectodermal cells, the primitive trophoblast, covers it except at one pole where the rapidly dividing cells have formed the "inner cell mass," which constitutes the beginning of the embryo.

While these changes take place, the ovum continues its passage into the uterine cavity, where it becomes implanted on the seventh or eighth day after ovulation. Various conditions may slow or obstruct the passage and cause nidation elsewhere, resulting in an ectopic pregnancy.

If the zygote splits very early (first 2 days after fertilization), each cell may develop separately its own placenta (chorion) and amnion (dichorionic diamniotic twins), which occurs 18% to 36% of the time. Most of the time, in monozygotic twins the zygote will split after 2 days, resulting in a shared placenta but two separate sacs (monochorionic diamniotic twins), occurring 60% to 70% of the time. In about 1% to 2% of monozygotic twinning the splitting occurs late enough to result in both a shared placenta and a shared sac (monochorionic monoamniotic twins). Later splitting of the zygote may result in incomplete separation, forming conjoined twins.

During the menstrual cycle, the ovarian hormones, estrogen and progesterone, act upon the endometrium, producing the premenstrual mucosa, which is sloughed during menstruation but remains when fertilization occurs. The pregravid endometrium gradually undergoes further changes to become the early decidua to which the blastocyst rapidly adheres once it has reached the uterus.

By the invasive capacity of its trophoblastic cells, the blastocyst sinks into the endometrium, which then closes over it and seals it from the uterine cavity, forming the decidua capsularis. The remaining decidua surrounding the blastocyst is called the *decidua basalis*, whereas the term *decidua vera* or *parietalis* designates the entire endometrium lining the uterus, except for the parts surrounding the blastocyst.

During the period of migration and implantation of the blastocyst, marked cellular proliferation has been taking place in the embryonic area. Three types of cells can be differentiated within the "inner cell mass." These constitute the three primary germ layers, the ectoderm, endoderm, and mesoderm.

From the ectoderm will derive the central nervous system, the epidermis, and certain skin appendages. The endoderm will furnish the epithelial linings and the glands of the gastroenteric and respiratory tracts. The mesoderm will give rise to the epithelium of the urinary and genital systems, the linings of the serous cavities, the various supporting tissues of the body, the blood, and the cardiovascular system.

After implantation, mesodermic cells grow out beneath the primitive trophoblast, which, by proliferation, forms villous projections into the surrounding decidua.

Each villus consists of a mesodermic core covered by two layers of trophoblastic cells. The outer cells have dark-staining nuclei and indefinite cell outlines. They are called *syncytial trophoblasts*. The more distinct cells of the inner layer are designated cytotrophoblasts or Langerhans cells. These decrease in number as pregnancy progresses and are difficult to find after the third month of gestation.

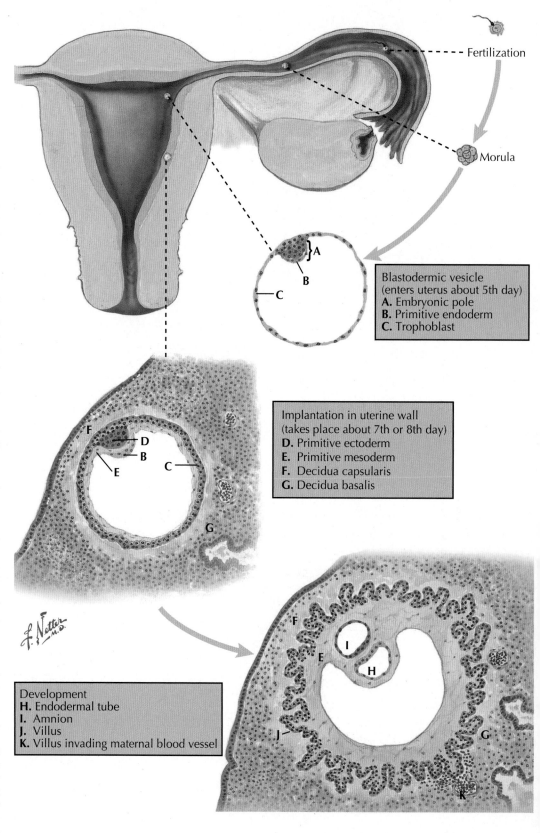

Fertilization

Morula

Blastodermic vesicle (enters uterus about 5th day)
A. Embryonic pole
B. Primitive endoderm
C. Trophoblast

Implantation in uterine wall (takes place about 7th or 8th day)
D. Primitive ectoderm
E. Primitive mesoderm
F. Decidua capsularis
G. Decidua basalis

Development
H. Endodermal tube
I. Amnion
J. Villus
K. Villus invading maternal blood vessel

Plate 12.2   Pregnancy

DEVELOPMENTAL EVENTS OF THE FIRST TRIMESTER

The first weeks following fertilization represent the most critical period for the success of a pregnancy. A high percentage (as high as 50%–60%) of fertilized oocytes do not result in pregnancies completing the first trimester of gestation. Despite the dramatic changes that the conceptus undergoes in the first 14 weeks of gestation, many patients are unaware of their pregnancy or delay seeking prenatal care. Emerging evidence suggests that during this period the foundations of a successful pregnancy and even the future health of the adult individual are set.

For the fertilized egg, zygote, and embryo, a number of events must occur. During the first trimester of gestation, the developing embryo implants in the endometrium (except in the case of ectopic pregnancies), the placental attachment to the mother is created, and the major structures and organs of the body are formed. About the 12th week of gestation, the placenta takes over hormonal support for the pregnancy from the corpus luteum. If this transition does not happen smoothly, the pregnancy can be lost. When the serum level of β–human chorionic gonadotropin (β-hCG) is greater than 1500 to 2000 mIU/mL, the level known as the *discriminatory zone*, transvaginal ultrasonography should visualize an intrauterine gestational sac in a normal, intrauterine, singleton pregnancy. If there is concern about the location or viability of the pregnancy, recent studies have advocated for a more conservative discriminatory zone before intervening (as high as 3500 mIU/mL).

Most patients do not have any specific signs or symptoms of implantation, although it is not uncommon to experience light bleeding at implantation or cramping during the first trimester. Clinical blood and urine tests (β-hCG) can detect pregnancy soon after implantation, which is as early as 6 to 8 days after fertilization. Home urine pregnancy tests normally cannot detect a pregnancy until at least 10 to 15 days after fertilization. Morning sickness occurs in about 70% of all pregnant women and typically improves after the first trimester. Some women will experience cramping during their first trimester, though this is usually of little concern unless there is meaningful bleeding as well. Symptoms of fatigue and breast fullness may occur relatively early in the course of gestation, and abdominal distention begins later in this trimester.

For the first 2 months of growth, the conceptus is referred to as an *embryo*. During this phase, the developing embryo is most sensitive to exposures to toxins, medications, radiation, and the effects of maternal condition that can disrupt the development process. Errors may result in major disruptions in structure or function of the fetus or the complete loss of the pregnancy. Later exposures to teratogens can result in a constellation of malformations related to the organ systems that are developing at that time; cardiovascular malformations tend to occur early in the embryonic period, and genitourinary abnormalities tend to result from later exposures.

Embryonic development is said to be complete when the embryo attains a crown-to-rump length of 30 mm (start of the fetal stage), corresponding in most cases to day 49 after conception. At the start of the third month of gestation, the risk of miscarriage decreases sharply and all major structures including hands, feet, head, brain, and other organs are present, and they continue to grow and develop. The fetal heart can be seen beating on ultrasonography, and the fetus bends its head and also makes general and startle movements. The gender of the individual may be seen as early as the 12th week. Brainstem activity has been detected as early as 54 days after conception, and the first measurable signs of brain electroencephalographic activity occur in the 12th week of gestation. If a genetic evaluation of the fetus is indicated, chorionic villus sampling may be performed between the 10th and 12th weeks of gestation or amniocentesis may be done between 15 and 20 weeks.

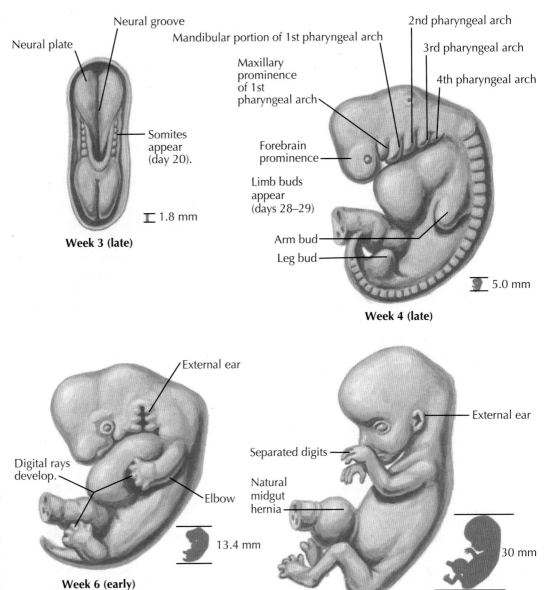

Neural plate · Neural groove · Somites appear (day 20).

1.8 mm

Week 3 (late)

Mandibular portion of 1st pharyngeal arch · Maxillary prominence of 1st pharyngeal arch · 2nd pharyngeal arch · 3rd pharyngeal arch · 4th pharyngeal arch · Forebrain prominence · Limb buds appear (days 28–29) · Arm bud · Leg bud

5.0 mm

Week 4 (late)

External ear · Digital rays develop. · Elbow

13.4 mm

Week 6 (early)

External ear · Separated digits · Natural midgut hernia

30 mm

Week 8

JOHN A. CRAIG—AD

Eyes closed · Intestines return to abdomen (week 10) · Sex distinguishable (week 12)

Early fetal period (week 8–week 16; CRL 5.0–14 cm)

CRL = crown-to-rump length

Plate 12.3

Reproductive System: VOLUME 1

Estrogen (estriol)

Progesterone (pregnandiol)

Chorionic gonadotropin

Weeks 14 16 18 20 22 24 26 28

The low levels of chorionic gonadotropin during this stage lessen breast tenderness and morning sickness.

Maternal blood volume and cardiac output increases 20%.

Colostrum is noticed at the 26th week of gestation.

Pregnancy loss at this period is associated with:

Thrombophilias

Placental inflammation, commonly along with chorioamnionitis

Cervical insufficiency

Digestive symptoms such as heartburn and constipation during this trimester are usually related to the enlarging uterus.

By the end of this trimester hemorrhoid and back pain may occur.

In this trimester more weight is gained to nourish the growing fetus.

DEVELOPMENTAL EVENTS OF THE SECOND TRIMESTER

The second trimester (14–28 weeks) is a time of growth and refinement of function; all major structures including hands, feet, head, brain, and other organs are present, and they continue to grow and develop. During this trimester, the risk of pregnancy loss dramatically lessens and levels of human chorionic gonadotropin plateau and often decline, easing many of the early adverse symptoms of pregnancy such as breast tenderness and morning sickness, though the enlarging uterus may now precipitate heartburn and constipation. (When a second-trimester pregnancy loss occurs, it is strongly associated with placental inflammation, often related to ascending infection and/or acute chorioamnionitis, though it may also occur because of aneuploidy, by thrombophilias, by cervical insufficiency, and others.) Any weight loss experienced in the first weeks of gestation is regained and further weight is gained to provide stores needed to provide nutrition for the growing fetus. Despite the relative lack of complications during the second trimester, early signs of later problems may first appear during this phase of pregnancy.

Although the fetus begins moving during the first trimester, it is not until the second trimester that movement of the fetus ("quickening") is felt. This typically happens around 20 to 24 weeks for first pregnancies and as early as 16 to 18 weeks for experienced mothers. Fetal waking and sleeping cycles become established and mimic those of the newborn, with the baby awake for about 6 hours a day.

Fetal and maternal changes are frequent during the second trimester: During this period, the fetus grows rapidly, weighing about 100 g and measuring 3 in. in length at 14 weeks to weighing roughly 900 g (2 lb) by the end of the second trimester. By 15 weeks gestation, the fetal heart pumps about 23 to 24 L of blood a day. Fetal viability (ability to survive apart from the mother) begins about 24 weeks, though neurologically intact survival at this stage is unlikely. There is an increase in maternal blood volume and cardiac output (20% greater) to feed the needs of the growing pregnancy. Toward the end of this trimester, maternal hemorrhoids and low back pain may make their appearance. Colostrum (the first form of breast milk) is present by 26 weeks of gestation. The placenta is fully functional, taking over the role of making estrogen and progesterone that had been performed by the corpus luteum. The fetus is making insulin and urinating, with fetal urine being a significant component of amniotic fluid. (The fetus will begin to outweigh the placenta sometime around the 16th week of gestation.) The teeth have formed inside the fetus's gums, and vernix and meconium make their first appearance. By the end of

Urinates
Sex is defined
Bone formation
Some facial expressions due to more developed muscles
Able to hear
Female fetus has uterus and vagina formed; the ovaries have between 6 and 7 million oocytes
Fetus can swallow
Development of lanugo
6 hours awake, 18 sleeping
Hair grows
Fingernails develop
Lungs produce surfactant
Response to sounds, pancreas produces insulin

Weeks 14 15 16 17 18 19 20 21 22 23 24 25 26 27 28

Fetus length from crown of the head to rump, in millimeters

250 — 1,000
210 — 820
160 — 630
120 — 460
87 — 320
— 200
— 110
— 45

Fetus's weight in grams

Length

Weight

Fetal "quickening" is felt earlier for experienced mothers

In 1st pregnancy, fetal "quickening" is usually felt in this period

Beginning of fetal viability

C. Machado —M.D.

the second trimester, fetuses hear and respond to external sounds.

By the early portion of the second trimester, the external genitalia have formed sufficiently that they can be recognized on ultrasonographic studies, distinguishing the fetus as male or female. It is also at this point that a female fetus will have the most egg cells of any point in her life. Oocytes peak at 6 to 7 million about 16 to 20 weeks gestation, declining to about 1 million at birth.

Screening for open neural tube and other defects (via measurement of maternal serum α-fetoprotein and other markers) is generally performed between 15 and 20 weeks. If a genetic evaluation of the fetus is indicated, an amniocentesis may be performed between the 15th and 20th weeks of gestation. It is generally during the second trimester that ultrasonographic screening for appropriate gestational age, fetal growth, and major fetal malformations is performed.

Plate 12.4

Pregnancy

DEVELOPMENTAL EVENTS OF THE THIRD TRIMESTER

During the third trimester (27–40+ weeks) the fetus continues to grow and develop, and maternal physiology changes in preparation for childbirth. It is most often during this phase of pregnancy that complications such as preeclampsia, bleeding, complications of diabetes or hypertension, abnormalities of growth or amniotic fluid, and preterm labor may emerge.

During the third trimester of gestation, the dramatic growth of the fetus continues as it attains its final birth weight and its organs prepare for function as an autonomous individual. Fetal fat accumulates to provide nutrition and insulation for the first few days of independent life, accounting for about 15% of fetal weight at term. By the 29th week, the fetus has 300 bones, though eventual fusion of more than 90 of these fetal growth plates following birth will leave the adult total of 206. At the beginning of this trimester, in the male, the testes descend into the scrotum under the guidance of the gubernaculum, which in the female become the round ligaments supporting the fundus of the uterus. Most babies will settle into their final birth presentation (cephalic, breech, or transverse) by about 36 weeks gestation.

Maternal blood volume increases by almost twice and cardiac output reaches its maximum. At term, 20% of maternal cardiac output goes to the uterus and placenta. Late in this trimester, changes in the collagen of the cervix prepare for dilation and effacement during labor and delivery. It is also in the latter portion of this trimester that the number of oxytocin receptors on the uterine muscle cells increases markedly and there is an increase in the number of intercellular gap junctions. These micropores between cells provide a mechanism to facilitate the organized and effective coordinated contractions necessary for successful labor.

Uterine contractions that have been present since conception become progressively stronger and more noticeable as the trimester progresses. These are the Braxton-Hicks contractions of late pregnancy and the contractions of labor and delivery. Amniotic fluid volume peaks at about a liter at 37 weeks.

As the uterus grows, displacement of the abdominal contents results in early fullness with meals, heartburn, and constipation. The growth also results in relocation of the maternal center of gravity, causing the mother to lean backward to compensate. This results in low back pain and the characteristic "duck waddle" of late pregnancy. When the fetal presenting part begins descent into the maternal pelvis (about 36 weeks gestation), causing a decline in fundal height, the patient experiences improved respiratory and gastric function but at the expense of greater pelvic pressure and a reduced bladder capacity.

Planning and preparation for breastfeeding should be undertaken during this trimester. No special physical preparation is needed for successful breastfeeding, but discussion, questions, and the acquisition of needed supplies (e.g., nursing bra) are best taken care of before delivery. Normal amounts of colostrum have been present from the beginning of this trimester, and some women experience breast leakage throughout this period.

For selected patients, "kick counts" may be used to assess the overall health of the fetus. In general, the detection of more than four fetal movements over the course of an hour indicates a healthy fetus. All patients should be encouraged to monitor their baby's activity levels and be evaluated for any prolonged reduction or absence in activity.

Because placental function declines after 40 weeks, testing of fetal and placental reserve through fetal non-stress testing, contraction stress testing, biophysical profiles, or measurements of fetal blood flow in various vessels may be indicated when there are complications of pregnancy or it extends beyond term.

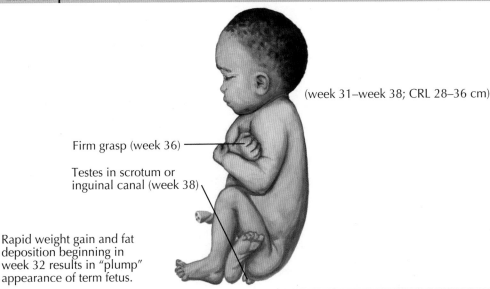

Late fetal period

(week 31–week 38; CRL 28–36 cm)

Firm grasp (week 36)

Testes in scrotum or inguinal canal (week 38)

Rapid weight gain and fat deposition beginning in week 32 results in "plump" appearance of term fetus.

Full-term fetus within the uterus

Placenta: fetal aspect

Umbilical cord

Amniochorionic membrane

Placenta

Plate 12.5

Reproductive System: VOLUME 1

DEVELOPMENT OF PLACENTA AND FETAL MEMBRANES

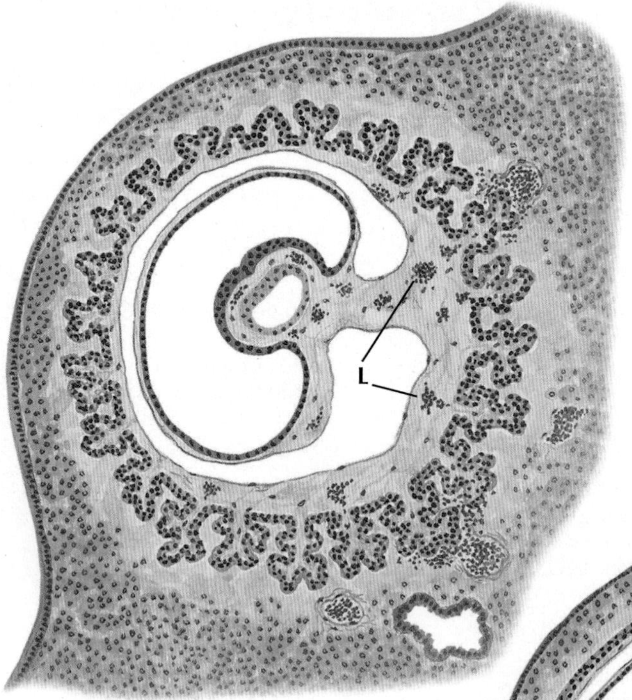

As the embryo grows, it must establish an efficient means of obtaining nutrients and eliminating waste products. It does this by establishing the placenta, an efficient interface between its vascular system and that of its mother. In addition, it must prevent rejection of the fetal allograft and secrete peptide and steroid hormones that modulate both maternal metabolism and fetal growth and development.

Trophoblastic cells have marked invasive capacities and grow into the walls of maternal blood vessels, establishing contact with the maternal bloodstream. In early pregnancy, trophoblastic cells frequently invade deep into the myometrium, but as pregnancy progresses, invasion is limited by profuse proliferation of decidual cells, which confine the trophoblastic invasion to the area just beneath the attachment of the growing placenta. In the rare instances when decidual cells fail to develop, implantation overlies an old scar, or there are defects in the development of the fibrinoid layer (Nitabuch layer), invasion of the uterine wall by chorionic villi is extensive. This can result in a placenta accreta, increta, or percreta.

In the recently implanted blastocyst, the rim of trophoblastic cells, with the underlying mesodermic stroma, constitutes the primitive chorion. At the same time, the amnion first appears as a small cavitation in the mass of proliferating ectodermal cells in the embryonic area. This cavity gradually enlarges and folds around the developing embryo, so that eventually the latter is suspended by a body stalk (the umbilical cord) in a closed bag of fluid (the amniotic sac).

During the early stage of development of the amnion, another vesicle appears in the embryonic area and for a time is much larger than the amnion. This is the yolk sac (not illustrated), the function of which in mammalian development is not known. As the embryo grows, the yolk sac decreases in size, until at term only a minute remnant can be found near the site of the cord attachment to the chorionic plate.

During the first 3 weeks after implantation, a luxuriant growth of the rudimentary villi over the entire blastodermic vesicle occurs, developing into a structure called the *chorion frondosum* or "leafy chorion." As the embryo, surrounded by the amnion, grows and protrudes more and more into the uterine cavity, the decidua capsularis and the underlying chorionic villi stretch and become flattened and atrophic. Most of the villi disappear from this region, which is then called the *bald chorion* or *chorion laeve.* Meanwhile the villi proliferate markedly in the highly vascular decidua basalis. Here the chorion frondosum persists and becomes a part of the fully developed placenta.

In rare cases the chorionic villi, beneath the decidua capsularis, do not undergo atrophy but establish vascular connections with the decidua vera, opposite the site of implantation, when the enlarging conceptus fills the uterine cavity. In this condition, called *placenta membranacea*, the entire chorion is covered with villi, and the thin placenta thus formed bleeds freely, does not separate spontaneously, and is difficult to remove manually during the third stage of labor.

The chorionic villi contain no blood vessels during the first 2 weeks of gestation, and the embryo has not yet developed a circulatory system. Nutrition is chiefly by osmosis. Toward the end of the third week, certain cells in the mesodermic stroma differentiate into blood islands, around which vascular walls soon appear. By branching and coalescence of these vessels, the entire chorion becomes vascularized. Meanwhile, a fetal heart and circulatory system have been developing. By the end of the fourth week, connections are made between the vessels of the chorion and those of the fetus, which have grown out through the body stalk, thus establishing a fetal-placental circulation.

Amnion enlarging and encircling the endodermal tube and fetal mesoderm. Blood islands (L) forming in mesoderm

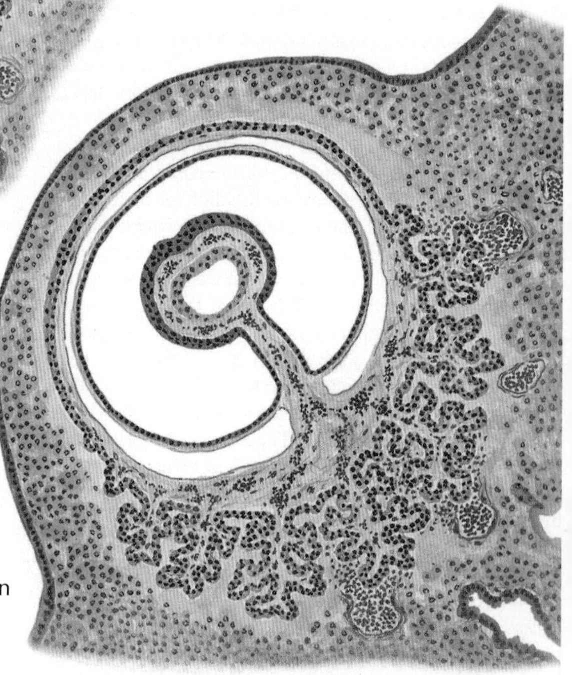

Amnion completely encircling the early fetus, which is attached only by the body stalk. Villi have atrophied to form chorion laeve and hypertrophied to form chorion frondosum. Blood islands coalescing to begin formation of fetal circulatory system

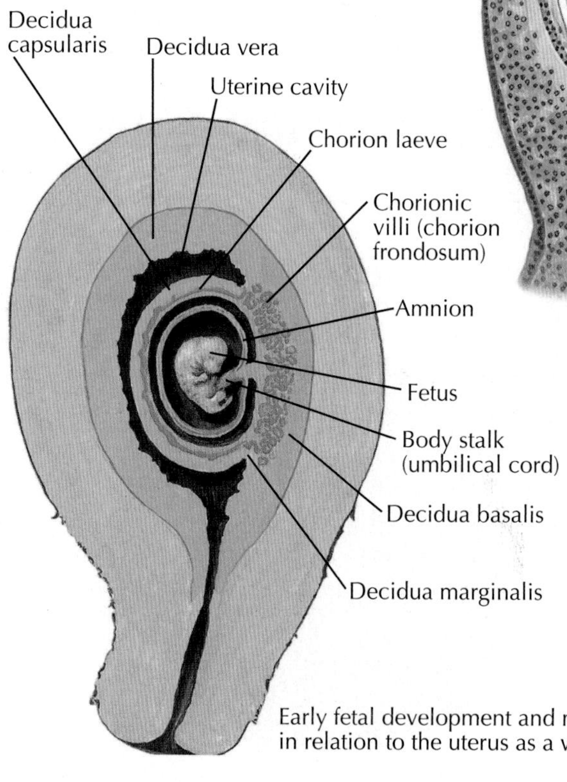

Decidua capsularis
Decidua vera
Uterine cavity
Chorion laeve
Chorionic villi (chorion frondosum)
Amnion
Fetus
Body stalk (umbilical cord)
Decidua basalis
Decidua marginalis

Early fetal development and membrane formation in relation to the uterus as a whole (schematic)

Plate 12.6

Pregnancy

CIRCULATION IN THE PLACENTA

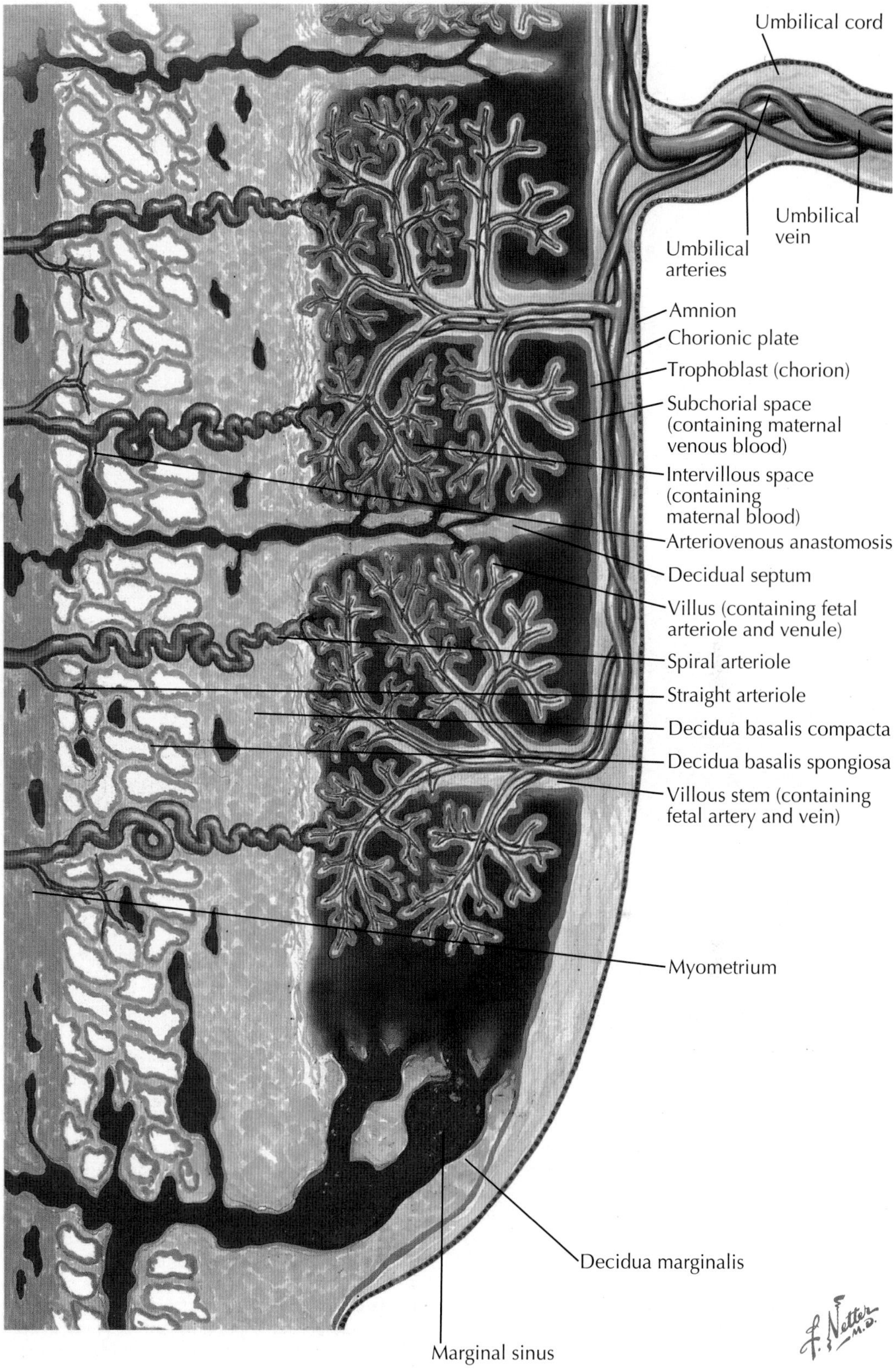

During the third week of gestation, the villi at the base of the placenta become firmly anchored to the decidua basalis. In later weeks the zone of anchoring villi and decidua becomes honeycombed with maternal vessels that communicate with the intervillous space. The spiral arteries in the decidua become less convoluted and their diameter is increased. This increases maternal blood flow to the placenta and decreases resistance. In response to the presence of the trophoblasts, the vascular endothelium is replaced by the trophoblast, and both the trophoblast and an amorphous matrix of fibrin and other constituents replace the internal elastic lamina and smooth muscle of the media. These changes are most marked in the decidual portion of the spiral arteries but extend into the myometrium as the pregnancy advances. The basal arteries are not affected.

The blood-filled lake in which the chorionic villi are suspended develops from the lacunae in the primitive trophoblast as it invades and opens up the maternal vessels of the decidua. Development of the maternal blood supply to the placenta is thought to be complete by the end of the first trimester of pregnancy (approximately 12–13 weeks). Abnormalities of this vascular process are found in women with fetal growth restriction and pre-eclampsia. (These abnormalities are thought to be due to defective invasion and may involve defects in protein expression.)

The villi absorb nutrients and oxygen from the maternal blood in the intervillous space, and these materials are transported to the growing fetus through the umbilical vein and its villous and cotyledon tributaries. Waste products for excretion into the maternal blood are brought from the fetus through two umbilical arteries, which are continuations of the fetal hypogastric arteries. These vessels terminate in the rich capillary network of the chorionic villi, where they are in close contact with the maternal bloodstream. (Terminal villi each contain three to five capillaries, forming capillary loops and occasional sinusoids.) The villi are oxygenated directly from the maternal blood and exhibit infarction whenever the maternal circulation around them ceases.

The details of the maternal blood flow through the placenta are not well understood. Observations indicate that the flow is much more rapid than was once believed and that the differences in the quality of blood in various areas of the placenta are quite marked. Currents and other dynamic factors probably cause these differences. The blood is more arterial toward the maternal aspect of the placenta, whereas in the subchorionic space it is venous in character. Although in most placentas the venous drainage is largely through the marginal sinus, part of the venous blood is returned to the uterine veins in the decidua basalis. The branching of the cotyledon stalks between the larger decidual septa divides the placenta to varying degrees into lobules, called *cotyledons*.

The marginal sinus is a large venous channel that courses beneath or through a gray ring of tissue formed by the membranes and the decidua marginata. It is not uncommon to find foci of obliteration, thrombosis, or rupture of the marginal sinus. This region is also the

most common site for various retrograde changes in the decidua and contiguous chorionic villi. These lesions have long been considered of little or no clinical importance, though specific data are lacking.

The placenta is not only an intrauterine organ of respiration, nutrition, and excretion for the growing fetus but is also a powerful endocrine gland in the physiologic economy of both mother and fetus. Within 10 days after fertilization, trophoblastic tissue, probably the Langerhans cells, has begun to produce chorionic

gonadotropic hormone, and by the end of the second month the placenta is the main source for elaborating estrogen and progesterone. Other hormones include human placental lactogen (also called *human chorionic somatomammotropin*), insulin-like growth factor, and other growth factors. The placenta is an important source of glycogen and cholesterol synthesis (important for fetal energy and hormone production), protein metabolism, and the elimination of lactate made by the placenta and fetus.

Plate 12.7

Reproductive System: VOLUME 1

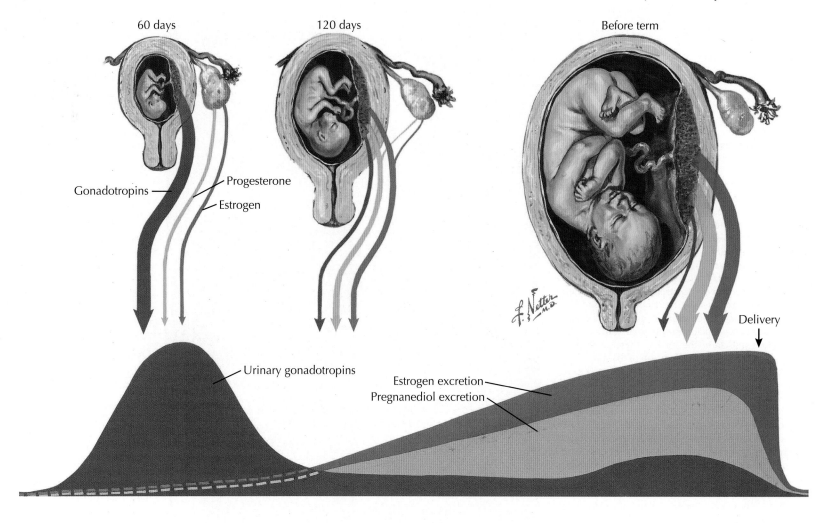

HORMONAL FLUCTUATIONS IN PREGNANCY

In addition to its function as the agent of transfer of gases and nutrients, the placenta has significant endocrine activity. It produces progesterone, which is important in maintaining the pregnancy; somatomammotropin (also known as *placental lactogen*), which acts to increase the amount of glucose and lipids in the maternal blood, estrogen, insulin-like growth factors, relaxin, and β-hCG. This hormonal activity is the main cause of the increased maternal blood glucose levels seen in pregnancy, which results in an increased transfer of glucose and lipids to the fetus but puts the mother at risk for developing clinical or overt diabetes.

The corpus luteum of the ovary secretes estrogen and progesterone until the fourth month of gestation in amounts only slightly higher than those produced after ovulation in the second half of the regular cycle. However, not later than the 60th day of gestation, the placenta begins to secrete these hormones in progressive quantities, which reach their maximum at the end of gestation. Chorionic gonadotropin rescues the corpus luteum from programmed demise and ensures that progesterone and estrogen are secreted in early pregnancy, until about 2 months of gestation when the placenta

takes on the role of producing sufficient progesterone and estrogen. Because of the marked production of estrogen and progesterone by the placenta, bilateral oophorectomy after the fourth month of pregnancy does not usually alter the course of gestation.

The site of formation of estrogen and progesterone in the placenta is the syncytial layer of the trophoblast. The production of progesterone by the trophoblast begins to decrease during the last month of gestation. This decrease is related to the cause of onset of labor, though the full nuances of the triggers of labor remain to be fully elucidated.

Chorionic gonadotropic hormone is secreted from the placenta soon after implantation, reaching its peak during the third month, after which its levels decrease, first sharply during the fourth and fifth months, then gradually leveling off until the end of gestation. Chorionic villi, specifically the syncytiotrophoblasts, are the site of production of this hormone. In addition to its role in promoting the continuing production of progesterone by the corpus luteum, it is thought that hCG affects the mother's immune tolerance of the conceptus. Because of its highly negative charge, hCG may repel the immune cells of the mother, protecting the fetus during the first trimester. It has also been hypothesized that hCG may be a placental link for the development

of local maternal immunotolerance. Chemically, it is a glycoprotein of a relatively large molecular size, composed of 244 amino acids with a molecular mass of 36.7 kDa. It is heterodimeric, with an α subunit identical to that of luteinizing hormone, follicle-stimulating hormone, and thyroid-stimulating hormone and a β subunit that is unique to hCG. A chemiluminescent or fluorometric immunoassay is used to detect β-hCG levels as low as 5 mIU/mL and allows quantitation of the β-hCG concentration.

In early pregnancy, the function of β-hCG seems to be aimed at keeping up the activity of the corpus luteum through interaction with the transmembrane receptor, resulting in continuing progesterone secretion, which is needed for the decidualization of the endometrium. After the fetus and placenta are well developed, the need for a corpus luteum, and therewith for this gonadotropic hormone, becomes less imperative.

The excretion rates of gonadotropins, estrogens, and pregnanediol vary to a great extent. The curves in the picture represent only an approximate graphic demonstration of the excretion changes during gestation rather than exact values at given times. For this reason, no scale has been entered. Not shown are the excretion values of adrenal cortical hormones, which are also increased during pregnancy.

Plate 12.8

Pregnancy

ECTOPIC PREGNANCY: TUBAL PREGNANCY

Ectopic pregnancy refers to the implantation of the embryo in any place outside the uterine cavity. According to the site of implantation, four kinds of ectopic pregnancy are distinguished: tubal, ovarian, abdominal or peritoneal, and cervical. Up to 2% of all reported pregnancies are ectopic, with the rate varying with age, race, and geographic location (highest in Jamaica and Vietnam). In one large series, 18% of patients presenting to the emergency department for pain or bleeding were ultimately found to have an ectopic pregnancy.

Tubal pregnancy is by far the most frequent of all ectopic pregnancies (96%). Here again, four types are recognized, depending on the portion of the tube in which the implantation takes place: interstitial (cornual), isthmic, ampullar, and infundibular. Although ampullar implantation has the highest incidence of tubal pregnancy, it is the interstitial form that is potentially the most serious from a clinical perspective.

The most important contributors to the occurrence and development of ectopic pregnancy are tubal damage or altered motility that causes the fertilized egg to be improperly transported, resulting in implantation outside the uterine cavity. The most common cause of tubal damage is acute salpingitis, with prior ectopic pregnancy or pelvic surgery contributing a small number of additional cases. In most of the remaining patients (50%), no risk factor is apparent. Abnormal embryonic development may play a role. Pelvic infections convey a sixfold increased risk; a prior ectopic pregnancy conveys a 10-fold increased risk, followed by prior female sterilization, increasing age (age 35–44, 3-fold greater rate than for women aged 15–24), non-White race (1.5-fold increased risk), assisted reproduction, cigarette smoking (30+/day, 3- to 5-fold increased risk), and endometriosis. Although intrauterine contraceptive devices markedly decrease the risk of ectopic pregnancy compared with use of no method of contraception, if pregnancy occurs with an intrauterine contraceptive device in utero, it is much more likely to be ectopic.

The early development of an ectopic pregnancy is the same as of an intrauterine gestation except for its location: the trophoblast possesses the same qualities and thus secretes chorionic gonadotropin, participating in the maintenance of the corpus luteum of pregnancy. This latter, in turn, elaborates enough estrogens and progesterone to induce all the maternal changes characteristic of the early stages of pregnancy. Initially, the level of chorionic gonadotropin is the same as in a normally developing pregnancy. The mother may manifest decidual transformation of the endometrium and slight enlargement and softening of the uterus, just as in uterine pregnancy.

The possibility of ectopic implantation must always be kept in mind. A good clue is the history of amenorrhea of several weeks, followed by bleeding (usually spotting) accompanied by abdominal pain, which may be slight or intense. The subjective complaints of early pregnancy may be mild or nonexistent, as in normal pregnancy. Physical examination may reveal the presence of a fullness in the adnexa or some irregular, sometimes

Sites of ectopic implantation

Interstitial · Tubal (isthmic) · Abdominal · Tubal (ampullar) · Infundibular (ostial) · Ovarian · Cervical

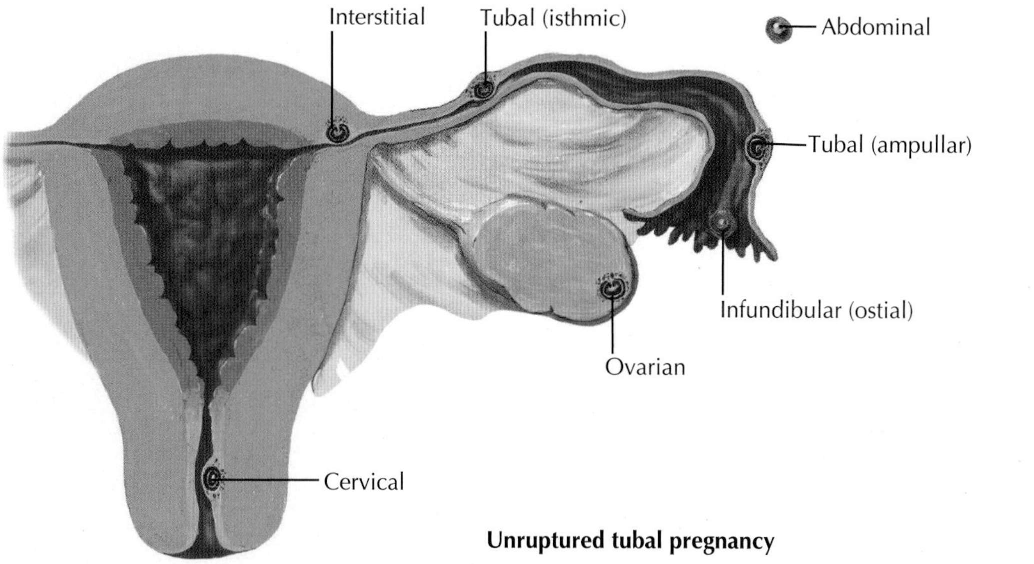

Unruptured tubal pregnancy

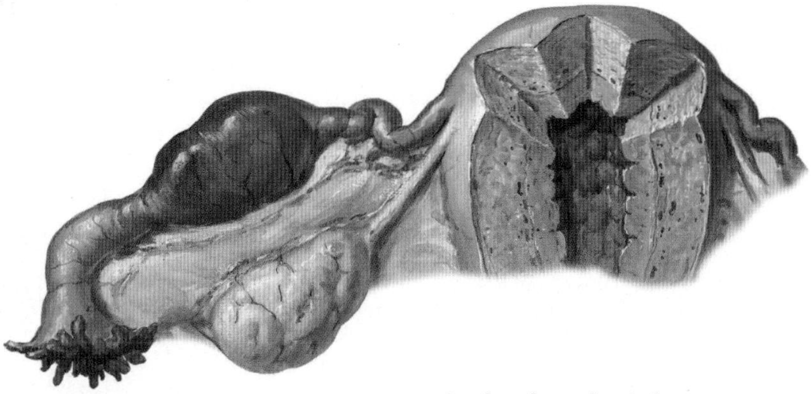

Chorion · Amnion · Fetus

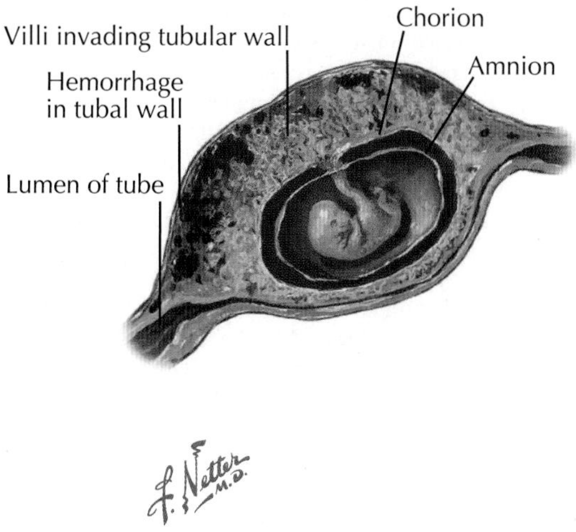

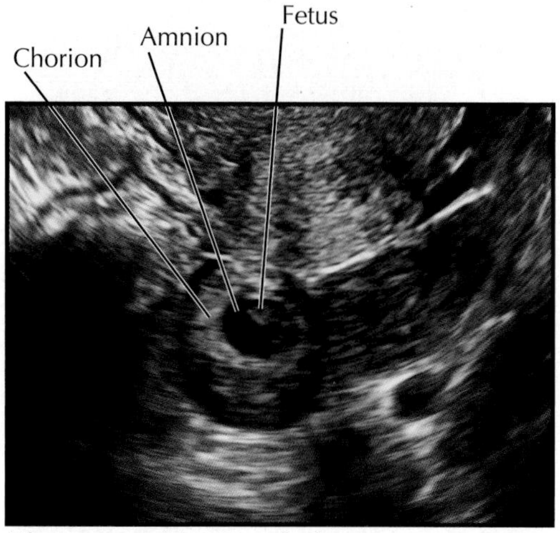

Ultrasonographic view of adnexa

Section through tubal pregnancy

Villi invading tubular wall · Chorion · Amnion · Hemorrhage in tubal wall · Lumen of tube

retrouterine, growth filling the cul-de-sac. Signs of hemorrhagic shock and peripheral collapse are seen when the intraperitoneal hemorrhage is severe. Transvaginal ultrasonography may document no gestational sac within the endometrial cavity and an adnexal mass. The finding of free fluid in the posterior cul-de-sac is common but not diagnostic. The finding of a fetal heartbeat in the adnexa is diagnostic.

Laboratory evaluations should include serial quantitative β-hCG levels (if the patient's condition permits).

(Levels lower than 3000 mIU/mL are found in about half of cases.) Normal pregnancies should demonstrate a doubling of serum β-hCG levels every 36 to 48 hours, whereas abnormal pregnancies will not. Serum progesterone (low) may be of diagnostic help if pregnancy is <6 weeks gestation. Almost 90% of patients with an ectopic pregnancy have levels less than 30 nM/L (10 ng/mL). A hematocrit of less than 30 mL/dL is found in about one-fourth of women with ruptured ectopic pregnancy.

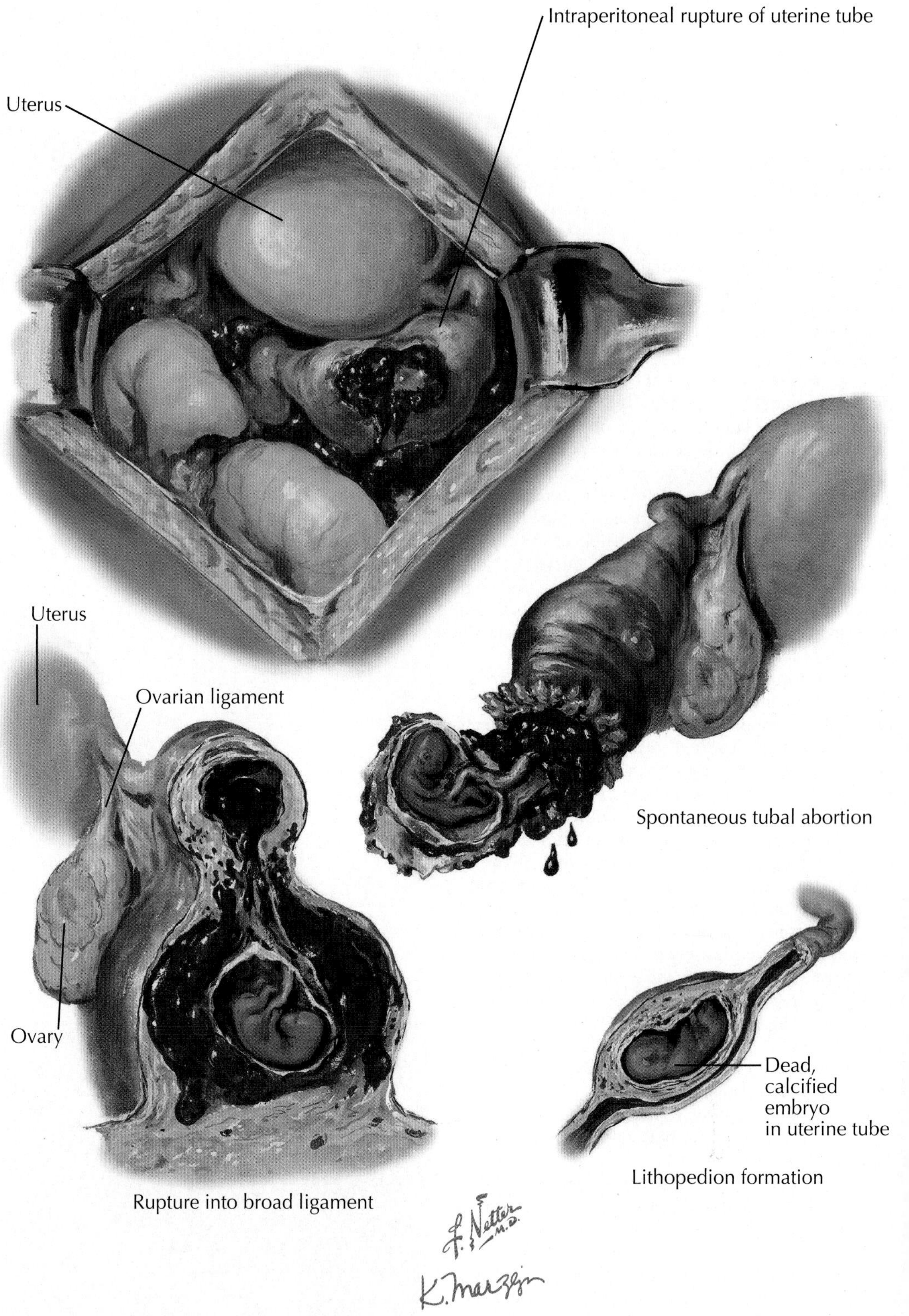

Plate 12.9

Reproductive System: VOLUME 1

Uterus

Intraperitoneal rupture of uterine tube

Uterus

Ovarian ligament

Spontaneous tubal abortion

Ovary

Dead, calcified embryo in uterine tube

Lithopedion formation

Rupture into broad ligament

ECTOPIC PREGNANCY: RUPTURE, ABORTION

Because the distensibility of the fallopian tube is limited, pregnancies that implant there generally cause symptoms or tubal rupture within 6 to 8 weeks after fertilization. Very rarely does a tubal pregnancy develop longer than into the fourth or fifth month without symptoms and signs that ultimately lead to the diagnosis. The most frequent outcome of tubal pregnancy is rupture through the tube into the peritoneal cavity. It usually occurs between the middle of the second and the end of the third month (menstrual age), but it may come earlier. A partial or total separation of the trophoblast from the tubal walls occurs, leading to death of the embryo. Blood extravasation and later extrusion of the embryo with blood clots into the peritoneal cavity follow, where they may slowly be absorbed, provided the hemorrhage was slight. The uterine decidua may sometimes separate as a whole and be eliminated as a decidual cast of the uterine cavity. Passage of the decidual cast can be confused with an early spontaneous abortion, and hence the passed tissue should be carefully examined for the presence of villi.

In many cases of tubal pregnancy, the trophoblast erodes the tubal wall. This leads to a tubal rupture, which is almost always accompanied by a serious, potentially catastrophic clinical picture of acute shock due to extensive hemorrhage into the peritoneal cavity. The time of tubal rupture varies with the site of implantation. If the embryo develops in the interstitial portion of the tube, rupture occurs relatively late, whereas nidation in the isthmic part results in rupture in the very early weeks because of the difference in the mass of musculature in the two parts of the tube. Rupture may take place spontaneously but may also occur following defecation, coitus, and vaginal examination. The consequences of a rupture after interstitial implantation are more serious because of the major vessels in this area.

In a few cases, rupture has taken place through the lower margin of the tube, where it is not covered by peritoneum and where the two folds of the broad ligament meet only loosely. In such instances, the tubal contents empty into the connective tissue of the mesosalpinx; that is, between the two peritoneal sheets. Here hematoma may develop, and the embryo will die, or a broad ligament pregnancy, also called *intraligamentary* or *extraperitoneal pregnancy,* may continue, depending on the degree of placental separation.

Although rupture of a tubal pregnancy or a tubal abortion with hemorrhage is a surgical emergency treated by laparoscopy or laparotomy, when an ectopic pregnancy is diagnosed early, medical therapy may be appropriate. Medical therapy may be considered for asymptomatic or mildly symptomatic patients. Methotrexate is generally used for chemical management of these patients. Methotrexate should not be used if the β-hCG level is higher than 15,000 mIU/mL, the adnexal mass is greater than 3 cm, or the patient's hemodynamic status is unstable. Patients with a history of active hepatic or renal disease, fetal cardiac activity demonstrated in the ectopic gestation, active ulcer disease, or significant alterations in blood count (white blood cell count <3000, platelet count of <100,000) are not candidates for this therapy.

All Rh-negative, unsensitized women with ectopic pregnancies should receive Rh immunoglobulin at a dosage of 50 μg if the gestation is of less than 12 weeks' duration and 300 μg if it is beyond 12 weeks.

Termination of tubal pregnancy by death of the embryo and its transformation into a lithopedion is a very rare event. Such a process may go on completely asymptomatically, with slow dehydration and mummification. This "missed tubal abortion," as it has been called, may be found only incidentally during laparotomy.

Hydatid mole formation and choriocarcinoma development have been observed in ectopic pregnancy but are extremely rare.

Plate 12.10

Pregnancy

Interstitial pregnancy

Uterus

Uterine tube

ECTOPIC PREGNANCY: INTERSTITIAL, ABDOMINAL, OVARIAN

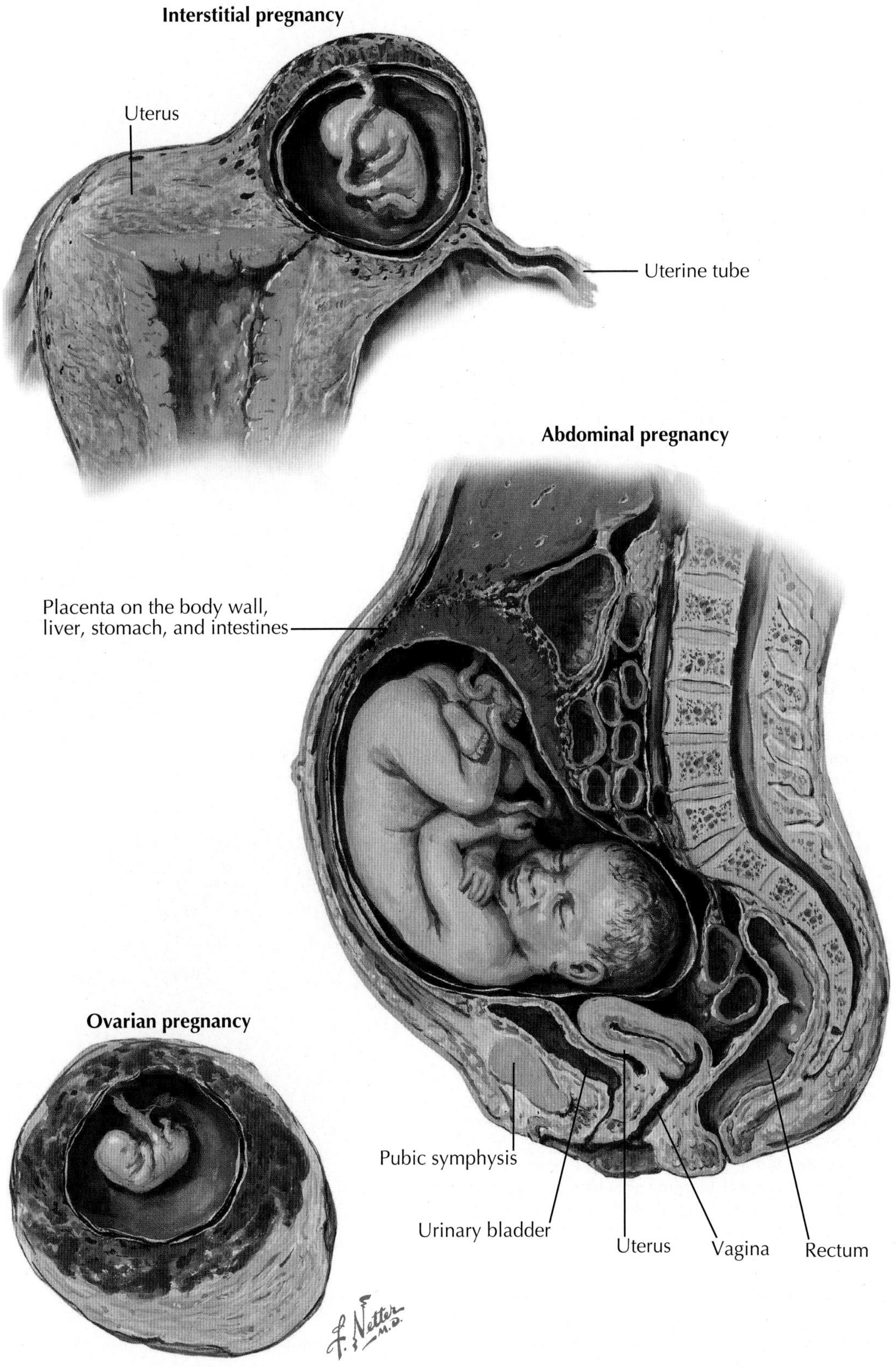

When, during the process of abortion or rupture, the trophoblast, after total separation, implants itself again somewhere in the peritoneum, as happens on rare occasions, it may grow and develop into a secondary abdominal pregnancy. The embryo in such cases may have remained in its original amniotic sac, or a new sac may have formed from the surrounding tissues. A secondary abdominal pregnancy may also result from a beginning tubal implantation that ruptured and became inserted between the leaves of the broad ligament. If the latter should rupture again, the embryo in the fetal sac may extrude into the peritoneal cavity, with the placenta remaining in the extraperitoneal position between the broad ligament sheets. In still more exceptional cases, the fertilized ovum may escape through the open end of the tube, attaching itself to the parietal or visceral peritoneum or the omentum, developing into a primary abdominal pregnancy. It has even been reported that an abdominal pregnancy has originated from a defect in the uterine wall, which had been filled and closed up by the omentum during the healing period after cesarean section. The remarkable feature of these abdominal pregnancies is that they may continue to near term before an occasion for diagnosis may even arise, even in the face of repeated ultrasonographic studies. The incidence of abdominal pregnancy is estimated to be roughly 1 in 10,000 live births.

Fetal salvage in these cases is the exception, though survival rates of more than 50% have been reported if the pregnancy progresses beyond 30 weeks gestation. When survival does occur, there is a much increased rate of fetal malformations, including facial or cranial asymmetry, limb defects, and central nervous system anomalies. Delivery must be by laparotomy, but such surgeries are associated with massive hemorrhage even when care is taken not to disturb the placenta. Because of the poor fetal and maternal outcomes associated with abdominal pregnancies, these pregnancies are generally interrupted as soon as the diagnosis is established.

Ovarian pregnancy is the rarest form of ectopic pregnancy. Although full-term ovarian pregnancies are on record, they more often eventuate in encapsulation and degeneration of the fetal mass. The diagnosis can be made only by finding ovarian structures around the amniotic sac upon microscopic study of the removed ovary. In a primary ovarian pregnancy, the oviduct and the broad ligament should not be involved.

In a low percentage of tubal implantations, the fertilized ovum may settle in the uterine end of the tube—its intramural or interstitial segment. In an interstitial pregnancy, owing to the greater muscular mass and vascularity, fetal growth may continue longer without rupture than in other types of tubal pregnancy. The danger resulting from rupture, however, is also greater, because the hemorrhage may be so profuse that it is

Abdominal pregnancy

Placenta on the body wall, liver, stomach, and intestines

Ovarian pregnancy

Pubic symphysis

Urinary bladder

Uterus

Vagina

Rectum

fatal within a very short time. Furthermore, the diagnosis of ectopic gestation in cases of interstitial pregnancies is more difficult in view of the lack of a mass in the tube by palpation or ultrasonography and an asymmetric uterine enlargement, which may be interpreted as a seemingly normal pregnancy or a bicornuate uterus.

Cervical pregnancy (not illustrated) has been observed in only a few cases. The cervical endothelium, not undergoing the typical progestational changes, is not adequately prepared to receive the trophoblast or

permit nidation. The placenta is attached to the cervical myometrium, and gestation advances not longer than into the third month, when abortion occurs. Some authors do not classify this condition within the ectopic pregnancies, but one should bear in mind that it shares with these anomalies all of the dangers connected with the difficulty of removing the placenta without serious hemorrhage. The low contractility of this portion of the uterus and the proximity of the uterine vascular supply increase the risk of hemorrhage even during curettage.

Plate 12.11

Reproductive System: VOLUME 1

ABORTION

Abortion is the loss or failure of an early pregnancy, and it is defined in several forms: complete, incomplete, inevitable, missed, septic, and threatened. A complete abortion is the termination of a pregnancy before the age of viability, typically defined as occurring at less than 20 weeks from the first day of the last normal menstrual period or involving a fetus of weight less than 500 g. Most complete abortions generally occur before 6 weeks or after 14 weeks of gestation. An incomplete abortion is the spontaneous passage of some, but not all, of the products of conception. A pregnancy in which rupture of the membranes and/or cervical dilation takes place during the first half of pregnancy is labeled an inevitable abortion. Uterine contractions typically follow, ending in spontaneous loss of the pregnancy for most patients. A missed abortion is the retention of a failed intrauterine pregnancy for an extended period. A septic abortion is a variant of an incomplete abortion in which infection of the uterus and its contents has occurred. It is a common cause of maternal death worldwide. A threatened abortion is a pregnancy that is at risk for some reason. Most often, this applies to any pregnancy in which vaginal bleeding or uterine cramping takes place but no cervical changes have occurred.

Estimates for the frequency of pregnancy loss are as high as 50% to 60% of conceptions and between 10% and 15% of known pregnancies. Most early pregnancy losses occur before 10 weeks of gestation, of which approximately 50% are caused by fetal chromosome abnormalities. Less than 2% of fetal losses are missed abortions. Septic abortions occur in 0.40 to 0.6 of 100,000 spontaneous pregnancy losses. Threatened abortions occur in 30% to 40% of pregnant women.

The clinical signs and symptoms of abortion manifest themselves with vaginal bleeding followed by uterine contractions and cervical dilation, but only 12% of patients with vaginal bleeding will have a pregnancy loss. Clinically, a distinction is made between threatened abortion and inevitable abortion. In the former, slight vaginal bleeding is seen, with or without feeble uterine contractions. The characteristic finding of this type of abortion is the absence of cervical dilation. Inevitable abortion is characterized by cervical dilation together with more severe vaginal bleeding and uterine contractions. In a fair number of cases of threatened abortion, pregnancy can proceed until full viability.

In inevitable abortion, uterine contractions become stronger as time progresses, bleeding becomes more severe, and the process ends by expulsion of the uterine contents. Abortion is called complete when the entire fetus, placenta, and membranes are eliminated. It is called incomplete when the fetus is expelled and all or part of the placenta or membranes remains inside the uterus. In the latter case, vaginal bleeding may continue as long as the placental parts are not removed spontaneously or by intervention.

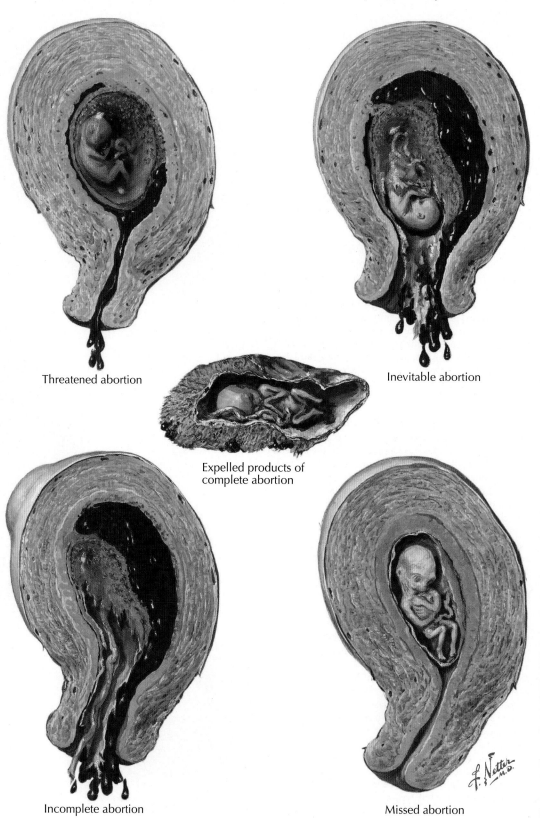

Threatened abortion

Inevitable abortion

Expelled products of complete abortion

Incomplete abortion

Missed abortion

In missed abortion, the fetus (if present) dies but the placenta is not detached from the uterine walls. In such cases the amniotic fluid is reabsorbed, and the fetus undergoes a process of dehydration and mummification.

Ultrasonography is useful in establishing the presence of a living embryo. Early pregnancy loss is defined as a nonviable, intrauterine pregnancy with either an empty gestational sac or a gestational sac containing an embryo or fetus without fetal cardiac activity within the first 12 6/7 weeks of gestation. The established tests for pregnancy, determining the presence of chorionic gonadotropins, are usually positive as long as any part of the placental tissue remains in contact with the maternal circulation and, after complete abortion, until the circulating chorionic gonadotropic hormones are completely eliminated. Although the presence of a living embryo is reassuring, it does not guarantee the successful outcome of the pregnancy.

Plate 12.12

Pregnancy

CERVICAL INSUFFICIENCY

The American College of Obstetricians and Gynecologists' definition of cervical insufficiency is "the inability of the uterine cervix to retain a pregnancy in the second trimester in the absence of clinical contractions, labor, or both." Cervical insufficiency is characterized by asymptomatic dilation of the internal os during pregnancy. This generally leads to dilation of the entire cervical canal during the second trimester with subsequent risk of rupture of the membranes and/or expulsion of the fetus. This affects 1/54 to 1/1842 pregnancies (variation resulting from uncertain diagnostic criteria). Although uncommon, it is thought to be involved with as many as 20% to 25% of all second-trimester pregnancy losses.

Cervical insufficiency may come from iatrogenic sources, most often damage from cervical dilation at the time of dilation and curettage or other manipulation, or damage caused by surgery (conization). Other possible causes include congenital tissue defect, uterine anomalies (uterus didelphys), and prior obstetric lacerations.

Generally cervical insufficiency is suggested by a history of second-trimester pregnancy loss accompanied by spontaneous rupture of the membranes without labor or rapid, painless preterm labor. The finding of prolapse and ballooning of the fetal membranes into the vagina without labor would strongly suggest cervical insufficiency. Cervical insufficiency must be differentiated from the presence of uterine anomalies, chorioamnionitis, and other sources of midpregnancy loss.

When the patient is at high risk for cervical insufficiency (generally by history) or cervical change is suspected, ultrasonography should be used to assess cervical length. Ultrasonography must also be performed before cervical cerclage to assess for abnormal fetal development. Although cervical length can be measured by ultrasonography, routine use of this has not proven to be an effective screening tool except in the face of a high-risk history. (Normal cervical length is approximately 4.1 cm [±1.02 cm] between 14 and 28 weeks and gradually decreases in length to 40 weeks, when it averages between 2.5 and 3.2 cm.) Signs of cervical funneling and cervical shortening are associated with an increased risk of preterm delivery, but management in the absence of other risk factors is unclear.

Currently the best screening technique remains frequent vaginal examinations beginning around the time of previous cervical change or the second trimester, whichever is earlier. Attempts to define or identify cervical insufficiency by hysterosonography, pull-through techniques with inflated catheter balloons, measurement of cervical resistance to cervical dilators, magnetic resonance imaging, and others have not gained clinical acceptance.

Treatment of cervical insufficiency is by cervical cerclage (placement of a concentric nonabsorbable suture close to the level of the internal cervical os) generally performed between 12 and 14 weeks of gestation. When the suture is placed vaginally, it is generally removed at 38 weeks of gestation. If labor occurs before this point and cannot be stopped, the suture should be removed immediately because of the risk of uterine rupture with

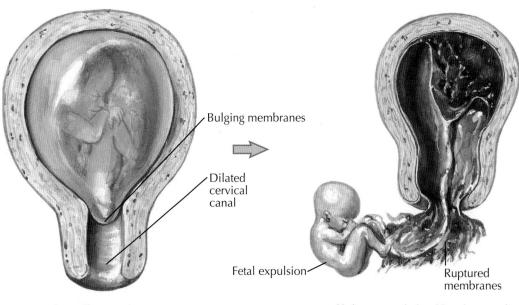

Cervical insufficiency becomes manifest in second trimester as dilation of cervical canal.

Bulging membranes

Dilated cervical canal

Fetal expulsion

Ruptured membranes

If left untreated, the dilated cervical canal may result in rupture of membranes and/or fetal expulsion.

Surgical management of cervical insufficiency (cerclage)

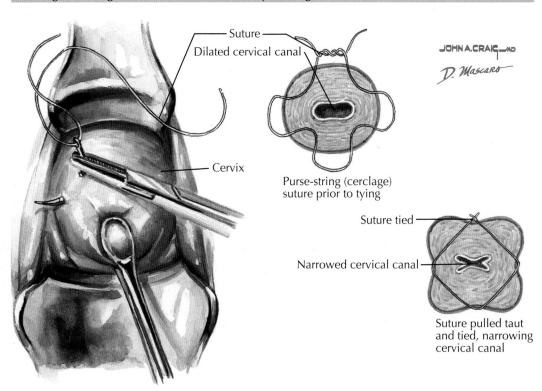

Suture

Dilated cervical canal

Cervix

Nonabsorbable purse-string suture placed around cervix at level of internal os

JOHN A. CRAIG—MD
D. Mascaro

Purse-string (cerclage) suture prior to tying

Suture tied

Narrowed cervical canal

Suture pulled taut and tied, narrowing cervical canal

an obstructed outlet. Cervical cerclage is occasionally performed transabdominally. When placed in this manner, these sutures are intended to remain permanently and they preclude vaginal delivery. The use of lever pessaries (such as the Smith-Hodge) has been reported to be associated with outcomes similar to those obtained by cerclage, but this modality is infrequently used and the data supporting the treatment is variable. Bleeding, uterine contractions, obvious infection, or rupture of the membranes are contraindications to cerclage. Because of

scarring after cerclage, some patients require cesarean delivery. With correct diagnosis and cervical cerclage, fetal survival increases from 20% to 80%.

Restriction of activity is often suggested, but evidence that this alters the outcome of pregnancy is lacking. After 24 weeks of pregnancy, bed rest may be the only therapy available because the risk of cerclage to trigger labor may outweigh the potential benefit. Prophylactic antibiotics and β-mimetics (tocolytics) have not been shown to be effective in prophylactic cerclage.

Plate 12.13

Reproductive System: VOLUME 1

MULTIPLE GESTATION

In roughly 3.4% of births in the United States, two or more fetuses coexist. This rate is rising, having done so by about 70% since 1980. In approximately 1/8000 to 1/10,000 births, there will be spontaneously occurring triplets. The rise in multiple births is thought to be due to the use of fertility drugs and other technologies and to an increased rate of childbearing in women older than 30, who are more likely to conceive multiples. In the United States, 36% of twin pregnancies and 77% of triplet and higher order pregnancies occur after infertility treatment.

The first weeks following fertilization represent the most critical period for the success of a pregnancy. Up to 50% of twin pregnancies identified in the early weeks will silently abort one fetus (with or without bleeding). It is also during this early period that the fertilized egg can split to form one or more "identical" (monozygotic) embryos. This occurs in about 4/1000 births. When more than one egg is released and fertilized during the same menstrual cycle (naturally or through assisted ovulation), fraternal (dizygotic) twins, triplets, or higher order multiples can result. Dizygotic twins are more common in mothers who are themselves a dizygotic twin.

Multiple gestations are responsible for a disproportionate share of perinatal morbidity and mortality, accounting for 17% of all preterm births (before 37 weeks of gestation), 23% of early preterm births (before 32 weeks of gestation), 24% of low-birth-weight infants (<2500 g), and 26% of very-low-birth-weight infants (<1500 g). Roughly 60% of twin gestations deliver before term, with rates rising with each additional fetus (e.g., 93% for triplets). Hospital costs for women with multiple gestations are on average 40% higher than for women with gestational age–matched singleton pregnancies because of their longer length of stay and increased rate of obstetric complications.

The possibility of a multiple gestation should be considered any time there is a discrepancy between uterine size (larger than expected) and gestational age or when multiple fetal heart tones are heard by auscultation or Doppler ultrasound study. Establishing the presence and number of fetuses early in gestation is important not only for family reasons but also because the presence of a multiple gestation increases the risk of gestational diabetes and other abnormalities. Multiple gestations also cause different levels of gestation-sensitive laboratory tests, such as maternal serum α-fetoprotein, which would be interpreted as abnormal in a normal, singleton pregnancy. Genetic amniocentesis may be considered for selected patients because twin gestations have twice the rate of abnormalities (monozygotic twin gestations have a 2%–10% rate). Furthermore, in multiple gestations, chorionicity can best be determined ultrasonically early in pregnancy by assessing the thickness of the dividing membrane between the gestational sacs; as pregnancy progresses, this distinction becomes more difficult.

To provide nutritional support for a multiple gestation, the mother should increase her caloric intake by roughly 330 kcal (twins) more than that normal for pregnancy. Appropriate iron and folic acid supplementation should also be ensured.

Perinatal morbidity and mortality for multiple gestations is two to five times higher than for singleton gestations. Preterm delivery is the most common cause of morbidity or mortality. Indeed, most twin pregnancies

TYPES OF TWINS

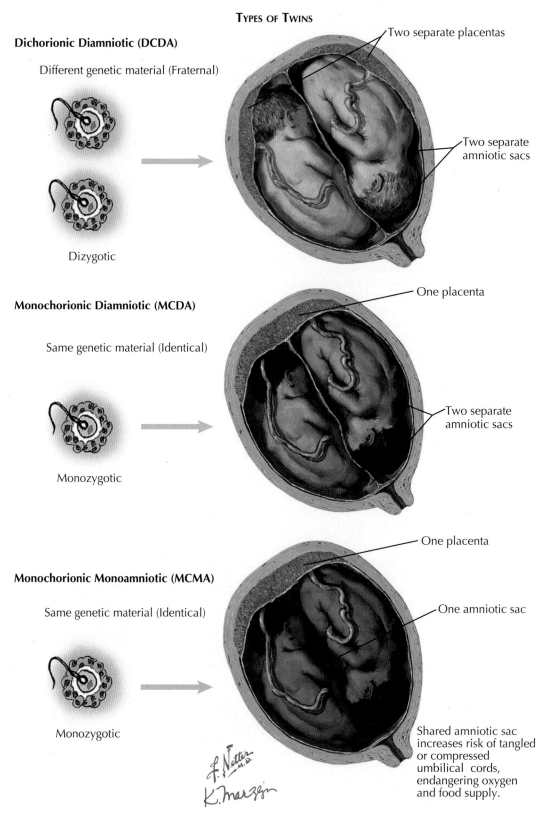

Dichorionic Diamniotic (DCDA)

Different genetic material (Fraternal)

Dizygotic

Two separate placentas

Two separate amniotic sacs

Monochorionic Diamniotic (MCDA)

Same genetic material (Identical)

Monozygotic

One placenta

Two separate amniotic sacs

Monochorionic Monoamniotic (MCMA)

Same genetic material (Identical)

Monozygotic

One placenta

One amniotic sac

Shared amniotic sac increases risk of tangled or compressed umbilical cords, endangering oxygen and food supply.

will deliver between 36 and 38 weeks of gestation. Other complications include intrauterine growth restriction (12%–47% vs. 5%–7% in singletons) or discordant growth, cord accidents, hydramnios, congenital anomalies (twofold increase), and malpresentation. Monozygotic twins have a 1% incidence of a monoamniotic sac that carries a 50% fetal mortality due to cord entanglement or conjoined twins. One-fifth of triplet pregnancies and one-half of quadruplet pregnancies result in at

least one child with a major long-term handicap, such as cerebral palsy. When matched for gestational age at delivery, infants from multifetal pregnancies have a nearly threefold greater risk of cerebral palsy.

Maternal complications of multiple gestation include abruptio placentae, placenta previa, preeclampsia, anemia, hyperemesis gravidarum, pyelonephritis, cholestasis, pulmonary edema, postpartum hemorrhage, and an increased operative delivery rate.

Plate 12.14

Pregnancy

PLACENTA: FORM AND STRUCTURE

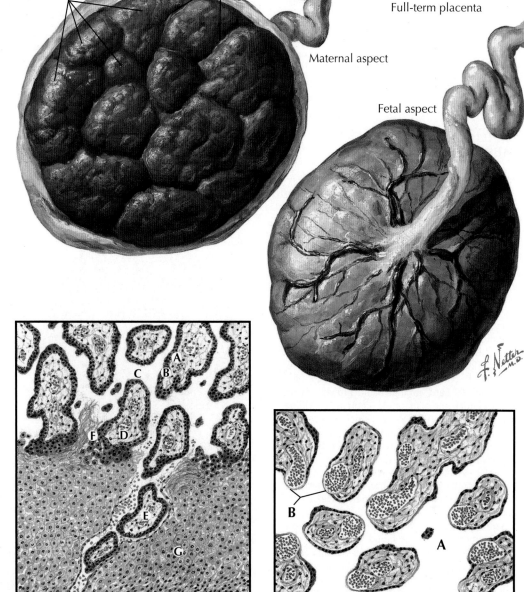

The normal placenta is depicted on this page, and some abnormal forms are shown subsequently. In the description, the characteristic features of both normal and abnormal forms have been integrated.

The placenta at term is flat, cakelike, round or oval, 15 to 20 cm in diameter, and 2 to 3 cm in breadth at its thickest parts. It weighs 500 to 600 g, or about one-sixth the weight of the fetus. Oversized placentas (placentomegaly) are found in cases of erythroblastosis and syphilis and sometimes without evident reasons. Numerous but of little apparent clinical importance are the many variations in placental shape, despite the fact that they may result from conditions such as retroplacental hemorrhage, abnormal nidation sites, and inadequate decidual blood supply.

The maternal aspect of the normal placenta is lobulated, because short decidual septa separate the major cotyledons. The lobulation may be accentuated, as in erythroblastosis, or obliterated for unknown reasons. The margin of the normal placenta, where decidua, chorionic plate, and fetal membranes meet, appears as a gray, opaque ring caused by the underfolding of membranes and the decidua marginata. It is here that the marginal sinus is usually found. This structure pursues a tortuous, irregular course around the margin of the placenta. It often becomes coiled and is difficult to open. Foci of obliteration, thrombosis, or rupture of the marginal sinus are not infrequently encountered. This sinus provides the major drainage of maternal blood from the hemochorionic interface. The underfolding of the membranes seldom exceeds 1 cm, but in cases of placenta circumvallata it might be quite extensive, and the underlying villi might have degenerated or become ischemic, resulting in a premature delivery of a stillborn fetus. However, even though the chorionic plate may be markedly decreased in size owing to an extensive underfolding, the chorionic villi are usually well vascularized, and this placental variety may have no clinical significance.

The color of a normal placenta is uniformly red except for the subchorionic regions and the spaces between the major cotyledons, which appear darker red, carrying blood that is more venous in character. Cross-sectioning of gently handled and properly fixed placentas exposes this difference and permits the recognition of intraplacental thrombosis and fibrin deposition quite frequently present in these venous areas. The fibrin depositions, incorrectly called "white infarcts," appear as white laminated nodules.

The normal placenta is of homogeneous spongy consistency. A few subchorionic nodules of fibrin and scattered flecks of gritty calcification are found frequently at term and have no recognized clinical or pathologic significance.

Section through deep portion of placenta—early gestation. A = villus, B = trophoblast, C = intervillous space, D = anchoring villus, E = villus invading blood vessel, F = fibrinoid degeneration, G = decidua basalis, H = gland

Appearance of placental villi at term. (A) Syncytial cell mass becoming trophoblastic embolus, (B) fetal blood vessel endothelium against a thinned syncytiotrophoblast, where they share a basal lamina. The cytotrophoblast has disappeared.

Microscopically, a villus of a normal placenta consists of a core of collagenous stroma containing well-filled capillaries; these often bulge from the surface of the villus, bringing the fetal blood very close to the maternal bloodstream, separated by only a thin layer of fetal capillary endothelium and the thinned, stretched-out cytoplasm of the syncytial cells. The nuclei of the syncytial trophoblasts tend to pile up on the surfaces of villi. These aggregations are called *placental giant cells*. They frequently are dislodged into the maternal circulation, where they form trophoblastic emboli to the mother's lungs and can be found in pulmonary capillaries during pregnancy and the puerperium. They never proliferate in the lungs and are apparently harmless. (Fetal cells have been documented in the maternal circulation many years after delivery.) These are not to be confused with amniotic emboli, which consist of the particulate matter of amniotic fluid. This material may gain entrance, though rarely, to the maternal circulation during labor and then may cause severe shock and maternal death.

Plate 12.15

Reproductive System: VOLUME 1

PLACENTA: NUMBERS, CORD, MEMBRANES

One placenta is the rule in singleton pregnancies. Occasionally, a bipartite placenta, consisting of two incompletely separated lobes with vessels extending from one lobe to the other before uniting with the umbilical vessels, may be encountered. Two parts, including the blood vessels, may also be completely separated by the fetal membranes and present a placenta duplex. In multiple pregnancy either more than one placental mass or one placenta, but with more than one amniotic sac, may be found. Monozygotic twins generally have two amnions but only one chorion (diamniotic monochorionic twins), which usually does not extend into the wall between the two sacs. Rarely are both twins in one amniotic sac (monoamniotic monochorionic twins), and these carry a 50% fetal mortality due to cord entanglement, growth restrictions, circulatory imbalances, or conjoined twining. Monochorionic twins who share a single placenta are also at risk for twin-to-twin transfusion syndrome. This syndrome is thought to result from an unbalanced net transfusion of blood between one twin and the other via placental vascular anastomoses. Despite a growing understanding of twin-to-twin transfusion syndrome, the exact pathophysiology remains to be elucidated.

Separated from the main placental mass, small accessory lobules of placental tissue occasionally may be situated in the membranes. The blood vessels from such lobules may join the vessels in the main placenta before entering the cord, or no such vascular connection may exist. The former condition is called *placenta succenturiata*, the latter *placenta spuria*. Postpartum hemorrhage and infection may occur if retention of an accessory lobe or lobule in the uterus has remained unrecognized. Careful search for torn vascular stumps on the cord and on the fetal aspect, which usually reveal such conditions, is therefore indicated.

The umbilical cord averages 55 cm in length. It is usually white, moist, and coiled. It is generally slightly longer in male than in female fetuses. It contains two arteries and one vein coiled around each other in a matrix of mucinous stroma called *Wharton jelly*. Microscopically, the cord is covered by one layer of cuboidal epithelium that is continuous at one end with the skin of the child and at the other with the lining of the amniotic sac. Two-vessel umbilical cords (1% of deliveries) are associated with a 20% increase in the risk of fetal anomalies. This condition is believed to be caused by atrophy of a previously normal artery, most often the left.

In cases of intrauterine infection, the umbilical vessel walls may appear yellow with purulent exudate, and their lumina may be obliterated with gray thrombi. When the fetus dies in utero, the cord and fetal membranes (but not the placenta) present postmortem changes comparable

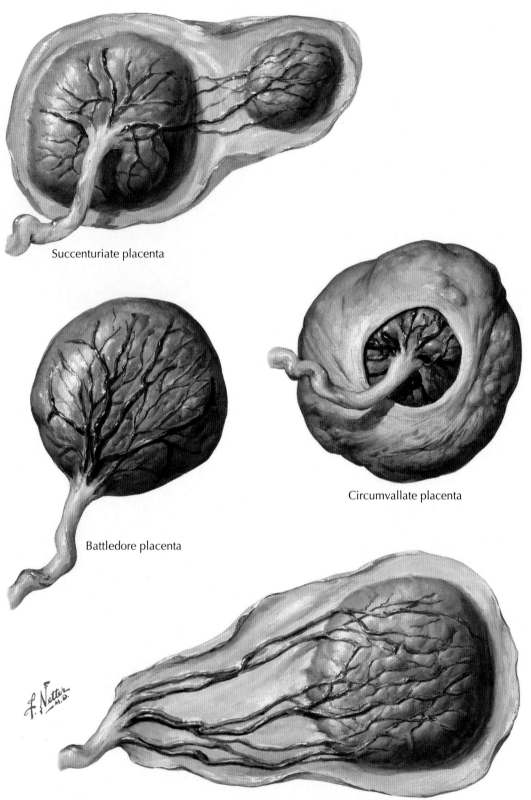

Succenturiate placenta

Battledore placenta

Circumvallate placenta

Velamentous insertion of cord

to those found in the fetus. Occasionally, an umbilical vessel ruptures, with formation of a hematoma in the cord, membranes, or chorionic plate, during the third stage of labor when such an event causes no harm.

The cord may be centrally or eccentrically attached to the placenta. Attachment over the marginal sinus (battledore placenta) or within the membranes (velamentous insertion) is rare. The umbilical vessels, in the latter case, divide before they reach the chorionic plate. If a low uterine implantation has occurred, and if the

membranes with the large umbilical branches have grown across the internal os (vasa previa), serious bleeding may occur during the last trimester or with rupture of the fetal membranes during labor.

The fetal membranes consist of the moist, glistening, transparent amnion and the slightly thicker yet transparent chorion to which adhere varying amounts of shaggy, usually vascularized decidua vera. In normal pregnancies, the delivered decidua vera is scanty and is apt to be present in patches.

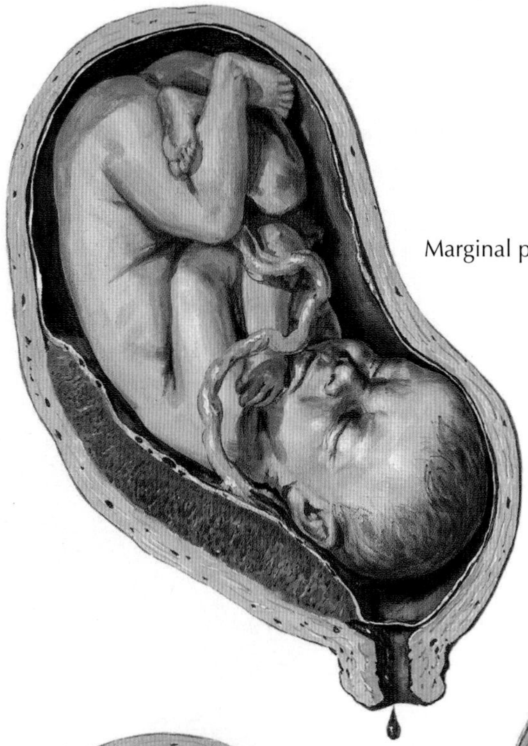

Plate 12.16

Pregnancy

PLACENTA PREVIA

Placenta previa refers to implantation of the placenta in the lower segment of the uterus, so that it partially or totally covers the internal os of the cervix. Placenta previa and abruptio placentae account for more than 85% of the cases of hemorrhage during the last trimester of pregnancy. This is associated with potentially catastrophic maternal bleeding and obstruction of the uterine outlet.

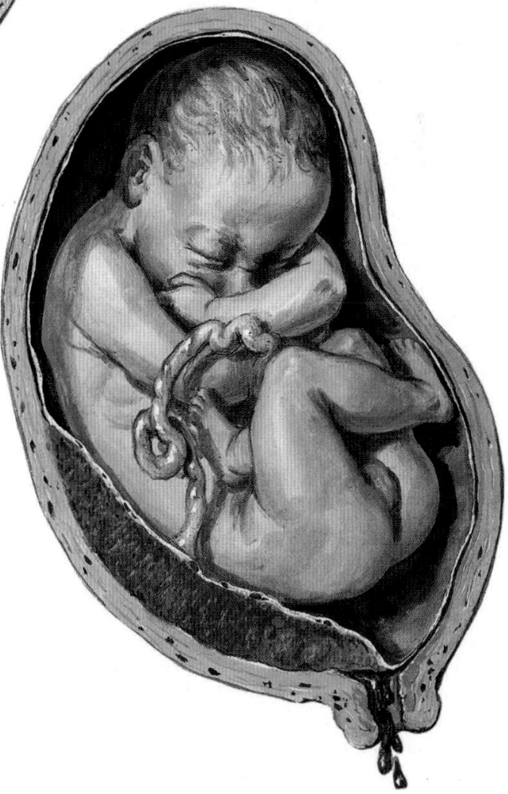

Placenta previa is classified into four types, according to the degree with which the placenta superimposes or encroaches on the internal os: total or central placenta previa, in which the internal os is covered entirely; partial placenta previa, in which the placenta partially caps the internal os (10%–90%); marginal placenta previa, in which only a small edge of the placenta is at the internal os; and low-lying, in which the placenta is located in the lower uterine segment but does not touch the cervical os. These degrees may vary with cervical dilation or gestational age.

Ultrasonographic studies indicate that the location of the placenta is subject to some degree of "migration" during the course of gestation. In addition, as the lower uterine segment elongates late in pregnancy, these relationships may change. Therefore the above classification of placenta previa is only relative, and it should be remembered that if a diagnosis is made of a particular type, it refers to the time of examination. In the partial and total varieties of placenta previa, a slight degree of separation of the placenta is inevitable when the lower segment of the uterus distends, and hence a certain degree of bleeding is bound to occur.

The incidence of placenta previa varies from 1 in 100 to 1 in 250 term deliveries. The condition is much more frequent in multiparas than in primiparas, in older patients (older than 35: 1%; older than 40: 2%), with a prior cesarean delivery (two- to fivefold increase), in smokers (twofold increase), following in vitro fertilization, and in multiple gestations.

Little is known regarding the etiology of the condition. It has been suggested that defective vascularization of the decidua, as the result of inflammatory or atrophic processes, may be a contributing factor for placenta previa. Under these circumstances, the placenta is forced to spread over a wide area to obtain sufficient blood supply. It is also possible that a multiplicity of factors contribute to lower implantation of the ovum with extension of the placenta toward the internal os.

The symptoms of placenta previa include painless hemorrhage (70% of cases), which usually appears after the seventh month of gestation. The hemorrhage may come at any time, without warning and even when the patient is asleep. It usually begins as a slight intermittent bleeding, but it may become profuse without any

Marginal placenta previa

Partial placenta previa

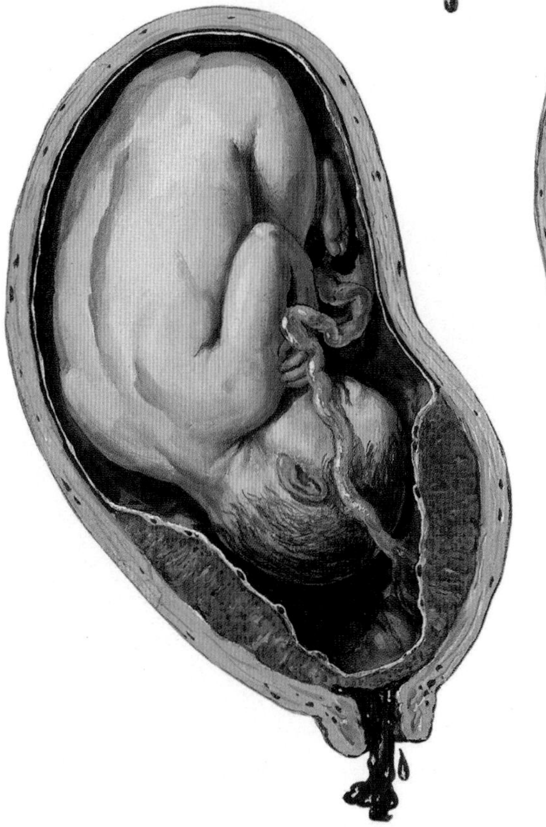

Total (central) placenta previa

notice. The mechanisms of bleeding in placenta previa are poorly understood. Separation of small areas and tears in the vessels may occur as the consequence of stretching of the uterine walls, especially the distended lower segment. The blood is maternal in origin.

The diagnosis is usually not difficult when the classic symptoms are present. Ultrasonography has replaced other imaging techniques and the classic "double set-up" (vaginal examination in the operating room so that an emergency operative delivery could be accomplished

should hemorrhage be precipitated). It is important to remember that any vaginal manipulation may precipitate extensive hemorrhage.

Because of the overstretched lower segment and abnormalities of placental attachment, profuse bleeding may occur even after the delivery of the fetus. The lower segment may be unable to contract sufficiently to check the bleeding. Placenta accreta occurs in 15% to 25% of cases of placenta previa, particularly in the presence of a previous cesarean section scar.

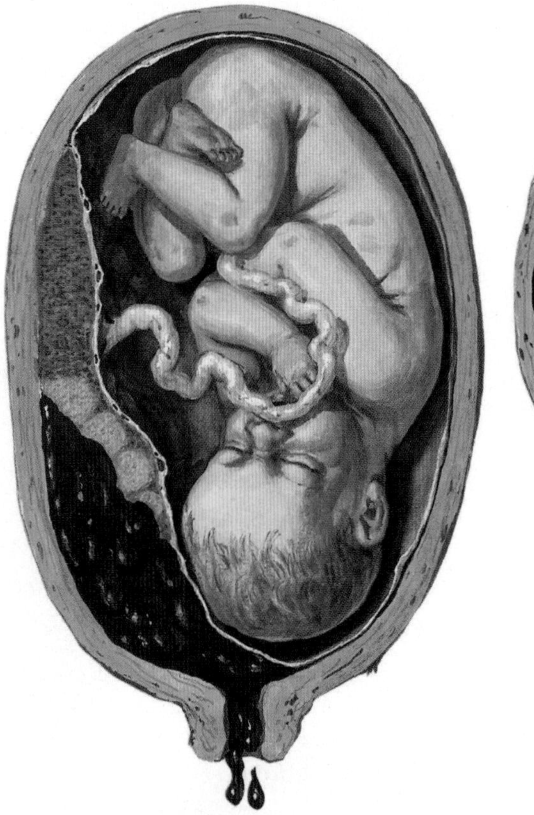

Plate 12.17

Reproductive System: VOLUME 1

ABRUPTIO PLACENTAE

The term abruptio placentae and its synonymous "premature separation of the normally implanted placenta" refer to separation of the placenta from its uterine attachment after the twentieth week of gestation. Prior to this period, detachment of the placenta is associated with abortion. Abruptio placentae is one of the major causes of hemorrhage in the last trimester of pregnancy. The bleeding from placental detachment may be external or internal. In the case of external bleeding, the blood dissects and insinuates itself between the placenta or its membranes and the uterine wall, escaping through the cervix. In the internal form, the bleeding remains concealed between the placenta and the uterine wall because of incomplete detachment of the placenta. The lower pole of the placenta frequently remains adherent to the uterine wall. When the entire placenta, or at least its lower pole, is detached, external bleeding is usually present. Another cause of concealed hemorrhage, even in the presence of complete separation, is the obstruction of the cervix by the presenting part. All of these factors may delay the diagnosis and thereby lead to serious consequences. Abruptio placentae is responsible for approximately 10% of all third-trimester fetal deaths.

The degree of separation of the placenta may assume various proportions, from small areas of separation to detachment of the entire placenta. Hence, the clinical manifestations may vary widely, according to the severity of the case and the amount of bleeding. Roughly two-thirds of cases are classed as severe. Many placentas with small areas of detachment may elude detection because of no or minimal clinical symptoms.

The immediate cause of the placental abruption is rupture of maternal vessels in the decidua basalis. Only rarely does the bleeding originate from the fetal side. Many cases are associated with preeclampsia or with other types of hypertensive diseases concomitant with pregnancy. It is thought that liberation of excessive amounts of thromboplastin and defibrination of the patient's blood are intimately connected with separation of the placenta. (Thrombin is also a potent uterotonic agent.) Other risk factors include a prior abruption (15% chance if one prior episode, 20%–25% for two or more prior events), smoking (2.5-fold risk), multiparity, alcohol abuse, cocaine use, polyhydramnios, maternal hypertension (5-fold risk), premature rupture of the membranes, external trauma, uterine leiomyomata, increased age or parity, and multiple gestation.

Abruptio placentae usually begins with a small hematoma between the decidua and the chorionic villi. This hematoma, in turn, increases the possibility of more bleeding and more separation. The uterus is unable to contract and stop the bleeding, as it does after delivery, because it still contains the products of conception. The clinical manifestations of abruptio placentae are usually quite characteristic: Sudden colic-like abdominal pain followed by extreme rigidity of the

External bleeding

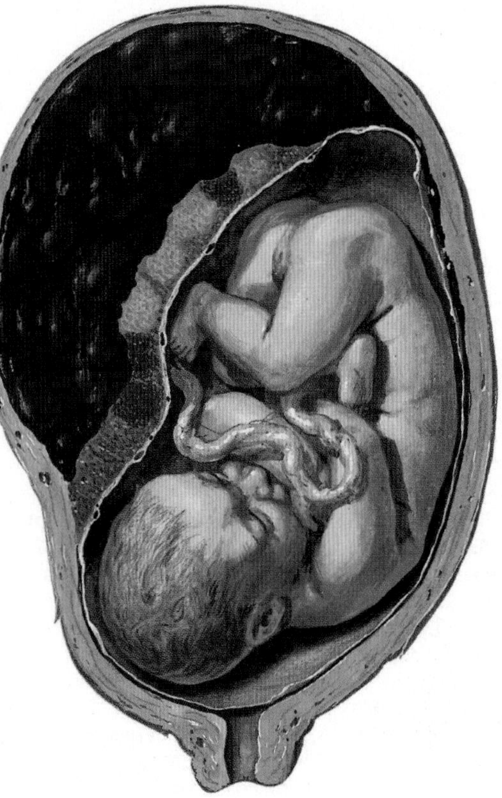

Internal (concealed) bleeding

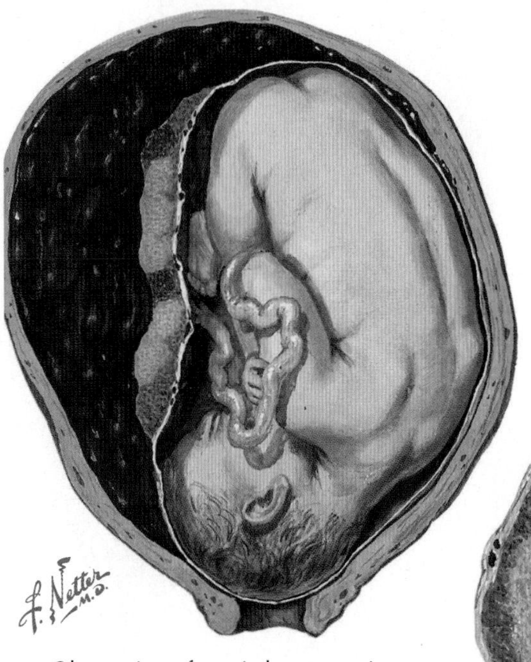

Obstruction of cervix by presenting part

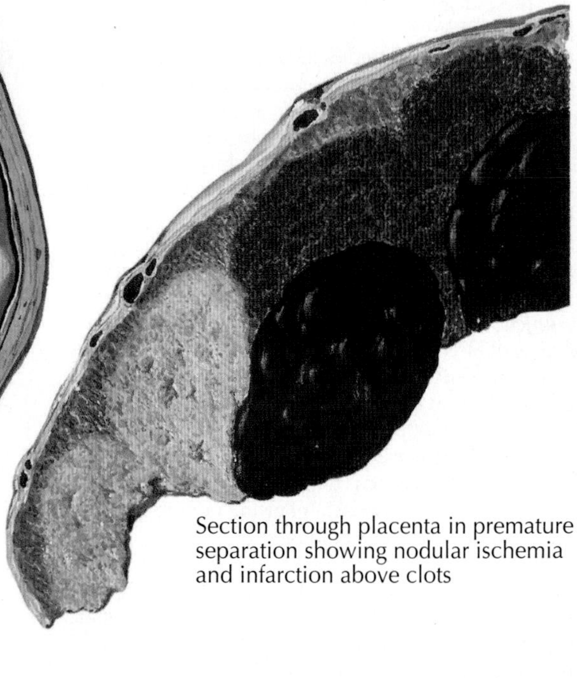

Section through placenta in premature separation showing nodular ischemia and infarction above clots

uterus, which presents a board-like consistency as a result of spasmodic contractions without any intermittent relaxation, is quite characteristic. If the placenta is completely or at least 50% separated, fetal heart activity may be nonreassuring or lost. Vaginal bleeding may or may not be present. Patients with extensive bleeding are often in severe shock, but the degree of shock is not proportional to the amount of bleeding. Occasionally, it is possible to suspect blood accumulation inside the uterus, when, despite its tetanic condition, a gradual

uterine enlarging is observed. Disseminated intravascular coagulation may accompany a severe abruption.

The management of abruptio placentae depends on the individual case. If fetal heart activity is present but compromised, immediate (emergent) cesarean delivery may be life-saving for both mother and baby. Lesser degrees of placental separation may be managed conservatively. If the cervix is soft, effaced, and somewhat dilated, rupture of the membranes may be sufficient to initiate labor and delivery of the baby.

Plate 12.18

Pregnancy

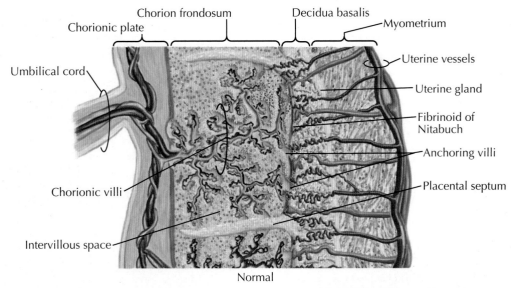

Normal

PLACENTA ACCRETA

Failure of the normal process of decidua formation results in a placental implantation in which the villi adhere directly to (accreta, 63%), invade into (increta, 15%), or pass through (percreta, 22%) the myometrium. One portion (partial) or all (total) of the placenta may be involved in this abnormality. The frequency of this abnormality is difficult to assess, and estimates vary with most authors placing the estimate close to 1 in 6000 births. Accreta appears to be increasing concomitant with the increasing cesarean section rate. Most pregnancies go to term with normal fetal development.

Placenta accreta (and other variants) occurs when there is abnormal decidua formation at the time of placental implantation as a result of imperfect development of the fibrinoid (Nitabuch) layer. This can also take place because of an abnormal site of placental implantation such as placenta previa, which is associated with 20% of placenta accretas, and/or uterine scars where normal decidual development may not occur (80%). The risk of an implantation abnormality with a placenta previa without previous uterine surgery is about 5% but increases with a history of previous surgery (to 15%–70% of cases). Previous cesarean delivery (0.03% after one up to 4.7% after more than five cesarean deliveries), multiparity (1 of 500,000 for parity <3, 1 of 2,500 for parity >6), older pregnant women, previous uterine curettage, previous uterine sepsis, previous manual removal of the placenta, leiomyomata, uterine malformation, prior abortion, and endometrial ablation all increase the risk of implantation abnormalities.

Often the first indication that an abnormality of placentation exists is the failure of the placenta to separate normally following the delivery of the fetus. Abnormally heavy bleeding following the delivery of the placenta (which may be heavy enough to be life-threatening) may also suggest an incomplete separation due to this condition.

Ultrasonography has been used to make the diagnosis before labor. Patients at elevated risk, such as those with a prior cesarean delivery and a low-lying placenta, may be studied by ultrasonography in an attempt to identify the absence of the subplacental hypoechoic zone or the presence of lacunar blood flow patterns. A "moth-eaten" appearance caused by multiple large, irregular intraplacental sonolucent spaces in a cotyledon adjacent to the involved myometrium is typical. The absence of these findings does not rule out this possibility. A low-lying placenta (near a previous uterine scar) noted in studies performed at less than 30 weeks may "migrate," leaving the cervix free at term in up to 90% of normal cases. If abnormal placental implantation is identified, plans for autologous blood donation and elective cesarean hysterectomy may be made.

Final diagnosis of this type of placental abnormality must be established histologically with the demonstration of the absence of the decidua basalis (replaced by loose

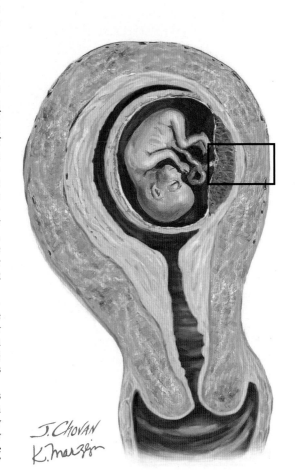

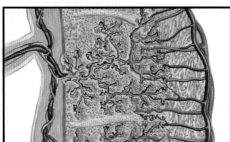

Accreta

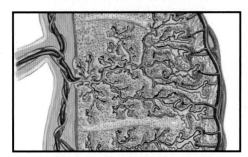

Increta

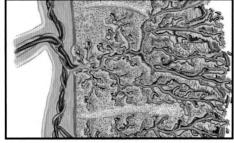

Percreta

connective tissue). In some cases, the decidua parietalis may be normal or absent and the villi may be separated from the myometrial cells by a layer of fibrin.

If a placenta accreta, increta, or percreta is suspected, aggressive fluid and blood support may be necessary. Oxytocin or other uterotonic agents should be used to promote uterine contractions after placental delivery (if accomplished). Life-threatening hemorrhage may occur; maternal mortality of as high as 2% to 6% has been reported for treatment by hysterectomy and up to 30% for conservative management. Coagulopathy secondary

to blood loss and replacement is common. Spontaneous rupture of the uterus before labor has been reported, and rupture of the uterus or inversion may occur during attempts to remove the placenta.

Most patients (60%) will require hysterectomy. If the invasion of the myometrium is incomplete and the bladder is spared, conservative management by uterine packing may be possible. Any time the diagnosis is considered, preparations for hysterectomy, including anesthesia, instruments, and adequate blood, should be ready before any attempt is made to free the placenta.

Plate 12.19

Reproductive System: VOLUME 1

COUVELAIRE UTERUS, AMNIOTIC FLUID EMBOLISM

Alexandre Couvelaire (1873–1948) described a pathologic condition that he called *uteroplacental apoplexy*, but which is better known as *Couvelaire uterus*. It is usually associated with premature separation of the placenta (abruptio placentae). The uterus, and occasionally the tubes and ovaries, becomes bluish or purplish in color and may resemble an ovarian cyst with a twisted pedicle. Occasionally, bloody fluid is found in the broad ligament and even in the peritoneal cavity. In severe cases, the uterus is unable to contract and remains atonic even after being emptied vaginally or by cesarean section. Disseminated intravascular coagulation and exsanguination are possible. Hysterectomy is often necessary to check the continuous bleeding from these atonic uteri.

The real cause of this condition is not well understood, except for the fact that it is usually associated with the severest form of abruptio placentae, particularly when the hemorrhage remains concealed. Because of the collection of blood behind the placenta, some authors believe that the blood infiltrates between the muscular fibers of the uterus, reaches the peritoneal surface, and eventually seeps into the peritoneal cavity. The intramuscular hemorrhage dissociates the muscular fibers and, probably through a toxic process, these fibers lose their contractile properties. Similar hemorrhage can be seen in the decidua overlying the muscular area that is infiltrated with blood. It has also been believed that the process is associated with consumption of clotting factors, frequently observed in cases of placental separation. The unclotted blood from the oozing area of placental implantation may infiltrate the surrounding decidua and uterine muscle, giving rise to the ecchymotic areas seen in Couvelaire uterus.

Maternal pulmonary embolism by amniotic fluid is a rare but frequently fatal complication of labor in which it has been hypothesized that amniotic fluid containing fetal squamous cells and hair enters the maternal vascular system and becomes lodged in the pulmonary vascular bed. Mechanical obstruction and anaphylaxis combine to produce an often fatal clinical course. The term *anaphylactoid syndrome of pregnancy* has been suggested but has not received wide acceptance. Clinically, the condition occurs more frequently in multiparas who develop tetanic contractions of the uterus after rupture of the membranes. The symptoms are usually observed near the end of the second stage and consist of dyspnea, cyanosis, disseminated intravascular coagulopathy, and peripheral circulatory failure. Death frequently follows within a few hours. Although the condition is rare (1 in 30,000 deliveries), it is one of the most common causes of maternal mortality in the United States and other developed countries.

The etiology and pathogenesis of this process are obscure. It is thought that the particulate matter of the amniotic fluid is forced into the venous channels of the uterus by powerful uterine contractions. Tears in the fetal membranes or placenta, separation of the placenta and open sinuses from placenta previa, and uterine rupture are cited as contributing causes that favor the dissemination of the amniotic fluid.

Although the condition can be diagnosed clinically, the diagnosis is generally supplemented by microscopic examination of the lung. Fetal ectodermal sloughed cells, vernix caseosa, meconium, and lanugo hair can

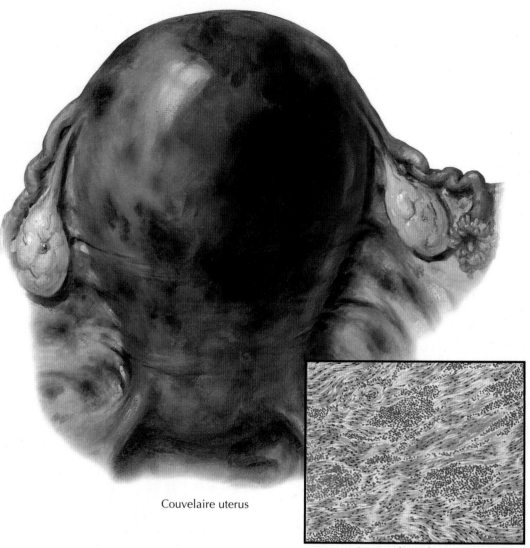

Couvelaire uterus

Section through myometrium showing disruption of muscle and interstitial hemorrhage

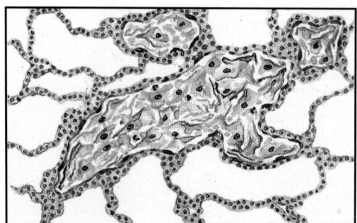

Amniotic emboli in vessels of lung

usually be seen in the pulmonary small arteries, arterioles, and capillaries of these patients; however, these may also be found in patients without the syndrome. Pulmonary infarction does not, as a rule, develop. Infiltration of polymorphonuclear leukocytes can be seen surrounding the embolic area.

Management consists of aggressive airway control and cardiovascular resuscitation (including myocardial support, inotropic agents and fluids, and high-concentration oxygen therapy). The use of vasopressors has been reported to be successful. Correction and support for clotting defects (blood and platelets, fresh-frozen plasma, and cryoprecipitate as indicated) may be necessary. In women who experience cardiac arrest before delivery, consideration should be given to perimortem cesarean delivery to improve newborn outcome. In those who have not experienced arrest, maternal considerations generally take precedence.

Plate 12.20

Pregnancy

Cross section through placenta showing fibrin deposits and thrombi

NODULAR LESIONS OF PLACENTA OTHER THAN TRUE INFARCTS

Although various kinds of nodules are found frequently in placentas at term, true infarcts are uncommon except in cases of preeclampsia or hypertension. Of the various placental nodules that can be differentiated from infarcts, the most common one is seen on the fetal aspect of the placenta. It is a firm, white mass, variable in size, which in cross section appears as a wedge-shaped, finely laminated, white or yellowish nodule just beneath the chorionic plate, to which it is usually attached. Frequently, a fresh blood clot appears at its periphery. This lesion, often multiple, has long been erroneously called a "white infarct." It may be found in other positions but with less frequency than beneath the chorionic plate. Microscopically, it consists of fine laminations of fibrin laid down parallel to the chorionic plate. Erythrocytes enmeshed in the fibrin network present various degrees of hemolysis. Often a few entrapped chorionic villi appear ischemic, but the sparsity of necrotic villi sharply differentiates this lesion from a true infarct. Fibrin deposits in placentas have no known clinical significance, but it is important to differentiate them from true infarcts.

Another common nodule that may appear anywhere in the placenta is composed of a dark-red blood clot. Microscopically, intraplacental clots may be divided into two main categories—thrombi and hematomas. In obstetric literature, both have been called "red infarcts" and "hematomas" at various times. A thrombus is an intravascular clot formed in the presence of circulating blood. It is built up in fine laminations of fibrin, platelets, and blood cells and originates usually from a small break in the continuity of the cells lining a vascular channel, which, in the case of the placenta, is usually the intervillous space. Deposits of fibrin may be remnants of incompletely absorbed thrombi formed in this manner.

The rupture of a blood vessel with hemorrhage and clotting of blood in tissues outside of the circulation results in placental hematomas. Placenta hematomas may be caused by the rupture of a fetal vessel in the umbilical cord, membranes, chorionic plate, or cotyledon stalk or within an area of infarction. The rupture of a maternal vessel within a decidual septum or in the decidual basalis can also result in a placental hematoma. Occasionally, rupture of the marginal sinus causes a large hematoma at the rim of the placenta. A hematoma may conceivably result from the rupture of a fetal vessel into the maternal circulation in the intervillous space, but this appears rare and difficult to document, although small transfers of fetal red blood cells do occur with some frequency. Undoubtedly, small rifts in the trophoblastic covering of villi occur, but these are

Intervillous thrombus

Fibrin deposit

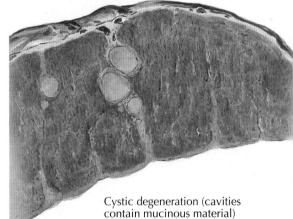

Cystic degeneration (cavities contain mucinous material)

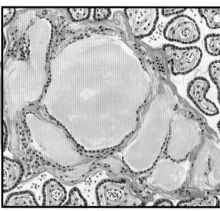

Cystic degeneration

promptly sealed off by fibrin deposition. When any incompatibility between the blood of the infant and that of the mother exists, fetal bleeding into the maternal circulation can lead to the production of antibodies in the maternal blood.

Another nodular lesion that may be confused grossly with infarcts is cystic degeneration. Small foci in decidual septa, and less frequently in trophoblastic cell columns, may liquefy and form cyst-like spaces filled with mucinous material resembling Wharton jelly. Microscopically, the absence of necrotic villi rules out infarction.

Chorioangiomas may closely resemble red infarcts grossly. They are rare lesions and can readily be distinguished microscopically from infarcts because of their neoplastic nature.

Fibrin deposits, thrombi, hematomas, and foci of cystic degeneration appear pathologically to be degenerative processes. Their etiology and clinical significance are unknown. Although minor degrees of these lesions are common in term placentas, they are far more numerous in certain cases of fetal death in utero, the cause of which often remains undetermined.

Plate 12.21

Reproductive System: VOLUME 1

GESTATIONAL TROPHOBLASTIC DISEASE

Four neoplasms of placental tissues are known, namely, chorioangioma arising from placental capillaries, hydatidiform (invasive) mole and choriocarcinoma arising from trophoblastic tissues, and placental-site trophoblastic tumor. Chorioangiomas are rare benign vascular tumors arising from the primitive chorionic mesenchyme, whose etiology is unknown. They are associated with increased maternal age, diabetes mellitus, and hypertension and are more common in multiple pregnancies. The tumor appears as a solitary, deep red, often-lobulated nodule in the placenta. It is of little clinical significance.

A hydatidiform mole consists of chorionic villi, which appear as grapelike clusters of vesicles. Moles are classified as being either complete, in which no fetus is present, or incomplete (partial), in which both fetus (generally abnormal) and molar tissues are present. The vesicles resemble youthful villi in that they are branching structures covered with two or more layers of trophoblastic cells, but they have no fetal blood vessels, and their stroma is only a loose-meshed matrix filled with clear gelatinous material. Molar pregnancy occurs in 1 of 1000 to 1500 pregnancies in the United States and as high as 10 per 1000 pregnancies in Asia. Molar pregnancies have the unique genetic attribute of a double contribution from the father: complete moles are mostly 46,XX all of paternal origin, though mitochondrial DNA of maternal origin remains; incomplete moles are most often triploid (69,XXY or 69,XXX) all of paternal origin.

The clinical manifestations are the same as those in normal pregnancy, except that the uterus enlarges more rapidly than usual and there are exaggerated symptoms of pregnancy. Diagnosis is facilitated by the passage of some grapelike vesicles, by the abortion of the mole, or a classic "snowstorm" appearance on ultrasonography. Molar pregnancies are associated with hypertension, preeclampsia, proteinuria, nausea, and vomiting (hyperemesis, 8%); visual changes, tachycardia, and shortness of breath are all possible. (Pregnancy-induced hypertension in the first trimester is virtually diagnostic.)

The treatment of molar pregnancies is surgical: evacuation of the uterine contents. This is most often accomplished via suction curettage. Because of the large size of some molar pregnancies and a tendency toward uterine atony, concomitant oxytocin administration is advisable and blood for transfusion should be immediately available. Once the uterus has been emptied, the patient should be closely followed for at least 1 year for the possibility of recurrent benign or malignant disease. Any change in the patient's examination, an increase in β-hCG titers, or a failure of the β-hCG level to fall below 10 mIU/mL by 12 weeks after evacuation should be evaluated. Serum hCG levels are generally monitored every 2 weeks until three consecutive tests are negative and then monthly for 6 to 12 months. Pregnancy should be prevented for about a year, because a rising titer in the nonpregnant woman may indicate the presence of choriocarcinoma.

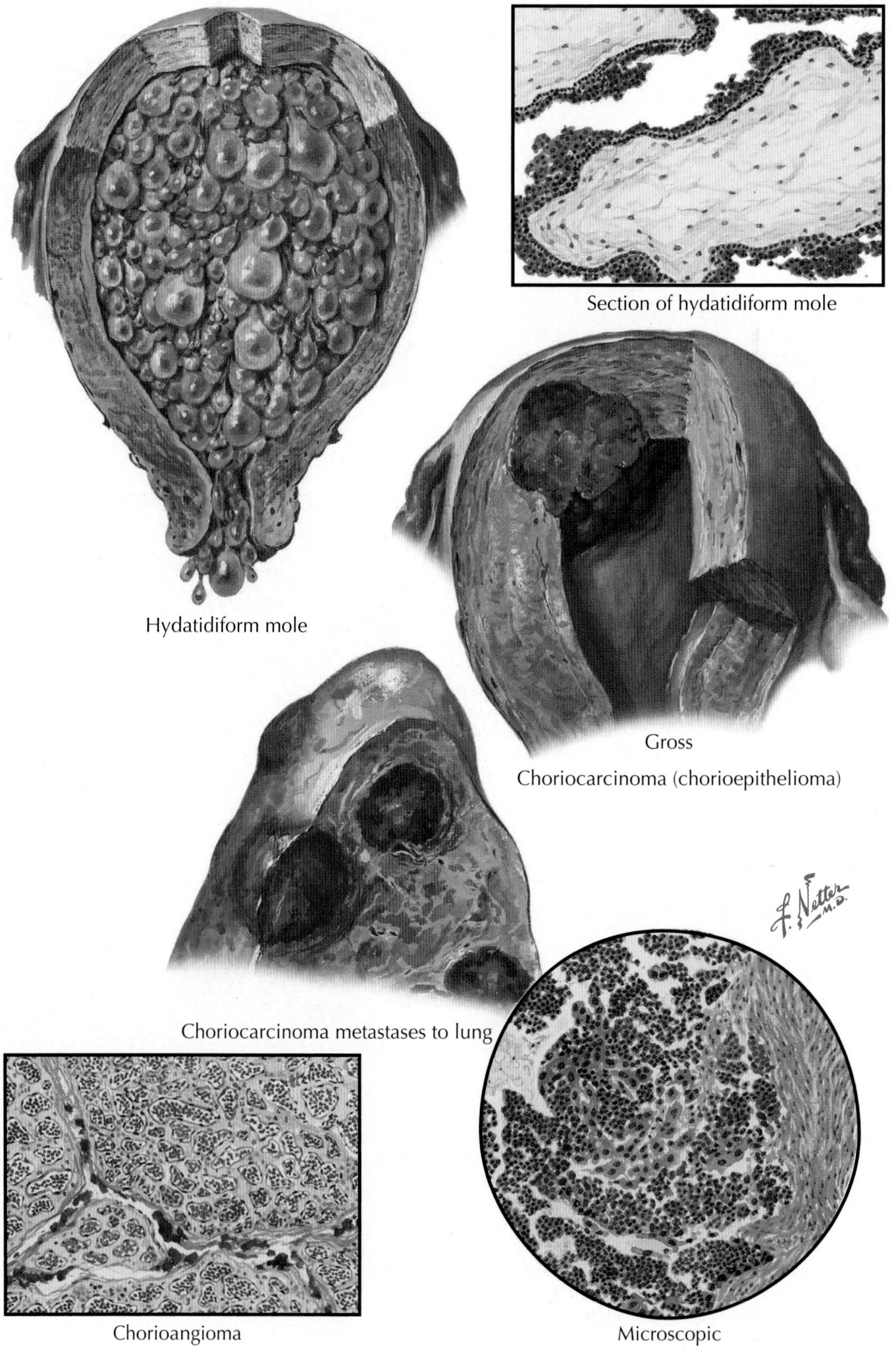

Hydatidiform mole

Section of hydatidiform mole

Gross

Choriocarcinoma (chorioepithelioma)

Choriocarcinoma metastases to lung

Chorioangioma

Microscopic

Gestational trophoblastic neoplasia is notable for the possibility of malignant transformation, although less than 10% of patients develop malignant changes. Choriocarcinoma, also called *chorioepithelioma*, is a rare but very malignant tumor that metastasizes early to the lungs. It is composed of both syncytial and cytotrophoblastic cells that do not form chorionic villi but grow destructively into the uterine wall. In about half of cases, it follows a hydatidiform mole; in the others, it follows an abortion or a term pregnancy or is, in rare instances, associated with a teratoma. Roughly 80% of molar pregnancies follow a benign course after initial therapy. Between 15% and 25% of patients develop invasive disease, and 3% to 5% eventually have metastatic lesions. The prognosis for patients with primary or recurrent malignant trophoblastic disease is generally good (>90% cure rate). Fewer than 5% of patients will require hysterectomy to achieve a cure for choriocarcinoma.

Plate 12.22

Pregnancy

Splanchnic nerves {
Greater
Lesser
Least
}

Celiac ganglion

Aorticorenal ganglion

Superior mesenteric ganglion

T7 spinal nerve (anterior ramus)

Sympathetic trunk and ganglia

T11 spinal nerve (anterior ramus)

Rami communicantes

Subcostal nerve (T12)

Inferior mesenteric ganglion

Intermesenteric (aortic) plexus

Superior hypogastric plexus

S1 spinal nerve (anterior ramus)

Hypogastric nerves

Pelvic splanchnic nerves

Inferior hypogastric (pelvic) plexus

Uterovaginal plexus

Pudendal nerve (S2, S3, S4)

Inferior anal (rectal) nerve

Lumbar splanchnic nerves

Iliohypogastric nerve (L1)

Ilioinguinal nerve (L1)

Vesical plexus

Dorsal nerve of clitoris

Posterior labial nerves

——— Sensory fibers from uterine body and fundus accompany sympathetic fibers via hypogastric plexuses to T11, T12 (L1?)

——— Motor fibers to uterine body and fundus (sympathetic)

·········· Sensory fibers from cervix and upper vagina accompany pelvic splanchnic nerves (parasympathetic) to S2, S3, S4

·········· Motor fibers to lower uterine segment, cervix, and upper vagina (parasympathetic)

– – – – Sensory fibers from lower vagina and perineum accompany somatic fibers via pudendal nerve to S2, S3, S4

- - - - - Motor fibers to lower vagina and perineum via pudendal nerve (somatic)

NEUROPATHWAYS IN PARTURITION

Control of pain during labor and delivery has become a major factor in obstetric practice, and pain has become a key element of assessment (vital sign) for all hospitalized patients. It is thus important to have an understanding of the topographic location and specialized functions of the neuroafferent pathways to all organs and structures involved in birth. The obstetrician often is faced with a need to maintain the uterine activity or to plan a coordinated augmentation of the expulsive forces in which the striated abdominal and intercostal muscles are involved, including the diaphragm.

The pain of labor is characterized as rhythmically increasing and fading pain that occurs synchronously with uterine contractions, coming every 3 to 4 minutes and lasting 30 to 40 seconds (but may occur more often). This pain is transmitted first over the sensory fibers from the corpus and fundus of the uterus (blue solid lines) to the large circumcervical ganglionic network (Frankenhäuser) and thence over the hypogastric nerves and the lower aortic postganglionic sympathetic fibers to the paravertebral sympathetic chain at the level of the second and third lumbar vertebrae. Continuing without synapse in a cephalic direction, these nerves traverse the gray rami of the 11th and 12th thoracic nerves and probably also the 1st lumbar nerve to enter the communicating system of these three dorsal root ganglia with the preganglionic afferent system in the lateral spinothalamic fasciculus of the spinal cord to the thalamic pain center and its cortical radiations. Whenever these pathways are interrupted by 11th and 12th paravertebral segmental block, by epidural 11th thoracic through first lumbar block, by ascending caudal block, or by saddle spinal block anesthesia, the labor contraction pain is alleviated.

The second component of labor pain is the backache associated with cervical dilation. These stimuli are transmitted through the parasympathetic system of the second, third, and fourth sacral nerves (blue dotted lines). The resulting sensation of sacral and sacroiliac discomfort has been interpreted as pain over the skin and fascia distribution of the somatic segmental branches of these nerves. Low saddle or spinal block, as well as the infrequently used caudal block, will relieve this pain.

The third component of childbirth pain is that transmitted from the stimulus of stretching the lower birth canal and the perineum. Pressure upon the bladder and rectum through the pudendal nerve or its perineal and hemorrhoidal branches may also be involved. This pain can be relieved by pudendal and perineal nerve block, anesthetizing the nerves indicated in the picture by the broken lines. These blocks, of course, also produce a flaccid paralysis of the perineal musculature, which, however, greatly facilitates operative or obstetric maneuvers

and provides analgesia for any reparative procedures that may be required following delivery.

Epidural anesthesia is commonly used for childbirth in the United States because it provides good analgesia with a wide margin of safety. Fewer than 1 of 100 women may experience a headache following an epidural anesthetic. Use of epidural anesthesia may be associated with reduced contraction frequency or strength or an impaired ability to push as effectively, so interventions such as oxytocin or operative delivery may become necessary.

Successful saddle or spinal anesthesia produces a more or less complete analgesia from the perineum and sacral plexus ascending to the 10th thoracic segment. The more heavily myelinated nerves of the lower abdominal musculature and, depending on the position of the patient and the timing of repositioning after injection of the anesthetic, the entire anterior roots continue to function and permit intentional cooperation of the individual by increasing the intraabdominal pressure required for pushing during delivery.

Plate 12.23

Reproductive System: VOLUME 1

LABOR

Labor is defined by rhythmic uterine contractions that result in progressive effacement and dilation of the cervix. Although labor is a continuous process, it is divided into three stages: First stage, from onset of labor to complete cervical dilation, although the exact time of onset is almost impossible to establish; second stage, from complete cervical dilation to the delivery of the fetus; and third stage, from fetal delivery to expulsion of the placenta. (Some add a fourth stage, recovery, which spans the time from delivery to 2 hours after.)

The physiologic changes that lead to the initiation of labor are many, complex, deeply interconnected, and incompletely delineated. The mean duration of human singleton pregnancy is 280 days (40 weeks) from the first day of the last menstrual period, though "term" is defined as between 259 to 293 days. The complex interaction of maternal signaling molecules (progestins and estrogens, prostaglandins, oxytocin, relaxin, nitrous oxide, and others), fetal molecules (cortisol, estrogen and others), and uterine distention reduce uterine contractile inhibition and induce an increase in uterine oxytocin and prostaglandin receptors, ion channels, and cellular gap junctions. The latter appear necessary to effect coordinated contractions that create a pressure gradient from the top of the uterus toward the cervix. Intrinsic slow and fast waves of myometrial cell depolarization become more and more effective in producing local, and then regional, muscle depolarization and contraction. Increasing pressure on the cervix causes stretch, neural signaling, and the local release of prostaglandins (predominately PGF$_{2a}$), which reinforces uterine contraction and oxytocin sensitivity in an ever-increasing positive feedback loop, eventually leading to the rhythmic contractions of labor. Despite the importance of this positive feedback loop, most researchers view the onset of labor as the loss of inhibition rather than an active process.

In humans, the timing of labor onset is thought to occur owing to changes in the fetal hypothalamic-pituitary-adrenal axis, increasing fetal cortisol, inducing placental enzymatic functions that downregulate inhibitory factors, such as progesterone. Placental estrogens up regulate myometrial gap junctions and uterotonic receptors (L-type calcium channels and oxytocin receptors) while placental and cervical production of prostaglandins increase, furthering the induction of their receptors and facilitating cervical ripening (PGE$_2$) and contractions (PGF$_{2a}$). The pivotal role these molecules play can be seen by the delay caused by the use of prostaglandin synthesis inhibitors such as nonsteroidal antiinflammatory drugs.

Oxytocin is the most potent endogenous uterotonic peptide and is important clinically in the management

of labor. Oxytocin levels, however, do not differ significantly in labor from those found in the weeks before labor begins (though fetal production does seem to increase). This reinforces the importance of the increase in number of oxytocin receptors in the myometrium (up to 200-fold) at term. In addition to oxytocin's myometrial effects, it also acts indirectly through enhancing amniotic and decidual prostaglandin synthesis.

Generally, the process of labor will result in a change of cervical dilation of about 1 cm/hr from 5 to 9 cm dilation. This rate of change can be affected by parity, the use of analgesics, active management of contractions,

fetal size, maternal height or weight, and other factors. The median time to dilate from 4 to 10 cm in nulliparas and multiparas is 5.3 hours and 3.8 hours, respectively. The median duration of the second stage of labor is 1.1 hours for nulliparas and 0.4 hours for multiparas, with 95% of women delivering by 3.5 and 2 hours, respectively. The average duration of labor for first-time mothers is approximately 9 hours, and it is 6 hours for multiparous women. The upper limit (95th percentile) of labor duration is roughly 18 and 13 hours, respectively. Criteria for the normal progress of labor remain unclear and controversial.

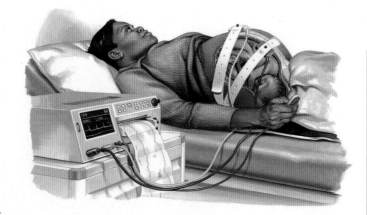

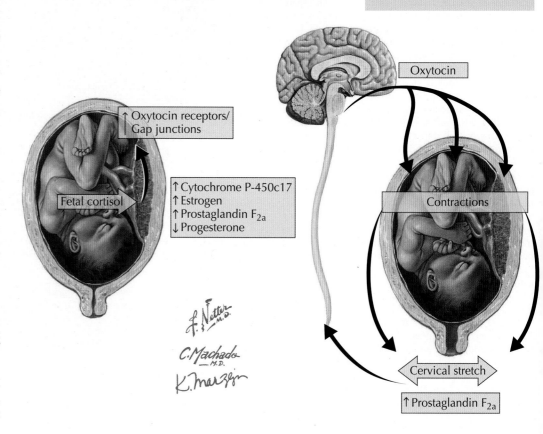

↑ Oxytocin receptors/ Gap junctions

Fetal cortisol

↑ Cytochrome P-450c17
↑ Estrogen
↑ Prostaglandin F$_{2a}$
↓ Progesterone

Oxytocin

Contractions

Cervical stretch

↑ Prostaglandin F$_{2a}$

Plate 12.24   Pregnancy

FETAL ASSESSMENT AND INTRAPARTUM MONITORING

Antenatal fetal assessment and testing is generally reserved for fetuses who appear not to be thriving or are at significant risk because of maternal or fetal factors identified during the pregnancy. Noninvasive testing is used to elicit signs of deteriorating status directed toward intervention and the prevention of mortality. Testing is based on the premise that marginal fetal oxygenation limits the fetus's ability to modulate heart rate in response to fetal movement or to the transient placental ischemia found during uterine contraction. In general, fetal heart rate should show acceleration to movement or contraction. Ultimately, the reduction of fetal morbidity and the improvement of neurologic outcome would be ideal, but objective studies to support the effectiveness of antepartum fetal testing are lacking. The mainstays of fetal assessment are the nonstress test (NST), contraction stress test (CST) or oxytocin challenge test (OCT), and biophysical profile (BPP) or modified biophysical profile (mBPP). Fetal kick counts are also employed to monitor fetal wellbeing but are generally not included in discussions of fetal assessment.

In general, each of the major fetal assessments are better at predicting health than fetal jeopardy; that is, they have more false-positive than false-negative tests (fetal death after a normal BPP is approximately 0.8 per 1000). The progression from NST to CST/OCT to BPP/mBPP represents both escalating degrees of complexity and invasiveness but also increasingly fine levels of discrimination in identifying fetuses at risk. (More than 60% of nonreactive NSTs may be false positives versus 0.6% false positives for BPP.)

A normal (reactive) NST has two or more accelerations (15 beats/min for 15 seconds) in a 20-minute period. Acoustic stimulation may also be used to startle the fetus and induce a heart rate increase. In the CST the occurrence of late decelerations occurring with 50% or more contractions (regardless of frequency) is "positive" and suggests fetal risk. The BPP is based on the NST, augmented by measures of fetal breathing movements, fetal activity and tone, and quantitation of amniotic fluid volume, rated on a 10-point scale (normal: 8–10/10, equivocal: 6/10, abnormal: ≤5/10). The pulsatile character of fetal blood flow in the umbilical cord or the middle cerebral artery may be used to assess the health of high-risk pregnancies, but these tests require special expertise to both perform and interpret. All testing must be viewed in the context of the clinical picture.

Although the use of electronic fetal monitoring during labor was adopted without the usual rigorous assessments of efficacy, sensitivity, or specificity, most labors in the United States undergo this monitoring. Electronic fetal monitoring devices track uterine activity and beat-to-beat fetal heart rate by either external means (tocodynamometry and Doppler ultrasonic

means) or by direct measurement (intrauterine pressure canula and fetal scalp electrode). The most accurate data are obtained by internal methods, but these are more invasive and require that the membranes have been ruptured and the cervix partially dilated.

During labor the primary measure of fetal status and reserve is the fetal heart rate pattern. The fetal monitoring device converts the time between fetal heart beats into beats per minute (fetal heart rate, FHR) and charts them on a continuous graph. This graph is classified based on

the baseline FHR, the variability of the FHR, long-term trends, and the presence of periodic accelerations and decelerations in relation to uterine activity using a three-tier classification system: Category I represents a normal tracing (predictive of normal fetal acid-base status), category II represents an indeterminate tracing that should prompt continued monitoring (observed at some point in 84% of tracings), and category III represents an abnormal tracing (associated with an increased risk of abnormal fetal acid-base status, 0.1% of tracings).

Antenatal testing

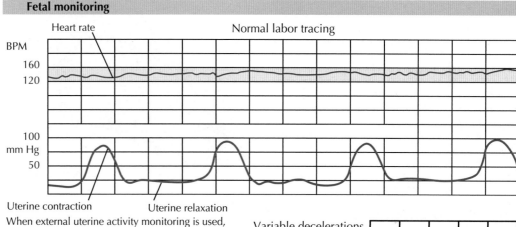

Nonstress test (NST)
Contraction stress test (CST)
Biophysical profile (BPP)

JOHN A. CRAIG—MD
C. Machado—M.D.

Fetal monitoring

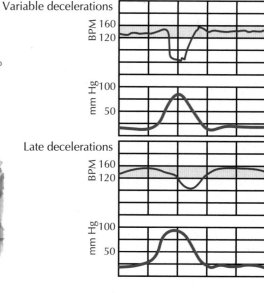

Heart rate — Normal labor tracing

When external uterine activity monitoring is used, the lower scale is dimensionless.

Uterine contraction — Uterine relaxation

Variable decelerations

Late decelerations

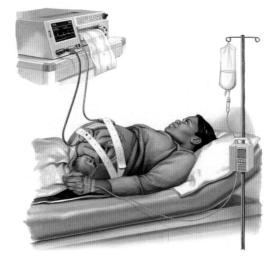

Plate 12.25

Reproductive System: VOLUME 1

CARDINAL MOVEMENTS

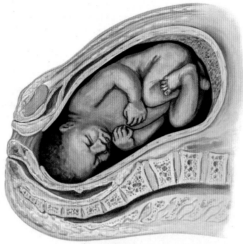

Engagement

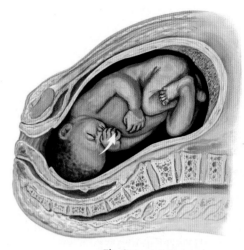

Flexion

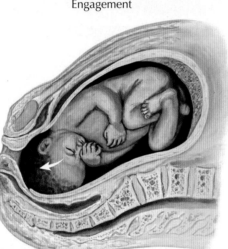

Descent

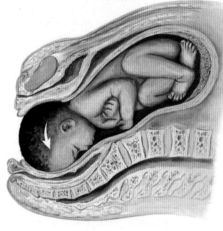

Internal rotation

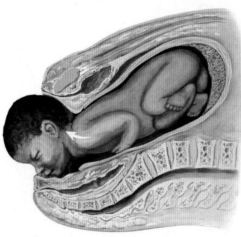

Extension

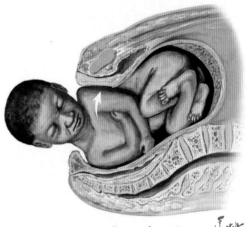

External rotation

NORMAL BIRTH

Successful delivery of the infant depends on the interaction of three variables: Power (uterine contractions), passenger (fetus), and passage (both bony pelvis and pelvic soft tissues). The fetus must also execute a series of maneuvers to allow passage through the maternal pelvis to the outside (cardinal movements). Abnormalities in any of the three variables, or in the completion of the cardinal movements, may result in a failure of the fetus to progress, necessitating either operative vaginal delivery (forceps or vacuum assist) or cesarean delivery.

At the time of presentation for early labor, the fetus is assessed for fetal lie, presentation, and position: Lie documents the relationship of the long axis of the fetus relative to the longitudinal axis of the uterus (longitudinal, transverse, or oblique), presentation refers to the fetal part that directly overlies the pelvic inlet, and position is the relationship of a particular portion of the presenting part (most often occiput or sacrum for cephalic or breech, respectively) to the maternal pelvis.

During the course of labor, the well-being of both mother and baby must be evaluated by periodic assessment of the mother's vital signs and the fetal heart rate. The latter may be accomplished by either intermittent auscultation after contractions or by continuous electronic fetal monitoring devices. The progress of the labor is monitored by periodic checks of cervical dilation and descent of the fetal presenting part. Some practioners choose to chart the patient's labor progress as a graphical representation (partogram) of the patient's cervical dilation over time; however, routine use of partograms has not been proven to significantly improve obstetric outcome.

Maternal hydration is most often maintained by intravenous fluids because of limited or absent gastric emptying that occurs during labor. (Many still allow the ingestion of liquids.) Amelioration of pain may be accomplished by systemic analgesics early in labor or by regional neuraxial anesthetics (such as epidural or caudal anesthetics) as labor progresses. Pudendal or local anesthetics may be used for terminal pain relief or to accomplish repairs.

Once the cervix is completely dilated, the fetus (in the vertex position) must descend though the vagina in a series of six cardinal movements ending in delivery. These are engagement, flexion, descent, internal rotation, extension, and external rotation. Engagement of the fetal head and some descent may occur before complete dilation has been accomplished. Engagement is defined as descent of the fetal biparietal diameter to below the pelvic inlet, identified clinically by the presence of the presenting part below the level of ischial spines (0 station). Flexion of the fetal head allows for the smaller diameters of the fetal head to present to the maternal pelvis. Descent is a necessity for the successful completion of passage through the vagina. Internal rotation, like flexion, facilitates presentation of the optimal diameters of the fetal head to the bony pelvis, most commonly rotating from transverse to either occiput

anterior (most common) or posterior. Extension of the fetal head occurs as it reaches the introitus and accommodates the upward curve of the birth canal at its distal end. External rotation occurs after delivery of the head as the head restitutes relative to the shoulders. These cardinal movements do not occur as a distinct series of discrete movements but rather as a group of movements that overlap as the fetus moves progressively toward delivery.

Following the delivery of the placenta, the uterus must contract to prevent maternal hemorrhage. To accomplish this, uterine massage as well as uterotonic agents such as oxytocin, methylergonovine maleate, or prostaglandins may be routinely used. Excessive blood loss at this or any subsequent time should suggest the possibility of uterine atony, retained placental or membranous material, uterine inversion, or unrecognized cervical, vaginal, or other laceration.

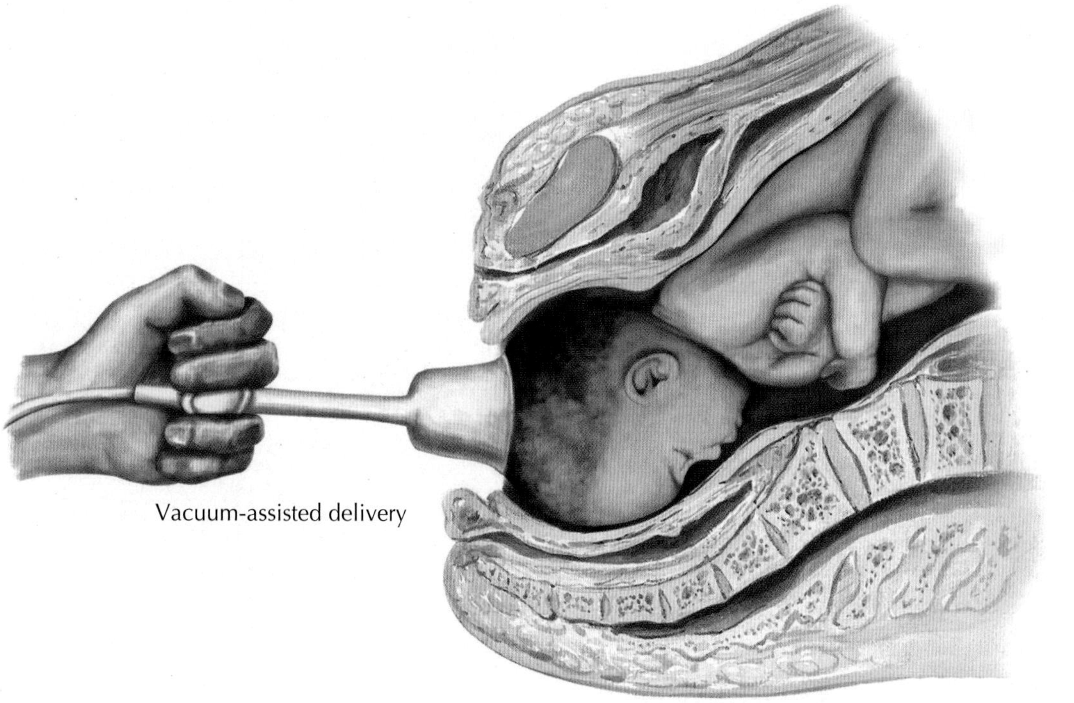

Plate 12.26

Pregnancy

OPERATIVE VAGINAL DELIVERY

Operative vaginal delivery is a method of assisting or expediting vaginal vertex delivery through the application of obstetric forceps or vacuum devices. Assisted or expedited vaginal delivery may become necessary because of maternal fatigue, prolonged second stage of labor, or certain types of maternal pulmonary, cardiac, neurologic disease, or perceived imminent fetal jeopardy during the second stage of labor. When there is evidence of a nonreassuring fetal status or acute fetal distress, operative vaginal delivery may provide a safer or more expeditious way of protecting fetal health. Roughly 3% of vaginal deliveries in the United States are assisted by operative delivery methods.

To perform either forceps- or vacuum-assisted delivery, the cervix must be completely dilated, the fetal presentation must be vertex, and position must be known (and relatively normal). The fetus must be fully engaged, the fetal membranes must be ruptured, and the patient must be able to cooperate with the delivery. Operative vaginal delivery is generally contraindicated when the gestational age is less than 34 weeks, there is fetal demineralization, or a clotting disorder is present. In addition, vacuum-assisted delivery is generally not done when there has been prior scalp sampling or multiple attempts at fetal scalp electrode placement.

For successful operative delivery, adequate maternal anesthesia or analgesia should be ensured in all but the most extreme circumstances. Whenever possible, the maternal bladder should be emptied (by catheter). The position of the fetal head must be ascertained by palpation of the sagittal suture and fontanelles. This can be supplemented by palpation of the fetal ear in some cases.

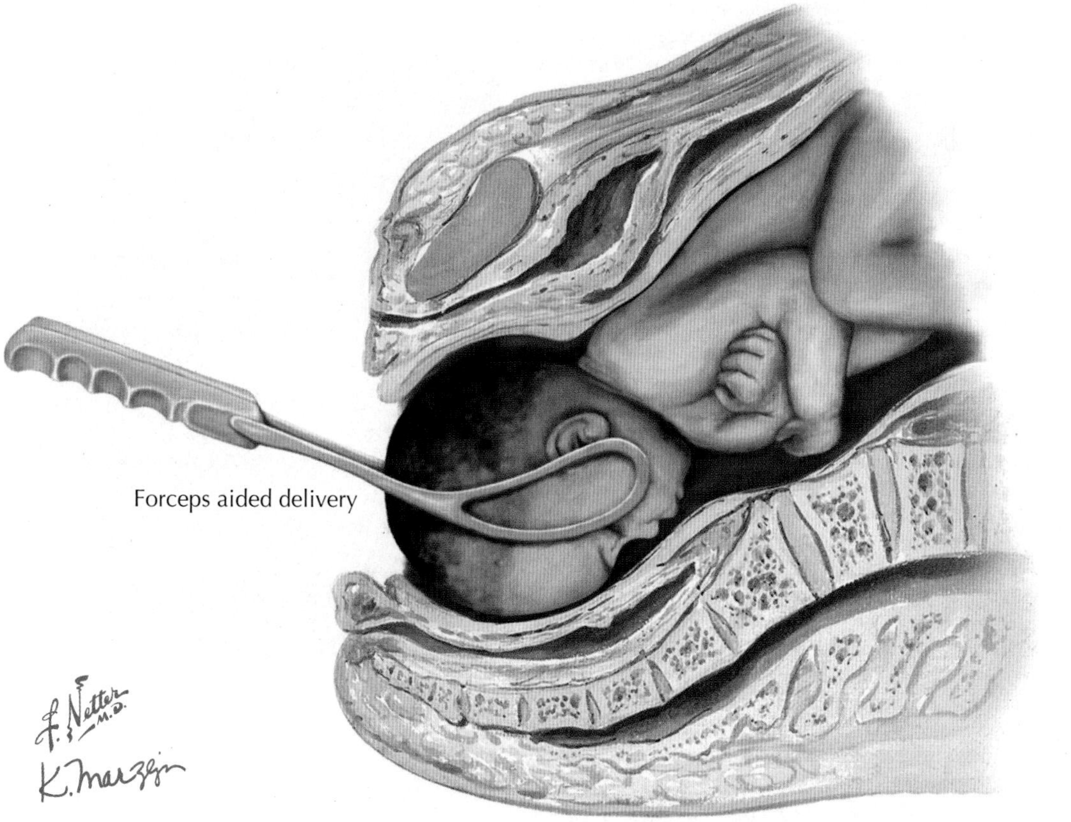

Current obstetric practice has rendered the challenging and difficult forceps deliveries of past eras exceedingly rare. Midforceps, applied when the vertex has not descended to the perineum and/or used for rotation of the fetal head when it is not in the direct occiput anterior position, are now used only in circumstances where there is an imminent threat to the well-being or survival of the fetus and a cesarean section cannot be done expeditiously. Outlet forceps or vacuum extraction, applied when the vertex is within 45 degrees of the occiput anterior and is on the perineum, is still used by experienced operators. There is no clear advantage of one modality over the other and the choice generally comes down to the particular preference and experience of the individual responsible for the delivery.

With either modality, it is critical that the device be carefully placed to avoid iatrogenic trauma to either mother or baby. It is also important that once placed, the device only be used to augment maternal expulsive efforts, avoiding both excessive force and extraneous movements that could result in maternal or fetal trauma: Owing to the fulcrum effect provided by

Vacuum-assisted delivery

Forceps aided delivery

forceps, uterine or vaginal wall lacerations can result, and rotational forces applied to the vacuum device can result in laceration or avulsion of the fetal scalp.

With either device, traction must be coordinated with maternal expulsive efforts. Traction begins in a horizontal or slightly downward (axis of the maternal pelvic canal) manner. To mimic the normal birth process, traction in the horizontal plane continues until the descending fetal head distends the vulva. As the fetal head further distends the vulva, the axis of traction is

gradually rotated upward, mimicking the normal extension process of the head as it rotates under the symphysis. Once the brow is palpable through the perineum, the device may be removed and the fetal head delivered by pressure on the perineum (modified Ritgen maneuver). The remainder of the delivery proceeds as with a spontaneous delivery. A 2017 systematic review concluded that available data do not support intrapartum extracranial pressure as a cause of fetal brain injury.

Plate 12.27

Reproductive System: VOLUME 1

OBSTETRIC LACERATIONS: VAGINA, PERINEUM, VULVA

Approximately 50% to 80% of women will sustain an obstetric laceration at the time of vaginal delivery. Traditionally a timely median or mediolateral episiotomy was believed to reduce the likelihood that such tears will be extensive. The role of routine episiotomy has come under question and fallen out of favor because despite prophylactic incisions, bad lacerations occur. The simplest type is a first-degree perineal laceration that extends posteriorly toward the anus through the vaginal epithelium and perineal skin. Occasionally, the inferior borders of the labia are also torn, and lateral retraction from the cut surface causes gaping of the wound. Bleeding may be brisk, but self-limited, although no vital structures have been damaged. It is important to make a thorough examination of the adjacent tissues to rule out the presence of occult damage elsewhere.

Second-degree lacerations involve the skin, vaginal epithelium, and the superficial muscles of the perineum but not the fibers of the external anal sphincter. They often extend upward along the sides of the vagina, producing a triangular defect because of retraction of the superficial perineal muscles. At the lower margin of a second-degree tear, the capsule of the external anal sphincter bulges upward into the wound. Concomitant lacerations of the anterior vagina, clitoris, prepuce, urethra, and labia are frequently present.

A third-degree perineal laceration (3% of deliveries) is a far more serious injury because of the threat of future interference with normal bowel function. In this instance the skin, vaginal epithelium, and perineal body are torn, and the external anal sphincter is ruptured anteriorly with retraction of its severed ends. Some authors distinguish three subgroups of third-degree laceration: 3a in which <50% of the external sphincter is damaged, 3b in which >50% of the external sphincter is damaged, and 3c in which both the external and internal sphincters are ruptured. Although the perineum receives the main expulsive force and is therefore more often lacerated, the incidence of damage to the anterior wall increases proportionately. Superficial epithelial wounds, perforation of the bladder, or even avulsion of the urethra may result.

A tear that includes the rectal mucosa or extends up the anterior rectal wall to compromise the internal sphincter is referred to as a *fourth-degree laceration* (1% of deliveries). Third- and fourth-degree lacerations commonly produce fecal incontinence if untreated and are slow to heal. The puckered scar tissue, which forms in wounds that heal by second intention in this area, is often painful.

Inspection of the cervix and upper vagina after delivery, regardless of the presence or absence of external wounds, should always be considered. Cervical lacerations originating at this time may be the source of problems, including postpartum bleeding and cervical insufficiency. If the tear extends to the vaginal fornices, as it often may, the end result may be dyspareunia or urinary incontinence due to

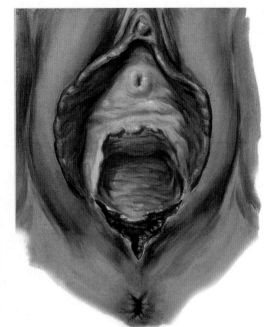

First-degree perineal laceration

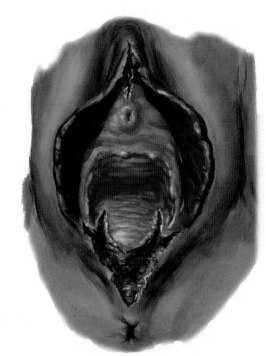

Second-degree perineal laceration plus tear of clitoris

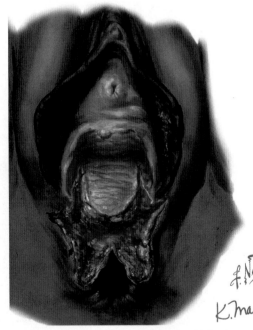

Fourth-degree perineal laceration and labial tear

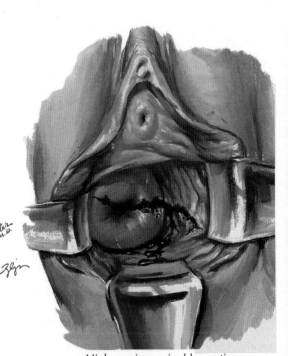

High cervicovaginal laceration

downward pull on the internal vesical sphincter. More acute symptoms are hemorrhage, hematoma, or infection followed by purulent leukorrhea.

The early and late clinical manifestations of all these injuries serve to emphasize the necessity of instituting prompt surgical treatment. Transfusions may be necessary to combat hemorrhage and shock if bleeding is significant. Sutures should be carefully and economically placed, which, in the difficult cases, usually requires the services of an assistant for

adequate exposure. Upon completion of the third stage of labor, all lacerations should be repaired. In the case of third- and fourth-degree lacerations, this means that the severed fibers of the rectal sphincters and their fibrous capsule are reunited and further strengthened by reapproximation with either an end-to-end or overlapping technique. Primary repair is always preferable because, in the event of failure, subsequent corrective procedures offer a much more limited prognosis.

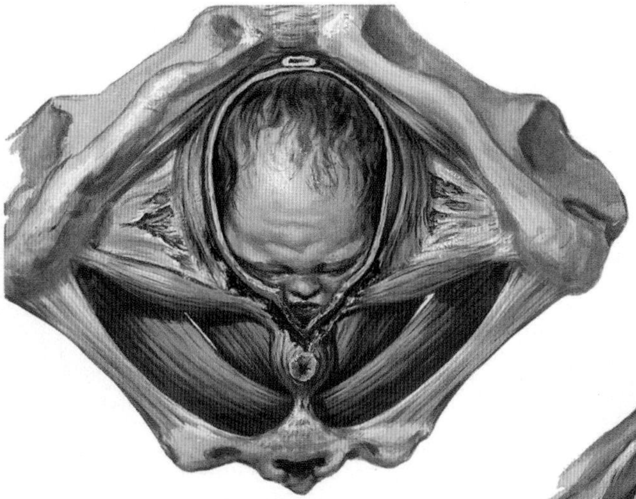

Plate 12.28

Pregnancy

OBSTETRIC LACERATIONS: FIBROMUSCULAR SUPPORT

The most common cause of direct injury to the vagina is childbirth. Before 1900, when most babies were delivered at home, these injuries were more frequent. Regardless of refinements in obstetric management and surgical technique, such accidents, both minor and major, continue to occur. A large number of variables in a delivery may account for this, including precipitous labor with sudden expulsion of the head, abnormal presentation or progress necessitating operative delivery, a large size baby, unusually friable maternal tissues, or an exaggerated lithotomy position. Vaginal lacerations are more common and more extensive in nulliparous women in whom the musculature of the birth canal and perineum has not previously been stretched.

In the cases illustrated, the infant's head has extended too soon, resulting in a near brow presentation, with increase in the diameter that must pass between the leaves of the pelvic sling at this level. The pressure thus exerted on the vaginal tube and its muscular supports has spread in several directions, but especially posteriorly toward the anus. The superficial muscles of the perineum, including the transverse perineal muscles, the upper margin of the external sphincter ani, and the more superficial fibers of the pubococcygei, have been ruptured to form a gaping wound. Some pressure has also been disseminated laterally, tearing the bulbocavernosi and shredding the thin inferior fascia of the urogenital diaphragm. Both urinary and fecal incontinence may result from such an injury. Infrequently, such lacerations are also associated with rectovaginal fistula formation, especially when damage to or frank laceration of the rectal mucosa goes unrecognized and unrepaired.

Because the vagina passes downward and forward in the interlevator cleft connected by musculofascial extensions to the pubococcygeus muscles on either side, downward traction on an infant's head impeded in midvagina may easily tear these connections as well as the interdigitating muscle fibers between the vagina and rectum. The vagina is completely separated from the rectum above the level of the external sphincter ani, and the separation continues laterally without damaging the major divisions of the pubococcygei. This injury occurs at about the level of the ischial spines and may be caused by an attempted forceps extraction.

A more severe laceration at approximately the same level, in addition to separating the pillars of the pubococcygei by rupturing their attachments to the lateral and posterior vagina, may tear the posterior puborectalis components, which give the principal support to the rectum and pelvic floor. The postpartum clinical effect of this is the development of a rectocele.

An aberrant application of forceps may cause a deep tear in the pubococcygeus muscle close to its origin on the inner surface of the superior pubic ramus. Damage of this type is difficult to recognize or repair at the time

Laceration of perineum and perineal musculature extending into external sphincter ani

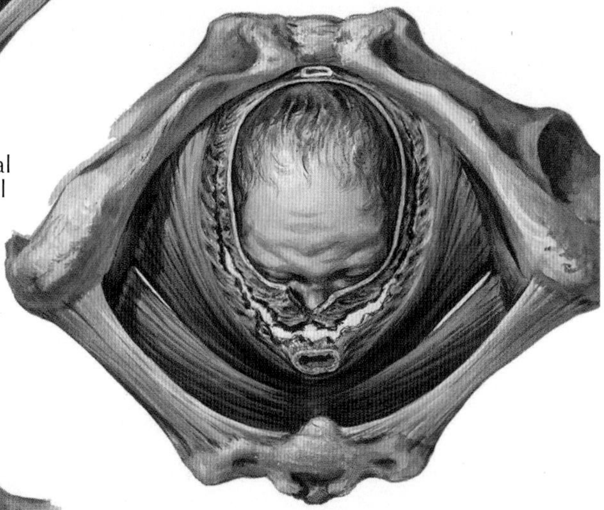

Laceration of the interdigitating (intercolumnar) fibers and fibromuscular visceral extensions due to separation of the pubococcygeus pillars and downward outward tension

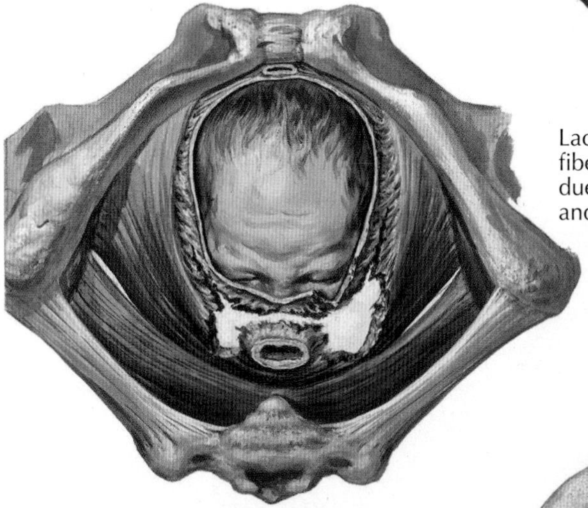

Laceration of the posterior portions of the pubococcygeus muscles and intercolumnar fibers

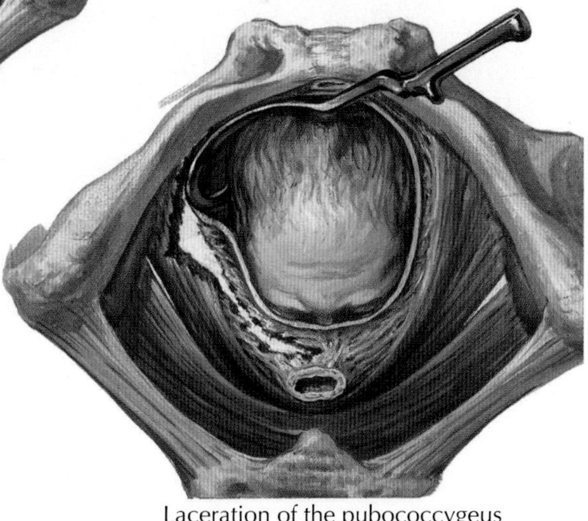

Laceration of the pubococcygeus close to its origin by blade of forceps

of delivery, and serious hemorrhage or hematoma formation may ensue. The tear often extends downward to separate the right lateral and posterior vagina from its supports and from the anterior rectal wall, with loss of almost an entire wing of the pelvic diaphragm. In the months following delivery, this may lead to varying degrees of prolapse of the pelvic viscera.

When forceps delivery was more commonly employed, rare cases of uterine rupture occurred during the process of placing the forceps blades or during forceps rotation. When forceps are used, and vaginal bleeding persists, the possibility of a lower uterine tear should be considered and evaluated by manual uterine exploration.

As with all surgical procedures, clear visualization, meticulous hemostasis, careful tissue handling, and tension-free, anatomically correct reapproximation of any tissues damaged are most likely to achieve a satisfactory outcome.

Plate 12.29

Reproductive System: VOLUME 1

Skin incisions for cesarean section

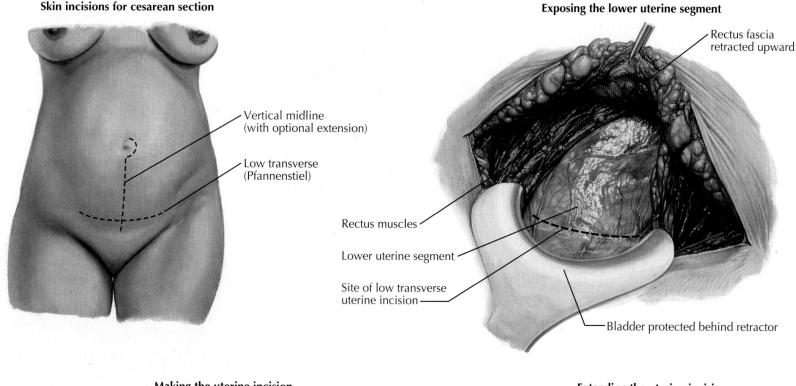

Vertical midline
(with optional extension)

Low transverse
(Pfannenstiel)

Exposing the lower uterine segment

Rectus fascia
retracted upward

Rectus muscles

Lower uterine segment

Site of low transverse
uterine incision

Bladder protected behind retractor

Making the uterine incision

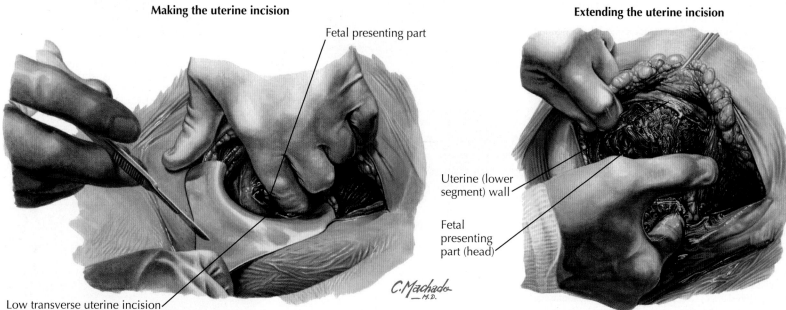

Fetal presenting part

Low transverse uterine incision

Extending the uterine incision

Uterine (lower
segment) wall

Fetal
presenting
part (head)

C. Machado
M.D.

CESAREAN DELIVERY

Cesarean delivery (or cesarean section) is the delivery of the fetus through surgical incisions in the mother's abdomen and uterus. It may be chosen to accomplish fetal delivery when it is impossible, impractical, or unsafe for the baby to be delivered vaginally. The rate of cesarean birth varies from 10% to more than 50% around the world, influenced by cultural factors and the availability of surgical care. In the United States the rate of cesarean births rose fivefold for the 20-year period ending in the early 1990s and is currently about 32%. The exact reasons for this are open to conjecture but concerns about liability, almost universal use of electronic fetal monitoring, increasing birth weight, and an increased number of repeat cesarean deliveries have all been argued.

Because cesarean delivery is a major surgical procedure, the rate of maternal mortality is roughly three- to fourfold higher than for vaginal delivery. Potential risks of cesarean delivery include a longer maternal hospital stay, an increased risk of respiratory problems for the baby due to iatrogenic prematurity, and greater complications in subsequent pregnancies, including increased risks of uterine rupture and placental implantation problems. The risks of placenta previa, placenta accreta, and the need for cesarean hysterectomy all increase with each succeeding cesarean delivery. Some have suggested that cesarean delivery decreases the risk of subsequent pelvic floor dysfunction and urinary incontinence, but analysis of stress urinary incontinence rates at 2 and 5 years after delivery has shown no difference based on the mode of delivery. At 3 months and 24 months after delivery, breastfeeding rates are also not altered by mode of delivery.

Cesarean delivery may be accomplished through either a lower abdominal vertical midline or transverse (Pfannenstiel) incision. Cesarean sections are not classified by the kind of abdominal incision made but rather as lower uterine segment (transverse or vertical) when the uterine incision is in the lower uterine segment or

Plate 12.30

Pregnancy

Delivering the fetal head

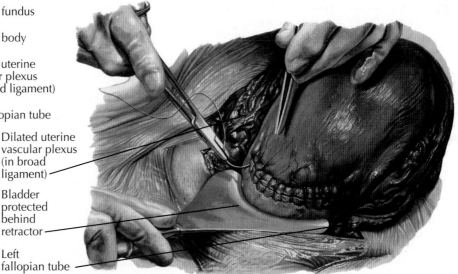

Fetal shoulder

Delivering the placenta

Placenta (fetal side)

Amnionic membranes

Umbilical cord

C. Machado
—M.D.

Exploring the uterine cavity (uterus exteriorized through skin incision)

Right fallopian tube

Uterine fundus

Uterine body

Dilated uterine
vascular plexus
(in broad ligament)

Left fallopian tube

Closing the uterine incision (uterus exteriorized through incision)

Dilated uterine
vascular plexus
(in broad
ligament)

Bladder
protected
behind
retractor

Left
fallopian tube

CESAREAN DELIVERY
(Continued)

classic when the incision is in the upper, contractile portion of the uterus. Patients with lower uterine segment cesarean deliveries may be candidates for future vaginal delivery because these incisions are less likely to rupture in labor. Patients with classic incisions and those who have had incisions of the upper uterus for other reasons (e.g., myomectomy, repair of uterine malformations, cornual resection) are at greater risk of rupture of the uterine scar before or during labor and are generally not advised to labor in subsequent pregnancies.

Recovery following cesarean birth is similar to that for other major abdominal surgeries, with a progressive return to full function expected over the subsequent 4 to 6 weeks.

Anesthesia for cesarean birth is generally provided by a regional neuraxial anesthetic. This allows for participation in the process by the mother and avoids sedation of the baby. When a general anesthetic must be used, as in emergency cases, rapid delivery of the infant may reduce the impact of anesthetic agents transferred from the mother's circulation.

Vaginal birth after cesarean section (VBAC) may be safe and effective in reducing maternal morbidity as well as cesarean section rates if careful maternal and

fetal monitoring is available as well as staff and facilities for emergency cesarean section. Approximately 60% to 80% of women planning VBAC will achieve a successful vaginal delivery. Although VBAC is appropriate for most women with a history of a low-transverse cesarean delivery, several factors increase the likelihood of a failed trial of labor, which in turn leads to increased maternal and perinatal morbidity. As the frequency of VBAC has increased, so has the number of cases of uterine rupture and other complications. As a result, many physicians and hospitals have discontinued the practice altogether, contributing to the increased rate of cesarean delivery and a decline in the VBAC rate to less than 10%.

Plate 12.31

Reproductive System: VOLUME 1

RUPTURE OF THE UTERUS

Rupture of the uterus may occur spontaneously, as with a previous cesarean section scar, uterine anomaly, or, rarely, an intact uterus, or it may be caused by trauma, including obstetric maneuvers such as forceps rotations. Spontaneous rupture of the intact uterus during pregnancy, without the patient being in labor, is an extremely rare occurrence. The cause usually lies within the uterus itself, as in the presence of adenomyosis or when the fetus is carried in a poorly developed horn of a bicornuate uterus. In these cases, the rupture occurs usually in the fundus, in contrast to ruptures during labor, which are usually in the lower segment.

Spontaneous rupture during labor is usually caused by difficult (obstructed) vaginal delivery or by unrecognized cephalopelvic disproportion. Transverse presentation requiring version, hydrocephalus, impacted tumors, and brow and face presentations are the most common factors in causing dystocia and contribute largely to spontaneous rupture of the unscarred uterus during labor.

Rupture of the uterus in a previous cesarean section scar occurs more frequently after classic cesarean section and T-shaped incisions (2%) than after the low cervical type. When vaginal delivery has been attempted in patients with a previous section, rupture occurs in 1% to 5% of cases, but the percentage is higher in the patients who have had more cesarean deliveries. Because this uterine rupture is more correctly a dehiscence of a previous incision, where scar tissue may have obliterated the major vessels supplying that area, in many instances little bleeding occurs, and the rupture may consequently remain silent for hours and days. The only sign that may be present is a slight abdominal tenderness on palpation of the region over the site of rupture. In some cases, herniation of the amniotic sac or of some fetal parts may be seen at operation. Although maternal mortality from uterine rupture is low, the reported perinatal death rate associated with uterine rupture ranges from 5% to 26%.

Rupture in the lower segment may extend to the fundus. The lateral sides are more frequently affected. The blood may enter the peritoneal cavity if the rupture opens the peritoneal sheath covering the uterus, or the blood may dissect between the sheets of the broad ligament, thus giving rise to retroperitoneal hematoma. In the latter case the bleeding may be checked temporarily because of the pressure of the clotted blood on the torn vessels.

Clinically spontaneous rupture of the uterus is heralded by a sharp "shooting" pain in the lower abdomen, which usually occurs at the height of an intense uterine contraction. Abdominal tenderness, particularly at the level of the lower segment, is a salient feature. Fetal

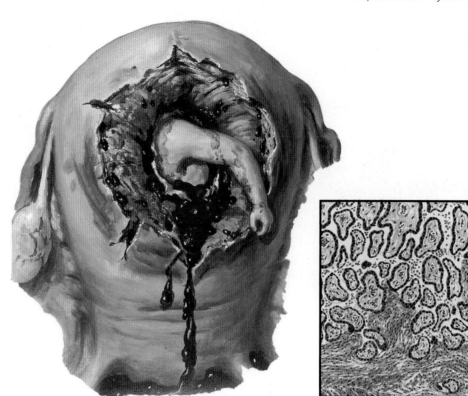

Rupture through scar of classic cesarean section

Placenta accreta

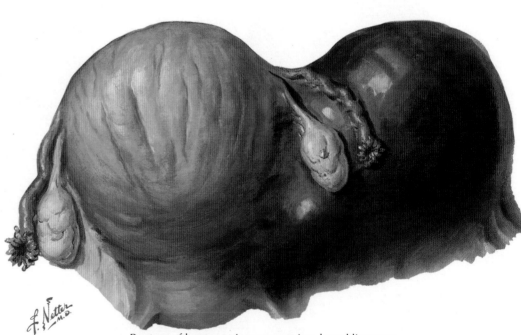

Rupture of lower uterine segment into broad ligament

heart beats and fetal movements may immediately cease. The fetus may be found in the abdominal cavity with the presenting parts out of the pelvis. It should be strongly suspected when the previously engaged presenting part is suddenly disengaged from the pelvis. This can be confirmed by bedside ultrasonography. The tear in the lower segment can sometimes be felt through the vaginal canal. Slight vaginal bleeding may or may not be present. Symptoms of shock may follow the episode, but the blood pressure may not fall precipitously.

Tachycardia is more frequent than hypotension. Many ruptures remain silent and unrecognized for several hours, the only signs being abdominal tenderness and vague abdominal pain.

Treatment is the same in all ruptures and consists of immediate laparotomy and delivery of the fetus. Cesarean hysterectomy is the method of choice for catastrophic ruptures, except when the patient is young and desires more babies, in which case attempts at repair may be worthwhile.

Plate 12.32

Pregnancy

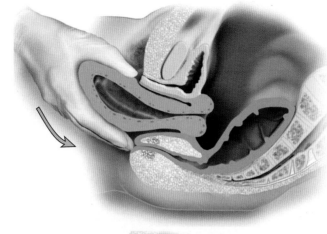

A. The fundus of the uterus is grasped by the operator's hand and gently pushed cephalward.

UTERINE INVERSION

Rarely, the uterus can be turned inside out immediately following the delivery of the placenta. Uncommon and most often iatrogenic (95%), this may be associated with catastrophic bleeding and cardiovascular collapse. Incomplete uterine inversion may also occur. (Rarely the condition has also been reported in nonpregnant patients with intrauterine pathology such as a pedunculated leiomyomata or large endometrial polyp.) The prevalence of uterine inversion is estimated to be about 1 in 3500 to 20,000 deliveries.

Inversion of the uterus can occur because of traction on the umbilical cord or downward pressure on the uterine fundus (Credé maneuver) to facilitate delivery of the placenta. This is more likely to occur with excessive force and a poorly contracted uterus or lower uterine segment. Abnormalities of placentation (placenta accreta, increta, or percreta) can increase the risk of this occurring because of the absence of separation of the placenta from the uterine wall in a normal manner. Risk factors for inversion include uterine atony secondary to multiparity (grand multiparity), uterine overdistention (multiple birth, polyhydramnios), a prolonged labor, prolonged oxytocin stimulation, muscle relaxant agents (such as $MgSO_4$), or rapid labor. Risk factors are present in less than 50% of cases.

The diagnosis of inversion of the uterus must be based on a high degree of suspicion. In some cases, a mass (the uterus) may be seen attached to or directly following the placenta as it delivers. More often, there is simply brisk bright red vaginal bleeding accompanied by bradycardia (due to vagal stimulation) and/or tachycardia, hypotension, and vascular collapse due to blood loss. The blood loss associated with uterine inversion can be catastrophic and is often underestimated. Significant blood loss occurs in almost 40% of cases. Uterine inversion must be differentiated from simple uterine atony following placental delivery, retained placental fragments or undiagnosed genital tract lacerations, which can generally be accomplished by simple clinical examination. Although ultrasonography may be used to verify the diagnosis, this is unnecessary and delays the implementation of therapy.

Uterine inversion is treated by rapid evaluation, fluid support, or resuscitation and calls for anesthesia assistance. A delay in treatment markedly increases the mortality rate. Specific treatment is carried out by the use of uterine relaxing agents to allow the replacement of the uterine fundus (may require general anesthesia with a relaxant agent such as halothane) and may require operative intervention (replacement or hysterectomy). Once the uterine wall has relaxed, gentle manual pressure on the fundus is used to displace it inward and upward until its normal position can be restored and the uterus returned to its normal configuration. Uterotonic agents are then used to obtain uterine contraction and hemostasis. Large-volume fluid replacement should be available and used liberally if there has been

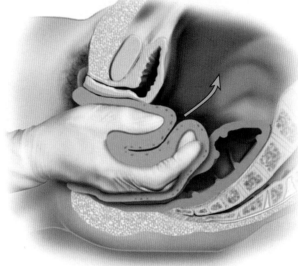

B. As the uterus is returned to the abdominal cavity, the body of the uterus must be allowed to revert to its normal configuration.

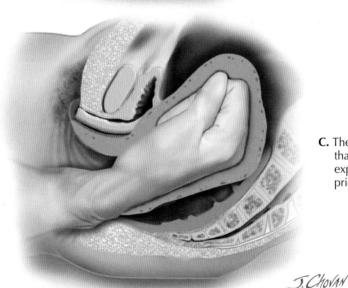

C. The examining hand is used to ensure that the fundus of the uterus is fully expanded into its normal position prior to the hand being removed.

J. Chovan

significant blood loss. If the placenta is still attached to the uterine wall, it should be left in place until after the uterine fundus has been reduced and returned to its normal location. Antibiotic prophylaxis should strongly be considered following the procedure.

If the uterine fundus cannot be repositioned vaginally through these maneuvers, immediate laparotomy is necessary (6%). This can allow simultaneous maneuvers from above and below. Traction on the round ligaments or a traction suture can sometimes be placed to assist

this effort. If a constriction ring is present and impeding replacement, the use of local anesthetics to break the muscular spasm or incision (generally along the posterior aspect of the uterus) may be needed. The possibility of hysterectomy to control bleeding must always be considered (3%).

Although unrecognized or untreated uterine inversion can end in hysterectomy, hemorrhagic shock, and cardiovascular collapse, if it is rapidly treated, the outcome is generally good.

Plate 12.33

Reproductive System: VOLUME 1

Urinary Complications of Pregnancy

Pregnancy leads to an increase in kidney size (1–1.5 cm in length), renal plasma flow (increases by up to 80%), and glomerular filtration rate (40%–50% above baseline). In most pregnant women, after the fourth month, the diameter of the upper third of each ureter has increased. The lumen, more than the wall, contributes to this amplification, which is most pronounced in the region over the brim of the pelvis and, as a rule, is more marked on the right side than on the left. The genesis of this ureteral expansion is due to several factors working together: pressure on the ureter and the kidney by the gravid uterus produces a mechanical effect. Structural changes in the ureteral wall have been recorded, and x-ray studies have led to the assumption that the musculature loses its tone. Dilation and increased tortuosity of the ureters have been produced in experimental animals by the administration of estrogens. This and the smooth muscle–relaxing effect of progesterone emphasize that mechanical, neurogenic, and hormonal factors work together in bringing about this physiologic pregnancy change, which, in the great majority of pregnant women, does not lead to any recognizable functional disturbances. Following delivery, the ureters rapidly return to normal size.

For reasons not known, however, the dilation may reach degrees that interfere with normal function. Every ureteral dilation is accompanied by a certain degree of stasis, which, in a retrograde fashion, may affect the renal pelvis. Functional examinations and pyelography have demonstrated that during pregnancy the excretion time is delayed and that the flow through the ureters slows down parallel to the tortuosity and enlargement of the ureter and the renal pelvis. These changes may cause the development of a marked hydroureter and hydronephrosis. In rare instances, all the consequences of hydronephrosis, such as flattened calyces and atrophy of the renal parenchyma may become manifest. Ultrasonography can be used to document and assess the degree of ureteral and renal dilation present.

Infection of the upper urinary collecting system is a frequent occurrence in cases of hydronephrosis. Pyelitis or pyelonephritis and ureteritis are relatively frequent complications of pregnancy. They may occur without extreme ureteral dilation, and the infection may not extend to the kidneys. The incidence of infection in the urinary tract is greater in the later stages of pregnancy than earlier ones. Pyelitis may become manifest only after delivery, possibly because of damage to the ureters.

Bacterial invasion of the ureteral mucosa is favored by ureteral dilation, urinary stasis, venous congestion, and edema. The exact route of infection in pyelonephritis in pregnant women has not yet been established. Bacterial invasion of the ureteral mucosa may occur through venous, lymphatic, or direct vesicoureteral reflux. The most frequent organism is bacterium *Escherichia coli,* which can be found in cultures of catheterized urine in more than 90% of cases.

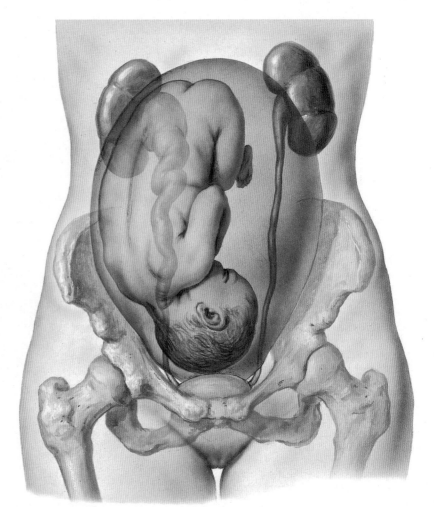

Dilation of right renal pelvis and ureter above pelvic brim

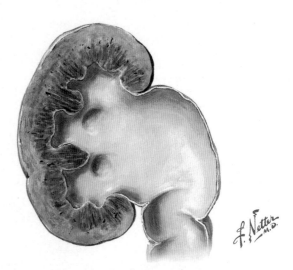

Kidney showing hydronephrosis

The diagnosis of urinary infection is easy in the acute or more severe cases and should not cause difficulties in the milder or subacute forms. Clean-catch urine examinations during prenatal care may reveal infections in an early stage, although for a definite diagnosis a fresh specimen obtained by catheterization is preferred. The characteristic symptoms include back pain in the lumbar region, fever (usually high), vomiting, frequent urination with the sensation of burning, and leukocytosis. Unless treated promptly and adequately, pyelonephritis not only constitutes a serious complication of pregnancy but also, because of its tendency to chronicity and recurrences, may produce irreversible renal changes that may cause renal insufficiency and hypertension.

Cystitis usually accompanies infection of the upper urinary pathways. The severity of cystitis varies from a mild form without ureteritis to extensive ulcerative cystitis and ureteritis. Cystitis and urethritis will generally prompt the classic symptoms of frequency, urgency, and dysuria.

Plate 12.34   Pregnancy

PREECLAMPSIA: SYMPTOMATOLOGY

Preeclampsia (once called toxemia of pregnancy) is a pregnancy-specific syndrome occurring after 20 weeks gestation through 2 weeks after delivery. It involves reduced organ perfusion, vasospasm, and endothelial activation and is characterized by hypertension, proteinuria, and other symptoms. Pregnancy can induce hypertension or aggravate existing hypertension. Edema and proteinuria (one or both) are characteristic pregnancy-induced changes, though proteinuria is no longer required to make the diagnosis. If preeclampsia is untreated, convulsions (eclampsia) may occur. Chronic hypertension may be worsened by being superimposed on pregnancy-induced changes. Severe cases may include hemolysis, elevated liver enzymes, and low platelet counts, labeled HELLP syndrome, which occurs in up to 20% of severe preeclampsia. Preeclampsia occurs in 5% to 8% of all births (250,000 cases per year) and results in 150 maternal deaths and 3000 fetal deaths per year. (Overall, hypertensive disease of some type occurs in approximately 12% to 22% of pregnancies, and it is directly responsible for 17.6% of maternal deaths in the United States.)

In the great majority of cases, the clinical manifestations of preeclampsia occur after the 20th week of gestation and disappear following delivery. Preeclampsia before 20 weeks gestation may occur with gestational trophoblastic neoplasia and antiphospholipid antibody syndrome. Another uncommon presentation for preeclampsia is in the postpartum period, when it has been reported to occur up to 14 days after delivery.

The earliest clinical signs of preeclampsia are often sudden and excessive weight gain, accompanied by a blood pressure higher than 140/90 mm Hg. Such weight gain reflects the retention of water and electrolytes. Eventually, pitting edema, particularly in the legs and face, develops. However, before the stage of pitting edema is reached, the interstitial space may accumulate large quantities of fluid. The normal average weight gain during pregnancy does not exceed 2.5 to 3 lb per month, and a greater weight gain should be suspected as abnormal water retention. Edema may precede hypertension, but for the clinical diagnosis of preeclampsia, the increased blood pressure is essential. In this respect the elevation of the diastolic blood pressure is more significant than that of the systolic, because it is the former which reflects the status of the peripheral resistance.

To make the diagnosis of preeclampsia there should be new onset of hypertension and proteinuria or the new onset of hypertension and significant end organ dysfunction with or without proteinuria after 20 weeks

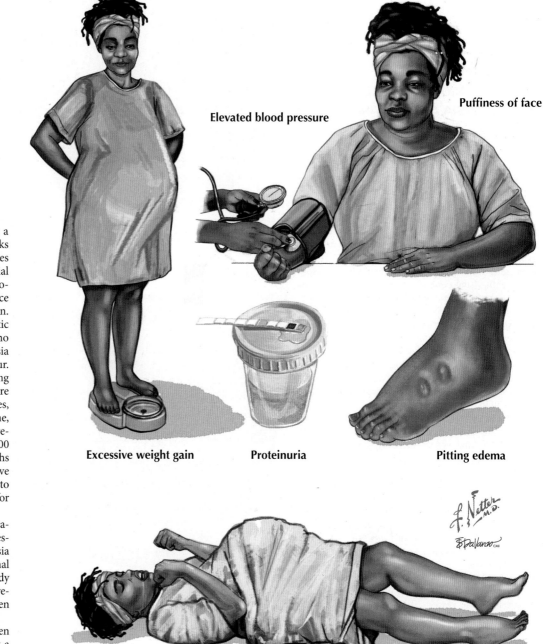

Clinical triad

Elevated blood pressure

Puffiness of face

Excessive weight gain   **Proteinuria**   **Pitting edema**

Convulsion in true eclampsia

of gestation or postpartum in a previously normotensive woman. These patients also have characteristic renal glomerular lesions (capillary endotheliosis) and increased vascular reactivity. They often manifest elevated liver enzymes, and thrombocytopenia. In the past, hypertension indicative of preeclampsia has been defined as an elevation of more than 30 mm Hg systolic or more than 15 mm Hg diastolic above the patient's baseline pressure; however, this has not proven to be a good predictor of outcome and is no longer part of the criteria for preeclampsia, although these patients do require close monitoring. The current threshold for blood pressure is systolic blood pressure ≥140 mm Hg or diastolic blood pressure ≥90 mm Hg on at least 2 occasions at least 4 hours apart. Eclamptic patients may undergo

convulsions with only moderate blood pressure elevation and only a slight degree of edema.

Conscientious, regular prenatal care is important to detect signs of preeclampsia as early as possible. The onset of preeclampsia may be insidious or abrupt. There may be a sudden progression into the convulsive phase, necessitating the termination of the pregnancy, thereby resulting in prematurity of the infant, which is the most frequent cause of perinatal mortality in preeclampsia. Preeclampsia predisposes to chronic hypertensive vascular disease, and the incidence of severe preeclampsia in subsequent pregnancies is increased. Multiple studies have demonstrated an association between a history of hypertensive disorder of pregnancy and future risk of hypertension and other cardiovascular disorders.

Plate 12.35

Reproductive System: VOLUME 1

PREECLAMPSIA: OPHTHALMOLOGIC CHANGES IN PREECLAMPSIA AND ECLAMPSIA

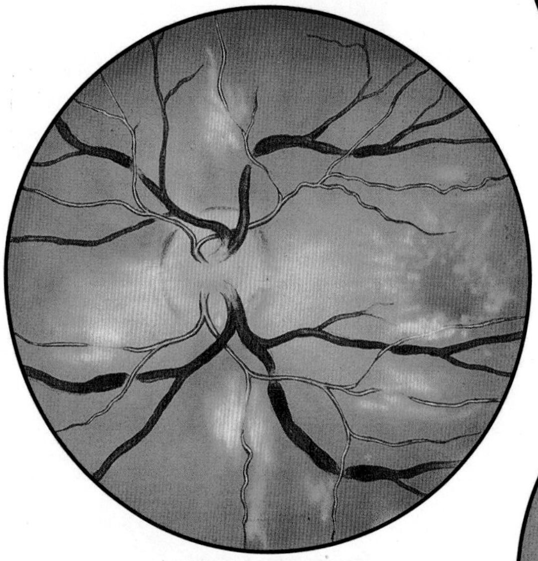

Visual disturbances are very frequent in eclampsia and preeclampsia and are symptoms of the severe end of the disease spectrum. (Ocular sequelae have been reported in up to one-third of cases.) They range from slight blurring of vision to various degrees of temporary blindness. Other symptoms have also been noted, including photopsias, scotomas, and diplopia. These disturbances are thought to be caused by the arteriolar spasm of the retinal vessels together with ischemia, edema, and sometimes retinal detachment. In some patients with visual changes in preeclampsia, a diffuse increase in macular thickness has been documented.

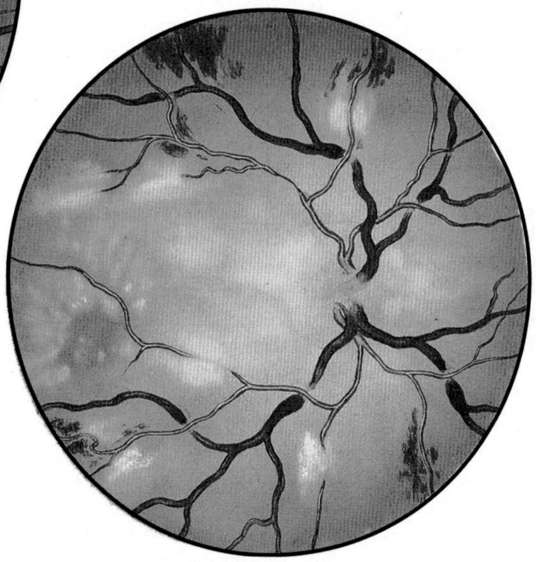

Examination of the eye grounds is of great help in the differential diagnosis between preeclampsia, eclampsia, and other hypertensive states coexisting with pregnancy. In preeclampsia, the first change in the retinal vessels consists of a spasm of the arterioles. The constriction is usually localized in certain areas of the retinal vessels. A series of sausage-linked or spindle-shaped constrictions may be seen in the terminal part of the retinal vessels or sometimes in the part close to the disk. The changes are seen more frequently in the nasal branches. Occasionally, all the retinal vessels are seen constricted to a marked degree.

To observe clearly the changes in these vessels, dilation of the pupils with atropine or an equivalent drug is essential. Comparison of the ratio of the diameter of the retinal arterioles to the retinal veins is informative. In normal individuals, the ratio of the arterioles to the veins is 2:3. In preeclampsia, this ratio may change to 1:2 or even 1:3, indicating extreme narrowing of the retinal arterioles.

Edema of the retina may be seen occasionally in preeclampsia and eclampsia, but it is much less frequent than spasm of the vessels. The edema usually appears first at the upper and lower poles of the disk and later progresses along the course of the retinal vessels. In rare instances, retinal edema becomes so intense that complete detachment of the retina occurs.

Hemorrhages and exudates are rarely seen in uncomplicated preeclampsia and eclampsia. They are more characteristic of chronic cardiovascular and renal diseases. Nerve fiber layer infarcts and vitreous hemorrhage secondary to neovascularization are also common. Despite this, most changes are reversible once preeclampsia resolves. Serous exudative retinal detachments may occur in severe preeclampsia or eclampsia. They tend to be bilateral, bullous, and associated with preeclampsia retinopathy changes. The underlying mechanism is most likely related to choroidal nonperfusion and resultant subretinal leakage. Most patients with serous detachments have resolution of symptoms within weeks after delivery.

Cortical blindness, although a rare complication, has been reported to cause vision loss in preeclampsia secondary to cerebral edema. This may result from vasospasm causing transient ischemia producing cytotoxic

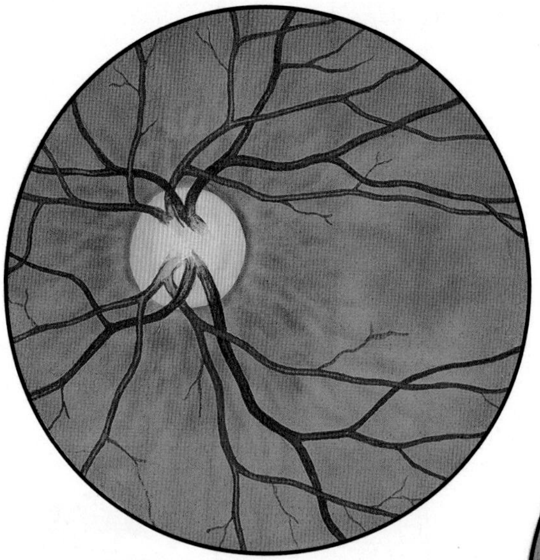

Normal

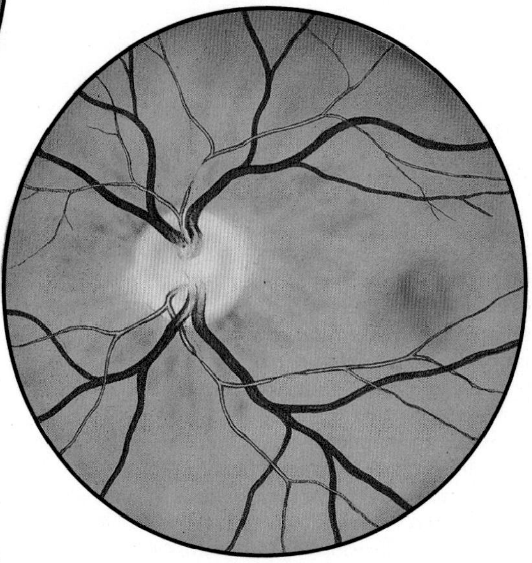

Eclampsia

Essential hypertension

Nephritis

edema. It is also possible that preeclampsia causes increased permeability from circulatory dysregulation, thus providing vasogenic edema. Resolution of the changes associated with preeclampsia and the resultant cerebral edema usually result in visual recovery.

In benign essential hypertension, examination of the eye grounds reveals a different picture. The retinal arterioles are more narrowed and tortuous, and they present the aspect of silver or copper wire. Arteriovenous nicking is very frequent in essential hypertension and rarely

seen in preeclampsia. Fresh and old exudates can be seen distributed in the retinal field, resembling cotton wool. In essential hypertension, hemorrhages are not frequently seen. In malignant hypertension and in chronic kidney diseases, besides the arteriolar changes described above, a great number of fresh and old exudates can be observed together with patches of old and fresh hemorrhages. Choking of the disk is so marked in these cardiovascular and renal conditions that delineation of its contours may become very difficult.

Plate 12.36

Pregnancy

Preeclampsia: Visceral Lesions in Preeclampsia and Eclampsia

Although preeclampsia and eclampsia are differentiated, depending on whether or not the patient has had a convulsion, the pathology of the two is essentially the same. Characteristic lesions frequently appear in the liver, kidneys, and brain, but they are inconstant in occurrence and may be absent even in severe cases with convulsions. Therefore they cannot be considered primary lesions but are probably the sequelae of the three constantly present features of the disease, namely, vasoconstriction, hypertension, and fluid retention.

In typical cases, the liver is swollen and mottled with small hemorrhages. Microscopically, the sinusoids around the smaller portal areas are plugged with fibrinoid material and surrounded by foci of hemorrhage and necrotic liver cells. Occasionally, midzonal necrosis is seen, but serial sections usually reveal continuity with larger periportal lesions. The condition may be widespread or may involve only a few subcapsular lobules.

Three types of renal lesions are associated with preeclampsia. The most common and characteristic one consists of narrowing of glomerular capillary lumina with thickening of the epithelial-endothelial glomerular membranes. This is known as *glomerular capillary endotheliosis* and results from swelling of endothelial cells. The afferent arterioles often appear to be stiff walled and are occasionally plugged with eosinophilic material. Obstruction of the blood flow through the glomerular tufts may cause anoxic degeneration of the distal tubules. Occasionally, this phenomenon proceeds to necrosis, in which case the lesion is called *lower nephron nephrosis*. In fatal cases of preeclampsia, moderate degeneration of tubular epithelium has been a frequent finding, but actual necrosis is rare. Another, but less common, renal lesion called *bilateral cortical necrosis*, results from severe vasoconstriction and necrosis of intralobular arteries, followed by symmetric bilateral infarction of renal cortical tissue. Although other diseases in which severe vasoconstriction plays a role have produced this renal lesion in both males and females, it has been found more frequently in cases of eclampsia than in any other condition.

The characteristic changes in the brain are edema and small foci of degeneration, both consequences of anoxia. After the onset of convulsions, petechial hemorrhages are common, and in fatal cases larger areas of hemorrhage and softening may appear. Preeclampsia and eclampsia account for more than 35% of all pregnancy-associated strokes. The capillaries and arterioles appear to be stiff walled and straight. More than the usual number are visible in microscopic sections, as though they had rolled out on the surface instead of being cut sharply by the microtome knife.

Edema of the subcutaneous tissues, lungs, and interstitial tissues of the viscera is present to varying extents in all cases. Likewise, small foci of degeneration and petechial hemorrhages are frequent, especially in the adrenals and myocardium.

All these lesions may be explained on the basis of widespread vasoconstriction, with significant elevations in total peripheral resistance, enhanced responsiveness to angiotensin II, and subsequent reductions in renal blood flow and glomerular filtration rate compared with

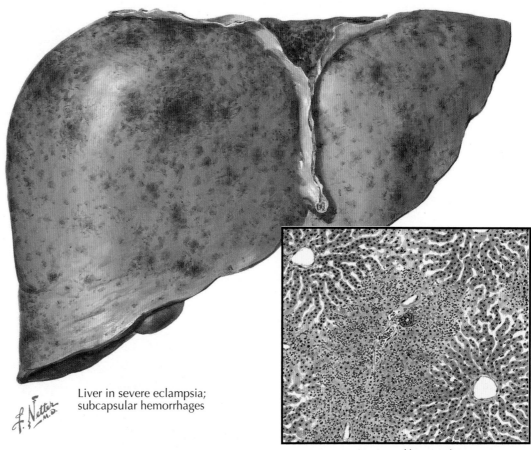

Liver in severe eclampsia; subcapsular hemorrhages

Section of liver with periportal necrosis

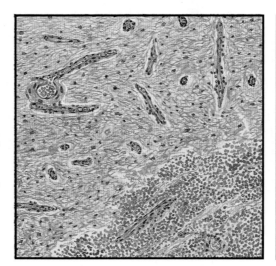

Hemorrhage and necrosis in brain

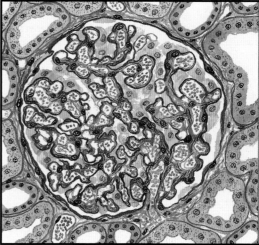

Fibrin deposition and swelling of epithelial cells in glomerulus

normal pregnancy. Although the physiologic mechanisms have been extensively studied during normal pregnancy in animal models, information regarding the mediators during preeclampsia has been limited because of the problems of performing studies during pregnancy. Although some animal models have been developed to study preeclampsia, information on the mechanisms involved in mediating the reduction in renal and hepatic function is lacking.

That severe vasoconstriction exists in this condition is evident from examination of the eye grounds and the renal as well as cerebral hemodynamics. Although the hypertension of preeclampsia resembles in many respects the malignant hypertension associated with renal disease, the renal lesions in the former condition seem to be the result rather than the cause of vasoconstriction. Several lines of experimental evidence support the hypothesis of a central role for the placenta in preeclampsia.

Plate 12.37

Reproductive System: VOLUME 1

Nodular ischemia of placenta

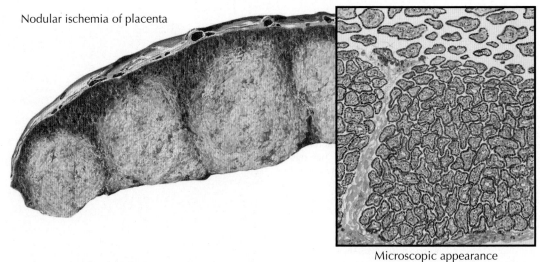

Microscopic appearance

PREECLAMPSIA: PLACENTAL INFARCTS

In patients with preeclampsia, there is shallow placentation and failure of the spiral arteries to remodel early in pregnancy leading to suboptimal uteroplacental blood flow and relatively hypoxic trophoblast tissue. As pregnancy advances, the placenta increasingly secretes antiangiogenic factors. These bind vascular endothelial growth factor and placental growth factor, which results in widespread maternal vascular inflammation, endothelial dysfunction, and vascular injury. Hypertension, proteinuria, and the other clinical manifestations of preeclampsia ensue. Despite these findings, there are no micro- or macroscopic placental lesions that are pathognomonic for preeclampsia.

Histopathologic studies have revealed close correlation between the occurrence of preeclampsia and conditions that are prone to cause a decrease in the maternal circulation to the placenta, to the decidua, or to both of these tissues. Obstruction of the maternal blood flow to one or more placental cotyledons causes true infarction of the involved areas. Unfortunately, the term *infarct* has often been used for a wide variety of nodular lesions in the placenta, and conflicting opinions have been expressed concerning the association of such lesions with preeclampsia.

True infarcts are usually found on the maternal aspect of the placenta but are often not visible until cross sections are made. They then appear as round or oval nodules of increased density and may be varying shades of red, yellow, or gray, according to their age. Microscopically, they consist of necrotic chorionic villi. Immediately after cessation of the maternal blood flow to a cotyledon, the intervillous spaces collapse. The part becomes pale and of increased density. This is called *nodular ischemia*. The areas with more venous blood beneath the chorionic plate and between the cotyledons are less affected than the centers of the nodules. If the fetus is alive, dilation and filling of the unobstructed villous capillaries ensue, and, thus, the part becomes congested and an acute red infarct is produced. If the fetus is dead, the infarct remains ischemic. In either case, as the villi become necrotic, the nuclei undergo karyorrhexis and karyolysis, the red cells become hemolyzed, and the entire area takes on a yellowish hue. A reaction zone of neutrophils forms at the margin between the dead and living tissue, appearing as a dense ring around the lesion. This is called the *subacute stage of infarction.*

Infarcts in the placenta do not heal by organization. No fibroblastic proliferation or budding of capillaries has been found in the many examples of old infarcts examined. Calcium is deposited at the periphery of the

Placental infarcts in progressive stages

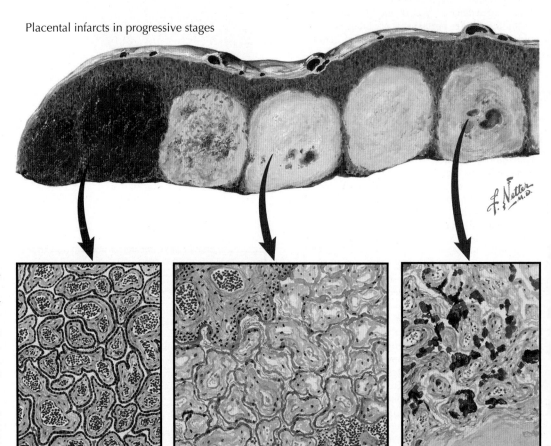

Acute (red) infarct. Intervillous spaces collapsed, villi compact. Villous capillaries dilated.

Subacute infarct. Necrosis of villi, hemolysis of villous blood, neutrophils at margin and in cotyledon stalk. Hemorrhage into infarct.

Healing infarct. Calcified areas, liquefaction in center.

lesions, which become gray or white as they age. The centers are prone to liquefy and become cystic.

Because cotyledon stalks bearing large fetal vessels are often included in the depths of large infarcts, the fetal circulation continues until necrosis of the supporting tissues causes rupture and hemorrhage of fetal blood into the necrotic area. If the hemorrhage is extensive, it may rupture retroplacentally and be a factor in the initiation of premature separation. This can also result in exposing the mother to fetal blood antigens such as Rh(D).

Studies carried out in the past several years have shown no significant difference between the placentas of pregnancies complicated with preeclampsia/eclampsia and control groups with regard to ischemic changes of the placenta. Endovascular trophoblastic plugs in the basal plate vessels may play an additional role in the development of ischemic lesions in preeclampsia/eclampsia, but these may also represent indirect evidence of the abnormal expression of certain adhesion molecules in this disorder.

Plate 12.38

Pregnancy

CAUSES OF DECREASED MATERNAL CIRCULATION

Various pathologic conditions may impede the maternal circulation to the placenta. They can be grouped as follows:

1. Diseases of the uterine vessels: (a) acute atherosis, (b) arteriolar sclerosis associated with essential hypertension, and (c) inflammation (angiitis) associated with chorioamnionitis.
2. Premature separation of the placenta associated with retroplacental hemorrhage or inflammatory exudation.
3. Conditions that may cause an increase in intrauterine pressure: (a) multiple pregnancy, (b) macrosomia, (c) polyhydramnios, and (d) hydatidiform mole.
4. Extensive thrombosis of the intervillous space or of the marginal sinus.
5. Death of the mother.

The most common cause of placental infarcts in cases of preeclampsia has been found to be acute atherosis of the decidual vessels. This lesion is manifested microscopically as a deposition of lipids, in the intima of decidual arterioles and endometrial arteriovenous lakes. Part of the material is doubly refractive under polarized light and occurs both extracellularly and inside lipophages. The lesions closely resemble acute fulminating atherosis in other settings. The process leads to marked intimal thickening and vascular occlusion. The lesions occur in the decidua vera, as well as in the basalis, but they do not involve to a comparable degree the vessels of the myometrium or other tissues in the body. Fat stains have not revealed the lesion in fetal vessels. Contiguous trophoblastic tissue seems to be a necessary factor in its pathogenesis. The lesions regress promptly after delivery. The cause of this condition is still unknown.

Although acute atherosis may be found in about 50% of all cases of preeclampsia by the use of fat stains on frozen sections of carefully selected decidua, the lesions have not been found in all cases of preeclampsia and do not constitute the only cause of maternal vascular obstruction. Another common cause of placental infarction is premature separation with retroplacental hemorrhage, the etiology of which is often undetermined. Moreover, inflammatory lesions associated with acute intrauterine infection during gestation occasionally spread through the walls of vessels and lead to thrombosis and occlusion. Furthermore, the blood flow to the placenta may be impeded by conditions that cause marked increase in intrauterine pressure, which, in turn, leads to overstretching of the uterine wall and collapse of the thin-walled decidual vessels. Although the higher incidence of preeclampsia in such cases lends support to the concept that decreased blood flow through the decidual vessels is a causative factor in preeclampsia, the actual proof of such diminished circulation has not yet been submitted.

Likewise, it is conceivable that extensive thrombosis of the intervillous space or of the marginal sinus would prevent adequate oxygenation of the placenta, because obstruction of the venous return elsewhere in the body frequently leads to infarction.

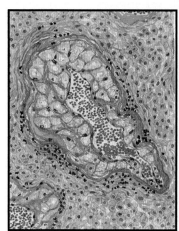
Lipophages in intima of vessel in decidua

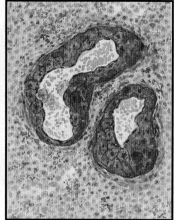
Lipid deposit in vessel (fat stain)

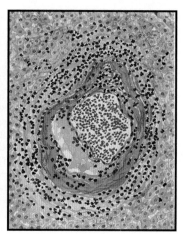
Atherosis and inflammatory reaction in vessel of decidua

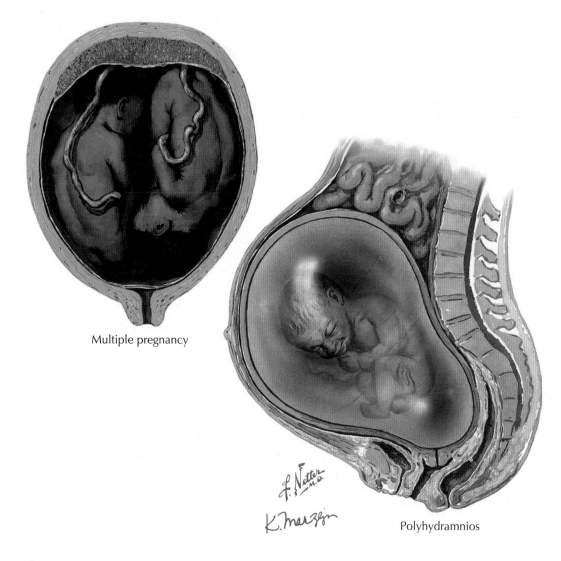
Multiple pregnancy

Polyhydramnios

When a patient has hypertension before the onset of pregnancy, the arterioles in the uterus and elsewhere in the body are usually hyalinized and have narrowed lumina. This lesion in itself seems to be insufficient to produce placental infarction, but it is an important contributing cause in those cases of essential hypertension in which preeclampsia is superimposed. In fact, a combination of two or more of the above conditions is the rule rather than the exception in cases of fatal preeclampsia or eclampsia.

Maternal death is listed as a cause of impeded blood flow to the uterus to emphasize the fact that, during the few minutes of continued fetal circulation after sudden maternal death, the earliest stages of placental infarction become manifest. Such cases present nodular ischemia of the entire placenta. Usually, a few foci of beginning engorgement of villous capillaries with fetal blood appear in some of the nodules. This constitutes the preliminary phase of acute hemorrhagic infarction of the placenta.

Plate 12.39

Reproductive System: VOLUME 1

INTRAUTERINE GROWTH RESTRICTION

Symmetric or asymmetric reduction in the size and weight of the growing fetus in utero, compared with that expected for a fetus of comparable gestational age, constitutes intrauterine growth restriction. This reduced growth may occur for many reasons, but most occurrences represent signs of significant risk of fetal death or jeopardy to the fetus. Some authors advocate identifying fetuses with growth between the 10th and 20th percentiles as having "diminished" growth and at intermediate risk for complications. Problems of consistent definition make estimates of the true prevalence of growth restriction difficult, but by most definitions it occurs in 5% to 10% of pregnancies.

The risk of intrauterine growth restriction increases with the presence of maternal conditions that reduce placental perfusion (hypertension, preeclampsia, drug use, smoking) or those that reduce the nutrients available to the fetus (chronic renal disease, poor nutrition, inflammatory bowel disease). Abnormalities of placental implantation or function can result in significant reduction in nutrient flow to the fetus. The risk is also higher at the extremes of maternal age: For women less than 15 years old the rate of low birth weight is 13.6% compared with 7.3% for women between 25 and 29 years old. When multiple gestations are excluded, the rate for women older than 45 years is greater than 20%. Multifetal pregnancies, especially higher order multiples, are at increased risk for growth restrictions. In most cases of growth restriction, no specific cause is identified.

Growth-restricted infants are at risk for progressive deterioration of fetal status and intrauterine fetal demise (twofold increased risk). (There is an 8- to 10-fold increase in the risk of perinatal mortality: growth restriction is the second most important cause of perinatal morbidity after preterm birth.) Long-term physical and neurologic sequelae are common. The risk of adverse outcome is generally proportional to the severity of growth restriction present.

Overt signs of significant fetal growth restriction may be absent until a significant reduction in growth has occurred. (Physical examination of the mother may miss up to two-thirds of cases; ultrasonography can exclude or verify growth restriction in 90% and 80% of cases, respectively.) Signs suggestive of growth restriction include a discrepancy between the externally measured size and what would be expected for the gestational age. On ultrasonographic examination, the fetus will show measures of long bone growth or abdominal or head circumference that are discordant with each other or those expected for the anticipated gestational age. Oligohydramnios may also be present. The early establishment of a reliable estimated date of delivery is critical to the accurate detection of a decelerated rate of fetal growth. The most accurate diagnosis will also be based on serial examinations that provide information about the growth of the individual fetus.

Intrauterine growth restriction must be distinguished from constitutionally small-for-gestational-age infants, who are not at increased risk. Asymmetric restrictions in growth argue against a constitutional cause. Early intrauterine insults are more likely to result in symmetric growth restriction, whereas later insults result in asymmetry. Similarly, intrinsic factors generally cause symmetric restriction; extrinsic factors generally cause asymmetric restriction. Growth restriction

resulting from intrinsic fetal factors, such as aneuploidy, congenital malformations, or infection, carry a guarded prognosis.

When intrauterine growth restriction is suspected or documented, enhanced fetal assessment and antenatal fetal testing (including nonstress testing, biophysical profiles, and/or contraction stress tests) should be planned. Doppler velocimetry of the umbilical arteries has been demonstrated to be strongly predictive of fetal

death when reversed or absent end diastolic flow occurs in the presence of intrauterine growth restriction. Patients at risk because of maternal disease should have early assessment of fetal growth (biparietal diameter, head circumference, abdominal circumference, and femur length) with frequent remeasurement as the pregnancy progresses. This may need to be done as often as every 2 to 3 weeks in severe cases. Careful fetal monitoring during labor is indicated for these infants.

Causes

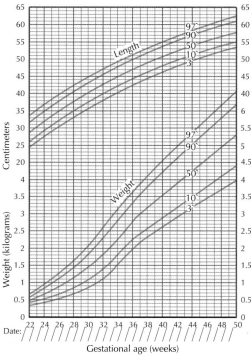

Maternal
Hypertension
Cardiovascular disease
Liver disease
Drugs
Inflammatory bowel disease
Hemoglobinopathy

Fetal
Congenital anomalies
Chromosomal abnormalities
Chronic fetal infection
Oligohydramnios

Placental
Placenta previa
Placental fibrosis
Placental infarction
Placentae abruptio
Chronic infection

Intrauterine growth restriction may occur in a symmetric or asymmetric manner. Evaluation of restriction is based on ultrasonic measurement of fetal head and abdominal circumferences compared with gestational age. Other antepartum tests are used to evaluate fetal health status.

Fetal-infant growth chart for preterm infants

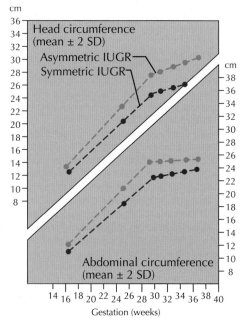

Plot growth in terms of completed weeks of gestation

Sources: Intrauterine weight—Kramer MS et al (ePediatr 2001): Length and head circumference—iklasson A et al (Acta Pediatr Scand 1991) and Beeby PJ et al (J Paediatr Child Health 1996): Postterm sections—CDC growth charts, 2000. The smoothing of the disjunction between the pre- and postterm sections generally occurs between 36 and 45 weeks.

Neonatal outcome

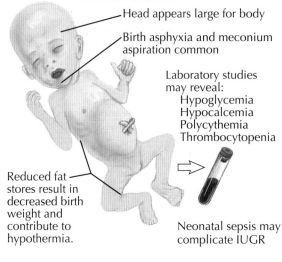

Head appears large for body

Birth asphyxia and meconium aspiration common

Laboratory studies may reveal:
Hypoglycemia
Hypocalcemia
Polycythemia
Thrombocytopenia

Reduced fat stores result in decreased birth weight and contribute to hypothermia.

Neonatal sepsis may complicate IUGR

Plate 12.40   Pregnancy

ERYTHROBLASTOSIS FETALIS (RH SENSITIZATION)

Isoimmunization of the mother to any dissimilar fetal blood group not possessed by the mother is possible. Historically the most common example is the Rh(D) factor. Erythroblastosis fetalis (hemolytic disease of the newborn) is characterized by sustained destruction of the fetal erythrocytes by specific maternal antibodies (immunoglobulin G, IgG), which cross the placenta to the fetus. What was once a common cause for fetal death has largely been eradicated by prophylactic maternal administration of immune globulin against the Rh(D) factor to those at risk. Despite this, D alloimmunization with serious sequelae in offspring still occurs.

Human red blood cells contain a complex group of inherited antigens, one of which is the Rhesus CDE antigen system, which consists of over 50 antigens. The genes for the CDE blood groups are inherited separately from the ABO groups and are located on the short arm of chromosome 1. One of the more important antigens of this group is Rh(D) factor. About 85% of all individuals are Rh(D)-positive and 15% are Rh(D)-negative. Any process that exposes the woman to blood carrying the D antigen including blood transfusion, miscarriage, ectopic or normal pregnancy, trauma during pregnancy, amniocentesis, and others can result in anti-Rh agglutinins being formed. The IgG antibodies can cross the placenta into the fetal circulation and result in the destruction of the Rh-positive fetal blood. Other isoimmunizations (most frequently Kell or Duffy antigens) can also result in similar effects on the fetus.

The three principal features of the disease are hemolytic anemia, icterus, and hydrops. The predominance of one or another of these manifestations in a given case depends mainly upon the degree of immunity in the mother's blood. When antibody titers are ≤1:8, no clinical intervention is required. When titers are ≥1:16 in albumin or 1:32 by an indirect Coombs test, amniocentesis, umbilical cord blood sampling, or Doppler velocimetry of the middle cerebral arteries should be considered. In severely affected fetuses, intrauterine transfusion may be required to prevent the full spectrum of hemolytic disease and hydrops.

In hydrops fetalis, the most severe form of the disease, the fetus often is born dead and macerated. Fluids accumulate in the serous cavities and body tissues. In severe cases marked hemolytic anemia may develop. The nucleated red cells may far outnumber the white blood cells. The viscera present many foci of extramedullary erythropoiesis, which is most characteristically seen in the lungs where the blood vessels in alveolar septa are filled with large erythroblasts.

In less severe cases the infant is born alive with less edema and milder anemia. Because the placenta is no longer available to transport bilirubin away, within a few hours icterus may develop as the red cells are destroyed, liberating hemoglobin for transformation into bilirubin more rapidly than the pigment can be eliminated by the liver. Icterus and anemia may gradually subside or may increase to cause death within a few days. In other cases, with fewer agglutinins in the infant's blood, the icterus may be mild, and only anemia (congenital anemia) may be manifested clinically. Most of these cases recover when exchange transfusion therapy is applied.

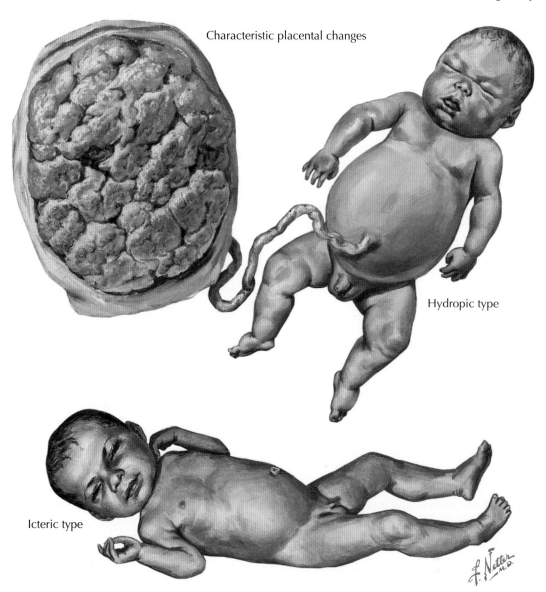
Characteristic placental changes

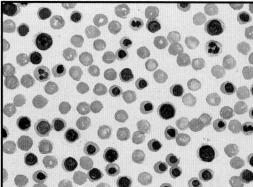
Hydropic type

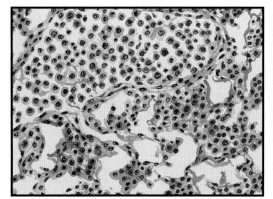
Icteric type

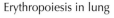
Erythropoiesis in lung

Blood smear showing erythroblastosis

In severe cases, the placenta is very large, excessively lobulated, pale, and edematous. Microscopically, the villi are swollen, edematous, and generously covered with trophoblasts, including occasional cytotrophoblastic cells even at term. The fetal blood is loaded with erythroblasts and other nucleated red blood cells. Intraplacental clots are frequent.

All patients should have their Rh type established and be tested for isoimmunization at the first prenatal visit. The gel microcolumn assay has gained widespread acceptance to replace the indirect Coombs test for this purpose. Those who are Rh-negative should receive D immune globulin after delivery, amniocentesis, fetal demise, miscarriage, ectopic pregnancy, or any other time exposure to Rh-positive cells may have occurred. Prophylactic administration between 28 and 30 weeks of gestation is also standard. With prophylaxis, the risk of isoimmunization is estimated to be 0.3%.

Plate 12.41

Reproductive System: VOLUME 1

Large, pale, boggy placenta

Macerated fetus

SYPHILIS

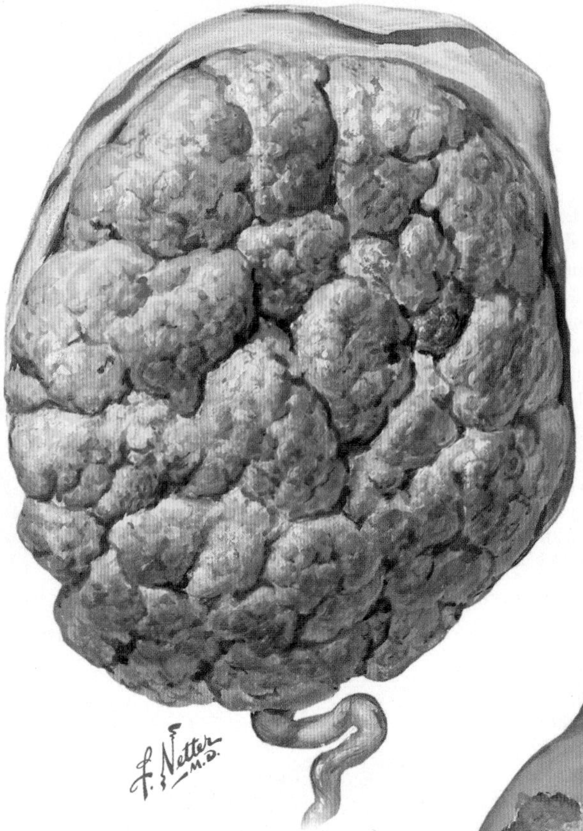

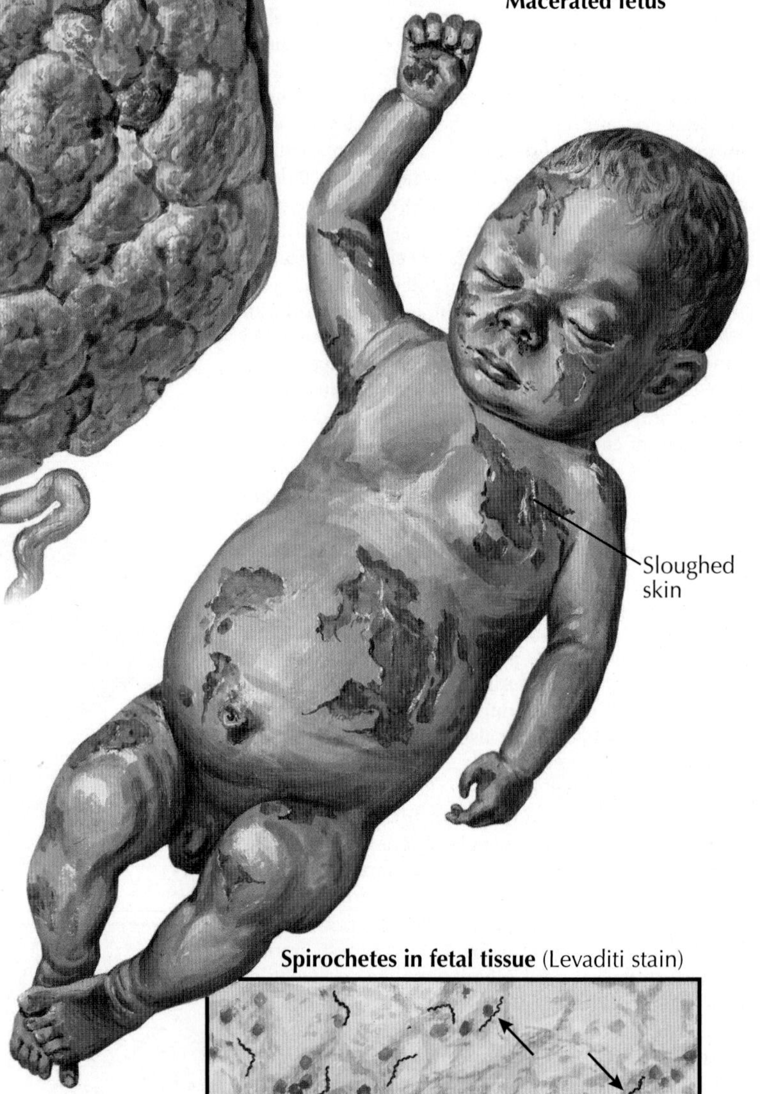

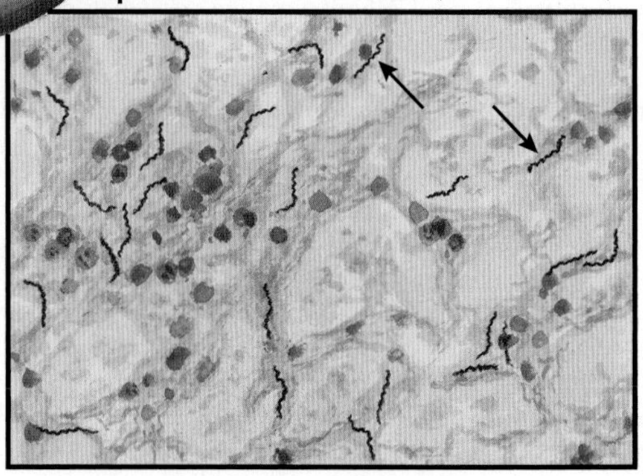

In many geographic regions, syphilis is still the most common cause of fetal death in the later months of gestation. In many developed countries, the number of primary and secondary syphilis cases has risen dramatically as a result of illicit drug use and the exchange of drugs for sex. Although less common in developed countries, the incidence of syphilis is high and increasing in many developing countries (and in the transitional economies of Eastern Europe and the former Soviet Union), particularly where HIV/AIDS is common. In the United States the rate of congenital syphilis is 0.33 cases per 100,000. Early maternal syphilis infection up to 4 years before pregnancy is associated with pregnancy loss (21%), preterm delivery (6%), and neonatal death (9%). Of infants born to mothers with primary or secondary syphilis, up to 50% will be premature, stillborn, or die in the neonatal period. In many cases, surviving children are born with congenital defects some of which may not be apparent for years.

The fetus is infected through the placenta from the mother. When an infected fetus is born alive, the symptomatology of congenital syphilis soon becomes manifest. Screening in the first trimester with nontreponemal tests such as rapid plasma reagin or Venereal Disease Research Laboratory test combined with confirmation of reactive individuals with treponemal tests such as the fluorescent treponemal antibody absorption assay is a cost-effective strategy. Those at risk should be retested in the third trimester. Because the development of automated treponemal enzyme immunoassays (a direct test that requires less manpower), many US laboratories have begun using a new algorithm for screening and diagnosis of syphilis: the use of treponemal-specific tests as first-line diagnostic screening, referred to as a "reverse" screening algorithm.

A syphilitic fetus, born in the fetal stage by abortion or later as a mature infant, is usually shorter than expected or otherwise growth restricted. When delivered alive or shortly after death in utero, the skin appears dry, brittle, and sometimes a lusterless gray. Vesicles may be found in various body regions. Rapid maceration, however, takes place when, as happens frequently, the fetus dies and remains in the uterus for a period of time, which may vary greatly. These external lesions should always prompt an autopsy, which will ascertain the diagnosis by the characteristic changes detectable in the internal organs. Inflammatory and degenerative changes are usually present in the liver, lungs, spleen, kidneys, and pancreas. Most characteristic are the bone changes, where the finding of an osteochondritis, with signs of disturbed ossification and deranged cartilage tissue, is considered pathognomonic. Efforts to demonstrate *Treponema pallidum (Spirochaeta pallida)* in the internal organs or bone are seldom successful in fetuses aborted during the first half of pregnancy. In later stages, particularly when the fetus is partially autolyzed, the viscera are usually flooded with organisms.

Sloughed skin

Spirochetes in fetal tissue (Levaditi stain)

No part of the placenta or fetal membranes seems to be impervious to the invasion of the *Treponema pallidum.* In untreated cases the placenta is enlarged, excessively lobulated, pale, and edematous. The cord and membranes show discoloration and other postmortem changes comparable to those in the macerated fetus. Microscopically, one finds diffuse inflammation of the placenta, increased fibrous stroma in the bloodless villi, and marked proliferation of the intima in the fetal vessels. Although these lesions are characteristic of syphilis, the only conclusive proof of the disease is the finding of the *Treponema* in the tissues (Levaditi stain).

In determining appropriate therapy, the stage of maternal infection, the length of fetal exposure, and physiologic changes in pregnancy that can affect the pharmacokinetics of antibiotics must all be considered. These decisions may be further complicated by allergy to penicillin or immunocompromise (HIV). Even with appropriate treatment, fetal infection may still occur in up to 14% of cases.

Plate 12.42

Pregnancy

PUERPERAL INFECTION

Puerperal infection generally refers to an infection of the genital tract in the postpartum period. For centuries, puerperal infection was the leading cause of maternal death, although this has changed dramatically with the advent of antibiotics. Maternal death rates associated with infection account for approximately 0.6 maternal deaths per 100,000 live births in developed countries—about 2% of maternal deaths there but 10% to 12% in resource-challenged settings. Endometritis is the most common form of postpartum infection, though other sources of postpartum infections include postsurgical wound infections, perineal cellulitis, mastitis, respiratory complications from anesthesia or underlying pulmonary disease such as asthma or obstructive lung disease, retained products of conception, urinary tract infections, and septic pelvic phlebitis. Overall, postpartum infection is estimated to affect 1% to 3% of normal vaginal deliveries, 5% to 15% of scheduled cesarean deliveries, and 15% to 20% of unscheduled cesarean deliveries.

The organisms responsible for the vast majority of puerperal infections are the anaerobic and aerobic nonhemolytic varieties of streptococci. These organisms are usually present in the birth canal, becoming pathogenic when carried to the uterine cavity during or after delivery.

Postpartum endometritis is typically a polymicrobial infection (70% of cases) involving a mixture of two to three aerobes and anaerobes from the genital tract. In most cases of endometritis, the bacteria responsible are those that normally reside in the bowel, vagina, perineum, and cervix. Commonly isolated organisms include *Ureaplasma urealyticum*, *Peptostreptococcus*, *Gardnerella vaginalis*, *Bacteroides bivius*, and group B streptococci. Other, though less frequent, organisms causing puerperal infection are *Staphylococcus albus* (*Micrococcus pyogenes*), anaerobic organisms, and the colon bacillus (*Escherichia coli*). *Chlamydia* has also been associated with late-onset postpartum endometritis.

Inadequate asepsis during labor and delivery, repeated vaginal examinations, and the use of contaminated materials are avoidable factors in the pathogenesis. Coitus late in pregnancy also has been considered to help disseminate inoculation and infection. Blood loss and trauma are considered the most frequent predisposing causes of puerperal infection. Trauma creates a portal of entry and produces a favorable environment for the development of virulent bacteria. Prolonged labor, particularly with early rupture of the membranes, retention of placental tissues, and major vaginal procedures producing vaginal and cervical lacerations, may initiate or foster puerperal infection.

The pathologic findings in puerperal infection are similar to those of any other wound infection. Following delivery of the fetus and placenta, the endometrium favors bacterial growth. Infection of vaginal lacerations may occur, but these are less frequent than endometritis. The appearance of the endometrium and its discharge vary according to the infecting organisms. It usually appears necrotic and yellowish green but may be black from decomposed blood. The inflammatory process may remain in the uterine cavity, spread to the parametrial tissues, or become widely disseminated. From the endometrium, the inflammatory process may extend along the uterine and other pelvic veins, resulting in

pelvic thrombophlebitis. Thrombophlebitis of the leg veins may also be seen. Extension of the inflammation through the lymphatic channels to the parametrial tissues and peritoneum results in parametritis, pelvic cellulitis, and peritonitis. Distant spread to lungs or liver may occur in the form of septic emboli and therewith cause septic infarcts and abscesses.

The diagnosis is usually made without difficulty. Fever occurring in the postpartum period, accompanied by lower abdominal tenderness, should be considered

to be a puerperal infection until proved otherwise. Extreme abdominal and uterine tenderness together with rigidity of the abdominal walls and absence of peristalsis are indicative of generalized peritonitis. The character and odor of the lochia may help in making the diagnosis and sometimes in recognizing the organisms. Some infections, notably those caused by group A β-hemolytic streptococci, may be associated with scanty, odorless lochia. Maternal mortality is highest when infection develops within 4 days after delivery.

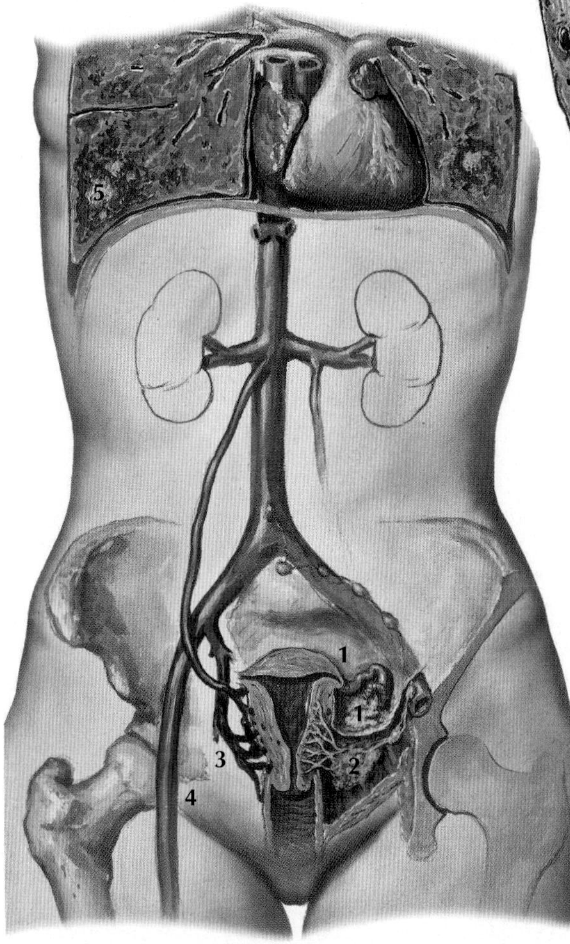

Septic endometritis

Dissemination of septic endometritis:
1. Peritonitis
2. Parametritis (via lymphatics)
3. Pelvic thrombophlebitis
4. Femoral thrombophlebitis
5. Pulmonary infarct or abscess (septic embolus)

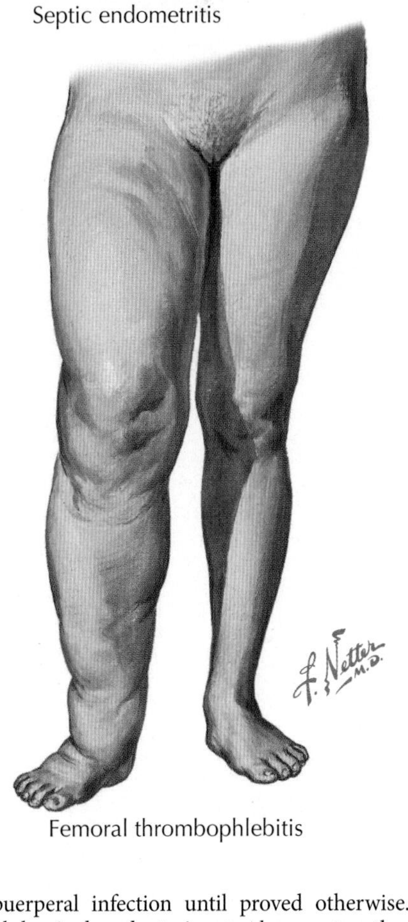

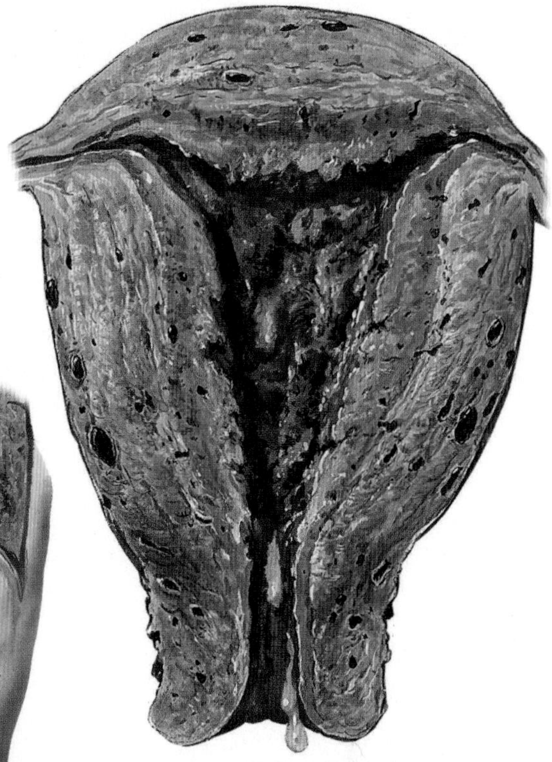

Femoral thrombophlebitis

BREAST

Plate 13.1

Reproductive System: VOLUME 1

Anterolateral dissection

Pectoralis major muscle (deep to pectoral fascia)

Axillary tail (of Spence)

Serratus anterior muscle

External oblique muscle

Suspensory ligaments of breast (Cooper)

Areolar glands

Areola

Nipple

Lactiferous ducts

Lactiferous sinus

Fat

Gland lobules

POSITION AND STRUCTURE

The breast is shown in its partially dissected state in the upper part of the plate and below in sagittal section. The size of the breast is variable, but in most instances it extends from the second rib through the sixth rib and from the sternum to the anterior axillary line, with an axillary tail in the outer and upper portions (axillary tail of Spence), which can be palpated along the outer border of the pectoralis major muscle. The mammary tissue lies directly over the pectoralis major muscle and is separated from the outer fascia of this muscle by a layer of adipose tissue, which is continuous with the fatty stroma of the gland itself.

Fatty deposits surround and intermix with the glandular elements and make up a significant portion of the breast structure, providing much of its bulk and shape. The ratio of fatty to glandular tissue varies among individuals and with the stage of life; with menopause, the relative amount of fatty tissue increases as the glandular tissue declines. A rich vascular and lymphatic network (discussed subsequently) supplies the breasts.

The sensory innervation of the breast follows the normal distribution of the dermatomes and is mainly derived from the anterolateral and anteromedial branches of thoracic intercostal nerves T_3 to T_5. Supraclavicular nerves from the lower fibers of the cervical plexus also provide innervation to the upper and lateral portions of the breast. Sensory enervation of the nipple is from the lateral cutaneous branch of T_4.

The center of the dome-shaped, fully developed breast in the adult female is marked by the areola mammae, a circular, pigmented skin area from 1.5 to 2.5 cm in diameter. The surface of the areola appears rough because of large, somewhat modified sebaceous glands, the glands of Montgomery, which are located directly beneath the skin in the thin subcutaneous tissue layer. The fatty secretion of these glands is said to lubricate the nipple. Bundles of smooth muscles in the areolar tissue serve to stiffen the nipple for a better grasp by the suckling infant.

The nipple or mammary papilla is elevated a few millimeters above the breast and contains 15 to 20 lactiferous ducts surrounded by fibromuscular tissue and covered by wrinkled skin. Partly within this compartment of the nipple and partly below its base, these ducts expand to form the short sinus lactiferi or ampullae in which the milk may be stored. These ampullae are the continuation of the mammary ducts, which extend radially from the nipple toward the chest wall, and from them sprout variable numbers of secondary tubules. These end in epithelial masses forming the lobules or acinar structures of the breast. The number of tubules and the size of the acinar

Sagittal section

Clavicle

2nd rib

Pectoralis major muscle

Pectoral fascia

Intercostal muscles

Intercostal vessels and nerve

Lung

6th rib

Suspensory ligaments of breast (Cooper)

Lactiferous duct

Lactiferous sinus

Gland lobules

Fat (subcutaneous tissue layer)

structures vary greatly in different individuals and at different periods in life. In general, the terminal tubules and acinar structures are most numerous during the childbearing period and reach their full physiologic development only during pregnancy and lactation. These epithelial structures constitute collectively the parenchyma of the gland. The stroma is composed of a mixture of fibrous and fatty tissue, and, in the absence of pregnancy and lactation, the relative amounts of fatty and

fibrous tissue determine the size and consistency of the breast.

The enveloping fascia of the breast is continuous with the pectoral fascia. It subdivides the glands into lobules and sends strands into the overlying skin, which, in the upper hemisphere, are known as the *suspensory ligaments of Cooper*. Because these strands are not taut, they allow for the natural motion of the breast but result in breast ptosis as these ligaments relax with age.

Plate 13.2

Breast

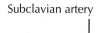

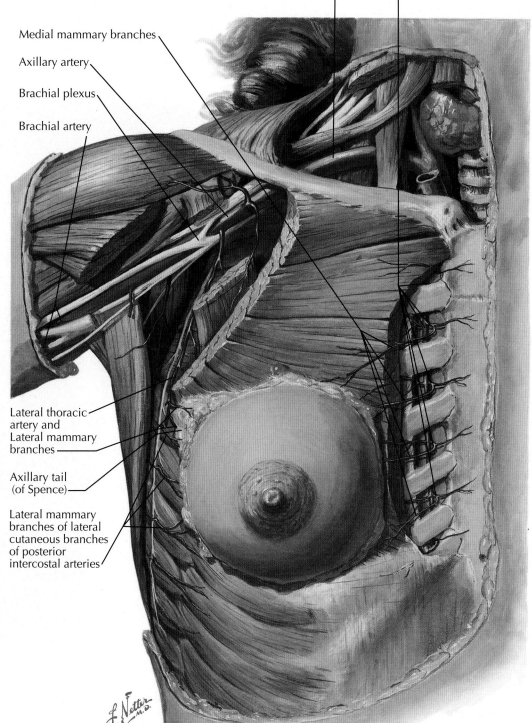

Internal thoracic artery and
its perforating branches

Subclavian artery

Medial mammary branches

Axillary artery

Brachial plexus

Brachial artery

Lateral thoracic
artery and
Lateral mammary
branches

Axillary tail
(of Spence)

Lateral mammary
branches of lateral
cutaneous branches
of posterior
intercostal arteries

BLOOD SUPPLY

The sources of the abundant vascular supply of the mammary gland are the descending thoracic aorta, from which the posterior intercostal arteries branch off; the subclavian artery, from which the internal mammary artery arises; and the axillary artery, serving the mammary gland through the lateral thoracic and sometimes through another branch, the external mammary artery. Additional blood may be supplied by branches from the thoracodorsal artery and the thoracoacromial artery, which is a short trunk that arises from the forepart of the axillary artery, its origin being generally overlapped by the upper edge of the pectoralis minor.

The intercostal branches of the internal mammary artery, the thoracic portion of which lies behind the cartilage of the six upper ribs just outside the parietal layer of the pleura, supply the medial aspect of the gland. The lateral cutaneous branches of the third, fourth, and fifth aortic intercostal arteries enter the gland laterally. The lateral cutaneous branches of the intercostal arteries penetrate the muscles of the side of the chest and then divide into anterior and posterior rami, of which only the anterior rami reach the mammary gland. The branches from the lateral thoracic artery, which descends along the lower border of the minor pectoral muscle, approach the gland from behind in the region of the upper outer quadrant. One of these branches (more developed in females than the other branches) is the external mammary artery, which turns around the edge of the pectoralis major muscle, where it could be seen in the picture if the breast were lifted up. An extensive network of anastomoses exists between the lateral thoracic artery and those vessels deriving from the internal mammary artery; the latter also anastomoses with the intercostal arteries, so that two or even three of the main sources supply many parts of the gland. The ramifications of all three main arteries form a circular plexus around the areola, which ensures the blood supply of the nipple and areola. The breast skin depends on the subdermal plexus for its blood supply. This plexus is in communication with underlying deeper vessels supplying the breast parenchyma, where a second plexus from the same main vessels is formed in the deeper regions of the gland.

A number of variations of this vascular distribution exist and should be considered to avoid the danger of necrosis; for example, in circular incisions around the nipple. The rich blood supply of the breast allows for a variety of surgical procedures, therapeutic or cosmetic,

to be performed while ensuring the viability of the skin flaps and breast parenchyma after surgery. This advantage can become a disadvantage by providing a point of systemic spread for infection or malignancy.

The veins follow the course of the arteries. Venous drainage is primarily into the axillary vein, with some blood draining into the internal thoracic vein. The axillary vein has an irregular anatomy, which complicates surgery under the arm. The surface veins encircle the nipple and carry blood to the internal mammary, axillary,

and intercostal veins, and to the lungs. These connections can allow breast cancer cells to travel to the lungs via these surface veins to form metastatic tumors. The intercostal veins join a complex network of vertebral veins in and around the spine, providing an additional path for cancer to spread to bone.

The veins draining the breast parenchyma are subject to inflammation and thrombosis as in other areas in the body. This can result in Mondor disease and thrombophlebitis, respectively.

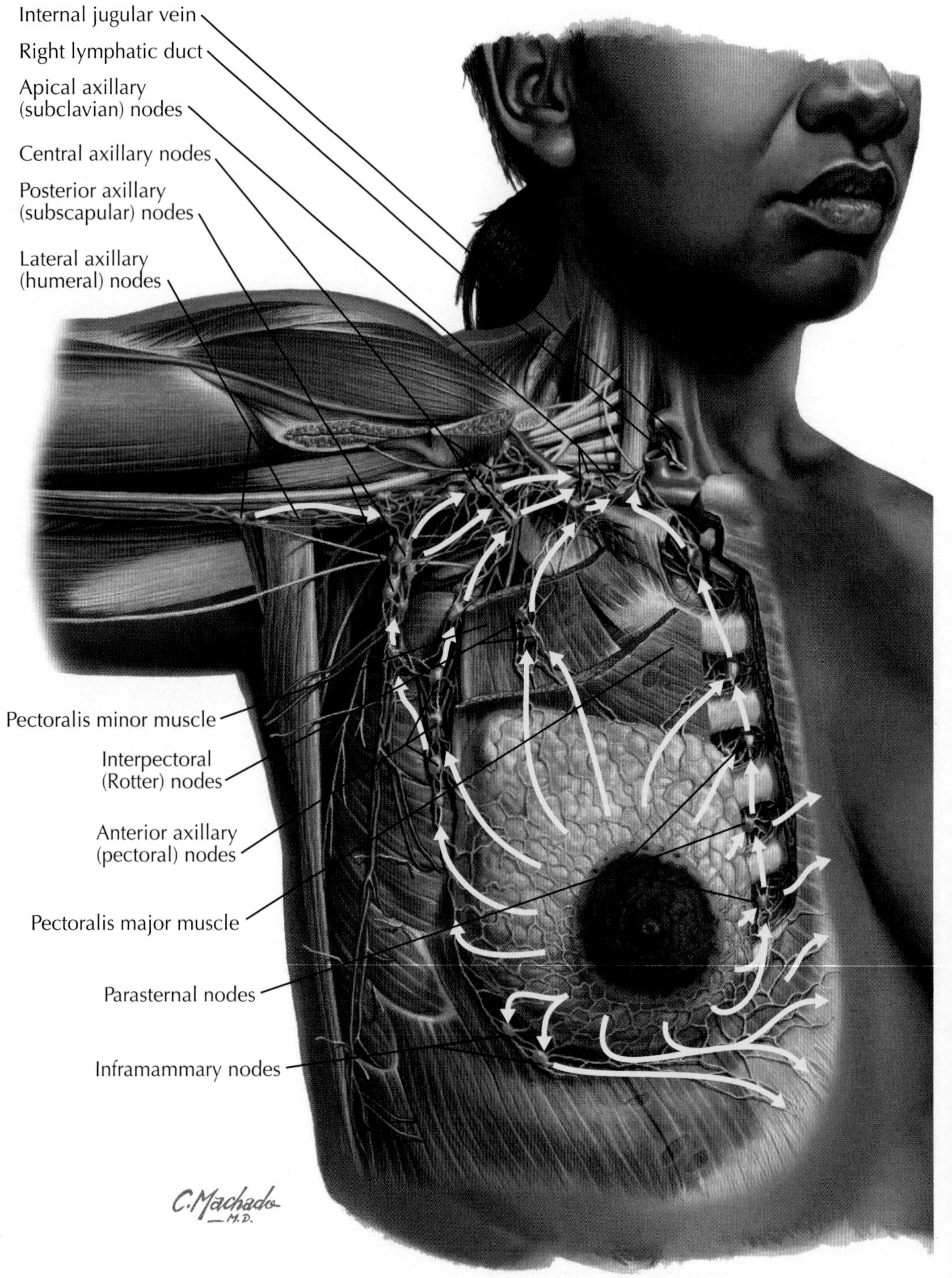

Plate 13.3

Reproductive System: VOLUME 1

Internal jugular vein

Right lymphatic duct

Apical axillary
(subclavian) nodes

Central axillary nodes

Posterior axillary
(subscapular) nodes

Lateral axillary
(humeral) nodes

Pectoralis minor muscle

Interpectoral
(Rotter) nodes

Anterior axillary
(pectoral) nodes

Pectoralis major muscle

Parasternal nodes

Inframammary nodes

C. Machado
_M.D._

LYMPHATIC DRAINAGE

The lymphatic drainage of the breast is complex. The mammary gland has a very rich network of lymph vessels, which is separated into two planes, the superficial or subareolar plexus of lymphatics and the deep or fascial plexus. Both originate in the interlobular spaces and in the walls of the lactiferous ducts. The lymph nodes that drain the breast are not linked in a straight line; instead, they are staggered, variable, and fixed within fat pads. This arrangement complicates lymph node removal during breast cancer surgery.

Collecting lymph from the central parts of the gland, the skin, areola, and nipple, most of the superficial plexus drains laterally toward the axilla, passing first to the anterior pectoral group of nodes, which are often referred to as the *low axillary group of glands*. The anterior pectoral nodes, four to six in number, lie along the border of the pectoral muscles adjacent to the lateral thoracic artery. The drainage passes thence to the central axillary nodes, which lie along the axillary vein, or to the midaxillary nodes. From there, the drainage is to the subclavian nodes at the apex of the axilla where the axillary and subclavian veins join. The axilla contains a varying number of nodes, usually between 30 and 60. Approximately 75% of the breast lymphatic drainage goes to these axillary regional nodes.

The deep fascial plexus extends through the pectoral muscles to Rotter lymph nodes, situated beneath the pectoralis major muscle, and thence to the subclavian nodes. This is known as *Groszman's pathway*. The rest of the fascial plexus, for the most part, extends medially along the internal mammary artery via the internal mammary nodes to the mediastinal nodes. Other paths of lymphatic drainage proceed from the lower and medial portions of the breast. One of these is the paramammary route of Gerota, through the abdominal lymphatics to the liver or subdiaphragmatic nodes. Another is a cross-mammary pathway, via superficial lymphatics to the opposite breast and opposite axilla. Metastases from one breast across the midline to the other breast or chest wall occur occasionally via this pathway. From the lower medial portion of the breast, some lymphatics of the fascial group drain, passing beneath the sternum, to the anterior mediastinal nodes situated in front of the aorta. Lymphatic drainage to the intercostal glands, which are located posteriorly along the vertebral column, and to subpectoral and subdiaphragmatic areas may also occur.

Lymph nodes play a central role in the spread of breast cancer. The axillary lymph nodes are particularly important, as they are among the first places that cancer is likely to metastasize from the breast. This cluster of lymph nodes is often referred to as level I nodes. (Level II nodes are located underneath the pectoralis minor muscle, and level III nodes are found near the center of the collarbone.) Other metastatic routes include lymphatics adjacent to the internal mammary vessels, allowing direct spread into the mediastinum.

Lymph drainage usually moves toward the most adjacent group of nodes: this is the basis for the concept of sentinel node mapping in breast cancer. In most instances, breast cancer spreads in a predictable way within the axillary lymph node chain based on the location of the primary tumor and the associated sentinel nodes. However, lymphatic metastases from one specific area of the breast may be found in any or all of the groups of regional nodes. Despite this observation, the concept of using a sentinel node to detect spread is still useful because in only about 3% of these females does the positive node occur outside of the axilla.

Plate 13.4

Breast

DEVELOPMENTAL STAGES

In a human newborn at birth, in the female as well as in the male, the mammary glands have developed sufficiently so that they appear as distinct hemispheroidal elevations, palpable as movable soft masses. This is especially prominent in postterm infants. Histologically, a number of branching channels with layers of lining cells and plugs of basal cells at their ends, the future milk ducts and glandular lobules, respectively, can easily be recognized histologically. In a great number of infants an everted nipple is observed, and in about 10% a greatly enlarged gland can be palpated, a condition that received the unfortunate name of mastitis neonatorum, though no signs of inflammation exist. These early glandular structures may produce a milklike secretion, the "witch's milk," starting 2 or 3 days after birth. All these neonatal phenomena in the breast are the result of the very intensive, maternal estrogen–driven developmental processes in the last stages of intrauterine life. The changes subside within the first 2 to 3 weeks of life. It is during this period that the breast undergoes marked involutional changes leading to the quiescent stage, which is characteristic of infancy and childhood. During these periods, the male and female glands consist of a few branching rudimentary ducts lined by flattened epithelium, surrounded by collagenous connective tissue.

For most girls, the first sign of puberty is usually the appearance of breast budding. In the United States this early breast change begins at an average age of 10.3 (±1.1, typically 8–13) years of age. The age of thelarche has been gradually decreasing for most girls (likely driven by nutrition), with some racial groups experiencing grater reductions than others, whereas the age of menarche has declined to a lesser extent.

With the onset of puberty and during adolescence, follicular ripening in the ovaries, in response to follicle-stimulating hormone of the anterior pituitary gland, is accompanied by an increased output of estrogen. In response to the latter, the mammary ducts elongate and their lining epithelium reduplicates and proliferates at the ends of the mammary tubules, forming the sprouts of the future lobules. This growth of ductal epithelium is accompanied by growth of periductal fibrous tissue, which is largely responsible for the increasing size and firmness of the adolescent female gland. During this period, the areola and nipple also grow and become pigmented.

With the onset of maturity—that is, when ovulation occurs and the progesterone-secreting corpora lutea are formed—the second stage of mammary development occurs. It is essentially concerned with the formation of the lobules and acinar structures. Although in the adult female, progesterone always asserts its influence when estrogen is simultaneously present, overwhelming experimental evidence indicates that this beginning unfolding of the lobules is a specific effect of progesterone. This

| Childhood | Puberty | Maturity |

gives the mammary gland the characteristic lobular structure found during the childbearing years. This differentiation into a lobular gland is finished approximately 1 to 1½ years after the first menstruation, but further acinar development continues in proportion to the intensity of the hormonal stimuli during each menstrual cycle and especially during pregnancies. Fat deposition and formation of fibrous stroma contribute to the increasing size of the gland in the adolescent period.

The predictable sequence of breast development brought on during adolescence forms one part of the sexual maturation scale (Tanner staging) that is used to assess the degree and sequence of pubertal development. In 1969 Marshall and Tanner defined five stages of breast development and pubic hair development that are combined and called Tanner, or pubertal, stages 1 through 5. For most girls, breast budding is the earliest sign of puberty and menarche is the latest.

Plate 13.5

Reproductive System: VOLUME 1

FUNCTIONAL CHANGES AND LACTATION

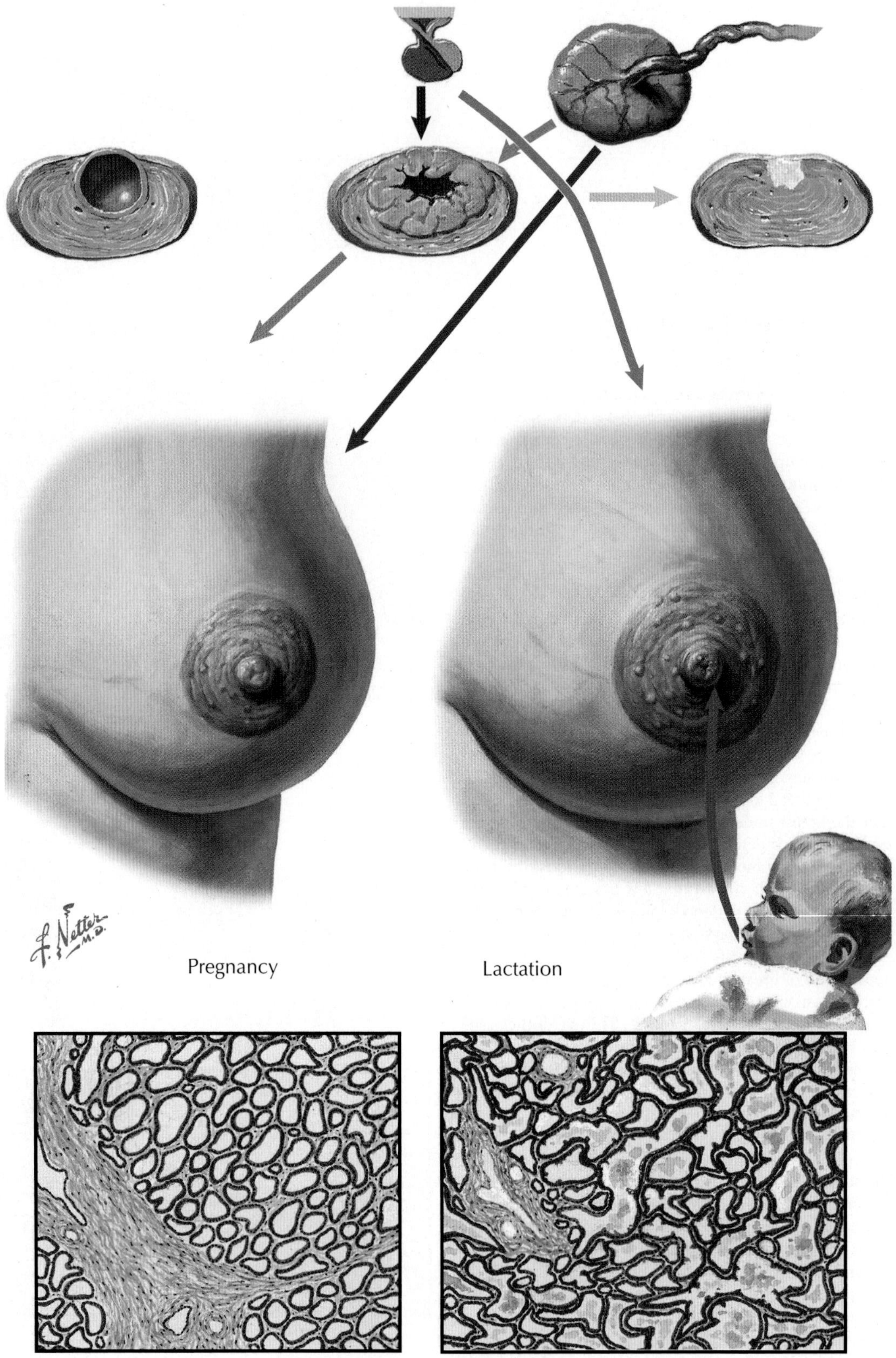

The maturational changes in hormones from the anterior pituitary gland and ovary are major factors in the development and functioning of the mammary gland. Follicle-stimulating and luteinizing hormones are indispensable for the production of ovarian estrogen and progesterone, which, in turn, control mammary gland development. These are necessary but not sufficient to prepare the breast for lactation.

The mammary gland of a nonpregnant female is inadequately prepared for secretory activity. Only during pregnancy do those changes normally occur that make milk production possible. In the first trimester of pregnancy, the terminal tubules sprouting from the mammary ducts proliferate to provide a maximum number of epithelial elements for future acinar formation. In the midtrimester, the reduplicated terminal tubules are grouped together to form large lobules. Their lumina begin to dilate, and the acinar structures thus formed are lined by cuboidal epithelium; occasional acini contain small amounts of colostrum secretion. In the last third of pregnancy, the acini formed in early and midpregnancy are progressively dilated. The high levels of circulating estrogens and progesterone during pregnancy are responsible for these alterations in the breast.

During pregnancy, as estrogen levels increase, there is a parallel hypertrophy and hyperplasia of the pituitary lactotrophs. An increase in prolactin occurs soon after implantation, concomitant with the increase in circulating estrogen. Circulating levels of prolactin steadily increase throughout pregnancy, peaking at about 200 ng/mL during the third trimester. This rise is in parallel with the continued increase in circulating estrogen levels over this time. Despite these elevated prolactin levels, lactation does not occur because estrogen inhibits the action of prolactin on the breast (most likely blocking interaction with the prolactin receptor).

Following childbirth, active secretion begins in the now maximally dilated acinar structures as a result of the stimulation by prolactin from the anterior pituitary gland and by the nursing of the infant. A day or two following delivery of the placenta, both estrogen levels and prolactin levels decline rapidly and lactation is initiated. Prolactin levels reach basal concentrations after 2 to 3 weeks in females who do not breastfeed. In nursing females, basal levels of prolactin decline to the nonpregnant range within 6 months after parturition; after each act of suckling, prolactin increases markedly, though transiently.

Lactation, starting 3 to 4 days after delivery, is stimulated and maintained through the mechanical act of sucking. In addition to prompting a pulse in prolactin, stimulation of the areola causes the secretion of oxytocin, which is responsible for the letdown reflex and ductal contraction that expels the milk. Therefore it is through these feedback mechanisms that suckling ensures further milk production.

Prolactin has not been shown to affect the macro- or microscopic changes in the gland. Its only function is to stimulate milk secretion after the tissues have

Pregnancy

Lactation

been previously adequately prepared (by estrogen and progestin). During consistent breastfeeding, follicular ripening and ovulation are suppressed for approximately 6 months.

The secretion of true milk takes place in the epithelial lining of the dilated acini by cuboidal or columnar cells with nuclei at their bases or tips. This epithelium rests on a narrow band of connective tissue that encloses thin-walled capillaries. Secretory globules and desquamated epithelial cells distend the acini and their afferent

channels. During the height of lactation, milk secretion and its storage account for one-fifth to one-third of the breast volume.

Nipple and breast stimulation can also increase prolactin levels in the nonpregnant female. Prolactin levels normally rise following ingestion of the noonday meal and may increase in response to exercise, sleep, and stress. For these reasons, prolactin levels normally fluctuate throughout the day, with maximal levels observed during nighttime sleep and in the early afternoon.

Plate 13.6

Breast

POLYTHELIA, POLYMASTIA, HYPERTROPHY

Congenital anomalies of the breast, such as agenesis or amastia, aplasia, or the absence of nipple and/or areola, are extremely rare. (Athelia or amastia is sometimes associated with Poland syndrome, consisting of absent chest wall muscles, absence of ribs 2–5, and deformities of hands or vertebrae.) An increase in the number of mammae or of nipples only is encountered somewhat more frequently. Both these conditions find ready explanation in the embryologic development of the breast. During the 6th to the 12th week of fetal life, the mammary glands first develop as solid down growths of the epidermis that extend into the mesenchyme from the axilla to the inguinal regions—the milk lines. Later, these ridges disappear, except in the pectoral area where the normal breast develops.

Accessory or supernumerary nipples (polythelia) occur in about 1% of males and 2% of females. These cases are sporadic; although familial polythelia is recognized, it is extremely rare. Most supernumerary nipples resemble a mole or birthmark and are only recognizable because of their anatomic location. Most often the supernumerary nipples are found 5 or 6 cm below the normal pair and toward the midline. They are usually not associated with significant amounts of underlying mammary tissue. Supernumerary nipples have been associated with an increased risk of genitourinary abnormalities, sporadic reports of malignancies, segmentation defect of the vertebrae, and other developmental abnormalities.

The accessory nipples without accessory mammary tissue are found anywhere in the course of the milk lines of the embryo. In the adult, this extends from the axillary to the inguinal regions. In the regions below the breast, the milk line runs medially to the normal nipple; above the breast it runs laterally toward each axilla. Supernumerary mammary glands (polymastia) situated laterally are more apt to be of considerable size and to undergo normal lactation compared with those situated medially. Bilateral axillary breasts that are of small size may develop during pregnancy and undergo lactation. They occur in approximately 1% to 2% of females of European descent and 5% to 6% of Asian females. Accessory breast tissue has been classified into eight levels of completeness from a simple patch of hair to a milk-bearing breast in miniature. This classification is based on the presence of glandular and fat tissue, a nipple, an areola, or tufts of hair.

Aberrant mammary tissue in the axilla without nipple formation is more prone to malignant change than is a supernumerary breast, in which the frequency of tumor occurrence is seemingly the same as with a normal single breast. Either benign or malignant tumors can occur in supernumerary or aberrant tissue.

Mammary hypertrophy is a common anomaly of the breast and affects both sexes. In females, the major forms of mammary hypertrophy are precocious or infantile hypertrophy and virginal or gravid hypertrophy

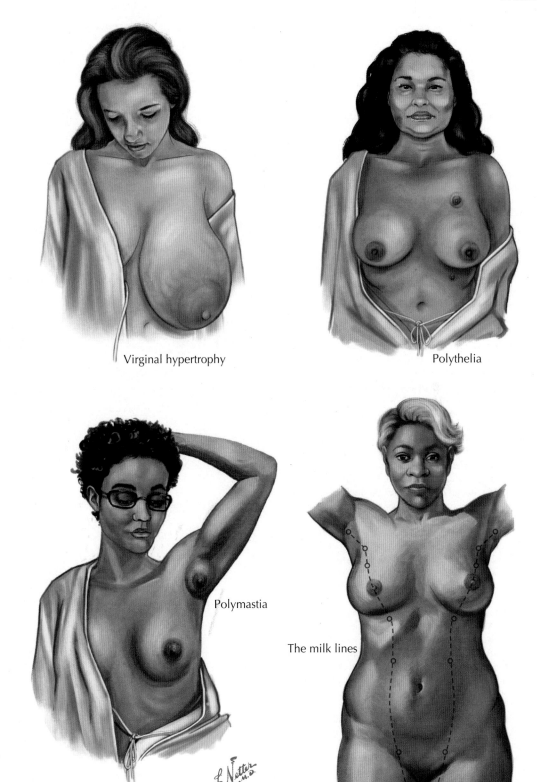

Virginal hypertrophy

Polythelia

Polymastia

The milk lines

occurring, respectively, in adolescent or pregnant females. Precocious mammary hypertrophy is associated with endocrine disturbances of the ovary. It is bilaterally symmetric and rarely of a marked degree. Virginal and gravid hypertrophies are of unknown origin and may be bilateral or unilateral, and the affected breast may grow to enormous size. The enlarging organs are composed of increased amounts of fibrous stroma with hypertrophied ducts, associated at times with lobular formation. The enlargement, once formed,

persists. When this type of hypertrophy occurs in teenage girls, it can have a deeply disturbing effect on a teenager's self-image and social development. The only effective treatment is reductive mammoplasty.

Some degree of asymmetry of breast development is common, with roughly 3% of patient examinations notable for asymmetric volume differences relative to the contralateral breast. This asymmetry represented a benign, normal variation unless an associated palpable abnormality is present.

Plate 13.7

Reproductive System: VOLUME 1

GYNECOMASTIA

Some degree of mammary hypertrophy is normally found in the male breast during adolescence. In two-thirds of all boys between the ages of 14 and 17 years, a button-shaped plaque of mammary tissue is palpated beneath the nipple. This is known as the *puberty node*. Although gynecomastia is usually bilateral, it can be unilateral. Normally, this involutes before the age of 21. Rarely, this adolescent growth of tissue may be two or three times its normal size and may be persistent. Sometimes it has been found so discrete and firm that the observers classified the enlargement as a benign fibroadenoma. Fat deposition without glandular proliferation is termed pseudogynecomastia.

Gynecomastia most frequently happens in newborn, pubertal, and older males. On palpation, the enlarged mammary gland may be the seat of increased tissue, both mammary and adipose, feeling like the normal female breast. Often a discrete, firm mass is felt, which is composed microscopically of increased amounts of periductal connective tissue surrounding mammary ducts containing hyperplastic epithelium.

Growth of the mammary gland during puberty is explained by changes in the endocrine environment characteristic of this age. Gynecomastia generally results from an imbalance in the estrogen-androgen balance, in favor of estrogen (stimulatory) over androgen (inhibitory), or increased breast sensitivity to a normal circulating estrogen level. Estrogens induce ductal epithelial hyperplasia, ductal elongation and branching, proliferation of the periductal fibroblasts, and an increase in vascularity just as they do in the female breast: the histologic picture is similar in male and female breast tissue after exposure to estrogen. The Leydig cells of the testes, long accepted to be the source of the androgens, also secrete estrogens. Most estrogen production in males is from the peripheral conversion of androgens (testosterone and androstenedione to estradiol and estrone, respectively) through the action of aromatase, mainly in muscle, skin, and adipose tissue. For this reason, overweight adolescent boys are more likely to undergo these changes or to have more marked changes than those of normal weight. The overall prevalence of adolescent gynecomastia ranges from 25% to 75%. It generally regresses within 2 years.

Gynecomastia in late adolescence and in the adult is, in many instances, associated with clinical endocrine disorders that result in estrogen excess or decreased androgens. Any endocrine disorder that results in hypogonadism, either primary, such as Klinefelter syndrome (46, XXY), or secondary, such as hypopituitarism due to an adenoma, can result in gynecomastia. Other causes include testicular and feminizing adrenal neoplasms. Hyperthyroidism is also associated with gynecomastia, which is thought to be related to a relative decrease in circulating free testosterone due to thyroid stimulated increases in sex hormone–binding globulin as well as increased peripheral aromatization. Genetic causes of gynecomastia include complete and incomplete forms of androgen insensitivity as well as certain types of congenital adrenal hyperplasia.

Gynecomastia in adult males is often multifactorial. Increased peripheral aromatization of testosterone to estradiol and the gradual decrease of testosterone production in the aging testes probably accounts for gynecomastia in older males. There are a number of medica-

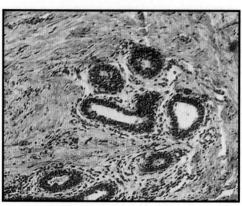

Hyperplastic duct epithelium and periductal stroma of prepubertal gynecomastia

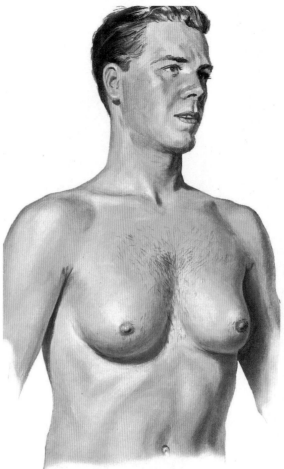

True gynecomastia (feminization)

Fibroadenomatous form of gynecomastia in adult

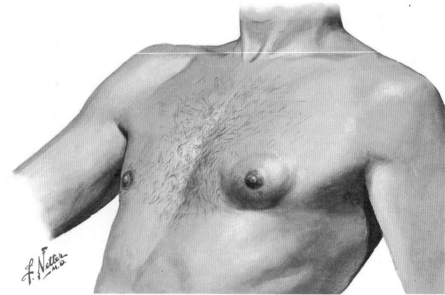

Fibroadenoma of one breast

tions associated with gynecomastia, including hormones like estrogen, some antibiotics like metronidazole, antihypertensives like spironolactone, antiulcer medications such as ranitidine, and psychoactive drugs like phenothiazines. Alcohol, especially if associated with cirrhosis, marijuana, methadone, and amphetamines, has also been associated with gynecomastia.

Rather frequently, gynecomastia is found in patients with testicular tumors (especially chorioepithelioma but also teratoma and interstitial cell tumors). Testicular

deficiency in all of its forms may be accompanied by gynecomastia of varying degrees. Mammary hypertrophy was originally described as an integral part of Klinefelter syndrome. Only when the underlying hyalinization process of the tubular apparatus of the testes in this condition starts late in puberty is gynecomastia a frequent but not obligatory phenomenon.

Simple mastectomy, performed through a curved incision following the margin of the areola, remains the most satisfactory treatment.

Plate 13.8

Breast

PAINFUL ENGORGEMENT, PUERPERAL MASTITIS

Painful engorgement of the breast is caused by vascular and lymphatic stasis. It usually occurs on the third or fourth day postpartum, before the onset of lactation. It also occurs when lactation, once established, is interrupted. The breasts are heavy, painful, warm, firm, and tender to palpation, with prominent axillary prolongations (axillary tail of Spence, part of the mammary gland that extends along the inferolateral edge of the pectoralis major toward the axilla). Fever rarely exceeds 1 or 2 degrees (°F) over normal. The overlying skin may be edematous and the nipple may be so flattened that the baby cannot grasp it. Pumping or manually expressing some breast milk can help reduce engorgement, allowing the baby to properly latch and nurse. The degree of engorgement usually lessens with each child; first-time mothers often have more engorgement than females who are nursing their second or subsequent children. In cases where lactation is being discontinued, the breasts should be firmly bound and ice packs and analgesics used as needed for pain relief.

Prevention of infectious mastitis consists of taking care to wash the hands well (and any other equipment used) before breastfeeding or breast manipulation. Additionally, the nipples and the infant's face should also be clean before each feeding.

Acute mastitis occurs more frequently during the first 4 months of lactation. Mastitis occurs in 2% to 10% of breastfeeding mothers in the United States, with more than half of these cases occurring in first-time nursing mothers. The portal of entry for the infectious organisms is usually a cracked or traumatized nipple allowing entry for organisms from the baby's nose and mouth. The signs of onset are fever, leukocytosis, unilateral tenderness, and a zone of induration. In some cases the infection progresses rather rapidly, and the body temperature may rise as high as 105°F to 106°F (40.5°C to 41°C). In such instances suppuration usually starts within 48 hours. Abscess formation can usually be avoided if antibiotic therapy is instituted promptly. For most cases, nursing need not be stopped. A tight binder supporting the breasts can improve symptoms, along with ice bags applied for analgesia. In suppurative cases, dicloxacillin therapy will treat the infection, but any abscesses formed should be evacuated. The choice of antibiotic should be adjusted based on the patient's history, allergies (if any), and the prevalence of methicillin-resistant *Staphylococcus aureus*. Ciprofloxacin, clindamycin, and trimethoprim/sulfamethoxazole are often effective against methicillin-resistant *S. aureus*. However, trimethoprim/sulfamethoxazole should be avoided in females breastfeeding infants below the age of 2 months.

According to the site of the mastitis, three types have been distinguished: the subareolar, the glandular, and the interstitial forms. In the subareolar type of infection,

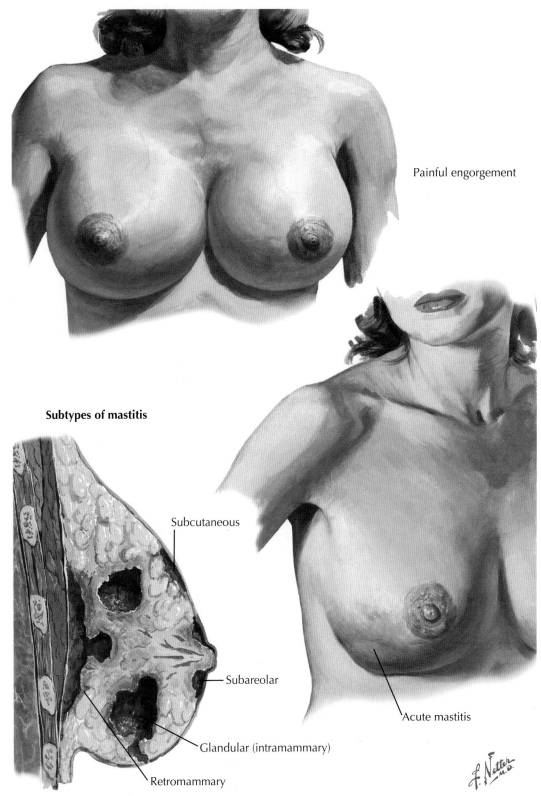

Painful engorgement

Subtypes of mastitis

Subcutaneous

Subareolar

Glandular (intramammary)

Retromammary

Locations of breast abscess

Acute mastitis

the abscess, when it forms, is confined to the area just beneath the nipple. In the glandular form, one or more lobes are involved, and the abscess may rupture spontaneously, giving rise to a sinus tract. In the interstitial form the fatty and connective tissues are involved, giving rise to a retromammary abscess overlying the pectoral fascia, as shown in the illustration. Once signs of suppuration have developed, efforts to localize the abscess by heat application should be made, and the abscess should be incised and drained. In some cases, a chronic

mastitis follows the acute condition. All symptoms and signs of acute mastitis may continue for weeks and months, although to a milder degree. Management of the chronic form is the same as for the acute.

Rarely, mastitis can occur in females who have not recently delivered as well as in females after menopause. Because inflammatory breast cancer has symptoms very similar to mastitis, the possibility that carcinoma may be masked or hide behind an abscess should be kept in mind.

Plate 13.9

Reproductive System: VOLUME 1

Clinical considerations

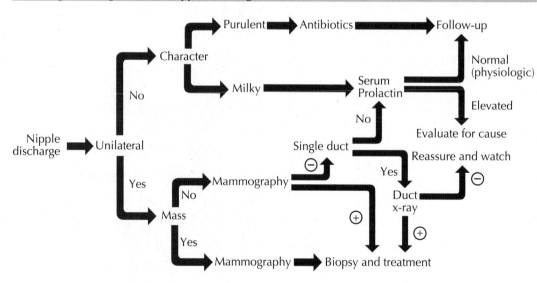

Character of discharge

Bloody
milky
purulent

Serous
serosanguineous

Presence
or absence
of a mass

Bloody
milky
purulent

Single or multiple
duct involvement

JOHN A. CRAIG—MD
D. Mascaro
K. Marzan

NIPPLE DISCHARGE

Nipple discharge is a distressing symptom that accounts for roughly one-third of breast complaints, second only to breast pain and breast mass. Between 50% and 80% of females will experience a discharge at some point in their life. Clinically significant nipple discharge is the spontaneous, continuous, or intermittent release of fluid from one or both breasts that may be milky, bloody, serous, serosanguineous, or cloudy; most physiologic discharge is white or green, clear, or yellow; serosanguineous or bloody nipple discharge is associated with malignancy in up to 50% of cases, but the color or clarity of the fluid cannot diagnose or rule out carcinoma.

When the discharge is bilateral, it is reasonable to presume that a systemic process is present. Galactorrhea (discussed subsequently) may be transiently present in females who have recently given birth, independent of breastfeeding. Periductal mastitis may also generate a purulent discharge.

Unilateral nipple discharge is most frequently limited to a single duct and reflects processes of a limited local scope. Benign ductal papilloma is the most common cause of single duct pathologic discharge (55%). These are an array of papillary cells that grow from the wall of the duct into its lumen. The discharge associated with these may be clear or grossly bloody. Rarely, these papillomas may contain atypia or ductal carcinoma in situ. Surgical excision is warranted if a palpable mass is present or if bloody discharge persists (for symptom relief).

Up to one-third of cases of unilateral nipple discharge are due to ductal ectasia. Ductal ectasia is characterized by distention of subareolar duct(s) with fibrosis and inflammation. Traditionally, the discharge associated with ductal ectasia is multicolored and sticky in character. Duct ectasia often resolves spontaneously, sometimes leaving a residual subareolar nodule that may be found on palpation.

The evaluation of unilateral nipple discharge begins with a history and a clinical examination with an attempt to elicit a sample of the discharge. This is done by gentle pressure at the periphery of the areola, milking any secretions toward the base of the nipple. A warm compress can facilitate the process. Attempts should be made to identify the duct(s) responsible for the drainage. Cytologic evaluation of the nipple discharge is associated with a false-negative result rate of almost 20% and is therefore of little value. A sample of the discharge viewed under

Management algorithm for nipple discharge

Nipple discharge → Unilateral → No → Character → Purulent → Antibiotics → Follow-up

Milky → Serum Prolactin → Normal (physiologic) / Elevated → Evaluate for cause

Yes → Mass → No → Mammography → Single duct → Duct x-ray → Reassure and watch

Yes → Mammography → Biopsy and treatment

the microscope, with or without a simple fat stain of the discharge, can confirm the physiologic character of the discharge as milk.

The possibility of a mass below the nipple or elsewhere in the breast should be evaluated by palpation of the breast and the axillary and supraclavicular regions. Following the clinical examination, mammography (of both breasts) is the next step in the evaluation in all but the most obvious of circumstances. When a specific duct has been identified, a ductogram or galactogram may be diagnostic. Ultrasonography of the periareolar area may demonstrate ductal ectasia or intraductal papillomas. Ultrasonography may identify lesions not visible on mammography and is a useful adjunct to mammography, especially for younger females.

Magnetic resonance imaging (MRI) of the breast is a relatively sensitive imaging modality with moderate specificity. In some institutions, it has become the preferred method of evaluation when mammography and ultrasonography fail to identify a cause for the nipple discharge. Availability, cost, and the required expertise limit this option. Ductoscopy, introduced in 1988, been advocated but does not have widespread availability or acceptance.

When ductal ectasia is thought to be the cause, surgical excision of the involved duct may be required for diagnosis and treatment. Approximately 25% of patients who undergo operations are found to have a malignancy. In only about 5% to 15% of cases of unilateral nipple discharge is the discharge due to breast cancer.

Plate 13.10

Breast

GALACTORRHEA

Galactorrhea is the spontaneous bilateral discharge of milky fluid from the nipples. (Many females, especially those who have given birth in the preceding 6 months, can express small amounts of milky fluid from one or both nipples, and this is not considered abnormal.) Galactorrhea is uncommon but reports vary from 1% to 30%, depending on the population studied. Although not inherently dangerous, galactorrhea can be the harbinger of significant underlying physiologic disruptions and, as such, deserves careful evaluation.

Because galactorrhea represents a symptom, multiple causes can result in the same clinical presentation. Pituitary adenoma or hypothyroidism can result in elevated prolactin levels, which can stimulate the breast parenchyma and result in milk secretion. Galactorrhea can also result as a side effect from pharmacologic agents. Most often this occurs with those drugs that affect dopamine or serotonin production or metabolism. (Some foods when consumed in excess can mimic this same process, notably licorice.) Some autoimmune diseases (sarcoid, lupus) or Cushing disease may result in the patient's symptoms. Chronic chest wall irritation such as from herpes zoster, breast stimulation, or breast irritation may result in the activation of neural pathways normally associated with physiologic milk production. Prolonged stimulation of these neural pathways can result in galactorrhea. Physiologic changes during pregnancy or after childbirth and/or nursing may lead to persistent milk secretion. Most pathologic processes that lead to galactorrhea result in an elevation of serum prolactin levels. This can be helpful in evaluating the source and threat posed by these symptoms.

Galactorrhea is often accompanied by other presenting complaints or conditions: one-third of patients with an elevated prolactin level experience amenorrhea or infertility. Prolonged hypogonadal amenorrhea resulting from hyperprolactinemia is associated with an increased risk of osteoporosis, vaginal and genital atrophic changes, dyspareunia, and libidinal dysfunction because of the associated endocrine disruption.

The evaluation of the patient with galactorrhea will, in part, be dictated by any associated symptoms suggestive of an underlying process. In the absence of other symptoms, measurement of serum prolactin levels begins the evaluation process. (Pregnancy should always be considered if menses are absent.) Prolactin should be measured in the fasting, resting state because eating and stress can increase levels. An elevated serum prolactin level suggests the need for radiologic evaluation of the pituitary. The preferred approach is computed tomography or MRI of the sella turcica. Unfortunately, there is a poor correlation between serum prolactin levels and the size of a pituitary lesion. Testing of visual fields may be indicated if there is a pituitary macroadenoma (≥10 mm).

When prolactin levels are low and imaging of the sella turcica is normal, observation alone may be sufficient. If observation is chosen, periodic reevaluation is required to check for the emergence of slow-growing tumors. Treatment with bromocriptine is recommended for

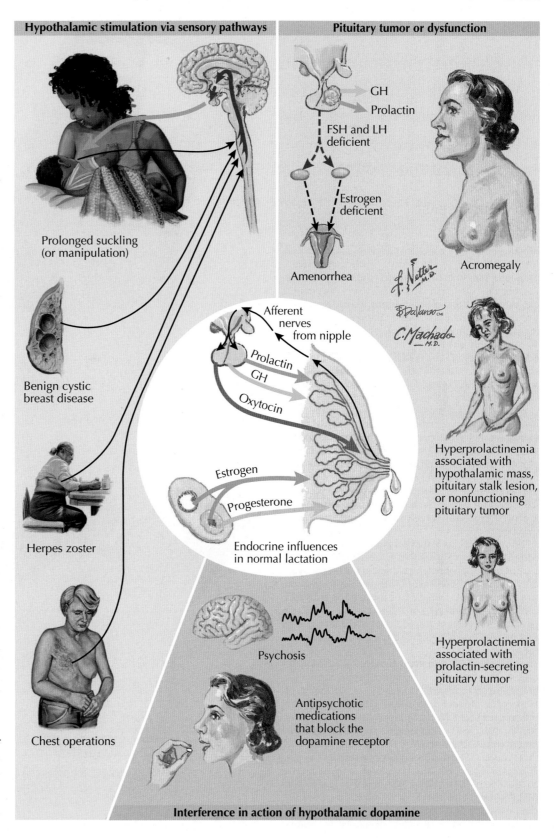

Hypothalamic stimulation via sensory pathways

Prolonged suckling (or manipulation)

Benign cystic breast disease

Herpes zoster

Chest operations

Pituitary tumor or dysfunction

GH
Prolactin
FSH and LH deficient
Estrogen deficient
Amenorrhea

Acromegaly

Afferent nerves from nipple

Prolactin
GH
Oxytocin

Estrogen

Progesterone

Endocrine influences in normal lactation

Hyperprolactinemia associated with hypothalamic mass, pituitary stalk lesion, or nonfunctioning pituitary tumor

Hyperprolactinemia associated with prolactin-secreting pituitary tumor

Psychosis

Antipsychotic medications that block the dopamine receptor

Interference in action of hypothalamic dopamine

patients who desire pregnancy, have distressing degrees of galactorrhea, or have macroadenomas. Unfortunately, medical therapy may be associated with nausea, orthostatic hypotension, drowsiness, or syncope, hypertension, or seizures, and bromocriptine therapy may interact with phenothiazines or butyrophenones.

Medical therapy is generally effective for patients with hyperprolactinemia. Prolactin levels should be measured every 6 to 12 months and visual fields reassessed yearly. The pituitary should be reevaluated every 2 to 5 years,

based on the initial diagnosis. The patient's symptoms may recur when medical therapy is discontinued.

Rapidly growing tumors, tumors that are large at the time of discovery, or those that do not respond to bromocriptine therapy may require surgical or radiation therapy. Surgery can often be accomplished via the transsphenoidal approach. Surgical therapy may result in complete loss of pituitary function requiring careful replacement and monitoring of other endocrine systems, including the thyroid and adrenal.

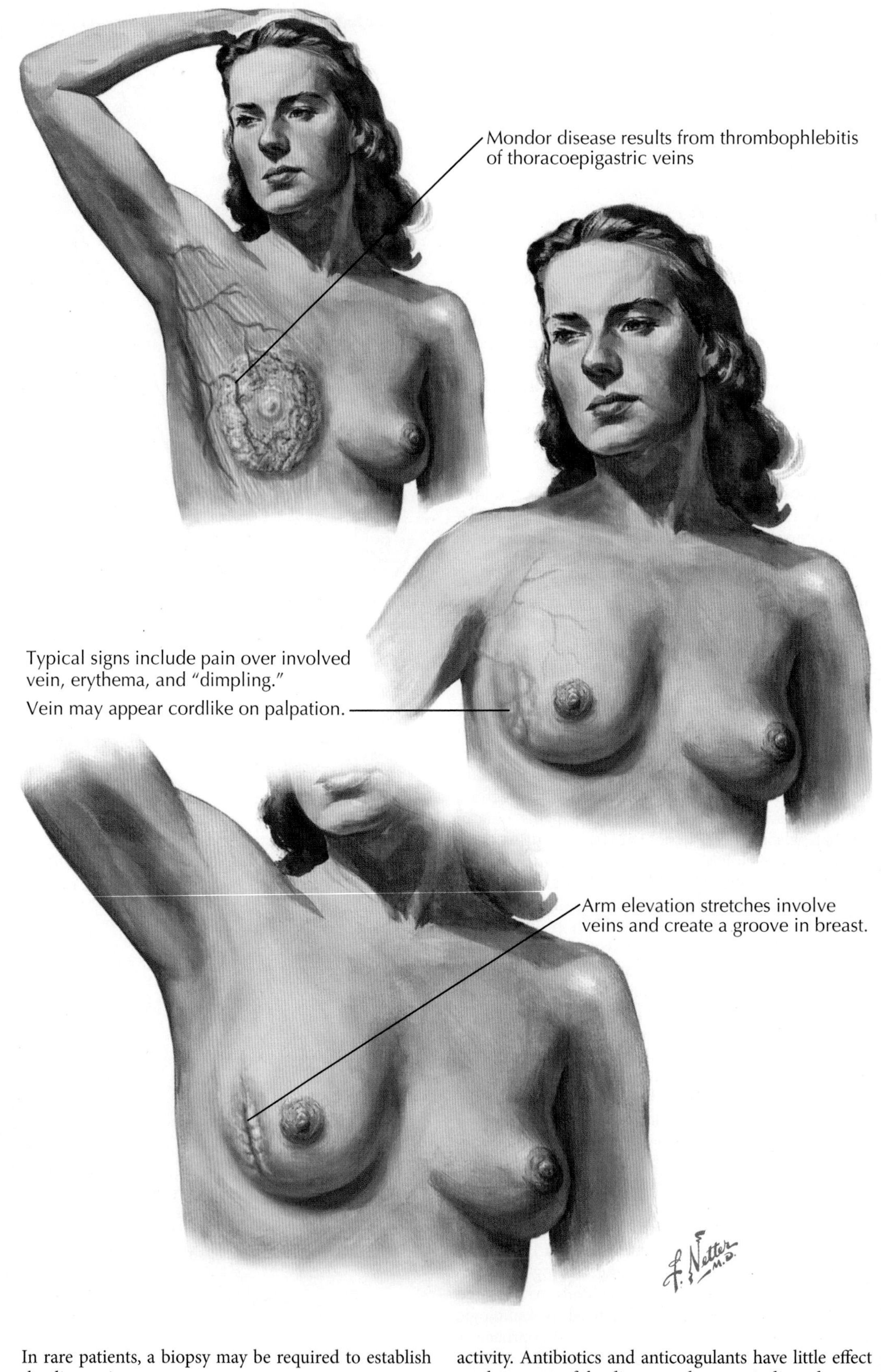

Plate 13.11

Reproductive System: VOLUME 1

MONDOR DISEASE

Mondor disease, or superficial angiitis, is a superficial thrombophlebitis of the breast, named after Henri Mondor (1885–1962), a French surgeon who first described the disease in 1939. This is a very uncommon clinical entity that may occur during the late reproductive or early menopausal years. The predominant age for patients with Mondor disease is between 30 and 60 years. This should not be confused with Paget-Schroetter disease, which refers to deep vein thrombosis of an upper extremity vein, including the axillary or subclavian vein, often following vigorous activity (though it can also occur spontaneously).

Breast phlebitis is most often linked to a recent pregnancy, trauma, or operative procedure but may occur spontaneously. It most often involves the thoracoepigastric veins of the breast and the lateral thoracic veins. Rarely, Mondor disease can present following augmentation mammoplasty, manifesting as temporary cords extending from below the breast toward the abdomen. This occurs in less than 2% of patients. In these patients, the cords appear at about 3 to 6 weeks, last a few months, and then usually disappear.

Thrombophlebitis of the breast veins usually presents with symptoms of pain that is acute and generally located in the upper outer quadrant of the breast. Typically, a thickened, tender cord with pain, erythema, and swelling is found. Dimpling of the skin or a distinct cord with erythematous margins may be found on physical examination. In addition, a shallow groove may be seen extending upward toward the axilla when the arm is raised.

Although these symptoms are typical of Mondor disease, they must be differentiated from those of a breast abscess or mastitis, ductal ectasia, carcinoma, or fat necrosis. Mondor disease can be distinguished from inflammatory cancer of the breast by the presence of sudden pain, early skin adherence, and progressive improvement, characteristics that are not present in these cancers. Scarring from previous surgery (biopsy, augmentation, or reduction) can result in thickening or a retraction of the overlying skin similar to that seen in Mondor disease but should be readily distinguished by careful history.

Mondor disease is generally diagnosed by history and physical examination. On physical examination there will be accentuation of dimpling or the formation of a groove over the affected vein. This often occurs when the ipsilateral arm is raised during physical examination. Mammography may be required to rule out other processes, but the diagnosis is generally established by physical examination and history. (On mammography, a beaded subcutaneous vein may be seen together with skin retraction. Rarely, the vein calcifies.) On ultrasonography, a tubular, hypoechoic structure corresponding to the thrombosed vein may be seen.

Mondor disease results from thrombophlebitis of thoracoepigastric veins

Typical signs include pain over involved vein, erythema, and "dimpling."

Vein may appear cordlike on palpation.

Arm elevation stretches involve veins and create a groove in breast.

In rare patients, a biopsy may be required to establish the diagnosis.

Mondor disease is benign and self-limited. The treatment of superficial thrombophlebitis of the breast is generally supportive: analgesics and heat reduce symptoms. The condition generally clears up on its own in 2 to 3 weeks, but it may take 6 weeks or longer to completely resolve. Although there is generally no restriction on physical activity, good mechanical support with a well-fitting bra or binder improves comfort during vigorous activity. Antibiotics and anticoagulants have little effect on the course of the disease and are not indicated.

Subcutaneous penile vein thrombosis (penile Mondor disease) has also been described, first in 1955. It appears suddenly as a generally painless indurations on the penile dorsal surface. The patient usually feels the superficial vein of the penis like a hard rope and presents with concerns or pain around this hardness. Its pathogenesis is unknown, although findings suggest that it might be of lymphatic origin.

Plate 13.12

Breast

BREAST IMAGING

In current medical practice, breast imaging is dominated by two modalities, mammography and ultrasonography, for screening and evaluation of suspicious breast lesions. MRI has demonstrated promise as an adjunct to traditional imaging for selected situations. Other modalities such as thermal imaging (thermography), molecular breast imaging (scintimammography), three-dimensional mammography (tomosynthesis), electrical impedance imaging (T-scan), and transillumination are either experimental or have not proven to be effective.

Mammography is the best mode of screening for early lesions currently available. Mammography can identify small lesions (1–2 mm), calcifications, or other changes suspicious for malignancy roughly 2 years before a lesion is clinically palpable. More than one-third of occult breast cancers have calcifications, making the otherwise undetected tumors visible through mammography.

Widespread use of mammography has been credited with reducing the mortality rate from breast cancer by up to 30%. Unfortunately, not all females receive appropriate screening on a regular basis. The most recent breast cancer screening guidelines recommend that mammography be performed every 1 to 2 years for females aged 40 to 49 years and annually thereafter. Most guidelines have dropped the suggestion to obtain routine baseline mammograms in females younger than 40 years. Most have recommended annual screening mammography and clinical breast examination for females aged 50 years and older. However, published and public controversy about the potential benefits and risks of screening mammography continues. The question of at what age, if ever, to stop mammography is also unresolved.

When the patient has a first-degree relative with premenopausal breast cancer, screening should begin roughly 5 years before the age at which the relative's cancer was diagnosed. For patients at increased risk for breast cancer (strong family history or genetic abnormality such as mutations of BRCA1 or -2), mammography should be augmented by MRI studies. MRI should not be used independently for screening because of its unacceptably high false-positive rate.

Mammography in younger females is more difficult to interpret than in older females because of the greater tissue density present during the reproductive years; breast cancers in this population are more easily missed for this reason. Overall, mammography is approximately 85% accurate in diagnosing malignancy, with a 10% to 15% false-negative rate. For this reason, it provides an adjunct to clinical impressions and the definitive procedure of biopsy but does not replace them. Roughly 10% of mammographic studies require additional views. Between 1% and 2% of screening studies necessitate histologic evaluation to establish a diagnosis. Total mammographic radiation exposure is minimal (<1 rad).

Ultrasonography has become a valuable tool for use along with mammography because it is widely available, noninvasive, and less expensive than other options. Originally, ultrasonography was primarily used as an effective method of differentiating cystic breast masses from solid breast masses, but it also provides valuable information about the nature and extent of solid masses and other breast lesions. Although ultrasound is less sensitive than MRI (detects fewer tumors), it has the advantage of costing less and being more widely available.

Breast ultrasonography is not routinely used for screening, but rather it is useful in the evaluation of palpable masses that are mammographically occult, in the evaluation of clinically suspected breast lesions in females younger than 30 years, and in the follow-up of abnormalities seen on mammography. Some studies have suggested that it may be helpful to use ultrasonography routinely with a mammogram when screening younger females or those with dense breast tissue. A large study evaluated the use of breast ultrasonography for screening and found that more breast cancers were found with the combined modalities compared with mammography alone, but the rate of false-positive studies and biopsies also was higher. Ultrasonography is generally acknowledged to be a highly operator dependent modality that requires a skilled practitioner, high-quality examinations, and state-of-the-art equipment.

Mammography

Position for craniocaudad projection

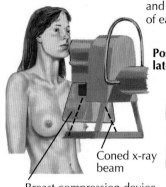

Usually two exposures at right angles (craniocaudad and lateral) are made of each breast.

Breast compression device

Position for lateral projection

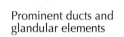
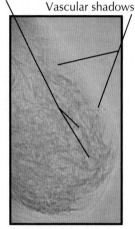

When additional breast and rib detail is needed, a mediolateral exposure is also made.

Position for mediolateral projection

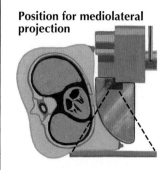

Coned x-ray beam

Breast compression device

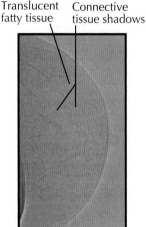

Translucent fatty tissue · Connective tissue shadows

Craniocaudad projection of normal fatty breast

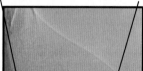

Prominent ducts and glandular elements

Vascular shadows

Lateral projection of normal dense glandular breast

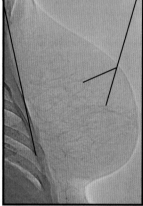

Rib detail shown in this projection

Connective tissue shadows

Mediolateral projection of normal breast

Ultrasonography

JOHN A. CRAIG—MD
C. Machado—M.D.

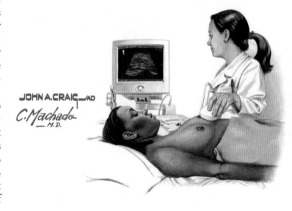

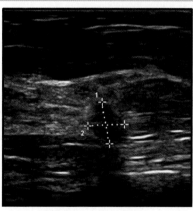

Cystic mass visible

Plate 13.13

Reproductive System: VOLUME 1

FIBROCYSTIC CHANGE: MASTODYNIA

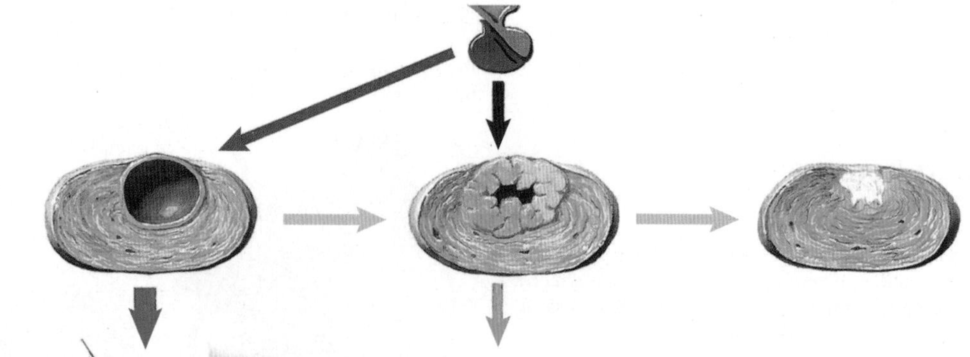

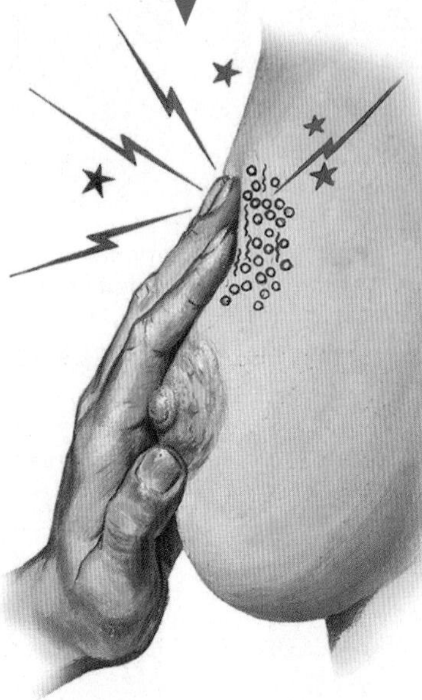

Fibrocystic change (previously called fibrocystic disease) is a nonspecific term that includes mastalgia (mastodynia), breast cysts, and nondescript lumpiness. These may occur in isolation or together. The breasts generally have a nodular and dense texture and are tender when palpated. Fibrocystic change is responsible for the most commonly reported breast symptoms, with up to 15% of affected females requiring treatment and up 70% of females experiencing breast pain at some point in their lives.

Mastalgia is the nonspecific term used for breast pain of any etiology. Mammary pain may occur in obese, pendulous breasts at or after the menopause when the weight of the breast stretches the suspensory ligaments and puts traction on the nerve fibers. These cases are not true mastodynia and are relieved by a supportive brassiere and by weight reduction. Another form of mammary pain, which does not arise in the parenchyma, is owing to intercostal neuralgia, which may complicate spondylitis, fatigue, or respiratory infections.

The most common cause of persistent breast pain is fibrocystic change. Breast pain can also arise from rapid hormonal change (especially a change that involves a rise in estrogen levels, such as starting birth control pills, hormone replacement, or pregnancy). In the absence of obvious pathologic changes, mastalgia has been attributed to caffeine consumption and high-fat diets, but hard data are lacking. Nongynecologic causes include dorsal radiculitis or inflammatory changes in the costochondral junction (Tietze syndrome), sclerosing adenosis, chest wall muscle spasms, costochondritis, fibromyalgia, and referred pain. Older patients may also suffer postherpetic neuralgia or neuritis following herpes zoster infections. This pain may mimic mastalgia.

The pain of fibrocystic change, at first present only in the premenstruum, becomes progressively more prolonged and more severe until it persists throughout the cycle. The breast affected is usually well developed. A swollen granular zone of increased density is felt, which is located far more frequently in the upper lateral quadrant than in other parts of the hemisphere. On compressing this swollen area with the examining fingers, pain is produced. The fibrocystic change is often bilateral. Definitive masses are generally not felt. Unilateral or localized pain suggests a pathologic process. Mammography may be indicated for other reasons but seldom directly assists in the evaluation of mastalgia.

When biopsied, the painful breast tissue is found to be more dense and fibrous than normal. The lobular tissue stands out as small pink dots in the dense white stroma, which encloses occasional small cyst formations. On microscopic examination, the lobules are stunted or irregular, with minute cystic dilations. Proliferating immature connective tissue, which stains poorly, surrounds the epithelial structures.

Mastodynia usually responds to medical therapy and to reassurance against the fear of cancer. General measures include analgesics, mechanical support (a well-fitting brassiere worn day and night), local heat, and reassurance. A reduction in methylxanthine intake is often beneficial. Premenstrual restriction of salt or fluids is recommended for selected patients. The role of

Schema of clinical syndrome: tender, granular swelling

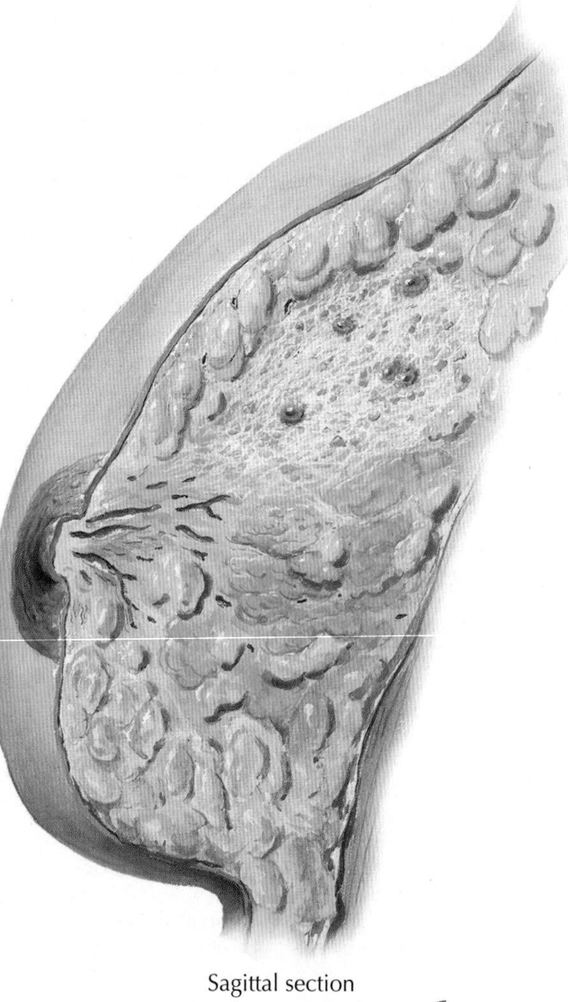

Sagittal section

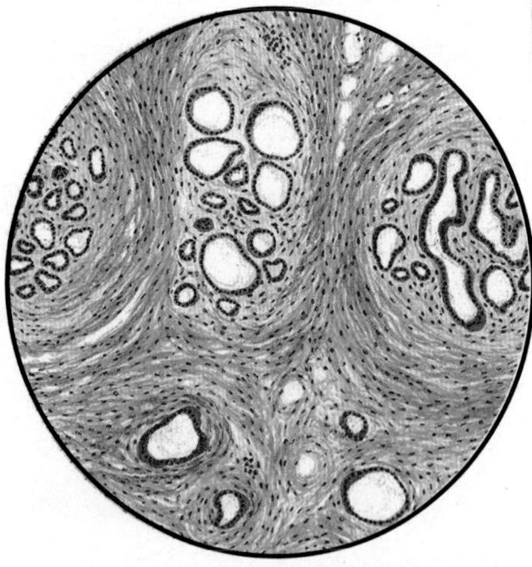

Microscopic aspect (stunted lobules in proliferating fibrous stroma)

vitamins A and E is unknown. Evening primrose and chasteberry have shown efficacy in limited trials but standardization of both therapy and active ingredients in varying preparations limits the ability to fully evaluate these as therapeutic options.

Combination oral contraceptives improve symptoms for between 70% and 90% of patients. In more resistant cases, treatment with spironolactone, danazol sodium (begun during menstruation or once pregnancy has been ruled out), or bromocriptine may be required. In

very selective patients, gonadotropin-releasing hormone agonists may be required. Diuretics must be used with care to avoid fluid and electrolyte disturbances. Bromocriptine may cause hypotension during the first several days of therapy. Care should also be exercised with patients who have compromised hepatic or renal function.

Whatever therapy is used, it remains essential to consider the possibility of cancer in all cases; however, breast pain is a rare symptom of breast cancer.

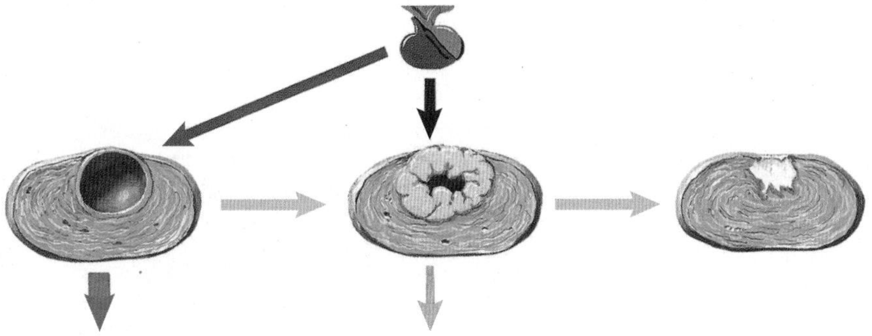

Plate 13.14

Breast

FIBROCYSTIC CHANGE: ADENOSIS

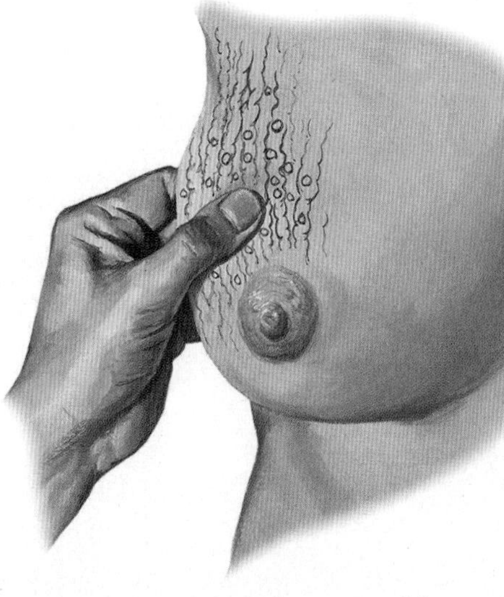

Stromal and ductal proliferation that results in cyst formation, diffuse thickening, cyclic pain, and tenderness are the hallmarks of fibrocystic change. The term fibrocystic change encompasses a multitude of different processes and older terms, including fibrocystic disease. It is the most common of all benign breast conditions, accounting for its linguistic demotion to change from the designation disease. To one extent or another, fibrocystic change affects 60% to 75% of all females. These changes are most common between the ages of 30 and 50 years, with only 10% of cases in females younger than 21 years. Methylxanthine intake has been proposed as a causative agent, but hard data are lacking. There is no evidence that oral contraceptives increase the risk of these changes. A family history of fibrocystic change is often present, but causality is difficult to establish.

The cause or causes of fibrocystic change are unknown, but it is postulated to arise from an exaggerated parenchymal response to hormones. A role for progesterone has been suggested based on the common occurrence of premenstrual breast swelling and tenderness. Other proposed sources for fibrocystic changes are altered ratios of estrogen and progesterone or an increased rate of prolactin secretion, but none of these has been conclusively established.

Adenosis is characterized by the occurrence in one or both breasts of multiple nodules varying from 1 mm to 1 cm in size, usually distributed about the periphery of the upper or outer hemisphere. The breasts affected tend to be small, dense, and edged like a saucer when grasped in the hand. Typical findings on physical examination include multiple cysts and mobile nodules intermixed with scattered bilateral nodularity, or a ropy thickening, especially in the upper outer quadrants of the breast. Pain and tenderness (which vary during the menstrual cycle) occur as in mastodynia, with the worst symptoms occurring just before menses. (The pain associated with fibrocystic change often radiates to the shoulders or upper arms.) Although pain is the most common complaint, up to 50% of cases of fibrocystic adenosis may be asymptomatic.

Fibrocystic changes appear in three steps: (1) proliferation of stroma, especially in the upper outer quadrants; (2) proliferation of the ducts and alveolar cells occurs, adenosis ensues, and cysts are formed; and (3) larger cysts are found and pain generally decreases. Proliferative changes may be extensive (although usually benign) in any of the involved tissues. Overall, the mammary tissue affected contains dense fibrous tissue, numerous minute cysts, and foci of epithelial proliferation. Lobule formation is much distorted. Some of the terminal tubules form solid plugs of basal cells, which, on cross section, appear as duct adenomas. Other tubules lead to greatly enlarged

Schema of clinical syndrome: cordlike and nodular with "saucer edge"

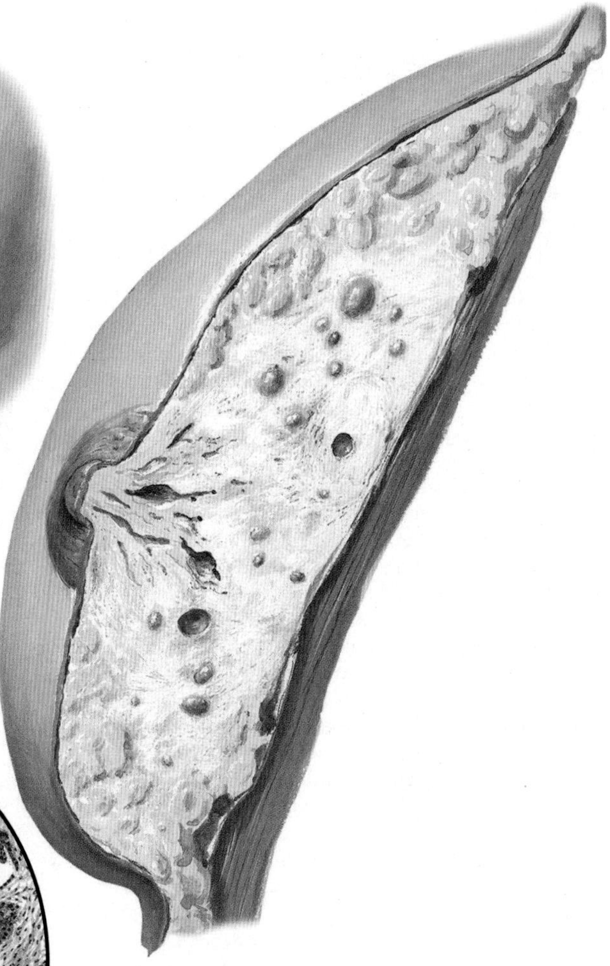

Appearance on cross section

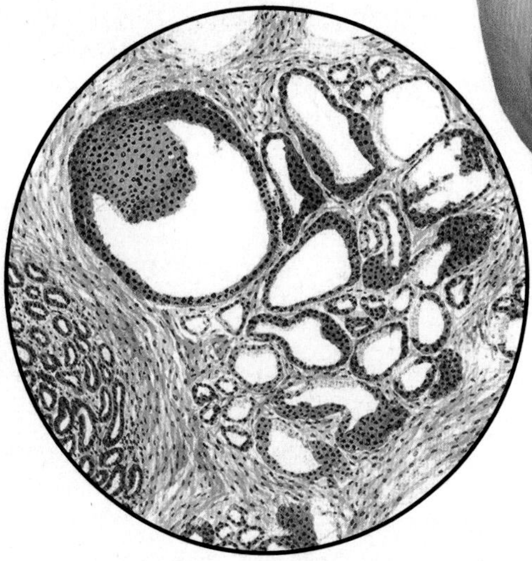

Dilated acini and epithelial proliferation

lobular structures, which are penetrated by dense strands of fibrous tissue giving the appearance of fibrosing adenoma. Differential diagnosis of adenosis from fibrosing adenoma is sometimes difficult, if not impossible, particularly if small, intraductal papillomas have developed in advanced cases of adenosis. Premenopausal age, multiplicity of more peripherally situated nodules, a brownish rather than a sanguineous discharge from the nipple, and the involvement of both sides of the breast favor adenosis.

Mammography may be used to assist with the diagnosis or to provide a baseline, but it is not necessary for diagnosis. Mammography is more difficult in younger females who predominantly have these complaints. As a result, ultrasonography may be of more help when imaging is deemed necessary. If the patient has a cystic breast mass, needle aspiration with a 22- to 25-gauge needle may be both diagnostic and therapeutic. Fine needle aspiration or core biopsy may be required if malignancy is suspected. When atypia is found in hyperplastic ducts or apocrine cells, there is a fivefold increase in the risk of development of carcinoma in the future.

Plate 13.15

Reproductive System: VOLUME 1

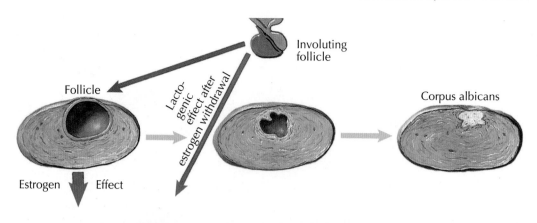

Involuting follicle

Follicle

Lactogenic effect after estrogen withdrawal

Corpus albicans

Estrogen   Effect

FIBROCYSTIC CHANGE: CYSTIC CHANGE

Cystic breast masses are frequently encountered in the clinical care of females. Sorting out those that represent a threat from those that may be followed conservatively is the challenge posed by the presence of cysts in the breasts. Some authors estimate that cysts form in the breasts of roughly 50% of females during their reproductive years. Roughly one in four females seek medical attention for some form of breast problem; often this takes the form of a palpable mass. The most common cause of a palpable breast cyst is fibrocystic change (found in 60%–75% of all females). Dilation of ducts and complications of breastfeeding (galactoceles, abscess) may also cause cysts.

The pathogenesis is not clear for the most common types of cyst formation. Cyclic changes in hormones induce stromal and epithelial changes that may lead to fibrosis and cyst formation. Cysts may be single or be found in clusters, with some up to 4 cm in diameter. Small cysts have a firm character and are filled with clear fluid, giving the cyst a bluish cast. Larger cysts may have a brown color resulting from hemorrhage into the cyst. Inspissated secretions or milk may form a cystic dilation of ducts (galactocele, ductal ectasia) that may be palpable as a cystic mass. Variable degrees of fibrosis and inflammation may be seen in the surrounding stroma. (Leakage of cyst fluid into the surrounding tissue induces an inflammatory response that may alter physical findings and imitate cancer.) The microscopic findings associated with breast cysts depend on the pathophysiologic changes involved.

In fibrocystic change, the cyst makes its appearance abruptly in a previously normal breast in which the parenchyma has been largely replaced by fat and is accompanied by a sticking or stinging sensation. A serous discharge from the nipple occurs in about 6% of the patients. On palpation a tense, movable, rounded mass is felt fluctuating between the fingertips of the right and left hands if the two hands alternately compress the mass. On transillumination, both the breasts and the tumor transmit the light readily. The cyst usually occupies a region midway between the nipple and the periphery of the breast.

On gross examination (when the cyst is exposed at operation), it has a characteristic blue dome that bulges into the subcutaneous fat. This cyst has a thin, fibrous wall, which may have an epithelial lining of duct cells resembling sweat gland epithelium. On opening the cyst, a smoky or cloudy straw-colored fluid is evacuated. Microscopically, the cyst wall is embedded in dense, fibrous mammary stroma. The gland is poor in acinar tissue.

The diagnosis and management of cystic masses in the breast are based on history, physical examination,

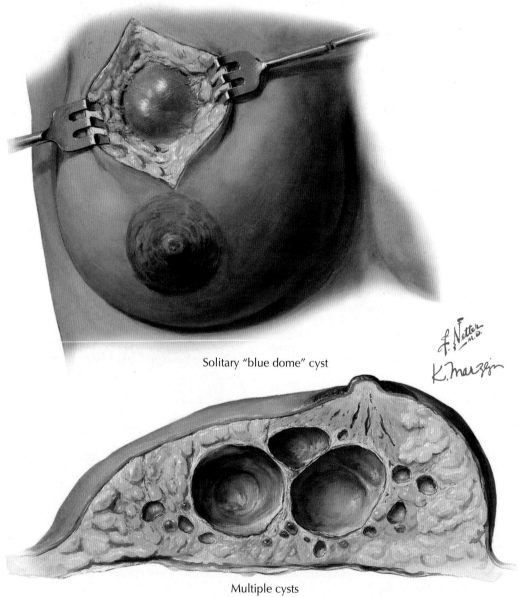

Solitary "blue dome" cyst

Multiple cysts

and aspiration, with the occasional adjunctive use of mammography and ultrasonography. (Ultrasonography is useful in differentiating solid and cystic breast masses, but it cannot be used to differentiate benign and malignant tissues.) Needle aspiration with a 22- to 25-gauge needle may be both diagnostic and therapeutic. If the cyst disappears completely and does not reform by a 1-month follow-up examination, no further therapy is required. Fluid aspirated from patients with fibrocystic changes is customarily straw colored. Fluid that is dark

brown or green occurs in cysts that have been present for a long time but is also innocuous. Bloody fluid requires further evaluation. Cytologic evaluation of the fluid obtained is of little value because of unacceptably high false-positive and false-negative results. After aspiration of a cyst, the patient should be rechecked in 2 to 4 weeks. Lack of complete resolution at the time of aspiration, recurrence of the cyst, or the presence of a palpable mass should prompt additional evaluation, such as fine-needle aspiration or open biopsy.

Plate 13.16

Breast

BENIGN FIBROADENOMA, INTRACYSTIC PAPILLOMA

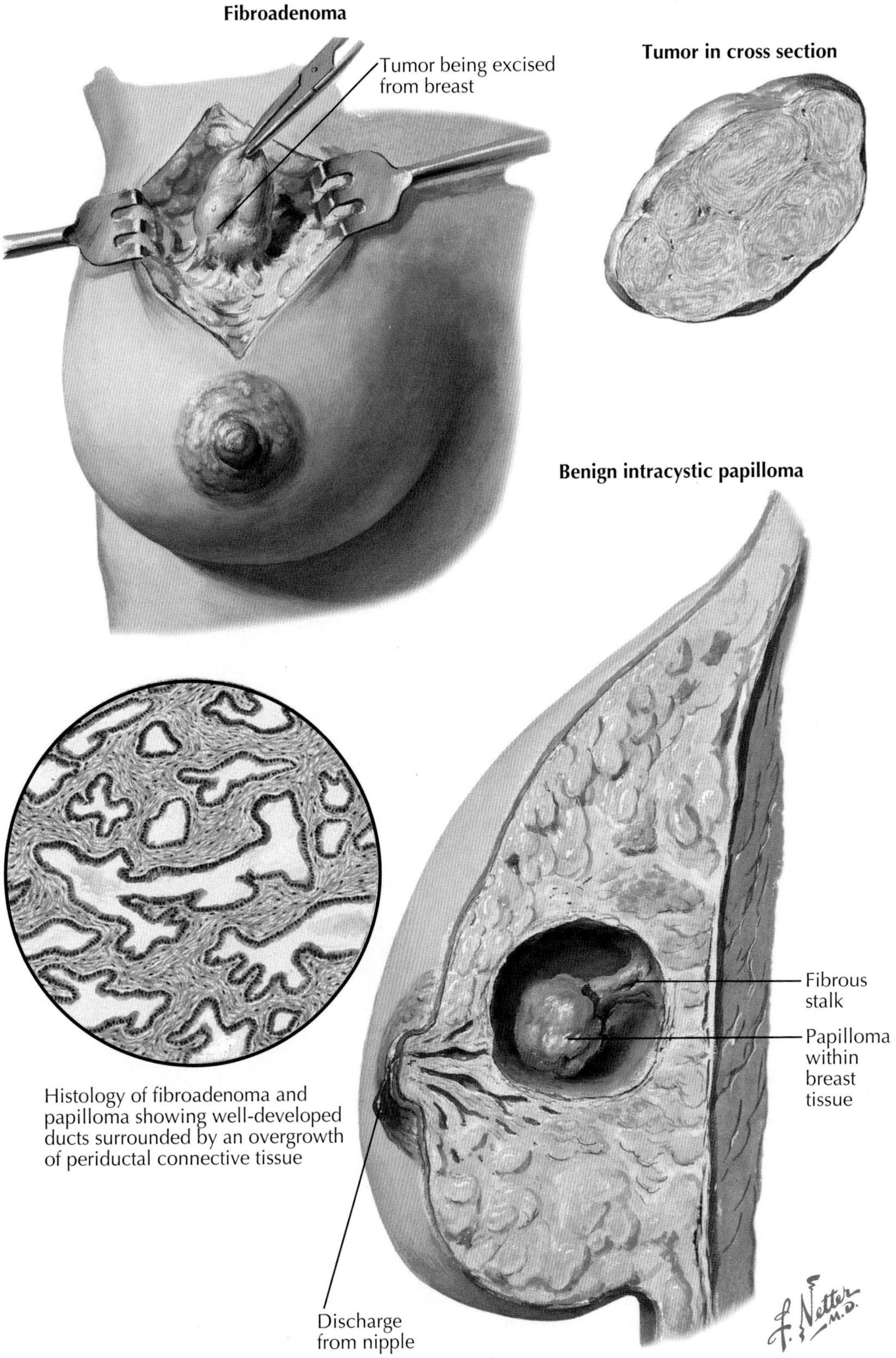

Fibroadenomas are the second most common form of breast disease and the most common breast mass. The peak incidence is from 20 through 25 years, with most patients younger than 30 years of age. More rapidly growing tumors may be found during adolescence. The tumors are twice as common in Blacks (30% of breast complaints), in patients with high hormone states (adolescence, pregnancy), and in patients receiving unopposed estrogen therapy.

Fibroadenomas are generally discovered as firm, painless, mobile, rubbery, solitary breast masses that may grow rapidly during adolescence or in high-estrogen states such as pregnancy or estrogen therapy. These tumors are generally discovered incidentally or during breast self-examination and average 2 to 3 cm in diameter, though they may grow as large as 6 to 10 cm. Multiple fibroadenomas are found in 20% of patients, and they are bilateral in 10% to 20% of patients.

The chief symptom is gradual enlargement of the mass over a period of months or years, the average duration being just under 3 years. On palpation, the tumor is firm, encapsulated, nodular, and freely movable. Mammography is generally avoided because of the typical patient age but can be diagnostic if needed. Breast ultrasonography can distinguish between solid and cystic masses, although it is often not required.

The structure of the tumor is lobular. A centrifugal nodule with sharply circumscribed, fleshy, and homogeneous character, usually spherical or ovoid in shape, characterizes them. Pink or tan-white fibrous whorls bulge from the surface when cut. Hemorrhagic infarcts are common. Microscopically, well-developed ducts are seen, surrounded by a marked overgrowth of periductal connective tissue. When this connective tissue is pale staining and loose and the epithelium of the ducts is compressed, the tumor is referred to as an *intracanalicular myxoma*. When the amounts of fibrous tissue and duct growth are more evenly balanced, the tumor is termed a fibroadenoma.

In early adolescence, in pregnancy, or toward menopause, when estrogen secretion is increased or dominant, the growth of fibroadenomas is more rapid. These are termed giant mammary myxomas. Malignant change is extremely rare and usually takes the form of fibrosarcoma occurring in the giant myxoma. After menopause, fibroadenomas tend to regress and become hyalinized but may remain unchanged or grow with estrogen therapy. The treatment is simple excision, which confirms the diagnosis and suffices for the cure.

Benign intracystic papillomas are soft epithelial growths occurring within a mammary duct or cystic acinar structure. They are about one-half as common as fibroadenomas and are usually found at or near the menopause, in the central zone of the breast. The duration of symptoms is variable, usually from 6 months to 5 years. The symptoms consist of either a sanguineous discharge from the nipple (in 50% of the cases) or a lump associated with moderate tenderness. The tumors are rarely of large size; they range in diameter from one to several centimeters. The larger ones are associated

with either retained bloody fluid within the cyst or malignant change, which occurs in about 10% of the cases. Multiple papillomas in one or both breasts are found in 14% of cases. On palpation, the benign papilloma is freely movable, soft, and either tense (cystic) or fluctuant.

Grossly, intracystic papillomas are encapsulated tumors in which epithelial tufts extend within the cavity and are bathed by varying amounts of serous or sanguineous fluid.

Smaller papillomas may be found in the neighboring ducts or through the ramifications of a group of ducts some distance from the main tumor. Microscopically, the arborescent epithelial outgrowths rest upon a fibrous stalk with an intact basement membrane. The treatment is simple excision, examination of the neighboring ducts for secondary papillomas, and excision of these where indicated. Recurrent tumors in elderly patients warrant simple mastectomy.

Fibroadenoma

Tumor being excised from breast

Tumor in cross section

Benign intracystic papilloma

Histology of fibroadenoma and papilloma showing well-developed ducts surrounded by an overgrowth of periductal connective tissue

Fibrous stalk

Papilloma within breast tissue

Discharge from nipple

Plate 13.17

Reproductive System: VOLUME 1

Giant myxoma

Section of breast tissue
containing tumor

Cyst
containing
myxoid
mass

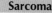

F. Netter M.D.

Clinical presentation
of tumor in right breast

Giant Myxoma, Sarcoma

A variety of fibroadenoma growing to immense size and occurring near the menopause was first described by the distinguished physiologist of the early 19th century, Johannes Müller, as "cystosarcoma phyllodes." This is a rare, predominantly benign tumor that occurs almost exclusively in the female breast. It represents less than 1% of all breast tumors. The duration of the growth extends over a period of 6 or 7 years, with rapid growth toward the end of this period, when these tumors can significantly increase in size in just a few weeks. The benign character of the growth is indicated by the absence of invasion of the skin or of the regional lymph nodes. The tumors are heavy, massive (>10 cm), lobulated growths with cystic areas. They have a sharply demarcated smooth texture and are typically freely movable. Their average weight is between 7 and 8 lb. Despite the size, the tumor remains movable and encapsulated, and the nipple is not retracted. Grossly, the tumor displays characteristics of a large malignant sarcoma, takes on a leaf-like appearance when sectioned, and displays epithelial cystic spaces when viewed histologically. Because most of these tumors are benign, the name may be misleading, leading to the preferred terminology of phyllodes tumor or giant myxoma.

The origin of these growths is in a preexisting intracanalicular myxoma. Dense fibrous tissue in whorls is separated by clefts from polypoid, fibrous, and epithelial masses projecting into cystic cavities. Under the microscope, the predominant component is myxomatous connective tissue with intervening dense fibrous strands. Most growths are benign, but some may be the seat of sarcomatous change in about 10% of cases, particularly when the tumor has existed for many years. These tumors are best treated by simple mastectomy with removal of the pectoralis fascia. Although these benign tumors often do not metastasize, they do have a reputation of growing aggressively and recurring locally. The malignant tumors metastasize hematogenously like other sarcomas. The histologic appearance does not always predict clinical behavior. Roughly 30% of patients with malignant phyllodes tumors will die of their disease. Other than surgery, there is no cure for phyllodes tumors, as chemotherapy and radiation therapy are not effective. Current studies do not support the use of adjuvant radiotherapy for patients with adequately resected disease.

Mammary sarcoma is relatively rare and represents between 1% and 2% of breast tumors. Many varieties of sarcomas, such as osteogenic, lympho-, myo-, lipo-, and myelosarcomas, have been described. In more than half of the cases, however, sarcomas of the mammary gland are of the fibrospindle cell–type arising in the

Giant myxoma. Microscopic view showing bland myxoid connective tissue containing uniform spindle cells.

Sarcoma

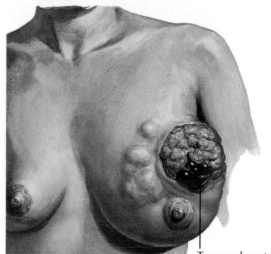

Tumor ulcerated through skin

Sarcoma. Microscopic view showing numerous crowded spindle cells with abnormal hyperchromatic nuclei.

stroma of the breast or from the stroma of preexisting fibroadenomas. The tumors, which may develop at any age but have their peak incidence between 45 and 55 years of age, are characterized by rapid growth, large size, and a firm consistency. Ulceration of the skin, with fungation, may occur. The tremendous size and the absence of axillary node involvement distinguish these growths from mammary carcinomas. Pain and rapid growth are the symptoms most commonly noted. A preexisting fibroadenoma may have been stationary

and asymptomatic for many years and then suddenly may become painful, giving rise to the rapidly growing and invading sarcoma.

Sarcomatous change has also been seen in benign myxomas. Grossly, the tumors are solid, fleshy growths, which may invade the pectoralis fascia. Microscopically, they are composed of tightly packed pleomorphic spindle cells. The treatment is radical mastectomy. The lungs are the most common metastatic site, followed by bone, heart, and liver.

Plate 13.18

Breast

Infiltrating carcinoma.
Seen in cross section of breast.

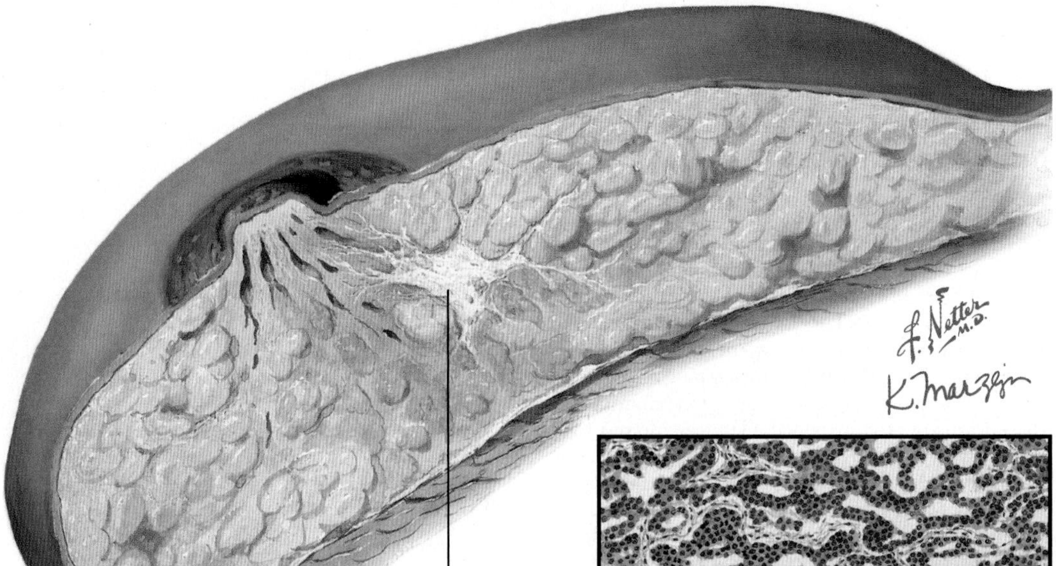

Stellate,
irregular
mass

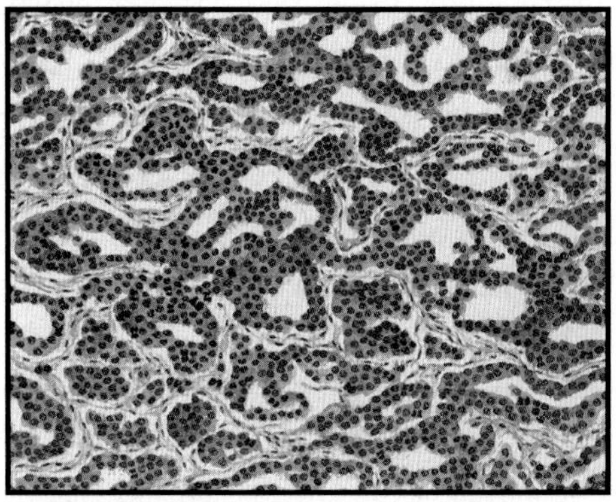

BREAST CANCER

Females in the United States have the highest incidence rates of breast cancer in the world. Worldwide, breast cancer is the second most common type of cancer after lung cancer and the fifth most common cause of cancer death. In the United States, breast cancer is the most common female cancer and the second most common cause of cancer death. The average lifetime risk of breast cancer for females in the United States is 12.4% (one in every eight females).

Approximately one-third of all forms of female carcinoma arise in the breast, and more than three-quarters of these are the infiltrating scirrhous type or lobular carcinoma. Breast cancer accounts for approximately 18% of cancer deaths and results in about the same number of deaths per year as auto accidents. The peak incidence is above 40 years of age, with 85% occurring after age 40 and 75% after age 50. Approximately 5% to 10% of breast cancers have a familial or genetic link.

The symptoms that bring the patient under examination are the discovery of the lump (55%–65% of cases), its increasing size, occasional fleeting pains or tenderness, and changes in the skin or nipple. Approximately 60% of palpable tumors are located in the upper outer quadrant of the breast. An abnormal mammogram without a palpable mass is the second most common cause for diagnosis (35%). One-quarter of all breast cancers are found during routine examination.

The major clinical findings on examination are the presence of a single lump in a breast otherwise normal to palpation in a patient more than 35 years old, the hard and irregular feeling of the tumor, the apparent nearness of the tumor to the examining fingers because of atrophy of overlying fat, the restricted mobility of the mass, and flattening or retraction of the skin or nipple on the affected side when arms or breast are manipulated. Excisional biopsy with or without radiographic control provides the only definitive diagnosis.

Grossly, mammary carcinoma is a dense, yellowish-white, stellate, indurated mass with a cut surface that is gritty and concave and that feels like an unripe pear. Unless secondarily infected, the growth is usually free of necrosis. It infiltrates the surrounding fatty and fibrous stroma of the breast. Microscopically, the tumor cells are of moderate size, with prominent hyperchromatic nuclei. The cells grow in small nests or in cords with prominent intervening fibrous tissue. In the more slowly growing cancers, the cells grow in scattered masses and tend to form acinar or tubular structures. In those more rapidly growing, the cells are scattered individually without histologic resemblance to normal structure.

The most common breast cancer histology is the infiltrating ductal carcinoma, accounting for about 75% of breast cancers. Scirrhous carcinoma is the most common subtype: well-demarcated hard nodules consisting of cords and nests of malignant ductal cells characterize it. Medullary and mucinous forms are also recognized.

Nipple retraction

Slow-growing form. Proliferation of duct cells with enlarged nuclei and irregular gland pattern.

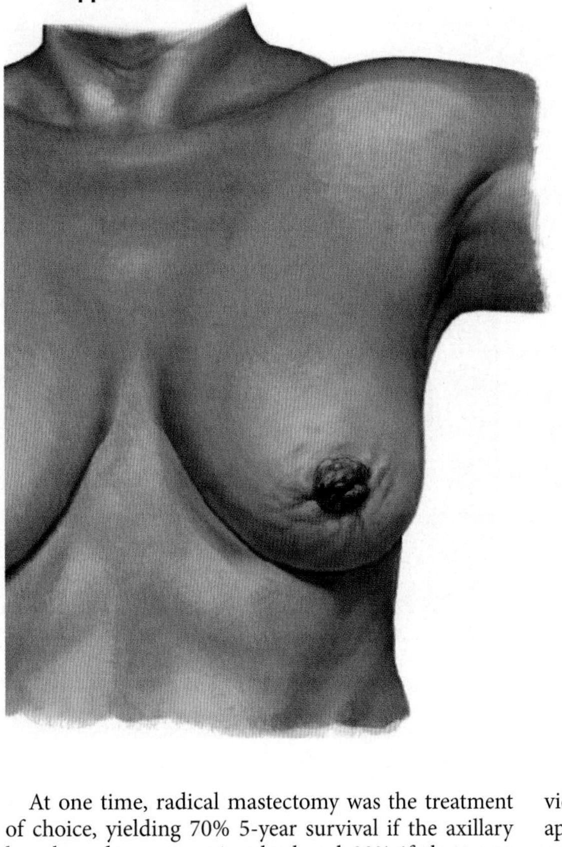

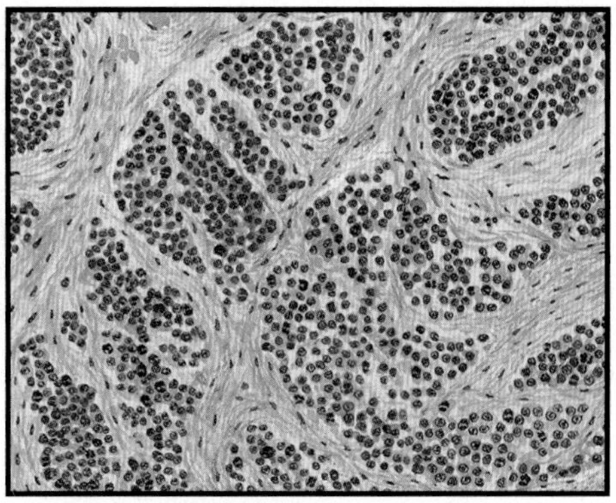

Rapidly growing form. Proliferation of duct cells with hyperchromatic nuclei in solid sheets and no glandular architecture.

At one time, radical mastectomy was the treatment of choice, yielding 70% 5-year survival if the axillary lymph nodes were uninvolved and 20% if there was lymph node involvement. This has given way to a much more nuanced approach that is dependent on a number of factors: the tumor's size; its inherent aggressiveness, as determined by the histology of the initial lesion; the presence of positive nodes; and the receptor status of the tumor. The major impetus for changes in management of breast carcinoma has come from a changing view regarding the biology of the disease. It has become apparent that many females with breast cancer have systemic disease at the time of initial diagnosis. The natural history of the developing breast carcinoma, with an average doubling time of 100 days, results in years of growth before its clinical discovery. Because occult vascular dissemination is likely to occur prior to diagnosis, treatment of breast carcinoma now relies upon both local and systemic therapy, without reliance on radical surgery.

Plate 13.19

Reproductive System: VOLUME 1

INTRADUCTAL AND LOBULAR ADENOCARCINOMA

The two main types of breast adenocarcinomas are ductal carcinomas (80%) and lobular carcinomas. Based on the tumor's histology, these are also sometimes classed as papillary adenocarcinomas; carcinomas with gelatinous, mucoid degeneration; or as a kind of intraductal carcinoma that forms plugs in preexisting ducts and circumscribed rings of carcinoma cells. These forms of circumscribed adenocarcinomas bulge outwardly from the chest wall rather than retract inwardly as in the infiltrating form. Skin adherence or ulceration and axillary node involvement occur much later in the course of the disease than in the ordinary scirrhous form. The tumors progress slowly to an immense size. The most common type of adenocarcinoma is ductal carcinoma, which begins in the cells of the ducts. Lobular carcinoma begins in the lobes or lobules and is more often found bilaterally than are other types of breast cancer. The cancer is classified based on the predominant histologic cells; however, several cellular patterns may be found in any one tumor.

In intraductal carcinoma in situ, the cellular abnormalities are limited to the ductal epithelium and have not penetrated the basement membrane of the duct. It is most common in females who are perimenopausal and postmenopausal. Because the disease does not produce a definitive mass, intraductal carcinoma in situ is not usually detected by palpation. The histologic diagnosis of intraductal carcinoma in situ includes a heterogeneous group of tumors with varying malignant potential. Carcinoma develops in approximately 35% of females with this disease within 10 years of initial diagnosis, and 5% to 10% of females will have a simultaneous invasive carcinoma in the same breast at the time of biopsy.

Unlike intraductal carcinoma in situ, lobular carcinoma in situ should not be treated as a cancer or cancer precursor but rather as a marker for an increased breast cancer risk. It has a much greater tendency to be bilateral and to present as multifocal disease. Three of four patients with lobular carcinoma in situ are in the premenopausal age group. The latent period to the development of invasive carcinoma is longer than with intraductal carcinoma in situ; often more than 20 years will elapse before infiltrating carcinoma develops. Approximately 20% of females with this disease eventually develop invasive breast carcinoma. Paradoxically, most of these subsequent carcinomas are ductal, not lobular.

In cases of infiltrating ductal carcinoma, nonuniform malignant epithelial cells of varying sizes and shapes infiltrate the surrounding tissue. The degree of fibrous response to the invading epithelial cells determines the firmness to palpation and texture during biopsy. Often the stromal reaction may be extensive. Approximately 10% of infiltrating ductal carcinomas are of a uniform histologic picture and are classified as medullary, colloid, comedo, tubular, or papillary carcinomas. In general, the specialized forms are grossly softer, mobile, and well delineated. They are usually smaller and have a more optimistic prognosis than the more common heterogeneous variety. Medullary carcinomas are soft, with extensive stromal infiltration by

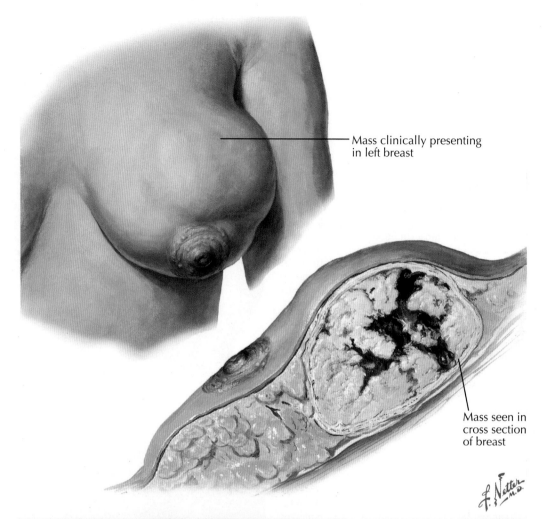

Mass clinically presenting in left breast

Mass seen in cross section of breast

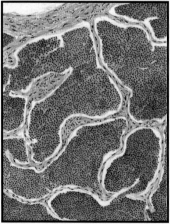

Papillary adenocarcinoma. Sheets of tumor cells with hyperchromatic nuclei from a large growth with papillary projections (*see cross section above*).

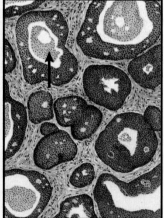

Duct cancer (comedocarcinoma). Nests of tumor cells with central foci of necrosis (*arrow*).

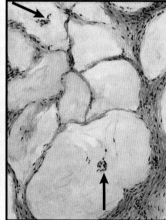

Gelatinous carcinoma. Clusters of malignant cells (*arrows*) embedded in thick gelatinous material.

lymphocytes and plasma cells. Colloid or gelatinous carcinomas have a similar soft consistency, with extensive deposition of extracellular mucin.

Infiltrating lobular carcinomas (8% of breast cancers) are histologically notable for the uniformity of the small, round neoplastic cells. Histologic subdivisions of infiltrating lobular carcinoma include small cell, round cell, and signet cell carcinomas. Often the malignant epithelial cells infiltrate the stroma in a single file fashion. This cancer tends to have a multicentric origin in the same

breast and to involve both breasts more often than infiltrating ductal carcinoma. On palpation, these growths feel boggy and semimovable and are dependent and heavy when the breast is moved upward. The papillary carcinomas may contain a cystic cavity with blood. The intraductal carcinomas form plugs (comedones), which may be expressed from the ducts. On cross section the gelatinous carcinomas contain a characteristic slimy, gray, mucoid material that spills from the tumor, which is honeycombed with this substance.

Plate 13.20

Breast

Inflammatory carcinoma

Inflamed skin

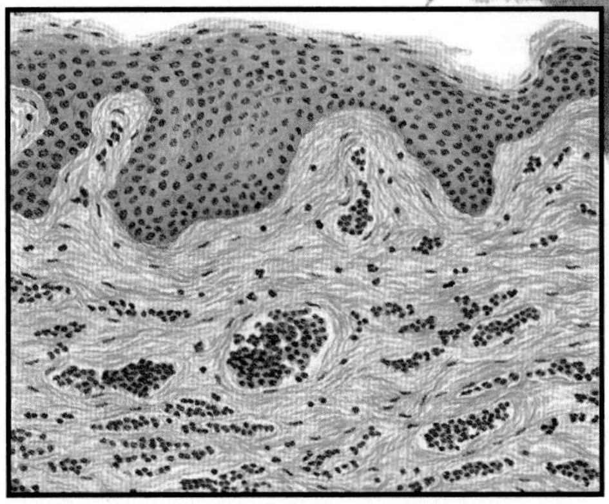

Inflammatory Carcinoma

Inflammatory or acute carcinoma, formerly designated as carcinomatous mastitis, is more often observed in patients with obese breasts or during pregnancy and lactation, from which is derived another older term, lactation cancer. Inflammatory carcinomas comprise approximately 0.5% to 2% of all breast cancers. This form is recognized clinically as a rapidly growing, highly malignant carcinoma, with infiltration of malignant cells into the lymphatics of the skin, which produces a clinical picture that simulates a skin infection. There is not a specific histologic cell type. In the TNM staging system for breast cancer, inflammatory cancer has its own classification, T4d, and by definition is staged as stage IIIb or above. (Stage IIIB breast cancers are locally advanced; stage IV breast cancer is cancer that has spread to other organs.) Because of the rapid growth of these tumors, the physical appearance of the breast is often different from that of patients with other stage III breast cancers.

Inflammatory breast cancer tends to be diagnosed in younger females compared with other breast cancers, and it occurs more frequently and at a younger age in Blacks than in Whites. Like other types of breast cancer, inflammatory breast cancer can occur in males but usually at an older age than females. There is some early evidence for an association between family history of breast cancer and inflammatory cancers, but more studies are needed.

The appearance of a rapidly widening area of inflamed skin usually occurs early in the disease and may precede the discovery of the underlying tumor. The dermal spread is caused by retrograde extension of the cancer cells through the lymphatics of the skin. The majority of cases are of the primary form; that is, when the patient has noted a small tumor in the breast or axilla only a few weeks prior to the appearance of inflammatory signs. The presence of the tumor in the secondary form antedates the skin inflammation by months. The tumor might already have reached a large size, or the skin changes may fall upon a mastectomy scar. The changes in the skin are characterized by a reddish or purplish discoloration and edema producing the characteristic orange peel effect. Multiple small nodules may also be present. The inflamed discoloration may extend up the neck and down the arm on the affected side, or across to the opposite breast and shoulder. A low-grade fever, enlarged axillary nodes, and an elevated leukocyte count, which may reach 15,000, accompany the carcinomatous invasion of the skin. Adenopathy may extend to the groin, and the skin over the abdomen may be inflamed; hence the term *erysipeloid* cancer has also been used. In a typical case the symptoms are usually less than 4 months in duration.

Tissue sections through a region with inflammatory cancer exhibit relatively few signs of acute inflammation. The paramount characteristic is the blockage of

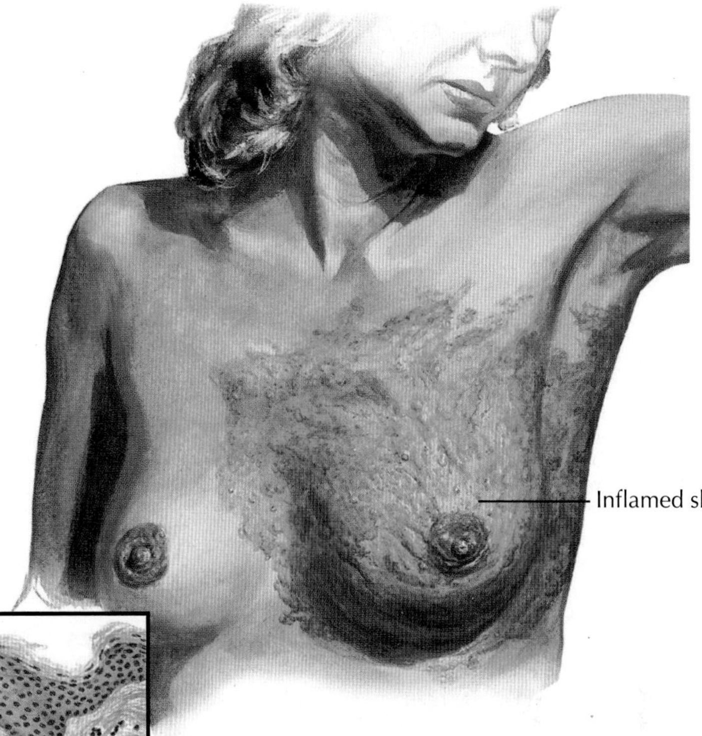

Invasion of dermal lymphatics

Recurrent cancer

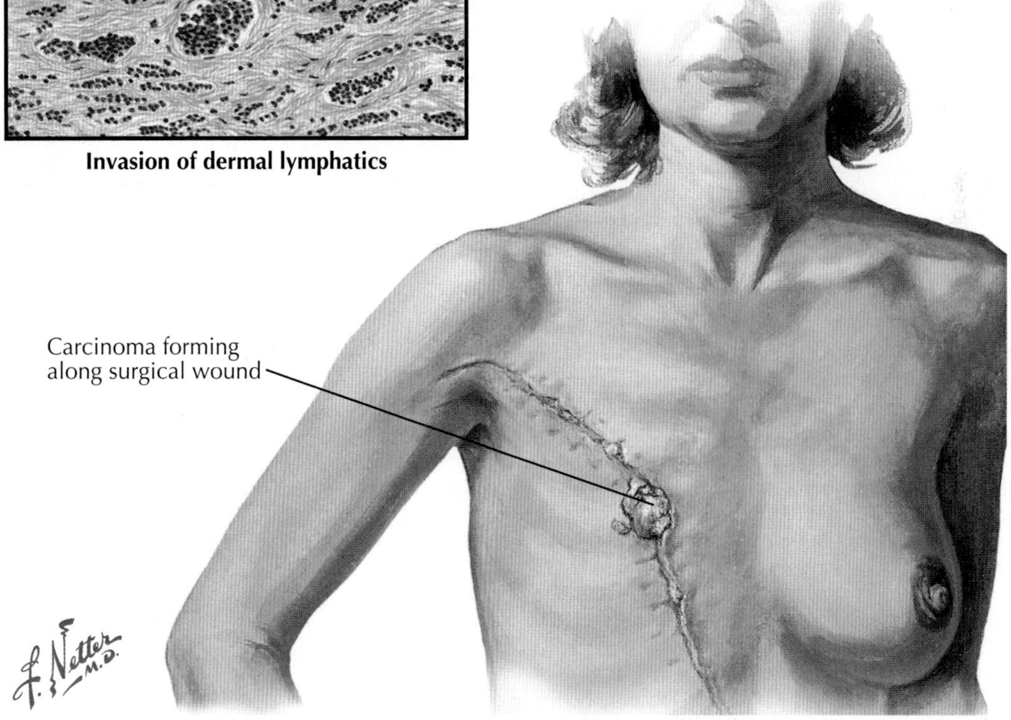

Carcinoma forming along surgical wound

lymphatics and superficial blood vessels with invading cancer cells. This same metastatic process into the subcutis is seen in preparations from a lenticular cancer, or carcinoma en cuirasse, where the invasion proceeds more slowly, more diffusely, and without edema.

Treatment consists of neoadjuvant chemotherapy, targeted surgery, radiation therapy, and hormonal therapy, but 5-year survival is only in the range of 30% to 75%, with recurrences common. This is significantly lower than for patients with other types of breast cancer. Neoadjuvant combination chemotherapy is generally the first treatment followed by targeted surgery. Additional treatments may include additional chemotherapy, hormonal therapy, or the recently added modality of special targeted therapy (such as trastuzumab) for patients whose tumors overexpress the HER-2 tumor protein.

Plate 13.21

Reproductive System: VOLUME 1

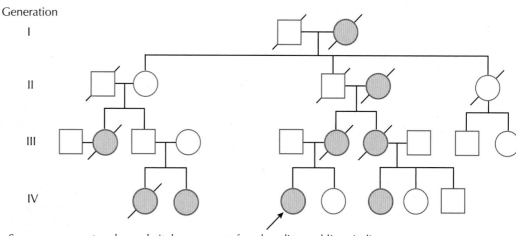

Squares represent males and circles represent females, diagonal lines indicate deceased, shaded individuals are affected, arrow indicates the proband.

HEREDITARY BREAST DISEASE

Approximately 5% to 10% of breast cancers have a familial or genetic link. In these families, breast cancer tends to occur at a younger age, and there is a higher prevalence of bilateral disease. The association between inherited breast and ovarian cancer has led to the term *hereditary breast ovarian cancer syndrome.*

Hereditary breast ovarian cancer syndrome is characterized by an early age of onset of breast cancer (often before age 50). In affected families, there is a family history of both breast and ovarian cancer and an increased chance of bilateral cancers or an individual with both breast and ovarian cancer. Pedigrees will demonstrate an autosomal dominant pattern of inheritance (vertical transmission through either the mother's or father's side of the family). Members of these families also have an increased incidence of tumors of other organs, such as the fallopian tube or prostate. Families with cases of male breast cancer and families of Ashkenazi Jewish ancestry are at increased risk for this syndrome (greater than 10-fold increase).

At least two genes have been found in which mutations can cause this pattern of inherited breast and/or ovarian cancer. It appears that germline mutations of the *BRCA1* tumor suppressor gene on chromosome 17q are responsible for a large proportion of these hereditary cancers. However, not all families in which hereditary breast or ovarian cancer is suspected are found to have mutations in either *BRCA1* or *BRCA2.* Having a single mutation in one of these genes does not appear to be sufficient to have a tumor develop. It is generally thought that mutations in both alleles, due to chemical, physical, or biologic environmental exposures, or chance errors in cell replication, must occur for tumor development. To date, hundreds of unique mutations have been identified in both *BRCA1* and *BRCA2,* most due to sporadic mutations unique to the individual or family. Specific recurring mutations have been found in individuals of Ashkenazi Jewish descent and persons from the Netherlands, Iceland, and Sweden. Mutations in the *BRCA* family of genes confer a lifetime risk of breast cancer that approaches 85%, though the risk of ovarian cancer is variable depending on the location of the mutation. The average lifetime risk of ovarian cancer is approximately 40% to 50%.

The *BRCA2* gene resides on chromosome 13, and the DNA sequence was determined in 1995. A female with a *BRCA2* gene mutation also has an 85% lifetime risk of breast cancer and a 15% to 20% lifetime risk of ovarian cancer. This mutation is associated with male breast cancer, conferring a 5% to 10% lifetime risk for a male with the mutation. *BRCA3* gene has been recently mapped to chromosome 8, but the details of any associated clinical syndrome have not yet been determined. Other rare syndromes carry increased risk of breast

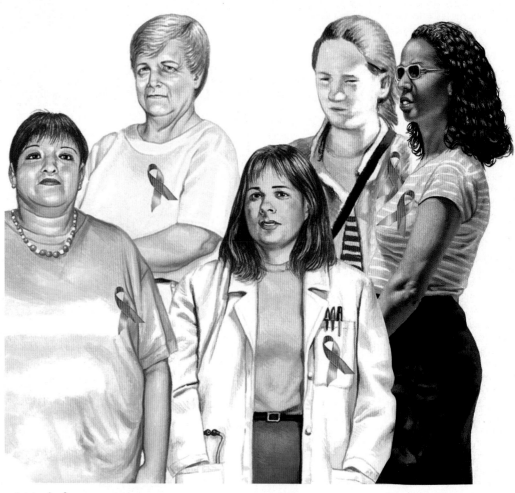

cancer such as Li-Fraumeni and Cowden syndromes, which are associated with pathogenic variants in the tumor protein p53 and phosphatase and tensin homolog tumor suppressor genes, respectively.

Presently, management recommendations for females with *BRCA* mutations vary from earlier and increased interval screening tests to prophylactic measures such as chemoprevention with tamoxifen, mastectomy, and oophorectomy. A task force has recommended breast self-examination beginning by age 20, annual or semiannual clinical examination beginning at ages 25 to

35 years, and annual mammograms beginning at ages 25 to 35 years. They made no recommendation for or against prophylactic surgery in these patients. Although there is good evidence suggesting that tamoxifen can significantly reduce the risk of breast cancer in females at high risk, there are still no conclusive data on the use of tamoxifen in a population of patients with a *BRCA* gene mutation. There are currently no effective screening techniques for the early detection of ovarian cancer. For this reason, some females at high risk choose to undergo prophylactic oophorectomy.

Plate 13.22

Breast

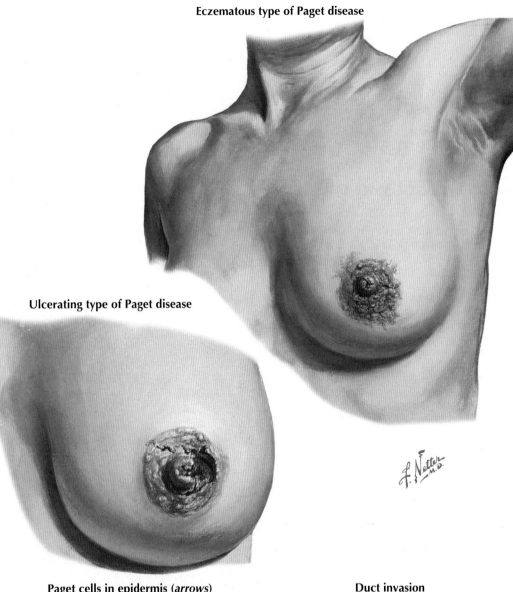

Eczematous type of Paget disease

PAGET DISEASE OF THE NIPPLE

In 1874, Sir James Paget described 15 females with chronic nipple ulceration who quickly developed cancer of the involved breast. Paget disease of the breast is rare, comprising between 1% and 2% of breast carcinomas. It is a malignant process that involves the nipple and areola. Rarely, it may also involve the skin of the vulva. This lesion has an innocent appearance that looks like eczema or dermatitis of the nipple. The clinical picture is produced by an infiltrating ductal carcinoma that invades the epidermis. Paget disease has an excellent prognosis.

Paget carcinoma is characterized by invasion of the nipple or areola and the mouths of the larger ducts by large malignant cells resembling those seen in transitional cell carcinoma of the mucous membranes elsewhere in the body. It is thought to arise in the dermo-epidermal junction from multipotent cells that can differentiate into either glandular or squamous cells. The average age at diagnosis is 62 for females and 69 for males. The duration of symptoms, which is approximately 3 years, and the symptoms, referable to the nipple, are characteristic clinical features of the disease. Paget disease is almost always associated with infiltrating or intraductal carcinoma in deeper parts of the breast (95% of cases). In most cases, involvement of the nipple precedes a definite tumor of the breast, but in a few instances the lump in the breast may be noted first. The disease is bilateral in less than 5% of the cases. Mammography is usually used to detect deeper lesions and lesions in the contralateral breast. In addition, a touch smear obtained by softening the crust with saline and gently scraping the surface often demonstrate the characteristic Paget cells.

The involved nipple has either a red granular appearance or is crusted and eczematous. After an interval of a few months, both the eczematous and the granular types undergo ulceration. Serum or blood oozes from the denuded region. A small amount of blood may be obtained on manipulation. In early stages, the zone immediately surrounding the nipple is indurated, whereas in later stages both the central zone and the periphery may be involved by a hard mass. Palpable axillary nodes are found in about 50% of the cases.

Grossly, besides the changes in the nipple, the larger ducts are dilated and filled with blood or inspissated secretion. Microscopically, large cells with deep staining or vesicular nuclei and pale-staining cytoplasm are found in the epidermis of the nipple. Mitotic figures are frequent. Dermal infiltrates of large neoplastic cells (Paget cells) are defining features of this condition. These cells have abundant clear cytoplasm with mucin and irregular prominent nucleoli. Most often, these cells arise from infiltrating ductal carcinoma. In cases where the cells in the nipple have infiltrated beyond the basement membrane, they invade both the larger ducts and the breast tissue.

Therapy is focused on treatment of the underlying malignancy and is most commonly surgical. When limited to the nipple, breast conservation may be

Ulcerating type of Paget disease

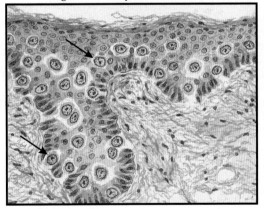

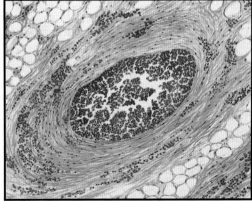

Paget cells in epidermis (*arrows*)

Duct invasion

possible. Adjunctive hormonal or chemotherapy is often recommended based on cell type and stage. Radiation therapy is a common adjuvant therapy following breast-conserving surgery.

The differential diagnosis from benign lesions of the nipple, such as keratosis and ulcers, depends largely on the discovery of a mass in the underlying tissue on palpation. Although biopsy of the nipple should

be avoided whenever possible, a study of the tissue becomes imperative in certain cases; for example, when the skin lesion does not heal within a matter of days under hygienic measures or on application of petrolatum. Even if the gland does not appear to be involved, it is important that the biopsy specimens obtained from such patients contain not only skin but also a representative portion of the mammary ducts.

Plate 13.23

Reproductive System: VOLUME 1

MALIGNANCIES OF MALE BREAST

Carcinoma of the male breast is a rare disease and represents only about 0.1% of all-site malignancy and is approximately 100 times less common than breast cancer in females, accounting for about 1% of all breast cancers. In the United States, male breast cancer accounts for fewer than 2000 cases per year and fewer than 500 deaths. The mean age at diagnosis is between 60 and 70 years, though males of any age can be affected with the disease. The average duration of symptoms before diagnosis is approximately 2 years. This long duration is probably explained by the disregard of this rudimentary organ by the male adult and by the examining physician. Predisposing risk factors are thought to include radiation exposure, estrogen administration, and diseases associated with hyperestrogenism, such as cirrhosis or Klinefelter syndrome. An increased risk of male breast cancer has been reported in families, with an increased incidence seen in males who have a number of female relatives with breast cancer and those in whom a *BRCA2* mutation on chromosome 13q is present. When there is a mutation in this gene, it confers a 5% to 10% lifetime risk for male breast cancer.

Because of the small amount of fatty stroma and glandular tissue in the male breast, ulceration of the skin or involvement of the nipple is an almost regular symptom of onset. Pain and trauma are often given as the reasons for consulting the doctor. The tumor is hard, irregular, and firmly attached to the overlying and underlying structures. Ulceration is common. The axillary lymph nodes are usually enlarged.

Differential diagnosis from gynecomastia can be made with fair certainty, taking the age of the patient into account. Nodular tumors in the middle-aged man should be excised and examined histologically. Even though a fibroadenoma, an intracystic papilloma, a lipoma or a benign epidermoid cyst usually leaves the skin over the nodule freely movable in contrast to carcinoma, and though these nodules are also softer than cancer, it is not recommended to exclude a malignant growth based only on these clinical signs.

On cross section, the neoplasm is firm, white, and infiltrating. A higher percentage of these growths are low-grade adenocarcinomas, probably arising in the developmental anomalies of the sweat glands or mammary epithelial structures. Pathologically, most carcinomas of the male breast resemble the infiltrating form found in the female breast, with infiltrating ductal cancer the most common tumor type. Lobular cancer has been described as well. Inflammatory carcinoma and Paget disease of the nipple have also been seen in males, but lobular carcinoma in situ has not. Lymph node involvement and the hematogenous pattern of spread are similar to those found in female breast cancer. The TNM staging system for male breast cancer is identical to the staging system for female breast cancer.

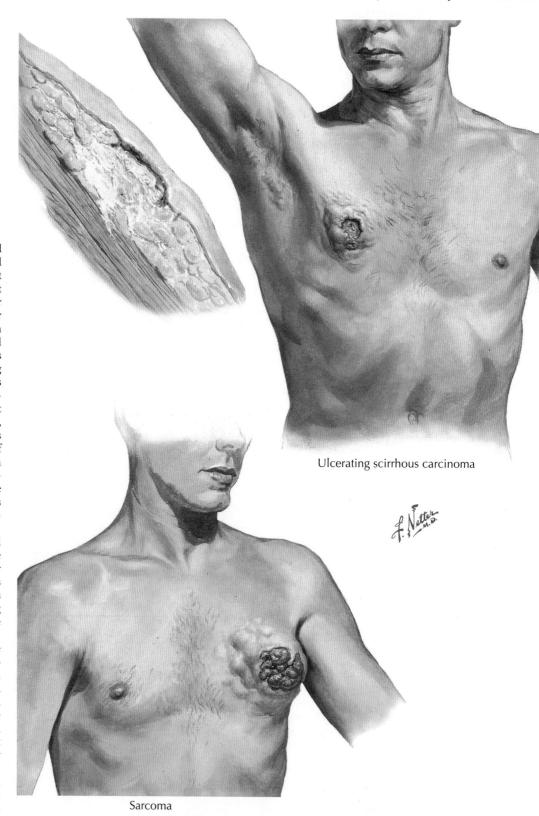

Ulcerating scirrhous carcinoma

Sarcoma

Overall survival is similar to that of females with similar stage breast cancers. The impression that male breast cancer has a worse prognosis may stem from the tendency of these tumors to be diagnosed at a later stage. Prognostic factors such as the size of the lesion and the presence or absence of lymph node involvement correlate well with prognosis. Whether ploidy and number of cells in S phase correlate with survival awaits more definitive data. Estrogen-receptor and progesterone-receptor status and erythroblastic oncogene B (ERBB2, formerly known as human epidermal growth factor receptor 2 or HER2) gene amplification are also being evaluated.

Although rare, various types of sarcomas of the male breast have been reported. Most are either fibrospindle or lymphosarcomas. These are rapidly growing tumors with early attachment to the overlying skin and are highly malignant. Simple mastectomy is employed. If lympho- or liposarcoma is disclosed by histologic examination, postoperative irradiation should be given.

SEX REASSIGNMENT

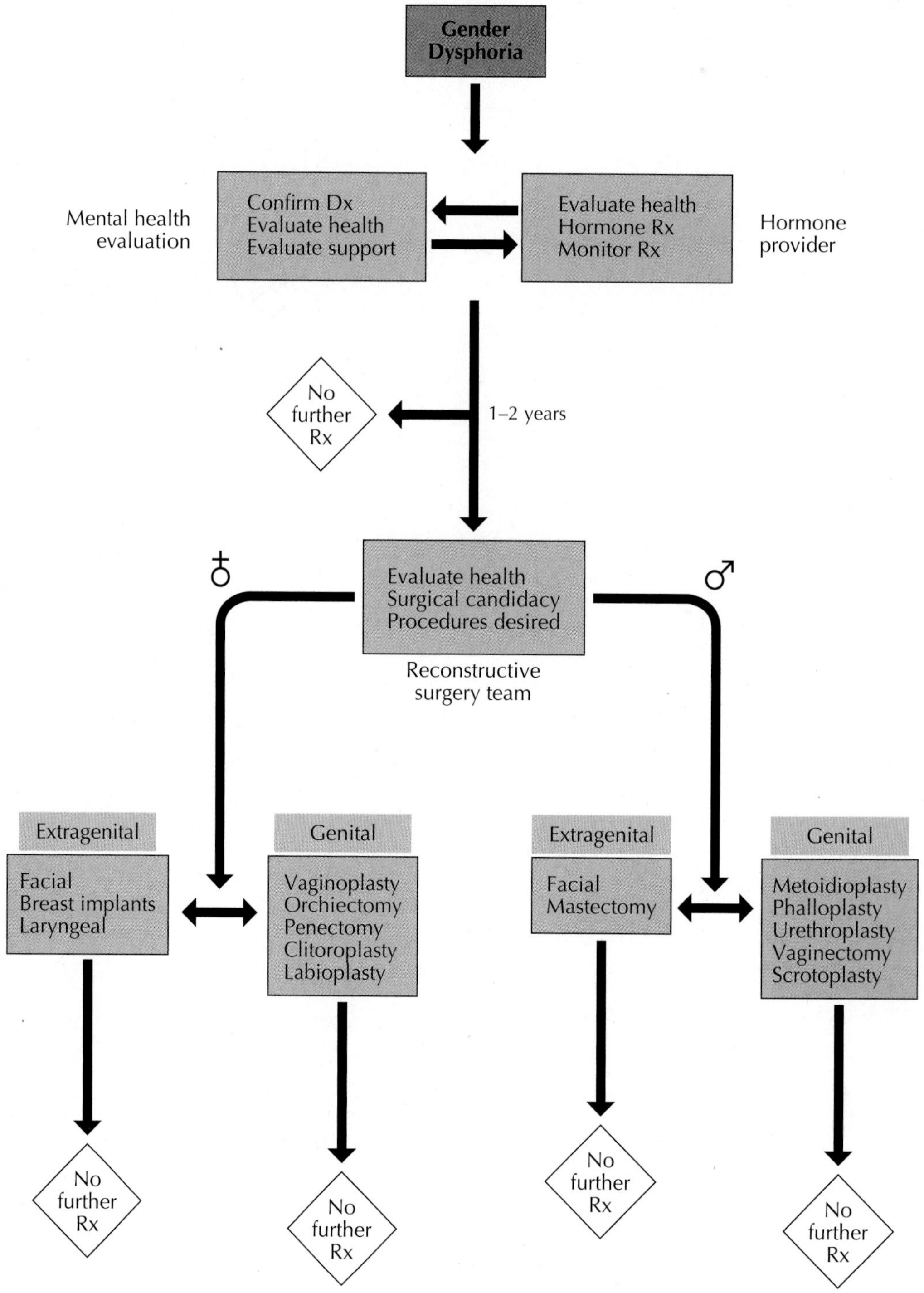

Plate 14.1

Reproductive System: VOLUME 1

GENDER DEFINITIONS

An individual's *sex* refers to their physiologic and biologic attributes, whereas the term *gender* relates to the socially constructed ideas about behavior and conduct that an individual holds. One's gender can include the properties of sex but, unlike sex, gender can be both fluid and ambiguous. Gender is generally considered a central characteristic of social organization. This distinction between sex and gender is a recent concept that gained prominence in mid-20th-century culture.

Gender identity refers to one's personal sense and identification of their particular gender and gender role in society. *Gender nonbinary* is an umbrella term that describes identities that are not solely male or female. *Gender expression,* or *gender presentation,* is one's behavior, mannerisms, interests, and appearance that are associated with femininity or masculinity. It is separate from sexual orientation and assigned birth sex. *Transgender* persons classically harbor a gender identity or gender expression that differs from their assigned sex at birth. *Transfeminine* is a term for someone who was assigned male at birth and has a predominantly feminine gender identity or presentation, and *transmasculine* is the equivalent term for one who was assigned female at birth and has a predominantly masculine gender identity or presentation. The opposite of transgender is *cisgender,* which describes individuals whose gender identity matches their assigned sex.

Gender dysphoria refers to the distress an individual feels owing to a mismatch between their gender identity and their sex assigned at birth. Gender dysphoria forms the basis for most cases of *gender reassignment* or *gender affirmation* medical and surgical treatments. *Transsexual* is a term to describe those individuals with gender dysphoria who desire to transition permanently to the gender with which they identify and who seek medical care to do so. A *trans man* describes a person who has transitioned from female to male and a *trans woman* refers to those who have transitioned from male to female.

The process of sex reassignment is a complex one that occurs in an organized, stepwise manner. The first step involves care from a mental health provider who specializes in gender health issues. The goals of this evaluation are to confirm the diagnosis of gender dysphoria, assess the patient's motivation and knowledge regarding gender affirmation treatments, evaluate the ability to give informed consent for treatments, and assess the patient's social support network and internal strength to manage the transition.

The second stage of care, often occurring in tandem with the first, involves referral to a hormone provider to begin hormonal treatment for managing secondary sexual characteristics, including body hair, muscle mass, and breast size. Females transitioning to males begin testosterone treatment and males transitioning to females begin estrogen therapy. The physical changes associated with these treatments can occur in as soon as 4 weeks but typically take several years to have their fully desired effect. In addition to altering physical appearance, hormone treatments can dramatically ease feelings of gender dysphoria. It is important that patients considering sex reassignment are medically healthy, because side effects of hormonal treatments include elevated blood pressure, weight gain, elevated liver enzymes, heart disease, polycythemia, thromboembolism, and infertility. It is generally recommended that patients take hormones for at least 1 year and live full time as their identified gender before proceeding with surgical procedures.

The third stage of gender affirmation is surgery to alter both extragenital and genital features to align with the desired sex. Extragenital surgery typically involves facial alterations and breast tissue removal or the placement of implants. Genital surgery for trans women involves orchiectomy, penectomy, labiaplasty, clitoroplasty, and vaginoplasty and is often described by the umbrella term vaginoplasty. The corresponding procedures for transmen include vaginectomy, urethral lengthening, scrotoplasty, metoidioplasty, and phalloplasty. Typically, only 10% of gender dysphoric patients proceed to complete this step as reassignment surgery is complex, irreversible, and can be costly. In addition, many dysphoric patients have adequate symptom relief with hormonal treatments alone. Approximately 1% of transgender patients will express regret after having sex reassignment surgery.

Plate 14.2

Sex Reassignment

SURGERY: MALE EXTRAGENITAL

The goal of extragenital procedures is to substantially improve gender incongruence. Extragenital surgery typically involves chest reconstruction ("top surgery") and facial alterations. Typically, chest surgery precedes fascial procedures because it has a larger effect on gender affirmation. Chest surgeries for female-to-male transgender patients have similarities to gynecomastia procedures for men, breast reduction surgery for women, and mastectomies for breast cancer. In addition, additional procedures involve contouring and reducing the chest wall, and repositioning the nipples and areola.

The most common chest masculinization procedure is the double incision technique with or without free nipple grafting. Buttonhole, keyhole, circumareolar, and inverted T are minimal incision, nipple sensation–preserving alternatives that may be used depending on breast anatomy. The double incision procedure is preferred in cases of large or sagging breasts and involves making a horizontal or U-shaped incision at the lower border of the pectoral muscle along the inframammary fold on each side. The skin is then lifted and the breast tissue and associated adipose tissue beneath it are excised. Resecting adipose tissue is critical in that 90% of the tissue composing the rounded contour of the breasts is fat interspersed in mammary tissue.

A circular incision is made to remove the nipple from the overlying breast skin. Excess breast skin is also excised to achieve a flat, dimple free chest wall that reflects the contours of the underlying pectoralis major and minor muscles. The nipple size is reduced to a 2 cm diameter and then replaced as a free nipple graft higher in the breast hemisphere that is sutured to the underlying vascularized tissue and covered with bolster sutures to improve graft take. Importantly, free-grafted nipples will lose most or all of their native sensation after surgery. Liposuction contouring can also be used to remove excess fat in the armpit area.

For reduction of smaller breasts, a subcutaneous mastectomy surgery that spares the skin, nipple, and areola is typically employed. These include the buttonhole, keyhole, circumareolar, and inverted T or anchor incisions. Typically, these incisions are made in the areolar borders along with smaller inframammary incisions, and underlying breast tissue is removed. The incised skin is then reattached at the border of the resized areola. With these techniques, the areola stays attached to its neurovascular pedicle, which improves viability and maintains nipple sensation. Other advantages include minimal scarring and faster healing time.

Facial masculinization surgery alters anatomic features to align more closely with gender identity. Typically, this involves altering facial features to be more prominent and angular. Surgically, this can entail reconstruction of the forehead, nose, upper lip, jaw, chin, and Adams apple or larynx prominence augmentation. Forehead augmentation is done to widen and flatten it with either implants or injectable materials that are molded in shape before hardening. Surgery on the nose involves cartilage or bone grafting to enlarge and broaden it. Alterations to chin anatomy, termed *mentoplasty*, is undertaken with osteotomy and implants. Similarly, jaw augmentation is performed with implants or fillers. Adam's apple or laryngeal prominence augmentation can be performed with fillers or with the use of rib cartilage grafts. Often, surgical and filler methods are combined to achieve desired changes. Hair transplantation is used to achieve **permanent masculine hair growth patterns that include sideburns, mustaches, and beards.**

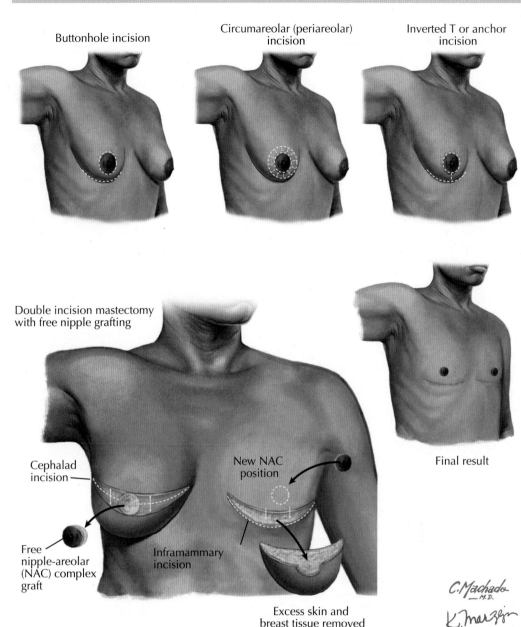

Chest reconstruction

Buttonhole incision

Circumareolar (periareolar) incision

Inverted T or anchor incision

Double incision mastectomy with free nipple grafting

Cephalad incision

New NAC position

Final result

Free nipple-areolar (NAC) complex graft

Inframammary incision

Excess skin and breast tissue removed

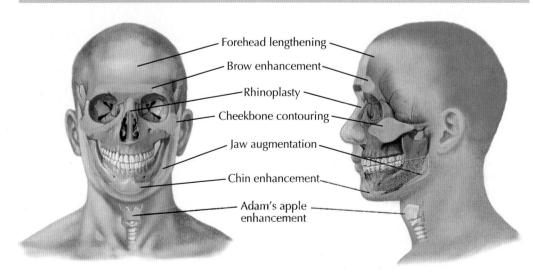

Facial masculinization

Forehead lengthening

Brow enhancement

Rhinoplasty

Cheekbone contouring

Jaw augmentation

Chin enhancement

Adam's apple enhancement

Plate 14.3

Reproductive System: VOLUME 1

SURGERY: MALE GENITAL—VAGINECTOMY, URETHRAL LENGTHENING, AND CLITORAL RECONSTRUCTION

Male genital gender affirmation surgery involves vaginectomy, urethral lengthening, scrotoplasty, perineal reconstruction, clitoral reconstruction, and phallus reconstruction. The two umbrella terms for transmasculine gender-affirming genitourinary surgery are *metoidioplasty*, where phallus reconstruction involves making the clitoris appear like a micropenis, and *phalloplasty*, where a free or pedicled flap is reconstructed into a proportional sized penis. Given the fluidity of gender and individualized surgical goals, a small number of patients will forego one or several key parts of their index gender affirming surgery. Secondary surgery involves penile and testis implant insertion.

Vaginectomy is often desired and is performed in conjunction with urethral lengthening procedures. It must be preceded by hysterectomy. Commonly the vagina is left in situ after deepithelialization or removal of the vaginal mucosa to eliminate secretions and the canal opening is closed with pursestring sutures. Tissues superficial to this closure include the neourethra (*pars fixa*) and the bulbospongiosus muscles along with adipofascial tissue, which are anastomosed in the midline to directly cover the neourethral suture line.

Urethral lengthening procedures are similar for metoidioplasty and phalloplasty. For metoidioplasty, urethral lengthening can be achieved with tubularization of neighboring endodermal and ectodermal labia minora tissue. The labia minora flaps are harvested with a U-shaped design or with ring-shaped tissue advancement. The ring flap is harvested by dissecting hairless tissue inferior to the vaginal introitus and positioning it lateral to the urethral meatus. This tissue advancement extends the neourethral opening from its native position to the glans clitoris. Dorsally the ring flaps are anastomosed superolaterally to the native urethral meatus with care taken to avoid obstructing Skene's gland ducts within the meatus. Ventral closure completes the urethral extension. Other techniques for urethral lengthening in metoidioplasty include combination labia minora and vaginal wall flaps with onlay grafts from genital skin or oral (buccal) mucosa. The reconstructed urethral segment for metoidioplasty has no name. For phalloplasty, there are two urethral segments: the pars fixa urethra is near identical to the lengthened segment in metoidioplasty; the *pars pendulans* urethra is the pendulous urethra within the free or pedicled flap used to create the phallus—a tube within a cylinder design.

In cases of planned metoidioplasty, the clitoris is enlarged with the preoperative use of testosterone. One technique for metoidioplasty includes clitoral skin removal/degloving and dorsal and ventral ligament release, with subsequent micropenis skin reconstruction with local labia minora and clitoral skin flaps. The preferred technique is metoidioplasty with clitoral skin preservation with ventral chordee release to avoid a dorsal dissection that could cause nerve damage as well as minimize risk of penile skin loss. The skin preservation technique also works well with the ring flap urethroplasty described previously.

For phalloplasty, the clitoris is completely deepithelialized to help with burial and dorsal nerve dissection. The clitoris, its neurovascular bundle, the ventral paired corporal bodies, and the ventral tubularized labia minora flaps (the pars fixa urethra) are transposed, buried, and fixed at the base of the reconstructed phallic shaft. The dorsal nerve is coapted to the lateral antebrachial nerve of the reconstructed neophallus. To obtain orgasm after phalloplasty, preservation of the contralateral dorsal nerve is crucial to allow the buried clitoris to be stimulated as the reconstructed phallus receives growing dorsal nerve axons within the lateral antebrachial cutaneous nerve bundle.

VAGINECTOMY, URETHRAL LENGTHENING, AND CLITORAL RECONSTRUCTION

Vaginectomy

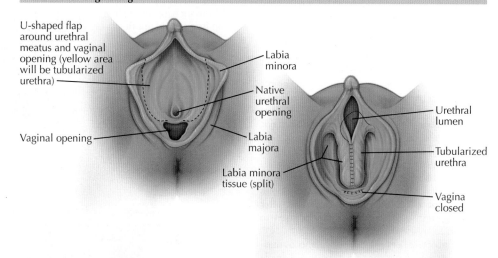

Closed vaginal opening

Vaginectomy. The vaginal canal is demucoalized and the remaining muscularis layer closed with serial rows of purse string suture.

Urethral lengthening

U-shaped flap around urethral meatus and vaginal opening (yellow area will be tubularized urethra)

Vaginal opening

Labia minora

Native urethral opening

Labia majora

Labia minora tissue (split)

Urethral lumen

Tubularized urethra

Vagina closed

Clitoral reconstruction

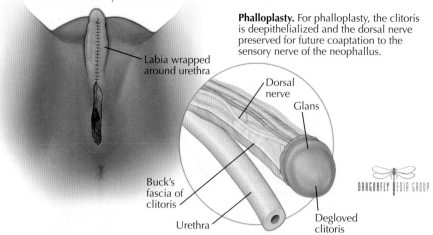

Metoidioplasty. For metoidioplasty, the clitoral skin is wrapped around the lengthened urethra to create a cylindrical shaft.

Labia wrapped around urethra

Phalloplasty. For phalloplasty, the clitoris is deepithelialized and the dorsal nerve preserved for future coaptation to the sensory nerve of the neophallus.

Dorsal nerve

Glans

Buck's fascia of clitoris

Urethra

Degloved clitoris

Plate 14.4

Sex Reassignment

METOIDIOPLASTY, PHALLOPLASTY, AND NEOSCROTUM FORMATION

Metoidioplasty and metoidioplasty neoscrotum

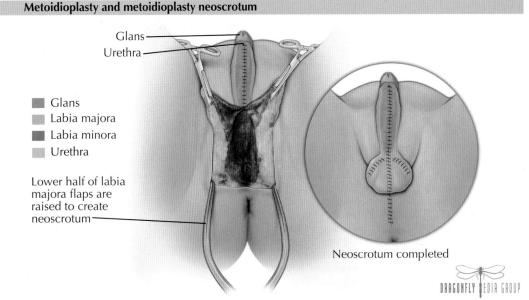

Glans
Urethra

■ Glans
▧ Labia majora
■ Labia minora
□ Urethra

Lower half of labia
majora flaps are
raised to create
neoscrotum

Neoscrotum completed

DRAGONFLY MEDIA GROUP

SURGERY: MALE GENITAL— METOIDIOPLASTY, PHALLOPLASTY, AND NEOSCROTUM FORMATION

The fashioning of a phallus that allows for standing micturition is a key surgical goal in transmasculine surgery. Two common approaches to phallus creation include metoidioplasty and phalloplasty.

Metoidioplasty involves creating a phallus using existing enlarged clitoral tissue. In its simplest form, a working microphallus is created by releasing the suspensory ligaments that connect the penis to the pubic bone. More complex metoidioplasties involve harvesting local vaginal tissue flaps to lengthen the urethra which is then channeled under the clitoral shaft skin to allow for an exit near the end of the microphallus. Nearby genital tissue can also be recruited to increase phallic girth. Phalloplasty employs larger flaps—both local and free—from the abdomen, thigh, forearm, or back, to create a neophallus. The radial forearm free flap is a popular choice for the neophallus due to pliable skin and adipose tissue, a reliable cutaneous nerve for coaptation to the recipient nerve, and robust vascularity from the radial artery, its venae comitantes, and branches of the cephalic vein that feed and drain the flap. The tubularized free flap is brought into the groin region after exposure of the recipient superficial femoral and saphenous vascular systems to allow for the anastomosis of the radial artery of the flap to the superficial femoral artery and the cephalic and comitantes veins of the flap to the recipient saphenous vein branches. The deep inferior epigastric vessels may also be used for this anastomosis. The dorsal nerve of the clitoris is coapted to the lateral antebrachial nerve of the forearm flap. Penis-like sensation is expected to develop in most radial forearm neophalluses.

For phalloplasty, the urethral lengthening techniques for extending the native urethra to the glans clitoris (par fixa urethroplasty) are similar to metoidioplasty. The main difference involves deepithelializing the clitoris, dissecting the dorsal nerve, and then translocating it to the mons pubis, where the phallus and its *pars pendulans* urethra (the neophallic urethral segment) will later be positioned. Creating the pars pendulans urethra varies widely based upon the type of flap used for phallic creation. Prefabricated tubularized grafts and combination flaps have been tried with varying success. The most common and reliable flap system employs the radial forearm free flap with a "tube-in-a-tube" design. This involves tubularization of a portion of the free flap used for phalloplasty followed by tubularization over the inner urethra, creating a tube-in-tube. In single stage phalloplasty, the pars fixa and pars pendulans urethrae are created simultaneously. In staged procedures, the pars fixa and pars pendulans are made separately. The most common staging is neophallus and pars pendulans urethroplasty followed 4 to 6 months later with pars fixa urethroplasty. Performing an initial pars fixa urethroplasty may be a preferred strategy in patients who are not sure if they prefer metoidioplasty or phalloplasty for their eventual surgical outcome. Phalloplasty can also be offered after metoidioplasty in patients with persistent dysphoria. Most patients who want and need phalloplasty favor single stage phalloplasty procedures.

Phalloplasty and phalloplasty neoscrotum

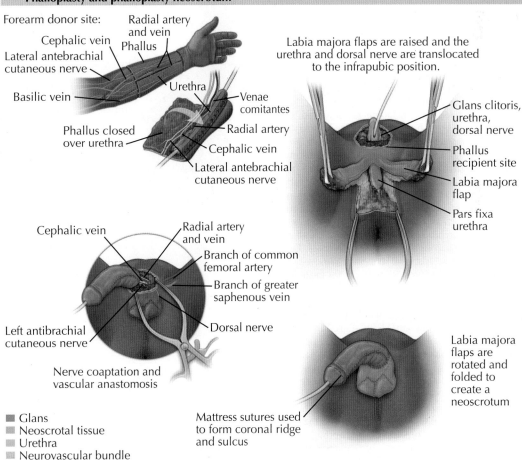

Forearm donor site:
Cephalic vein
Lateral antebrachial
cutaneous nerve
Radial artery
and vein
Phallus
Urethra
Basilic vein
Phallus closed
over urethra
Venae
comitantes
Radial artery
Cephalic vein
Lateral antebrachial
cutaneous nerve

Labia majora flaps are raised and the
urethra and dorsal nerve are translocated
to the infrapubic position.

Glans clitoris,
urethra,
dorsal nerve
Phallus
recipient site
Labia majora
flap
Pars fixa
urethra

Cephalic vein
Radial artery
and vein
Branch of common
femoral artery
Branch of greater
saphenous vein
Dorsal nerve
Left antibrachial
cutaneous nerve
Nerve coaptation and
vascular anastomosis

Labia majora
flaps are
rotated and
folded to
create a
neoscrotum

■ Glans
▧ Neoscrotal tissue
□ Urethra
▨ Neurovascular bundle

Mattress sutures used
to form coronal ridge
and sulcus

Neoscrotum creation or scrotoplasty techniques generally involve creating a pouchlike scrotum employing adjacent labia majora tissue. Most commonly, labia majora rotational advancement flaps are used. Inferolateral incisions are made on each side around the labia majora tissue, and each flap is elevated and advanced. The flap tips are then folded superomedially and sewn to complete the scrotoplasty. Penile and testicular prosthetic implants are placed separate from the metoidioplasty and phalloplasty procedures, typically

6 months (testicular implants) and 12 months (penile implants) postoperatively. For metoidioplasty, the labia majora flaps are smaller than for phalloplasty to create a more proportionally sized scrotum.

Perineal reconstruction involves multilevel closure over the deeper tissue including the vaginectomy site and the urethral suture line. The first layer is the bulbospongiosus layer followed by more superficial adipofascial tissue and inner thigh skin, resulting in a flat, masculine-appearing perineum without labial tissue.

Plate 14.5

Reproductive System: VOLUME 1

Surgery: Female Extragenital

Top surgery for male to female gender affirmation seeks to increase breast size and alter chest shape. Transgender females tend to have broader chests and larger, thicker pectoral muscles, along with smaller nipples and areolas and a shorter distance between nipples and inframammary folds. These differences are minimized through feminizing breast surgery, breast augmentation, and mammoplasty and chest construction. These are typically performed together in a single-stage procedure. Incisions employed for feminizing breast surgery included inframammary, periareolar, transaxillary (in the armpit), or transumbilical (belly button) and are chosen to minimize scar exposure. Breast implants, currently consisting of either saline-filled or silicone-filled, are usually placed either behind the existing breast tissue (subglandular) or under the pectoralis major muscle (submuscular). Fat grafting from the abdomen can also be considered to complete desired contour changes and further round out breast appearance. In addition to breast augmentation with implants or fat, breast lifts are popular to create a fuller look.

Many facial features, including the forehead, eyes, jaw, cheeks, and brow, have well recognized associations with gender. Facial feminization surgery involves procedures to change the shape of the face to look more feminine. The hairline and forehead are altered to create a smaller surface area. In general, the bony ridge above the eye sockets tends to be more pronounced in men than women. In addition, female foreheads tend to be higher, smoother, and more rounded. To feminize the forehead, the forehead bone is cut, removed, reshaped, and replaced to accommodate these differences. Excess eyelid skin characteristic of males is removed with blepharoplasty procedures. Rhinoplasty for facial feminization generally involves reducing the size and angularity of the nose as well as narrowing it. To shorten the distance between the nose base and the upper lip, lip lifts create a shorter, more curled lip. Lips can also be enlarged with implants or fillers or by using fat grafts. The wider lower male jaw can be reduced and narrowed by bone sculpting procedures. Masculine chins are generally longer than feminine chins and tend to be more squarely shaped. To shorten and narrow the chin, genioplasty procedures involve a horizontal cut in the chin bone with a removal of a wedge of bone. As the laryngeal prominence or Adam's apple is more protuberant in men, tracheal shave procedures of the laryngeal cartilage can reduce its size. Feminine hairlines tend to be lower on the forehead than masculine hairlines. Hairline lowering surgery involves incisions made at the hairline, followed by scalp elevation, advancement, and fixation to the bone with excision of excess forehead skin. Typically, the suture line is placed near but not at the hairline to reduce its visibility. To fill in balding areas of the head and temple characteristic of males, hair transplantation from areas of thicker head hair to the balding and thinning areas of the head are often performed. Skin-tightening surgery, such as face-lifts, provides other options to smooth skin.

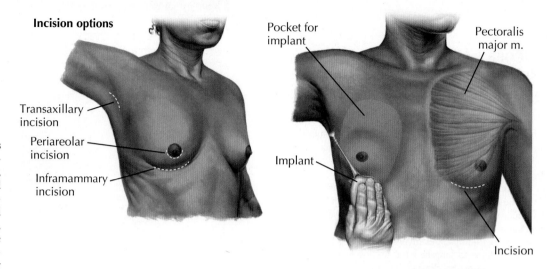

Chest reconstruction

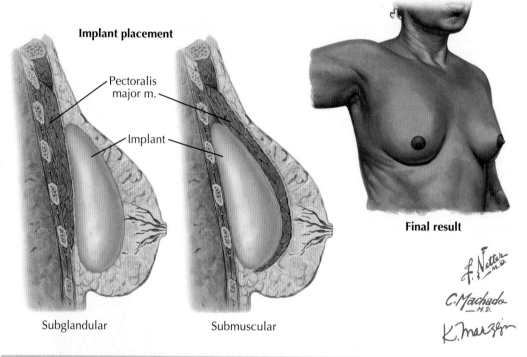

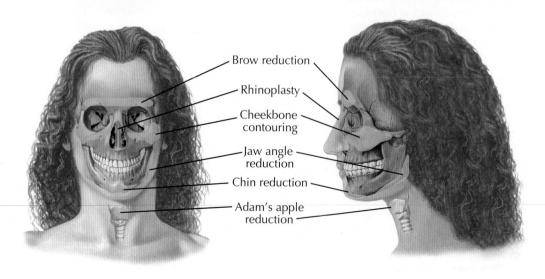

Facial feminization

Plate 14.6

Sex Reassignment

SURGERY: FEMALE GENITAL—ORCHIECTOMY, PENECTOMY AND URETHRECTOMY

The umbrella term used to describe the series of female genital reassignment ("lower" or "bottom") procedures is *vaginoplasty*. It involves penectomy, orchiectomy, urethrectomy, clitoroplasty, and labiaplasty.

Transgender patients commonly begin the process of surgical gender affirmation with simple orchiectomy, or removal of the testicles. The early removal of testosterone-producing testicles in the transgender process also simplifies the hormone replacement process by lowering the amount of estrogen supplementation needed. Orchiectomy involves a midline scrotal raphe incision under anesthesia and involves excision of the testes and associated epididymides and vasa deferentia along with the remainder of the infrainguinal spermatic cords bilaterally. Typically, the testes and associated tissues are dissected intact, and the spermatic cord clamped and ligated with permanent suture near the external inguinal ring. The cord structures are then divided, the tissue excised, and the proximal spermatic cord stump inspected for adequate hemostasis. The scrotum incision is closed with absorbable suture.

Penectomy begins with a circumcising incision and degloving of the penis. Sufficient distal mucosal collar skin is left with the glans to allow for a clitoral hood to be fashioned later. The skin dissection is maintained in the avascular plane between Dartos and Buck's fascia to the base of the penis. The bulbospongiosus muscle is also excised entirely to further debulk the tissue. The dorsally located neurovascular bundle, which supplies blood and sensation to the glans penis, is preserved and dissected off the paired corporal cavernosal tissue. The penile corporeal bodies are divided proximally at the level of the pubic symphysis and the tunica albuginea of the proximal ends oversewn for hemostasis. The remaining intact penile shaft skin is preserved and inverted to later line the neovagina.

At the time of penectomy, urethrectomy is undertaken to fashion a shortened urethra that allows for urination while sitting. During disassembly of the penis, the corpus spongiosum body harboring the urethra is dissected free of the paired corpus cavernosal bodies and retained. The excess spongiosal tissue in the bulbar region of the spongiosal body is excised from the urethra, debulked and tapered to prevent a periurethral bulge in the future anterior vaginal canal. Once the clitoroplasty and labiaplasty have been performed, the urethra is then matured by trimming, shortening, and placing it posterior to the neoclitoris. It is sutured in place with ventral spatulation to prevent meatal stenosis. A Foley catheter is maintained postoperatively until the vaginal packing is removed.

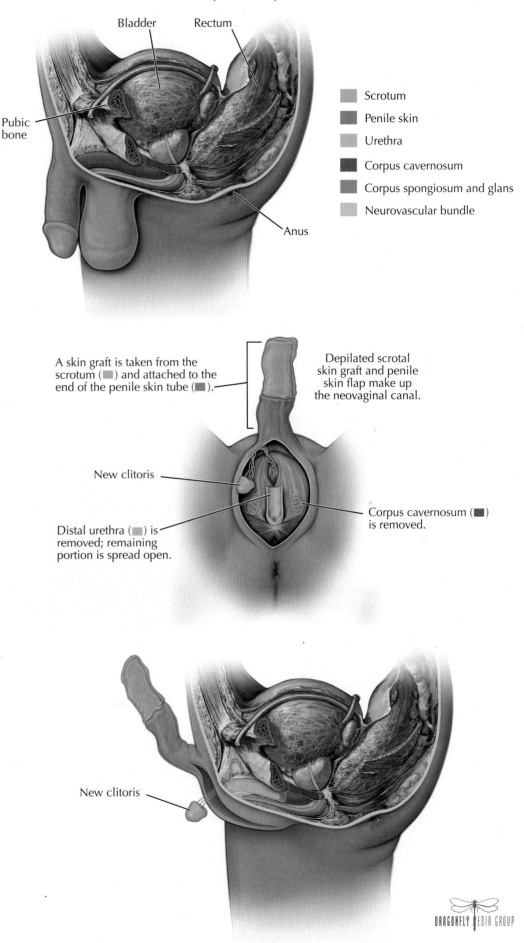

ORCHIECTOMY, PENECTOMY, AND URETHRECTOMY

Bladder Rectum

Pubic bone

Anus

- Scrotum
- Penile skin
- Urethra
- Corpus cavernosum
- Corpus spongiosum and glans
- Neurovascular bundle

A skin graft is taken from the scrotum (▪) and attached to the end of the penile skin tube (▪).

Depilated scrotal skin graft and penile skin flap make up the neovaginal canal.

New clitoris

Distal urethra (▪) is removed; remaining portion is spread open.

Corpus cavernosum (▪) is removed.

New clitoris

Plate 14.7

Reproductive System: VOLUME 1

CLITOROPLASTY, LABIAPLASTY, AND VAGINOPLASTY

Clitoroplasty

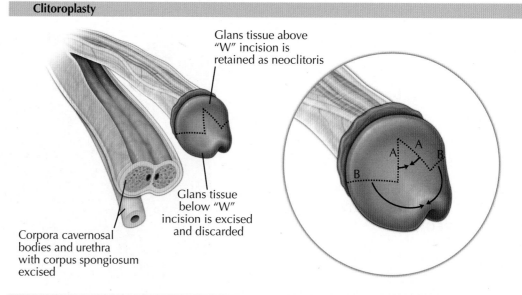

Glans tissue above "W" incision is retained as neoclitoris

Corpora cavernosal bodies and urethra with corpus spongiosum excised

Glans tissue below "W" incision is excised and discarded

SURGERY: FEMALE GENITAL— CLITOROPLASTY, LABIAPLASTY, AND VAGINOPLASTY

Once the male organs are removed or debulked, female genital reconstruction can begin. Clitoroplasty involves revising the penile glans and accordioning the neurovascular bundle such that the clitoris is placed above the corporeal stumps and sutured to the pubic symphysis. The large male glans penis undergoes surgical reduction to create a smaller neoclitoris. Glans reduction is typically performed using a "W" incision in the midglans in which the tissue ventral to the incision is excised and the glans tissue dorsal to the incision is retained. Clitoroplasty then continues by rolling the wings of the "W"-shaped glans to the midline ventrally. The dorsal collar of the remaining circumcised penile glans skin is then folded over the top of the neoclitoris to reconstruct the clitoral hood. The lateral collars of the redundant penile glans skin are brought to the midline underneath the clitoris and sutured together to complete the clitoroplasty. The placement of the clitoris on the pubic symphysis guides the subsequent placement of the spatulated urethral meatus within the vaginal vestibule.

For labiaplasty, the feminine vulva requires the recreation of both labia minora and labia major to shroud the vaginal vestibule. The dorsal labia minora is fashioned out of penile shaft dorsal collar skin as described earlier. The inferolateral labia minora are created with dorsal bulbar urethral tissue and by folding the periurethral tissue on either side of the vestibule to create flaplike tissue ridges. The labia majora are created out of the remnant scrotal tissue after its excess is removed, typically leaving a "U"-shaped incision to close and allow for their creation. Importantly, scrotal skin has abundant hair follicles, which is not a desired feature within the vulvar vestibule, and scrotal hair electrolysis should be undertaken in advance of vaginoplasty for optimum results.

By far the most challenging step in vaginoplasty surgery is the creation of a neovaginal canal. Several different approaches have been taken to create a functional neovagina: primary vaginoplasty using local penile and scrotal skin flaps and grafts, intestinal vaginoplasty using ileal or colon bowel segments to gain larger and greater vaginal canal depth, and peritoneal flap vaginoplasty. With all approaches, access to the potential space between the rectum and urethra is created by removal of the bulbospongiosus muscles and identification and division of the perineal body and levator muscles within the perineum. Great care must be given to avoid rectal or urethra injury. This dissection is carried proximally until the retroperitoneum is identified and the depth of dissection reaches 13 to 14 cm. With primary vaginoplasty, the newly created vaginal canal is lined with several local tissues including inverted penile skin and harvested scrotal skin along with a perineal skin flap. The skin lining the vagina is thinned and hair removed from it by electrolysis or laser. The penile skin flap and scrotal skin graft are typically sutured together over a dilator model, followed by inversion and insertion into the previously dissected canal. An opening is made in the inverted penis skin flap to bring out the neoclitoris. The perineal skin flap is then advanced into the neovagina ventrally.

Alternatives to primary vaginoplasty with local skin are intestinal and peritoneal flap vaginoplasty. Intestinal

Labiaplasty and vaginoplasty

The penile-scrotal skin tube is turned inside-out and inverted into the space between the bladder and prostate, and the rectum.

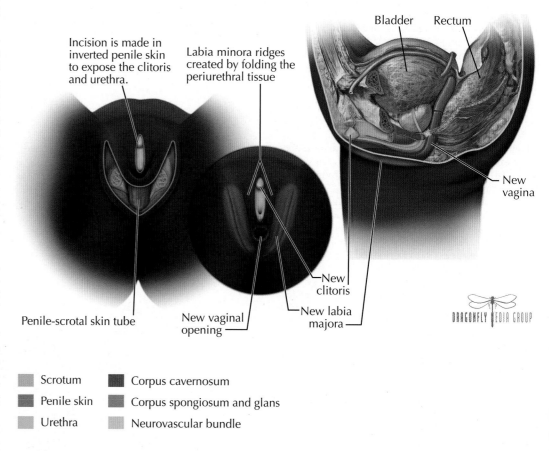

Incision is made in inverted penile skin to expose the clitoris and urethra.

Labia minora ridges created by folding the periurethral tissue

Bladder   Rectum

New vagina

New clitoris

New labia majora

Penile-scrotal skin tube

New vaginal opening

�en Scrotum	▪ Corpus cavernosum		
▪ Penile skin	▪ Corpus spongiosum and glans		
▪ Urethra	▪ Neurovascular bundle		

substitution with sigmoid colon or small intestine were initially favored given their proximity to the pelvis, hairless nature, and self-lubrication qualities. However, intestinal neovaginas have fallen out of favor given the large amount of mucous production, the morbidity associated with the bowel harvest, and chronic foul odor. Peritoneum is a strong tissue that is highly available, lacks donor site morbidity, and is hairless. It can be harvested intraabdominally using laparoscopic and robotic techniques—approaches that can also aid in the

neovaginal canal dissection. Harvested peritoneal flaps are sewn to the inverted penile skin flap, obviating the need for scrotal skin grafts. After neovagina creation, a vaginal packing is left in place postoperatively and removed 1 week later, after which patients begin dilating the neovagina regularly and continue with lifelong dilations. Unique vaginoplasty complications include wound dehiscence of the labial closure (15%–30%), rectal and urethral injures (1%), urethra-neovaginal fistula (1%–2%), and vaginal stenosis (5%–10%).

Section 1 Development of the Genital Tracts and Functional Relationships of the Gonads

Aatsha PA, Arbor TC, Krishan K. Embryology, sexual development. [Updated 2022 Sep 8]. In: StatPearls [Internet]. Treasure Island (FL): StatPearls Publishing; 2023. https://www.ncbi.nlm.nih.gov/books/NBK557601/

Garcia-Alonso L, Lorenzi V, Mazzeo CI et al. Single-cell roadmap of human gonadal development. Nature. 2022;607:540-547.

Section 2 Penis and Male Perineum

Baskin LS. Hypospadias and urethral development. J Urol. 2000;163 (3):951-956.

Baskin LS, Shen J, Sinclair A, et al. Development of the human penis and clitoris. Differentiation. 2018;103:74-85.

Burnett AL, Nehra A, Breau RH, et al. Erectile dysfunction: AUA guideline. J Urol. 2018;200:633.

Lue TF. Erectile dysfunction. N Engl J Med. 2000;342(24):1802-1813.

Section 3 Scrotum and Testis

Borawski JM. Sexually transmitted diseases. In: Partin A, Dmochowski R, Kavoussi L, Peters C, Wein A, eds. Campbell-Walsh Urology. 12th ed. Elsevier; 2021:1251-1272.

Link RE, Tang N. Cutaneous diseases of the external genitalia. In: Partin A, Dmochowski R, Kavoussi L, Peters C, Wein A, eds. Campbell-Walsh Urology. 12th ed. Elsevier; 2021:1273-1306.

Turek PJ. Male reproductive physiology. In: Partin A, Dmochowski R, Kavoussi L, Peters C, Wein A, eds. Campbell-Walsh Urology. 12th ed. Elsevier; 2021:1390-1410.

Section 4 Seminal Vesicles and Prostate

Aaron L, Franco OE, Hayward SW. Review of prostate anatomy and embryology and the etiology of benign prostatic hyperplasia, Urol Clin N Am. 2016;43:279-288.

Nguyen HT, Etzell J, Turek PJ. Normal human ejaculatory duct anatomy: a study of cadaveric and surgical specimens. J Urol. 1996;155: 1639-1642.

Polackwich A, Shoskes D. Chronic prostatitis/chronic pelvic pain syndrome: a review of evaluation and therapy. Prostate Cancer Prostatic Dis. 2016;19:132-138.

Turek PJ. Seminal vesicle and ejaculatory duct surgery. In: Graham SD, ed. Glenn's Urologic Surgery. 6th ed. Lippincott, Williams & Wilkins; 2004:439-445.

Section 5 Sperm and Ejaculation

Godart ES, Turek PJ. The evolution of testicular sperm extraction and preservation techniques. Fac Rev. 2020;9:2.

Krausz C, Riera-Escamilla A. Genetics of male infertility. Nat Rev Urol. 2018;15:369-384.

Masters V, Turek PJ. Ejaculatory physiology and dysfunction. Urol Clin North Am. 2001;28:363.

Smith JF, Turek PJ. Ejaculatory duct obstruction. Urol Clin North Am. 2008; 35:221-227.

WHO Laboratory Manual for the Examination and Processing of Human Semen. 5th ed. Cambridge University Press; 2010.

Yatsenko AN, Turek PJ. Reproductive genetics and the aging male. J Assist Reprod Genet. 2018;35:933-941.

Section 6 Vulva

American College of Obstetricians and Gynecologists. ACOG Practice Bulletin No. 215. Vaginitis. Obstet Gynecol. 2020;135: e1-17.

American College of Obstetricians and Gynecologists. ACOG Practice Bulletin No. 224. Diagnosis and management of vulvar skin disorders. Obstet Gynecol. 2020;136:e1-14.

American College of Obstetricians and Gynecologists. ACOG Committee Opinion No. 345. Vulvodynia. Obstet Gynecol. 2006;108: 1049-1052.

Section 7 Vagina

Leung J, Abrams JY, Maddox RA, Godfred-Cato S, Schonberger LB, Belay ED. Toxic shock syndrome in patients younger than 21 years of age, United States, 2006–2018. Pediatr Infect Dis J. 2021;40(3):e125-128.

Section 8 Uterus and Cervix

American College of Obstetricians and Gynecologists. ACOG Practice Bulletin 11. Management of endometriosis. Obstet Gynecol. 2010;116:223-236.

American College of Obstetricians and Gynecologists. ACOG Practice Bulletin No. 218. Chronic pelvic pain. Obstet Gynecol. 2020;135:e89-109-605.

Section 9 Fallopian Tubes

Curry A, Williams T, Penny ML. Pelvic inflammatory disease: diagnosis, management, and prevention. Am Fam Physician. 2019;100(6):357-364.

Section 10 Ovaries

American College of Obstetricians and Gynecologists. ACOG Practice Bulletin No. 174. Management of adnexal masses. Obstet Gynecol. 2016;128:e210-26.

American College of Obstetricians and Gynecologists. ACOG Practice Bulletin No. 194. Polycystic ovary syndrome. Obstet Gynecol. 2018;131:e157-71.

Section 11 Ovum and Reproduction

Bagshawe A, Taylor A. ABC of subfertility. Counselling. BMJ. 2003;327(7422):1038-1040.

Carson SA, Kallen AN. Diagnosis and management of infertility: a review. JAMA. 2021;326(1):65-76.

Olatunji O, More A. A review of the impact of microfluidics technology on sperm selection technique. Cureus. 2022;14:e27369.

Rowell P, Braude P. Assisted conception. I—general principles. BMJ. 2003;327(7418):799-801.

Turek PJ. Practical approach to the diagnosis and management of male infertility. Nat Clin Pract Urol. 2005;2:1-13.

Section 12 Pregnancy

American College of Obstetricians and Gynecologists. ACOG Practice Bulletin No. 181. Prevention of Rh D alloimmunization. Obstet Gynecol. 2017;130:e57-70.

American College of Obstetricians and Gynecologists. ACOG Practice Bulletin No. 183. Postpartum hemorrhage. Obstet Gynecol. 2017;130:e168-86.

American College of Obstetricians and Gynecologists. ACOG Practice Bulletin No. 193. Tubal ectopic pregnancy. Obstet Gynecol. 2018;131:e91-103.

American College of Obstetricians and Gynecologists. Practice Bulletin No. 205. Vaginal birth after previous cesarean delivery. Obstet Gynecol. 2019;133:e110-27.

Section 13 Breast

American College of Obstetricians and Gynecologists. Practice Bulletin No. 126. Management of gynecologic issues in women with breast cancer. Obstet Gynecol. 2012;119:666-82.

American College of Obstetricians and Gynecologists. Practice Bulletin No. 164. Diagnosis and management of benign breast disorders. Obstet Gynecol. 2016;127:e141-56.

American College of Obstetricians and Gynecologists. Practice Bulletin No. 179. Breast cancer risk assessment and screening in average-risk women. Obstet Gynecol. 2017;130:e1-16.

American College of Obstetricians and Gynecologists, with the Committee on Genetics and the Society of Gynecologic Oncology. Practice Bulletin No. 182. Hereditary breast and ovarian cancer syndrome. Obstet Gynecol. 2017;130:e110-26.

Section 14 Sex Reassignment

Bustos VP, Bustos SS, Mascaro A, et al. Regret after gender-affirmation surgery: A systematic review and meta-analysis of prevalence. Plast Reconstr Surg Glob Open. 2021;9(3):e3477.

Heston AL, Esmonde NO, Dugi DD 3rd, Berli JU. Phalloplasty: techniques and outcomes. Transl Androl Urol. 2019;8:254-265.

McEvenue G, Xu FZ, Cai R, McLean H. Female-to-male gender affirming top surgery: a single surgeon's 15-year retrospective review and treatment algorithm. Aesthetic Surg J. 2018;38:49-57.

Van Boerum MS, Salibian AA, Bluebond-Langner R, Agarwal C. Chest and facial surgery for the transgender patient. Transl Androl Urol. 2019;8:219-227.

Yilmaz KB, Narter KF. Transgender surgery: a review article. J Urol Surg. 2021;8:227-233.